COMPREHENSIVE FINANCIAL PLANNING STRATEGIES for DOCTORS and ADVISORS

Best Practices from Leading Consultants and Certified Medical Planners™

Testimonials

Written by doctors and healthcare professionals, this textbook should be mandatory reading for all medical school students—highly recommended for both young and veteran physicians—and an eliminating factor for any financial advisor who has not read it. The book uses jargon like "innovative," "transformational," and "disruptive"; all rightly so! It is the type of definitive financial lifestyle planning book we often seek, but seldom find.

LeRoy Howard; MA, CMP™ candidate
Financial Advisor
Fayetteville, North Carolina

"I taught diagnostic radiology for over a decade. The physician-focused niche information, balanced perspectives and insider industry transparency in this book may help save your [financial] life."

Dr. William P. Scherer; MS
Barry University
Fort Lauderdale, Florida

"This book was crafted in response to the frustration felt by doctors who dealt with top financial, brokerage and accounting firms. These non-fiduciary behemoths often prescribed costly wholesale solutions that were applicable to all, but customized for few; despite ever changing needs. It is a must-read to learn why brokerage sales-pitches or Internet resources, will never replace the knowledge and deep advice of a physician focused financial advisor, medical consultant or collegial Certified Medical Planner™ *financial professional."*

Parin Khotari; MBA
Whitman School of Management
Syracuse University, New York

"In today's healthcare environment, in order for providers to survive they need to understand their current and future market trends, finances, operations, and impact of Federal and state regulations. As a healthcare consulting professional for over 30 years supporting both the private and public sector, I recommend that providers understand and utilize the wealth of knowledge that is being conveyed in these chapters. Without this guidance providers will have a hard time navigating the supporting system which may impact their future revenue stream. I strongly endorse the contents of this book."

Carol S. Miller; BSN, MBA, PMP
President-Miller Consulting Group
ACT IAC Executive Committee Vice-Chair at-Large
HIMSS NCA Board Member

"This is an excellent book on financial planning for physicians and health professionals. It is all inclusive yet very easy to read with much valuable information. And, I have been expanding my business knowledge with all of Dr. Marcinko's prior books. I highly recommend this one, too. It is a fine educational tool for all doctors."

Dr. David B. Lumsden; MD, MS, MA
Orthopedic Surgeon
Baltimore, Maryland

"There is no other comprehensive book like it to help doctors, nurses and other medical providers accumulate and preserve the wealth that their years of education and hard work have earned them."

Dr. Jason Dyken; MD, MBA
Dyken Wealth Strategies
Gulf Shores, Alabama

"I plan to give a copy of this book written—"by doctors and for doctors"—to all my prospects, physician and nurse clients. It may be the definitive text on this important topic."

Alexander Naruska; CPA
Orlando, Florida

"Health professionals are small-business owners who need to apply their self-discipline tactics in establishing and operating successful practices. Talented trainees are leaving the medical profession because they fail to balance the cost of attendance against a realistic business and financial plan. Principles like budgeting, saving and living below one's means, in order to make future investments for growth, asset protection and retirement possible, are often lacking. This textbook guides the medical professional in his/her financial-planning life journey from start to finish. It ranks a place in all medical school libraries and on each of our bookshelves."

Dr. Thomas M. DeLauro; DPM
Professor and Chairman, Division of Medical Sciences
New York College of Podiatric Medicine

"Physicians are notoriously excellent at diagnosing and treating medical conditions. However, they are also notoriously deficient in managing the business aspects of their medical practices. Most will earn $20–30 million in their medical lifetime, but few know how to create wealth for themselves and their families. This book will help fill the void in physicians' financial education. I have two recommendations: (1) every physician, young and old, should read this book; and (2) read it a second time!"

Dr. Neil Baum; MD
Clinical Associate Professor of Urology
Tulane Medical School, New Orleans, Louisiana

"I worked with a Certified Medical Planner™ on several occasions in the past, and will do so again in the future. This book codified the vast body of knowledge that helped in all facets of my financial life and professional medical practice."

Dr. James E. Williams; DABPS
Foot and Ankle Surgeon
Conyers, Georgia

"This is a constantly changing field for rules, regulations, taxes, insurance, compliance and investments. This book assists readers, and their financial advisors, in keeping up with what's going on in the healthcare field that all doctors need to know."

Patricia Raskob; CFP®, EA, ATA
Raskob Kambourian Financial Advisors
Tucson, Arizona

"I particularly enjoyed reading the specific examples in this book which pointed out the perils of risk ... something with which I am too familiar and have learned (the hard way) to avoid like the Black Death. It is a pleasure to come across this kind of wisdom, in print, that other colleagues may learn before it's too late; many, many years down the road."

Dr. Robert S. Park; MD
Robert Park and Associates Insurance
Seattle, Washington

"Although this book targets physicians, I was pleased to see that it also addressed the financial planning and employment benefit needs of nurses; physical, respiratory and occupational therapists; CRNAs, hospitalists and other members of the health care team....highly readable, practical and understandable."

Nurse Cecelia T. Perez; RN
Hospital Operating Room Manager
Ellicott City, Maryland

"Personal financial success in the PP-ACA era will be more difficult to achieve than ever before. It requires the next-generation of doctors to rethink frugality, delay gratification and re-define the very definition of success and work-life balance. And, they will surely need the subject matter medical specificity and new-wave professional guidance offered in this book. This book is a "must read" for all health care professionals, and their financial advisors, who wish to take an active role in creating a new subset of informed and pioneering professionals known as Certified Medical Planners™."

Dr. Mark D. Dollard; FACFAS
Private Practice
Tysons Corner, Virginia

"As healthcare professionals, it is our Hippocratic duty to avoid preventable harm by paying attention. On the other hand, some of us are guilty of being reckless with our own financial health—delaying serious consideration of investments, taxation, retirement income, estate planning and inheritances until the worry keeps one awake at night. So, if you have avoided planning for the future for far too long, perhaps it is time to take that first step toward preparedness. This in-depth textbook is an excellent starting point—not only because of its readability, but because of the team's expertise and thoroughness in addressing the intricacies of modern investments—and from the point of view of not only gifted financial experts, but as healthcare providers, as well ... a rare combination."

Dr. Darrell K. Pruitt; DDS
Private Practice Dentist
Fort Worth, Texas

"This text should be on the bookshelf of all contemporary physicians. The book is physician-focused with unique topics applicable to all medical professionals. But, it also offers helpful insights into the new tax and estate laws; fiduciary accountability for advisors and insurance agents; with investing, asset protection and risk management, and retirement planning strategies with updates for the brave new world of global payments of the Patient Protection and Affordable Care Act (Obamacare) 2014. Starting out by encouraging readers to examine their personal "money blueprint" beliefs and habits, the book is divided into four sections offering holistic

life cycle financial information and economic education directed to new, mid-career and mature physicians.

This structure permits one to dip into the book based on personal need, to find relief, rather than to overwhelm. Given the complexity of modern domestic healthcare, and the daunting challenges faced by physicians who try to stay abreast of clinical medicine and the ever-evolving laws of personal finance, this textbook could not have come at a better time."

Dr. Philippa Kennealy; MD, MPH
The Entrepreneurial MD
Los Angeles, California

"Physicians have economic concerns unmatched by any other profession, arriving ten years late to the start of their earning years. This textbook goes to the core of how to level the playing field quickly, and efficaciously, by a new breed of dedicated Certified Medical Planners™. With physician-focused financial advice, each chapter is a building block to your financial fortress."

Thomas McKeon; MBA
Pharmaceutical Representative
Philadelphia, Pennsylvania

"Excellent Resource—This textbook is written in a manner that provides physician practice owners with a comprehensive guide to financial planning and related topics for their professional practice in a way that is easily comprehended. The style in which it breaks down the intricacies of the current physician practice landscape makes it a 'must read' for those physicians (and their advisors) practicing in the volatile era of healthcare reform."

Robert James Cimasi; MHA, ASA, FRICS, MCBA, CVA, CM&AA, CMP™
CEO-Health Capital Consultants, LLC
St. Louis, Missouri

"Rarely can one find a full compendium of information within a single source or text, but this book communicates the new financial realities we are forced to confront; it is full of opportunities for minimizing tax liability and maximizing income potential. We're recommending it to all our medical practice management clients across the entire healthcare spectrum."

Alan Guinn
The Guinn Consultancy Group, Inc.
Cookeville, Tennessee

"Dr. David Edward Marcinko; MBA, CMP™ and his team take a seemingly endless stream of disparate concepts and integrates them into a simple, straight forward and understandable path to success. And, he codifies them all into a step-by-step algorithm to more efficient investing, risk management, taxation and enhanced retirement planning for doctors and nurses. His text is a vital read—and must execute—book for all healthcare professionals and physician-focused financial advisors."

Dr. O. Kent Mercado; JD
Private Practitioner and Attorney
Naperville, Illinois

"Kudos—The editors and contributing authors have compiled the most comprehensive reference book for the medical community that has ever been attempted. As you review the chapters of

interest and hone in on the most important concerns you may have, realize that the best minds have been harvested for you to: Plan well... Live well"

Martha J. Schilling; AAMS®, CRPC®, ETSC, CSA
Shilling Group Advisors, LLC
Philadelphia, Pennsylvania

"I recommend this book to any physician or medical professional that desires an honest no-sales approach to understanding the financial planning and investing world. It is worthwhile to any financial advisor interested in this space, as well."

David K. Luke; MIM, MS-PFP, CMP™
Net Worth Advisory Group
Sandy, Utah

"Although not a substitute for a formal business education, this book will help physicians navigate effectively through the hurdles of day-to-day financial decisions with the help of an accountant, financial and legal advisor. I highly recommend it and commend Dr. Marcinko and the Institute of Medical Business Advisors, Inc. on a job well done."

Ken Yeung; MBA, CMP™
Tseung Kwan O Hospital
Hong Kong

"I've seen many ghost written handbooks, paperbacks and vanity-published manuals on this topic throughout my career in mental healthcare. Most were poorly written, opinionated and cheaply produced self-aggrandizing marketing drivel for those agents selling commission based financial products and expensive advisory services. So, I was pleasantly surprised with this comprehensive peer-reviewed academic textbook; complete with citations, case examples and real-life integrated strategies, by and for, medical professionals. Although a bit late for my career, I recommend it highly to all my younger colleagues ..... Its credibility and specificity stands alone."

Dr. Clarice Montgomery; PhD, MA
Retired Clinical Psychologist

"In an industry known for one-size-fits-all templates, and massively customized books, products, advice and services; the extreme healthcare specificity of this text is both refreshing and comprehensive."

Dr. James Joseph Bartley
Columbus, Georgia

"My brother was my office administrator and accountant. We both feel this is the most comprehensive textbook available on financial planning for healthcare providers."

Dr. Anthony Robert Naruska; DC
Winter Park, Florida

COMPREHENSIVE FINANCIAL PLANNING STRATEGIES for DOCTORS and ADVISORS

Best Practices from Leading Consultants
and Certified Medical Planners™

Edited by

Dr. David Edward Marcinko, MBA, CMP™
Prof. Hope Rachel Hetico, RN, MHA, CMP™

Foreword by Jason Dyken MD, MBA, CWS®

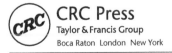

CRC Press
Taylor & Francis Group
Boca Raton London New York

CRC Press is an imprint of the
Taylor & Francis Group, an **informa** business

A PRODUCTIVITY PRESS BOOK

CRC Press
Taylor & Francis Group
6000 Broken Sound Parkway NW, Suite 300
Boca Raton, FL 33487-2742

First issued in hardback 2019

© 2015 by Taylor & Francis Group, LLC
CRC Press is an imprint of Taylor & Francis Group, an Informa business

Library of Congress Cataloging-in-Publication Data

Comprehensive financial planning strategies for doctors and advisors : best practices from leading
  consultants and certified medical planners / edited by David Edward Marcinko and Hope Rachel Hetico.
    p. ; cm.
  The trademark symbol appears after the word "planners" at the end of the subtitle.
  Includes bibliographical references and index.
  ISBN 978-1-4822-4028-3 (hardcover : alk. paper)
    I. Marcinko, David E. (David Edward), editor. II. Hetico, Hope R., editor.
  [DNLM: 1. Physicians--economics. 2. Practice Management--economics. 3. Risk Management. W 79]

R728.5
331.2'81362172--dc23   2014034118

Visit the Taylor & Francis Web site at
http://www.taylorandfrancis.com

and the CRC Press Web site at
http://www.crcpress.com

Exordium

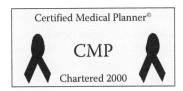

Certified Medical Planner©

CMP

Chartered 2000

Comprehensive Financial Planning Strategies for Doctors and Advisors: Best Practices from Leading Consultants and Certified Medical Planners™ will shape the physician-focused financial planning landscape for the next generation of Health 2.0 medical professionals and their financial advisors.

WHY NOW?

We created this innovative textbook because the healthcare industry is rapidly changing and the financial planning ecosystem has not kept pace. Traditional insurance-commission and sales-driven generic advice is yielding to a new breed of deeply informed fiduciary advisor and educated consultant, or Certified Medical Planner (CMP™). The Internet and social media of the last decade demonstrate that medical providers are becoming accustomed to the need for knowledgeable advice. And financial planning is set to be transformed by "market disruptors" that will soon make an impact on the $2.8 trillion healthcare marketplace for those financial advisors serving this sector.

We are at the leading edge of this positive disruption—also known as niche-based Financial Planning 2.0—that over time will see today's command-controlled financial services industry becomes a wide open academic marketplace. And a growing cadre of specialty entrants is poised to shake up the industry, drawing billions of dollars in revenue from traditional broker-dealer organizations while building lucrative new markets.

For example, an iMBA Inc survey points to the growing need for financial advisors to serve current and future medical professionals thanks to their eagerness to seek premium financial planning solutions from non-traditional sources and providers, like the online Certified Medical Planner™ charter designation program. The industry is ripe for a shakeup, and physician-focused financial planning will soon have its own new brands. We aim to be among the first movers and top tier names in the industry.

HOW WE ARE DIFFERENT?

Comprehensive Financial Planning Strategies for Doctors and Advisors: Best Practices from Leading Consultants and Certified Medical Planners™ will change this niche industry sector by following eight important principles.

First, we have assembled a world-class editorial advisory board and independent team of contributors and reviewers and asked them to draw on their experiences in contemporaneous healthcare-focused financial planning. Like many of their physician and nurse clients, each struggles mightily with decreasing revenues, increasing costs, automation, SEC scrutiny, and higher physician–client expectations in today's competitive financial advisory and technological landscape. Yet their practical experience and physician-focused education, knowledge, and vision are a source of objective information, informed opinion, and crucial information to all consultants working with doctors and medical professionals in the financial services field.

Second, our writing style allows us to condense a great deal of information into one book. We integrate bullet points and tables, pithy language, prose, and specialty perspectives with real-world examples and case models. The result is an oeuvre of integrated financial planning principles vital to all modern physicians and allied healthcare professionals.

Third, to the best of our knowledge, this is the first peer-reviewed book of its type, as we seek to follow traditional medical research and journal publishing guidelines for best practices. We present differing viewpoints, divergent and opposing stakeholder perspectives, and informed personal and professional opinions. Each chapter has been reviewed by one to three outside independent reviewers and critical thinkers. We include references and citations, and although we cannot rule out all biases, we strive to make them transparent to the extent possible.

Fourth, our perspective is decidedly from the physician-client side of the equation. More specifically, as consultants to medical professionals, we champion the physician-investor over the financial advisor. And to the extent that both sides ethically succeed, we hope all concerned "do well—by doing good." This is unique in the fee and commission-driven financial services industry. Much like the emerging patient-centered care initiative in medicine, we call it client-centered advice.

Fifth, it is important to note that deep specificity and niche knowledge is needed when advising physicians and healthcare providers. And so we present information directly from that space, and not by indirect example from other industries, as is the unfortunate norm. Medical case models, healthcare industry examples, and anecdotal insights from the *Overheard in the Doctor's Lounge* and *Overheard in the Advisor's Lounge* features are also included. Finally, personalized financial planning for all medical professionals is our core and only focus.

Sixth, this textbook represents an academic template for about 25% (125/500 credit hours) of the Certified Medical Planner™ chartered professional online certification program curriculum. It is useful for those studying, auditing, or considering matriculation for this prestigious designation mark.

Seventh, we include a glossary of terms specific to the text, a list of comprehensive advice sources, and three illustrative physician-specific financial plan examples additionally available by separate order.

Finally, as editors, we prefer engaged readers who demand compelling content. According to conventional wisdom, printed texts like this one should be a relic of the past, from an era before instant messaging and high-speed connectivity. Our experience shows just the opposite. Applied physician-focused personal financial planning literature from informed fiduciary sources is woefully sparse, just as a plethora of generalized Internet information makes that material less valuable to doctor clients.

A SEMINAL WORK

Rest assured that *Comprehensive Financial Planning Strategies for Doctors and Advisors: Best Practices from Leading Consultants and Certified Medical Planners*™ will become a seminal book for the advancement of personal financial planning and related personal micro-economic principles in this niche ecosystem. In the years ahead, we trust these principles will enhance utility and add value to your book. Most importantly, we hope to increase your return on investment by some small increment.

If you have any comments or would like to contribute material or suggest topics for future editions, please contact me.

Professor Hope Rachel Hetico
Managing Editor

Target Market and Ideal Readers

Comprehensive Financial Planning Strategies for Doctors and Advisors: Best Practices from Leading Consultants and Certified Medical Planners™ should be in the hands of all

- Allopathic (MD), osteopathic (DO), and podiatric physicians (DPMs); dentists (DDS and DMD); nurses (RNs-LPNs), advanced nurse practitioners (ANPs), and physician assistants (PAs); physical therapists (PTs), doctors of chiropractic (DCs); CRNAs, and DVMs; occupational therapists (OTs), physical and speech therapists, and related assistants and allied healthcare providers.
- Medical, law, graduate, and nursing school students, interns, residents, and fellows as well as new, mid-life, and mature healthcare practitioners of all types!
- Financial Advisors (FAs), registered investment advisors (RIAs), Certified Financial Planners® (CFPs), wealth managers (WMs), chartered financial analysts (CFAs), chartered life underwriters (CLUs), insurance agents, stock-brokers, bankers, attorneys, registered financial consultants (RFCs), certified public accountants (CPAs), enrolled agents (EAs), investment advisors (IAs), and all other financial intermediaries, consultants, and product salesman of all stripes, degrees, and general designations.
- Retail, discount, wholesale (on-ground and online) brokerage firms, and wirehouses as well as hedge and mutual fund managers and hospital and healthcare entity endowment fund managers.
- Fraternal financial services organizations like the American College of Financial Services in Bryn Mawr, Pennsylvania; Certified Financial Planner Board of Standards (CFP-BOD) in Washington, DC; the College for Financial Planning (CFP) in Centennial, Colorado; and the National Association of Personal Financial Advisors (NAPFA) in Arlington Heights, Illinois, etc.
- All undergraduate, graduate, and business schools and universities with related certification conferring education programs and investing or insurance-related diplomas, adult learning, and CEU programs.

Dedication

It is an incredible privilege to edit Comprehensive Financial Planning Strategies for Doctors and Advisors: Best Practices from Leading Consultants and Certified Medical Planners™. *One of the most rewarding aspects of my career has been the professional growth acquired from interacting with medical colleagues and legal and financial services professionals of all stripes. The mutual sharing and exchange of ideas stimulates the mind and fosters advancement at many levels.*

For example, we take pride and inspiration from pioneering medical and financial planning colleagues such as John Stephens, MD, MBA, CFA®, CFP®; Erik Thurnher, MD, CFP®; Joel Greenwald, MD, CFP®; Douglas G. Burnette, MD, CFP®; Jeff Davenport, MD, CFP®, Ralph Broadwater, MD, CFP®, AIF®; Carolyn McClanahan, MD, CFP®; Richard Mata, MD, MS, CMP™ [Hon]; Stanley S. Zelman, DDS, CFP®; Jeffery Hochstein, DDS, CFP®; John N. Carmody, DDS, CFP®; Robert J. Mallin, DDS, CFP®; James M. Belcher, DDS, CFP®; Gregory Kasten, MD, MBA, CFP®; Harold Whittman, DDS, CFP®; Joseph Ellis, DPM, EA, CFP®; Brent W. Bost, MD, MBA, CPA; Jeffrey J. Rockefeller, DPM, MBA, CFP®; and James Winston Phillips, MD, JD, MBA, LLM.

Of course, creating this text was a significant effort that involved all members of our firm. Over the past year, we interfaced with numerous outside private and public companies—as well as the Internet blogosphere—to discuss its contents. And although impossible to list every person or company that played a role in its production, there are several other people we wish to thank for their support and encouragement: Kristine Mednansky— senior editor business improvement (healthcare management), Karen Sober—editorial assistant, Kari Budyk—senior project coordinator, and Richard O'Hanley—CRC Press (Taylor & Francis Group).

Finally, we acknowledge this text would not have been possible without the support of our families whose daily advocacy encouraged all of us to completion. It is also dedicated to our clients, all Certified Medical Planners™, adult learners, and the contributing authors who crashed the development life cycle in order to produce time-sensitive material in an expedient manner. The satisfaction we enjoyed from working with them is immeasurable.

Any accolades are because of them…. All defects are my own.

Dr. David Edward Marcinko; MBA, CMP™
Norcross, Georgia, USA

Contents

SECTION I   For All Practitioners

SECTION II   For New Practitioners

SECTION III   For Mid-Career Practitioners

Editorial

EDITOR-IN-CHIEF

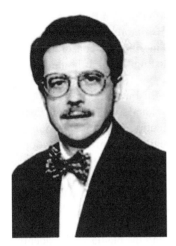

Dr. David Edward Marcinko is a next-generation apostle of Nobel Laureate Kenneth Joseph Arrow, PhD, as a healthcare economist, administrative and technology futurist, risk manager, and former board-certified surgeon from Temple University in Philadelphia. In the past, he edited eight practice-management books, three medical textbooks and manuals in four languages, five financial planning yearbooks, dozens of interactive CD-ROMs, and three comprehensive healthcare administration dictionaries. Internationally recognized for his clinical work, he is an honorary distinguished visiting professor of surgery at the Marien Hospital, Aachen, Germany, who provides litigation support and expert witness testimony in state and federal court, with medical publications archived in the Library of Congress and the Library of Medicine at the National Institutes of Health (NIH). His thought leadership essays have been cited in journals such as *Managed Care Executives, Healthcare Informatics, Medical Interface, Plastic Surgery Products, Teaching and Learning in Medicine, Orthodontics Today, Chiropractic Products, Journal of the American Medical Association, Podiatry Today, Investment Advisor Magazine, Registered Representative, Financial Advisor Magazine, CFP™ Biz (Journal of Financial Planning), Journal of the American Medical Association* (JAMA.ama-assn.org), *The Business Journal for Physicians,* and *Physician's Money Digest* and by companies and professional organizations like the Medical Group Management Association (MGMA), American College of Medical Practice Executives (ACMPE), American College of Physician Executives (ACPE), American College of Emergency Room Physicians (ACEP), Health Care Management Associates (HMA), and PhysiciansPractice. com and by academic institutions such as the UCLA School of Medicine, Northern University College of Business, Creighton University, Medical College of Wisconsin, University of North Texas Health Science Center, Washington University School of Medicine, Emory University School of Medicine and the Goizueta School of Business at Emory University, University of Pennsylvania Medical and Dental Libraries, Southern Illinois College of Medicine, University at Buffalo Health Sciences Library, University of Michigan Dental Library, and the University of Medicine and Dentistry of New Jersey, among many others. Dr. Marcinko also has numerous primary and secondary editorial and reviewing roles to his credit.

Dr. Marcinko earned his undergraduate degree from Loyola University, Maryland, completed his internship and residency at the Atlanta Hospital and Medical Center, is Fellow of the American College of Foot and Ankle Surgeons, earned his business degree from the Keller Graduate School of Management (Chicago), and his financial planning diploma from Oglethorpe University (Atlanta). He was a licensee of the Certified Financial Planner® Board of Standards for a decade and holds the Certified Medical Planner™ designation (CMP™). He earned Series #7 (general securities), Series #63 (uniform securities state law), and Series #65 (investment advisory) licenses from the National Association of Securities Dealers (NASD) and Financial Industry Regulatory Authority (FINRA), and he held a life, health, disability, variable annuity, and property-casualty license from the state of Georgia. Dr. Marcinko was also co-founder of an ambulatory surgery center that was sold to a public company. He has been a Certified Physician in Healthcare Quality (CPHQ), a certified American Board of Quality Assurance and Utilization Review Physician (ABQAURP), a medical-staff vice president of a general acute care hospital, an assistant residency director, a founder of a computer-based testing firm for doctors, and president of a regional physician practice-management corporation in the Midwest. He was a member of the American Health Information Management Association (AHIMA) and the Healthcare Information and Management Systems Society (HIMSS) and the Microsoft Professional Accountant's Network (MPAN), the Microsoft Health User's Group (MS-HUG), and a registered member of the U.S. Microsoft Partners Program (MPP). Dr. Marcinko was also a website engineer and beta tester for Microsoft Office Live Essentials program. As president of a privately held physician practice management corporation in 1999, he consolidated 95 solo medical practices with $150 million in revenues for a pre-IPO listing. In 2011, he joined the Physician Nexus Medical Advisory Board.

Dr. Marcinko is chief executive officer for the Institute of Medical Business Advisors, Inc. The firm is headquartered in Atlanta and works with a diverse list of individual and corporate clients. It sponsors the professional Certified Medical Planner™ charter designation program and counsels maverick physicians transitioning into alternate careers. As a nationally recognized educational resource center and referral alliance, iMBA and its network of independent professionals provide solutions and managerial peace-of-mind to physicians, healthcare organizations, and their consulting business advisors. He also helped developed medical, business, and graduate and undergraduate school curriculum content for the American College of Physician Executives (ACPE), Medical Group Management Association (MGMA), and the American College of Healthcare Executives (ACHE). A favorite on the lecture circuit, Dr. Marcinko is often quoted in the media and frequently speaks on related topics throughout this country and Europe in an entertaining and witty fashion. He is a popular authority on transformational business strategies across a pantheon of related industries. He is also a social media pioneer and publisher of the *Medical Executive Post*, an influential syndicated Health 2.0 interactive blog forum.

As an award-winning journalist, media broadcaster, speaker, public health ambassador, financial planning, and economics consultant, Dr. Marcinko is available to colleagues, clients, and the press at his corporate office in Atlanta, Georgia.

MANAGING EDITOR

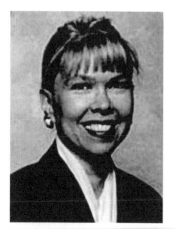

Professor Hope Rachel Hetico received her bachelor's degree in nursing (BSN) from Valpariso University, and her master of science in healthcare administration (MHA) from the University of St. Francis, in Joliette, Illinois. She is the author or editor of a dozen major textbooks and is a nationally known expert in managed medical care, medical reimbursement, case management, health insurance, utilization review, National Association of Healthcare Quality (NAHQ), Health Education Data Information Set (HEDIS), and The Joint Commission (TJC) Clinical Quality Measures (CQMs) and regulations.

Prior to joining the Institute of Medical Business Advisors as chief operating officer, Ms. Hetico was a hospital executive, financial advisor, insurance agent, Certified Professional in Healthcare Quality (CPHQ), and distinguished visiting assistant professor of healthcare administration for the University of Phoenix, Graduate School of Business and Management in Atlanta. She was also the national corporate director for Medical Quality Improvement at Abbey, and then Apria Healthcare, a public company in Costa Mesa, California.

A devotee of health information technology and heutagogy, Ms. Hetico is responsible for leading the website www.CertifiedMedicalPlanner.org to the top of the exploding adult educational marketplace, expanding the online and on-ground CMP™ charter designation program, and nurturing the company's rapidly growing list of medical colleagues and financial services industry clients.

Professor Hetico recently completed successful consulting engagements as ACO clinical integration coordinator for Resurrection Health Care Preferred in Chicago and as performance improvement manager for Emory University and Saint Joseph's Hospital in Atlanta. She is currently on assignment for Presence Health Partners, the largest Catholic health system in Illinois.

PROJECT MANAGER

Mackenzie Hope Marcinko is a computer science, linguistics, and business management intern from the University of Pittsburgh. Founded in 1787, the university is a healthcare informatics and technology pioneer and one of the nation's most distinguished members of the Association of American Universities. It perennially ranks as one of the top public universities in total sponsored research funding and is among the top 10 recipients of funding from the National Institutes of Health (NIH).

EXECUTIVE DIRECTOR

Ann Marie Miller; RN, MHA, is the project manager for the Institute of Medical Business Advisors Inc. and the Certified Medical Planner™ online professional education and certification designation program, Norcross, Georgia.

ACADEMIC DEAN AND PROVOST

Eugene Schmuckler; PhD, MEd, MBA, CTS, is the consulting psychologist for the Institute of Medical Business Advisors, Inc. and the Certified Medical Planner™ online professional education and certification designation program, Norcross, Georgia.

NORTH AMERICAN AMBASSADOR

Rachel Pentin-Maki; RN, MHA, is a former Intensive Care Unit (ICU) and Telemetry Unit (TU) manager, nursing school instructor, and Finnish Rest Home BOD member, Lantana, Florida.

INTERNATIONAL AMBASSADOR

Keung Chi [Kenneth] Yeung; MBA, CMP™, is a hospital administrator and financial consultant for the Tseung Kwan O Hospital, Hong Kong. He speaks English, Cantonese, Mandarin, and Chinese.

About the Book Cover

This colorful vector-graphic silhouette depicts doctors, nurses, and allied healthcare professionals seeking deep client-centered and collaborative financial advice from a fiduciary-focused consultant or Certified Medical Planner™.

Foreword

Healthcare professionals who wrongly believe that a generalist financial advisor or a one-size-fits-all approach to personal financial planning is adequate for their needs must change this mindset immediately and read this comprehensive textbook.

Why? An industry sea-change of technology, transparency, and specialization is upon us, and *Comprehensive Financial Planning Strategies for Doctors and Advisors: Best Practices from Leading Consultants and Certified Medical Planners*™ is important enough to lead the way! There is no other comprehensive book like it to help doctors, nurses, and other medical providers accumulate and preserve the wealth their years of education and hard work have earned them.

For example, the increasing complexities of the Patient Protection and Affordable Care Act's delivery system with its emerging and global Accountable Care Organization (ACO) reimbursement models, along with new tax laws and investing vehicles, risk management, compliance legalities and cyber-technology, and revised retirement, asset protection, and estate planning issues of the "new economic normal" all mandate that standard advice for the masses—promoted by the sales-orientated financial services industry purveyors of the past—be severely challenged by modern physicians and financial advisors.

In fact, all healthcare professionals and their financial advisors need to focus on our specific industry and use this resource to understand the integrated principles of contemporary financial planning. And they should be merged with the specific economic life cycle needs of medical providers. Indeed, this unique book created *by doctors and for doctors* helps colleagues and their advisors understand why they are so different and why they require a new array of thought-leading techniques and strategies to achieve personal goals and objectives.

The text is a masterful collection of academic and peer-reviewed research and writing, with real-world experiences, case studies, and models with references, all blended with traditional and innovative information specific to the business of health care. It serves as a fiduciary's guide to help doctors develop a comprehensive financial plan that focuses on their unique needs. It is indeed transformative. Some even call it the next generation of financial planning for health professionals—version 2.0—because it assists them in creating a legacy, after a life of service, to *pay-it-forward*.

As an internist and now a wealth management specialist for more than a decade—who is also married to an orthodontist—my informed opinion is to read *Comprehensive Financial Planning Strategies for Doctors and Advisors: Best Practices from Leading Consultants and Certified Medical Planners*™ to become educated, then enlightened, and finally fiscally stable over time.

In summary, congratulations to the editor and team who produced this revolutionary textbook. I highly recommend it. "Read it and financially reap."

Jason Dyken; MD, MBA, CWS®
Certified Wealth Strategist®
Dyken Wealth Strategies
Gulf Shores, Alabama

Preface

In my 20 years of medical practice and 15 years as a financial advisor, I observed that physicians are particularly disadvantaged when it comes to anything regarding finance. Most doctors and health-care providers have enough on their mind practicing their specialty and keeping up with technology, compliance and practice trends that planning for their financial future is often forgotten. Financial planning and good investment practices require a solid background of how companies work in the "real world" and an awareness of how they function within the economy. These economic essentials are vital to understanding business, as are principles like budgeting, risk management, cash flow analysis, fiscal benchmarking, and rudimentary accounting that are presented in this book. Yet physicians have economic concerns that are different than most people.

- First, they enter the workforce about a decade later than their nonmedical contemporaries, leaving fewer productive years and beginning with enormous medical school debt levels.
- Second, they tend to marry and have children later in life, often postponing their offspring's educational funding and their own retirement planning.
- Third, family members often erroneously think of them as affluent, seeking their financial assistance.
- Fourth, health reform and managed care have reduced remuneration just as governmental scrutiny has burdened practices with costly IT, privacy rules, and PP-ACA regulations.
- Fifth, a three-decades-long bull market in bonds and equities is over, and if the current "new-normal" prevails—meaning a 4.5% real annualized rate of return on equities and a 1.5% real rate on bonds—wealth accumulation for all will be reduced going forward.
- Sixth, physicians lack financial management expertise, especially after changes in the tax code, electronic connectivity initiatives, various new practice risks, healthcare reform and the PP-ACA, and so on.

Accordingly, informed advice from a medically focused advisor, or Certified Medical Planner™, is vital. And construction of a comprehensive financial plan, with an Investment Policy Statement (IPS), that acknowledges the impact of health reform and the PP-ACA is now almost an essential requirement for success.

Traditionally, a well-conceived financial plan consisted of tax reduction planning, various insurance matters, investing, portfolio management, retirement, and estate planning. For modern physicians of the Health 2.0 Era, however, these disciplines, and many more, must be incorporated into the mix in a managerially and psychologically sound manner not counterproductive to individual components of the plan. As a sobering caveat, the integration of these protean disciplines is no longer an academic luxury but a pragmatic survival imperative recognized by the contemporary Certified Medical Planner™ and corporate sponsors at the Institute of Medical Business Advisors, Inc. The following two examples are illustrative.

- Recall the sad tale of Dr. Debasis Kanjilal, the pediatrician from New York who, in 2000, put more than $500,000 into the dot.com company InfoSpace on the advice of Merrill Lynch's star analyst Henry Bloget. Is it any wonder that when the company crashed, the analyst was sued, banned for life from the securities industry, and Merrill settled out of court? As a matter of public record, other analysts, such as Mary Meeker of Morgan Stanley, Dean Witter and Jack Grubman from Salomon Smith Barney/Citigroup, were involved in similar debacles. Would passage of Senate bill HR 1000, also known as the

Pension Security Act (PSA) creating the category of *Fiduciary Advisor* for qualified participants such as those with 401(k) plans, have prevented this mischief by adding stockbrokers to ERISA's list of prudent experts?

- Now, reflect a moment on medical colleagues willing to securitize their practices a few years later and cash out to Wall Street servitude for riches not rightly deserved. Where are firms such as MedPartners, Phycor, FPA, Coastal Healthcare, and a host of others now? A recent survey of the Cain Brothers Physician Practice Management Corporation Index of publicly traded PPMCs revealed a market capital loss of more than 99% since inception. Would niche-educated and physician-focused financial advisors (the Certified Medical Planner™ professional designation did not yet exist) have been able to avoid this calamity?

Want more proof this book is sorely needed? Just remember the sub-prime mortgage crisis of 2008, recognized and acted upon almost exclusively by contributor Michael J. Burry, MD. And don't forget the financial impact of the Patient Protection and Affordable Care Act (PP-ACA) that is finally rolling out through 2016; it is both pervasive and invasive to virtually all Americans and medical providers, with detractors and advocates on both sides.

Of course, financial planning and personal economics is always challenging because chaos is the constant element of life. It is even more so for physicians, who face the reality that medical care is becoming a commodity in the United States. Even the late Dr. C. Everett Koop, MD opined that although Americans have no constitutional right to healthcare, the perception of one is so strong that the country is likely to have a socialized system some time in the near future. With our national agenda dominated by terrorism, the threat of biological and chemical warfare, bioengineering and the ethical concerns of human cloning, electronic medical records, mobile health and ICD-10, technological advancements, para-professional practitioners, and health network hacking and cyber-insecurity, it is unlikely that significant governmental financial assistance to physicians will take place anytime soon. In fact, many opine that over the next few years, reimbursement rates set by the Center for Medicare and Medicaid Services (CMS) could further erode by another 15–20% after full implementation of the PP-ACA.

Individual provider and personal circumstances also change as the domestic healthcare milieu is in constant flux. Comprehensive financial planning for medical professionals is truly a journey and not a destiny. Progress toward personal and practice goals are the objective, not some composite index, annualized rate of return, or stock price.

Therefore, for physicians and health professionals to survive, economic and financial competency are required in the new order. Hopefully, the requisite material to begin the task has been codified for them, and their advisors, in *Comprehensive Financial Planning Strategies for Doctors and Advisors: Best Practices from Leading Consultants and Certified Medical Planners™*.

And so, if there is some financial issue not specifically addressed in this book, fear not! The sub-niche topic you seek will likely be covered in a future iMBA Inc. textbook or online at the Medical Executive-Post (www.MedicalExecutivePost.com). Join our more than 750,000 readers and subscribers today. A subscription is fast, free, and secure.

Dr. David Edward Marcinko, MBA, CMP™
Certified Medical Planner™
Editor-in-Chief

Introduction for Condensed Reading and Review

Comprehensive Financial Planning Strategies for Doctors and Advisors: Best Practices from Leading Consultants and Certified Medical Planners™ is written in prose form with a value proposition that is solely for medical professionals and their financial advisors. Uniquely, it is written by and for doctors and those financial advisors with intimate knowledge of the healthcare industrial complex. We use nontechnical jargon without the need to document every statement with a citation from the literature. This allows a large amount of information to be condensed into a single and practical book. It also allows the reader to comprehend an important concept in a single reading session with a deliberate effort to include current information. The interested reader is then able to research selected topics. Overlap of material is reduced, but important concepts are reviewed for increased understanding.

The textbook itself is divided into four life-cycle sections, with 24 logically progressive yet stand-alone chapters by 24 contributing experts integrated by our editorial staff.

Section I commences with the seldom discussed topic of behavioral finance and economics, integrated with holistic and life cycle financial planning, as the physiological and psychological divide is professionally examined by a physician, psychiatrist-securities analyst, and psychologists for the benefit of financial advisors. Chapter 2 gives an overview of physician job recruitment and employee retention, while Chapter 3 reviews student debt, medical education costs, and dwindling-to-flat health worker compensation. Chapter 4 is on the economics of fringe benefit plans for employed doctors and medical professionals, including stock options of a public healthcare entity or hospital. Chapter 5 is on fundamental micro-economic topics and money management principals followed by personal financial benchmarks and budgeting for young medical professionals. Chapter 6 concludes with a review of financial statements for a proto-typical medical practice with cash flow analysis that is basic to both profitable operations and investing.

Section II begins with Chapter 7 on insurance strategies for doctors, their possessions and practices, and seamlessly flows into Chapter 8 on modern medical risk management issues of current import well beyond malpractice liability. Chapters 9 and 10 are conjoined in that the personal tax reduction strategies outlined in the former are carried over into medical office practice accounting strategies in the later. Chapter 11 reviews investment products, concepts, and vehicles from the perspective of Modern Portfolio Theory (MPF), the Capital Asset Pricing Model (CAP-M), and the Arbitrage Pricing Theory (APT). Chapter 12 concludes by reviewing the complexities of protective trusts and more complex asset protection planning for physicians.

Section III gives a rare insider's look at investment banking and the actual Wall Street order and trading process, including an insider's look at the murky world of high-frequency trading (HFT) in Chapter 13. Chapters 14 and 15 explore the covert world of hedge funds and related market neutral funds, respectively. Chapter 16 discusses commercial real estate as an asset class, while Chapter 17 explores the emerging concept of the independent medical practice as another distinct portfolio class for physician owners. The section concludes with both traditional and new concepts of the retirement planning life cycle specifically for healthcare professionals in Chapter 18.

Section IV starts with a discussion on professional portfolio construction (Chapter 19), followed by Chapter 20 on investment policy statement construction (IPS) for individual physicians and major hospital endowment funds. Chapter 21 contemplates the emotional and financial implications of divorce and other special lifestyle situations. Chapter 22 reports on the legal and contracting needs for medical practice sales and succession planning. Chapter 23 reviews modern estate planning strategies and previews the "ethical-will" concept first imagined by physicians and just now being noted by financial advisors. Chapter 24 rightly concludes the book with a discussion on choosing the financial consultant that is the best fit for the medical practice environment and modern health-care provider. It offers a unique emphasis on industry obfuscation practices, fees, commissions, and automated processes as well as thoughts on credentials, training, licensure, and education.

Regardless of background, readers of all types should use this book in the following way.

First, read the Front Matter. Browse through the Table of Contents and the entire book *in toto*. Next, slowly read chapters of specific interest to your professional efforts or life-cycle stage. Then, extrapolate portions that can be implemented as pertinent strategies helpful to your own personal situation or professional advisory setting. Finally, use the book as an actionable reference for review and return to it time and again … and stay current with our related interactive blog forum: www. MedicalExecutivePost.com … to learn and enjoy!

In conclusion, as you read, study, and reflect on this challenging new-era textbook, remember the guiding philosophy of Eric Hoffer: *"In a time of drastic change; it is the learners who will inherit the future. The learned find themselves equipped to live in a world that no longer exists."*

Hope Rachel Hetico
Managing Editor
Mackenzie Hope Marcinko
Project Manager

About the Institute of Medical Business Advisors, Inc.

iMBA Inc. is a leading physician executive, medical practice, hospital and healthcare institutional educator, economics and medical valuation consulting firm, and focused provider of textbooks, CD-ROMs, handbooks, templates, tools, dictionaries, and on-site and distance learning for the health administration, financial management, and health policy space. iMBA Inc. leverages opportunity, seeks change, and helps clients to maximize revenue and increase profits. Projects are completed under Non-Disclosure or Non-Circumvention Agreements. We protect the confidentiality of clients, their projects, our recommendations, and their future ongoing plans.

Recently, iMBA Inc. released two major organizational textbooks under the CRC Press (Productivity Press) imprimatur:

- *Hospitals and Healthcare Organizations* (*Management Strategies, Operational Techniques, Tools, Templates and Case Studies*) 2013
- *Financial Management Strategies for Hospitals and Healthcare Organizations* (*Tools, Techniques, Checklists and Case Studies*) 2014

So this text represents the next iMBA initiative into the personal financial planning niche space for physicians and all medical professionals. By integrating the above, iMBA Inc. provides an online asynchronous teaching platform for financial advisors, healthcare accountants, management consultants, and adult learners seeking the professional charter and certification designation known as Certified Medical Planner™.

The firm also serves as a national resource center and referral alliance providing financial stability and managerial peace of mind to struggling physician clients. As competition increases, iMBA Inc. is positioned to meet the collaborative needs of medical colleagues and institutional clients today and well into the disruptive medical and financial services sector and future participatory ecosystem.

iMBA Inc., Corporate Communication Subsidiaries:

PHYSICIANS: www.MedicalBusinessAdvisors.com
PRACTICES: www.BusinessofMedicalPractice.com
HOSPITALS: http://www.crcpress.com/product/isbn/9781466558731
CLINICS: http://www.crcpress.com/product/isbn/9781439879900
BLOG: www.MedicalExecutivePost.com

Notices

DISCLAIMER NOTICE

The information presented in *Comprehensive Financial Planning Strategies for Doctors and Advisors: Best Practices from Leading Consultants and Certified Medical Planners*™ is presented for general informational and educational use only. Prior to engaging in the type of activities described, you should receive independent counsel from a qualified relevant professional. Care has been taken to confirm the accuracy of the information presented, but we offer no warranties, expressed or implied, regarding its currency and are not responsible for errors or omissions or for any consequences from the application of this information. Examples are generally descriptive and do not purport to be accurate in every regard. They are blinded and not all inclusive. The financial services sector and healthcare industry is evolving rapidly, and all information should be considered time sensitive.

Although sponsored by the Institute of Medical Business Advisors, Inc., we maintain an arm's-length relationship with the independent authors and firms who carried out research and prepared the book. The goal of iMBA Inc. is to be unbiased to the extent possible and to promote protean professional perspectives and opinions.

HOLD-HARMLESS NOTICE

This publication is designed to provide information in regard to the subject matter covered. It is not intended to constitute business, insurance, financial planning, technology, legal, accounting, tax, retirement, medical practice management, succession, estate planning, or any other advice. It is sold with the understanding that the editors, authors, reviewers, and publishers are held-harmless in these matters. Examples are generally descriptive and do not purport to be accurate in every regard. The physician-focused financial planning space for medical professionals is evolving rapidly and all information should be considered time sensitive. If advice or other assistance is required, the services of a competent professional person should be sought.

Modified from a *Declaration of Principles* jointly adopted by

- Committee of the American Bar Association
- Committee of Publishers and Associations

FAIR USE NOTICE

Comprehensive Financial Planning Strategies for Doctors and Advisors: Best Practices from Leading Consultants and Certified Medical Planners™ contains URLs, blog snippets, links, and brief excerpts of material obtained from the Internet or public domain, the use of which has not always been specifically authorized by the copyright owner. We are also making such material from our own other books available to advance the understanding of related issues and for the general purpose of reporting and educating. Moreover, we use modern crowd-sourcing methods as well as contributions from our blog forum, www.MedicalExecutivePost.com. We believe this constitutes a "fair use" of any copyrighted material as provided by section 107 of the U.S. Copyright Law. In accordance with Title 17 U.S.C. Section 107, the material is distributed to those who have expressed an interest in text purchase. Moreover, all register®, trade™, service (SM), and copyright© marks are the intangible intellectual property of their respective owners. Mention of any specific product, service, website domain, or company does not constitute endorsement. No compensation was obtained for including the same.

ABOUT INTERNET CITATIONS

Comprehensive Financial Planning Strategies for Doctors and Advisors: Best Practices from Leading Consultants and Certified Medical Planners™ uses uniform resource locators (URLs) to direct readers to useful Internet sites with additional references. However, host entities frequently reorganize and update sites, so URLs can change rapidly. Citations for this text are therefore "live" when published, but we cannot guarantee how long they will remain so, despite our best efforts to keep them current.

Acknowledgments

Creating this interpretive text was a significant effort that involved all members of our firm. Over the past year we interfaced with various public resources such as state governments, the federal government, Federal Register (FR), the Centers for Medicare and Medicaid Services (CMS), and the U.S. Department of Health and Human Services (DHHS), as well as numerous private firms, professionals, and our Internet blog readers to discuss its contents, *Comprehensive Financial Planning Strategies for Doctors and Advisors: Best Practices from Leading Consultants and Certified Medical Planners*™, and helped make it a success!

David Edward Marcinko
Hope Rachel Hetico
Mackenzie Hope Marcinko
Ann Marie Miller

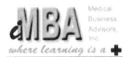

Institute of Medical Business Advisors, Inc—Corporate Headquarters
Peachtree Plantation—West
Suite # 5901 Wilbanks Drive
Norcross, Georgia, USA 30092-1141
770.448.0769 (phone)
Email: MarcinkoAdvisors@msn.com
Email:AdviceForDoctors@Outlook.com
Internet: www.MedicalExecutivePost.com

Contributors

Dr. Dennis Bethel
Bethel Investment Group
Web: http://www.bethelinvestmentgroup.com
Web: http://www.nesteggrx.com
Email: Dennis@nesteggrx.com

Dr. Dennis Bethel received his medical degree from the University of Minnesota. He worked for many years as a full-time emergency medicine physician, but the increasing administrative burdens of medicine spurred his real-estate investment career. With nearly a decade of multifamily real estate experience, Dr. Bethel now focuses on large commercial multifamily acquisitions across multiple markets. The purpose of his educational website is to help medical professionals become knowledgeable of this asset class (www.nesteggrx.com). Today, he believes physicians should consider income-producing multifamily real estate and diversify a portion of their investment portfolio outside the volatile world of the stock market.

Dr. Gary L. Bode; CPA, MSA, CMP™ [Hon]
President - Gary L. Bode MSA CPA PC
2999 Singletree Court
Leland, NC 28451
Phone: (910) 399-2705
Web: www.GaryBodeCPA.com
Email: info@garybodecpa.com

Dr. Gary L. Bode was the chief financial officer (CFO) for a private mental healthcare facility and previously the chief executive officer (CEO) of Comprehensive Practice Accounting, Inc. in Wilmington, North Carolina. The firm specialized in providing tax solutions to medical and dental professionals. Dr. Bode was a board-certified practitioner and managing partner of a multi-office medical group practice for a decade before earning his master of science degree in accounting (MSA) at the University of North Carolina. He is a nationally known forensic health accountant, financial author, educator, and speaker. His areas of expertise include producing customized managerial accounting reports, practice appraisals and valuations, restructurings and innovative financial accounting, as well as proactive tax positioning and tax return preparation for healthcare facilities. Currently, Dr. Bode is chief accounting and valuation officer (CAVO) for the Institute of Medical Business Advisors, Inc. and chief executive officer and founder of Gary Bode MSA CPA, PC. He presents at medical associations throughout the country, with numerous book chapters in texts like *The Business of Medical Practice, Hospitals and Healthcare Organizations* and the *Financial Management Strategies for Hospitals and Healthcare Organizations* by the Institute of Medical Business Advisors, Inc.

Dr. Michael J. Burry
Retired-Founder - Scion Capital Group
20400 Stevens Creek Boulevard
Suite 840
Cupertino, CA 95014

Dr. Michael J. Burry is a hedge fund manager and physician who founded Scion Capital LLC, which he ran from 2000 until 2008. Dr. Burry was one of the first investors in the world to recognize and invest in the impending subprime mortgage crisis. Author Michael Lewis profiled him in his 2010 book *The Big Short: Inside the Doomsday Machine*, and he was featured in Gergory Zuckerman's 2009 book *The Greatest Trade Ever: How John Paulson Bet against the Markets and Made $20 Billion*. Dr. Burry attended UCLA for his undergraduate degree, graduated from Vanderbilt School of Medicine, and did his residency in neurology at Stanford Hospital. He left the medical profession in 2000 and started Scion Capital, which would eventually make millions for investors by investing in undervalued stocks and then betting heavily against subprime mortgages in advance of the 2008 financial crisis. In April 3, 2010, op-ed for the *New York Times*, Burry argued that anyone who studied the financial markets carefully in 2003, 2004, and 2005 could have recognized the growing risk in the subprime markets. He faulted federal regulators for failing to listen to warnings from outside a closed circle of advisors. He has presented at medical associations throughout the country and authored textbook chapters for the iMBA, Inc. As of 2015, he was still managing his own investments.

Dr. Gary A. Cook; EJD, MSFS, CLU®, RHU, ChFC, CFP®, CMP™ [Hon]
Internet Pipeline, Inc.
5454 Jaclyn Lane
Bethlehem, PA 18017

Dr. Gary A. Cook earned a degree in mathematics at the Indiana University of Pennsylvania and a master of science degree in financial services at the American College in Bryn Mawr Pennsylvania, as well as Chartered Life Underwriter® and Registered Health Underwriter. As an accredited Estate Planner, he taught courses in that discipline as well as insurance, business, and finance planning and is past president of the Chester Country Estate Planning Council. He earned his executive juris doctorate at Concord Law School of Kaplan University and is a professional author, sought-after public speaker, and television guest for the Insurance Broadcast System, Inc. He is also a member of the Society of Financial Service Professionals, the Financial Planning Association, and the Association for Advanced Life Underwriting. Formerly, Dr. Cook was an assistant vice president, advanced market support, for AIG Life Insurance Companies (USA). He was also content manager for COSS Development Corporation. Today, he is product manager and advanced sales specialist for Internet Pipeline, Inc. of Charlotte, North Carolina. Dr. Cook has presented at financial and medical associations throughout the region and has contributed several book chapters for the Institute of Medical Business Advisors, Inc.

Dr. Jeffrey S. Coons; PhD, CFA®
Manning & Napier Advisors, Inc.
1100 Chase Square
Rochester, New York 14604
Phone: (585) 325-6880
Fax: (585) 325-9085

Dr. Jeffrey S. Coons is the co-director of Research at Manning and Napier Advisors, Inc. with primary responsibilities focusing on the measurement and management of portfolio risk and return relative to client objectives. This includes providing analysis across every aspect of the investment process, from objectives setting and asset allocation to ongoing monitoring of portfolio risk and return. Dr. Coons is also a member of the Investment Policy Group, which establishes and monitors secular investment trends, macroeconomic overviews, and the investment disciplines of the firm. Dr. Coons holds a doctoral degree in economics from Temple University, graduated with distinction from the University of Rochester with a bachelor or arts in economics, holds the designation of Chartered Financial Analyst, and is one of the employee-owners of Manning and Napier.

Perry D'Alessio; CPA
D'Alessio Tocci & Pell LLP
Certified Public Accountants and Business Advisors
20 West 36th St. 10th Floor
New York, New York City 10018
Phone: (212) 244-6166
Fax: (212) 695-2951
Web: www.DaleCPA.com
Email: www.dalecpa.com

Perry D'Alessio has 20-year experience in public accounting. He specializes in the taxation of closely held businesses and their owners as well as high wealth individuals. He has a broad range of experience that includes individual, corporate, partnership, fiduciary, estate, and gift taxation. Business development has also been a focus. Particularly in the healthcare and fitness industry, he worked with successful entities whose emphasis was on growth through development of strategic relationships and unit building. Mr. D'Alessio earned his bachelor of business administration degree in accounting at Baruch College and currently is a Certified Public Accountant in New York. He is a member of the American Institute of Certified Public Accountants (AICPA) and the New York State Society of Certified Public Accountants (NYSSCPA). He served on several New York State Society tax committees including PCAOB and HealthCare. Mr. D'Alessio presents at financial and medical associations throughout the region, and he authored a book chapter in the *Financial Management Strategies for Hospitals and Healthcare Organizations* for the Institute of Medical Business Advisors, Inc.

Dr. Charles F. Fenton III; FACFAS, JD CMP™ [Hon]
Law Offices: Suite # 101
1145 Cockrell Court
Kennesaw, Georgia, 30152-4760
Phone: (404) 233-4350
Fax: (404) 231-0853

Dr. Charles F. Fenton is a board-certified surgeon from Temple University who received his law degree as class valedictorian from Georgia State University and practices in Atlanta, Georgia. His clients include physicians involved in audits and recoupment actions as well as disputes with insurance or managed-care companies. He is a contributing author to many books on healthcare law and medical practice as well as many other medico-legal publications for physicians and the Bar. Currently, he is chief legal officer for the Institute of Medical Business Advisors, Inc.

Lawrence E. Howes; MBA, CFP®, CMP™ [Hon]
Sharkey, Howes and Javer, Inc
720 S. Colorado Blvd.
Suite # 600 - South Tower
Denver, CO 80246-1919
Phone: (303) 639-5100
Fax: (303) 759-2335
Web: www.SHWJ.com

Lawrence E. Howes is a principal in Sharkey, Howes and Javer, Inc. in Denver, Colorado. He earned his undergraduate degree in management and an MBA at Regis University. He has served on the Institute of Certified Financial Planners National Committee on Communication, Government Affairs, and Education and drafted the legislative application for the first Investment Advisory Law in the state of Colorado. Currently, he is on the State Department of Treasury Investment

Advisory Committee and the Securities Commissioner's legislative subcommittee on financial planning and investment advisory regulation for the same state. Mr. Howes writes for the *Journal of Financial Planning*, *Financial Advisory Practice* and *Financial Planning* magazine, among other consumer publications. He is a practice management consultant to investment advisory and legal firms, across the United States, and program leader for the Colorado and New Mexico Bar Associations.

Anju D. Jessani; MBA, APM
Divorce with Dignity Mediation Services
42 Main Street, 2nd Floor
Clinton, NJ 08809
Phone: (908) 303-0396
Web: www.DWDMediation.org

Anju D. Jessani is a divorce mediator and founder of the firm Divorce with Dignity. She received her Association for Conflict Resolution education from the Center for Family and Divorce Mediation in New York and her practical education through the Hudson County Court's Mediation Program in New Jersey. Currently, she serves on the New Jersey Administrative Office of the Courts' Parenting Time Committee. She is an editor for *The Children's Advocate*, an Advanced Practitioner Member of the Association for Conflict Resolution, and an Accredited Mediator by the New Jersey Association of Professional Mediators. Ms Jessani contributes to numerous professional journals and media talk shows. She holds an MBA from the Wharton School and a BA from Rutgers University. Prior to founding Divorce with Dignity, she was a manager with Price Waterhouse and a vice president with J.P. Morgan.

Alexander M. Kimura; MBA, CFP®, CMP [Hon], AIF®
Argosy Wealth Management
21250 Hawthorne Boulevard, Suite 560
Torrance, CA 90503 USA
Phone: (424) 212-4949

Alexander M. Kimura graduated with honors from Harvard University. He earned an MBA from the Anderson School of Management at UCLA and began his Wall Street career at Morgan Stanley, one of the nation's preeminent investment banking firms. He received specialized training from Renaissance Trust on charitable tax planning strategies and is an adjunct faculty member at UCLA, teaching an extension course on pensions and other retirement benefit plans. Mr. Kimura was also senior financial advisor for the Financial Network Investment Corporation.

Dr. Bradley Klontz; PsyD, CSAC, CFP®
Financial Psychologist and Managing Partner
OCCAM Asset Management, LLC
P.O. Box 529
Kapaa, HI 96746
Web: www.YourMentalWealth.com
Email: btklontz@aol.com

Dr. Bradley Klontz, is a financial psychologist (PsyD), Certified Substance Abuse Counselor (CSAC), and Certified Financial Planner®. He is an associate professor of Personal Financial Planning at Kansas State University, a Fellow of the American Psychological Association, and a former president of the Hawaii Psychological Association. Dr. Klontz has coauthored four books on the psychology of money: *Mind over Money* (Broadway Business, 2009), *Wired for Wealth* (HCI, 2008), *The Financial Wisdom of Ebenezer Scrooge* (HCI, 2005, 2008), and *Facilitating*

Financial Health: *Tools for Financial Planners, Coaches,* and *Therapists* (NUCO, 2008). His fifth book, *Financial Therapy: Theory, Research and Practice,* was published in 2014. Dr. Klontz's work has been featured on ABC News' *20/20* and *Good Morning America* and in *USA Today, The Wall Street Journal, New York Times, Washington Post, Los Angeles Times, Time, Kiplinger's, Money Magazine,* NPR, and many other media outlets and professional magazines and journals, including his Mind Games: Your Client column for *On Wall Street* magazine and his *Mind over Money* blog for *Psychology Today.*

Dr. Ted Klontz; PhD
Financial Psychologist and Co-Founder
Klontz Consulting Group
P.O. Box 529
Kapaa, HI 96746
Web: www.YourMentalWealth.com
Email: ted@klontzconsulting.com

Dr. Ted Klontz, is co-founder of Your Mental Wealth and Klontz Consulting Group. With 40 years of counseling experience, he is recognized as a pioneer in the emerging field of financial psychology specializing in specific behavioral change. Dr. Klontz has an extensive national private consulting practice, working with individuals, couples, families, businesses, and organizations. As a financial psychologist (PsyD), he is the author of six books, a published researcher, a professional speaker, trainer, workshop designer and facilitator, and trouble-shooter. His corporate work is focused on assisting in strategic planning, productivity, succession, and employee retention issues. His clients include/have included the U.S. Defense Department, financial professionals, collegiate and professional athletes, entertainers, high wealth/profile individuals, and families. Dr. Klontz is well known for the development and customized application of unique tools and techniques for helping change troublesome behaviors. He appears frequently in expert roles in local, national, and international media.

Dr. Brian J. Knabe; CFP®, CMP™
Savant Capital Management
190 Buckley Drive
Rockford, IL 61107
Phone: (815) 227.0300
Fax: (815) 226.2195
Web: www.SavantCapital.com
Email: BKnabe@savantcapital.com

Dr. Brian J. Knabe, is a financial advisor and a member of the Savant Capital Management advisory team. He routinely meets with clients, advisors, portfolio managers, and planners in order to develop comprehensive planning, investment, and tax strategies. Dr. Knabe is also a clinical assistant professor in the Department of Family Medicine with the University of Illinois. He is a member of the American Academy of Family Physicians, the Illinois State Medical Society, and the Catholic Medical Association. Dr. Knabe is a magna cum laude graduate of Marquette University with an honors degree in biomedical engineering. He earned his medical degree from the University of Illinois College of Medicine and attended the University of Illinois for his family practice residency, where he served as chief resident. Dr. Knabe is a Certified Medical Planner™ and a Certified Financial Planner® who earned a diploma in financial planning from Marquette University. Dr. Knabe often speaks to financial service and medical associations throughout the country. He has authored book chapters for the Institute of Medical Business Advisors, Inc.

Timothy J. McIntosh; MBA, MPH, CFP®, CMP™ [Hon]
SIPCO - Strategic Investment Partners, LLC
1100 NE Loop 410, Suite 636
San Antonio, Texas 78209
Phone: (800) 805-5309
Web: www.SIPLLC.com
Email: tmcintosh@sipllc.com

Timothy J. McIntosh is chief investment officer and founder of SIPCO. As chairman of the firm's investment committee, he oversees all aspects of major client accounts and serves as lead portfolio manager for the firm's equity and bond portfolios. Mr. McIntosh was a professor of finance at Eckerd College from 1998 to 2008. He is the author of *The Bear Market Survival Guide* and *The Sector Strategist*. He is featured in publications such as *The Wall Street Journal, New York Times, USA Today, Investment Advisor, Fortune, MD News, Tampa Doctor's Life,* and *St. Petersburg Times.* He has been recognized as a Five Star Wealth Manager in *Texas Monthly* magazine and continuously named as Medical Economics' "Best Financial Advisors for Physicians" since 2004. He is also a contributor to SeekingAlpha.com, a premier website of investment opinion. Mr. McIntosh earned a bachelor of science in economics at Florida State University, a master of business administration (MBA) at the University of Sarasota, a master of public health degree (MPH) at the University of South Florida, and is a Certified Financial Planner® practitioner. His previous experience includes employment with Blue Cross/Blue Shield of Florida, Enterprise Leasing Company, and United States Army Military Intelligence.

J. Christopher Miller; JD
Law Offices of J. Christopher Miller, PC
11800 Amber Park Drive, Suite 130
Alpharetta, Georgia 30009
Phone: 678-746-2900
Web: www.NorthFultonWills.com
Email: cmiller@northfultonwills.com

J. Christopher Miller, is an estate planning and business law attorney in Alpharetta, Georgia. He frequently conducts seminars on the formation of limited liability companies and trusts addressing special needs issues. Chris earned his bachelor's degree and his juris doctor at Emory University, Atlanta, Georgia. He was admitted to the State Bar of Georgia in 2000 and is a member of the Atlanta Bar Association's Section of Estate Planning and Probate.

Shikha Mittra; MBA, CFP®, CRPS®, CMFC®, AIF®
President - Retire Smart Consulting LLC
103 Carnegie Center
Suite #300 A
Princeton, NJ 08540
Phone: (609) 955-3456
Fax: (609) 520-8731
Web: www.RetireSmartConsulting.com
Email: info@retiresmartconsulting.com

Shikha Mittra has two decades of industry experience working with physicians, dentists, and top-level executives in both public and private sector businesses and foundations, bagging several awards for her work. She was rated one of the top financial planners in the country from 2006 to 2013. As a Certified Financial Planner®, she is also a Chartered Mutual Fund Counselor®, Chartered Retirement Plan Specialist®, and Certified Cash Balance Consultant. Ms Mittra is adjunct professor of finance and business at Rutgers University, New Brunswick, New Jersey, a Regional Board Member of the National Association of Personal Financial Advisors NAPFA (2011–2013). Board of Trustees of Financial Planning Association of New Jersey Chapter (2008–2011), and an Advisory Board Member of the *Journal of Financial Planning* (2008–2009). *Medical Economics* listed her as a best financial advisor for doctors in 2012. Ms Mittra is also an Accredited Investment Fiduciary® helping employers reduce their fiduciary liability by following global fiduciary standards of care in managing their retirement plans.

Thomas A. Muldowney; MSFS, ChFC®, CFP®, CLU®, CRC®, AIF®, CMP™
Savant Capital Management
Chairman of the Board and Principal
190 Buckley Drive
Rockford, IL 61107
Phone: (815) 227.0300
Fax: (815) 226.2195
Web: www.SavantCapital.com
Email: tmuldowney@savantcapital.com

Thomas A. Muldowney has 35 years of experience in the banking, investment, insurance, and financial services industries. He taught at Rock Valley and Sauk Valley Community Colleges and served as a contributing author for the Elder Law Portfolio Series published by the Law and Business Division of Wolters and Kluwer through Aspen Publishers. His topics included financial planning for the elderly and postmortem estate planning. Mr. Muldowney earned a bachelor of arts degree at Rockford College and a master's degree in financial services (MSFS) at the American College. He is a Chartered Life Underwriter® (CLU®), Chartered Financial Consultant® (ChFC®), Certified Retirement Counselor® (CRC®), Certified Financial Planner® (CFP®), Certified Medical Planner™ (CMP™), and an Accredited Investment Fiduciary® (AIF®). Mr. Muldowney is an active member of professional organizations such as the National Association of Personal Financial Advisors (NAPFA), the Financial Planning Association (FPA), and the Society of Financial Service Professionals (FSP). Since 2004, he has represented Savant on *Medical Economics* magazine's list of "Top 150 Best Financial Advisers for Doctors." He has presented at financial and medical associations and authored several publications for the Institute of Medical Business Advisors, Inc. Mr. Muldowney is also on the TD Ameritrade Advisory Panel, a board member of the Discovery Center Museum, chair of the Finance Committee and board member for the St. Anthony Medical Center Foundation, chair of the Investment Committee and treasurer of the Boylan Education Foundation Board of Directors, and is on the Board of Trustees for Rockford College.

Dr. Eugene Schmuckler; PhD, MEd, MBA, CTS
Institute of Medical Business Advisors, Inc
Academic Dean and Consulting Psychologist
Certified Medical Planner™ Online Education Program
Suite # 5901 Wilbanks Drive
Norcross, Georgia 30092
Phone: (770) 448-0769
Web: www.CertifiedMedicalPlanner.org
Email: MarcinkoAdvisors@msn.com

Dr. Eugene Schmuckler was the coordinator of behavioral science at the Georgia Public Safety Training Center and is a licensed psychologist. He is on the board of directors of the Association of Traumatic Stress Specialists and is a Certified Trauma Specialist. Dr. Schmuckler is an international speaker and author, with publications translated into Dutch and Russian. He is a consulting psychologist and director of Behavioral Finance for the Institute of Medical Business Advisors, Inc. and the academic dean for the Certified Medical Planner™ online designation and professional certification program. He frequently writes for the Institute of Medical Business Advisors, Inc. Dr. Schmuckler earned his MBA and PhD at Louisiana State University.

Dr. Kenneth Shubin-Stein; CFA®
Spencer Capital Management, LLC
10 East 53rd Street, 22nd Floor
New York, NY 1002
Phone: (212) 287-1569
Fax: (212) 504-8172
Web: www.SpencerCapital.com

Dr. Kenneth Shubin-Stein is the founder and portfolio manager of Spencer Capital Management and the chairman of Spencer Capital Holdings. He is a former director of Public Prep and a former director and chairman of MRV Communications. Dr. Shubin-Stein is an adjunct professor at the Columbia University Graduate School of Business co-teaching Advanced Investment Research with Cheryl Strauss Einhorn. Prior to joining Spencer Capital Management, Ken Shubin-Stein was a financial analyst at Promethean Capital Management in Manhattan and co-founder of Compo Asset Management, LLC, a U.S.-based equity value investment partnership. Previously, he was a medical technology analyst for the Abernathy Group in New York, an investment management firm specializing in the medical and technology sectors. Dr. Shubin-Stein completed his surgical internship at the Mount Sinai Medical Center in New York and is a graduate of the Albert Einstein College of Medicine. His undergraduate degree, in dual concentrations, is from Columbia College. He is a Chartered Financial Analyst®. His charity foundation, Crutches-4-Kids (C4K), was co-founded in 2009 with his twin sister Beth Shubin-Stein, MD and Christopher Ahmad, MD, who is head team physician for the New York Yankees. In 2011, Crutches-4-Kids was officially honored at Yankee Stadium by New York Yankees pitcher CC Sabathia and Starter for its extraordinary efforts providing crutches to impoverished and disabled children around the world.

Dr. Dimitri A. Sogoloff; MBA
President/CEO
Horton Point LLC
120 West 45Th Street 4th Floor
New York, New York 10036

Dr. Dimitri A. Sogoloff leads a seeding/incubation platform of emerging systematic managers trading liquid markets. The quantitative hedge fund seed capital, operational infrastructure, risk management, oversight, and product distribution capability (managed accounts, single manager funds, and institutional platforms) offers talented systematic traders with proven ability to generate uncorrelated alpha. Like other hedge fund seeders, Horton Point LLC looks to capitalize on the difficult fund-raising climate for those who invest in highly liquid securities via strategies that are uncorrelated to mainstream markets. Dr. Sogoloff graduated from Columbia University Medical School, from Columbia University Business School with an MBA in finance, and with a bachelor of science degree from the Columbia University—FU Foundation School of Engineering and Applied Science. Dr. Sogoloff is past co-founder and president of Alexandra Investment Management, LLC.

Stephen P. Weatherby; CFP®
Sharkey, Howes and Javer, Inc
720 S. Colorado Blvd.
Suite # 600 - South Tower
Denver, CO 80246-1919
Phone: (303) 639-5100
Fax: (303) 759-2335
Web: www.SHWJ.com
Email: Stephen@shwj.com

Stephen P. Weatherby joined Sharkey, Howes and Javer in 2012. Previously, he was a personal financial counselor with Military Health Net providing financial education and counseling to the United States Military at various worldwide locations from 2008 to 2012. He earned a bachelor of science degree at Texas Tech University in family financial planning, a program consistently viewed as the nation's premier program of its kind. Mr. Weatherby has been a Certified Financial Planner® professional since 2007.

Section I

For All Practitioners

The vast majority of physicians and medical professionals major in one of the hard science while in college; biology, engineering, chemistry, mathematics, computer science or physics, and so on. Few take undergraduate courses in finance, business management, securities analysis, accounting, or economics; although this paradigm is changing with modernity. These courses are not particularly difficult for the premedical baccalaureate major, they are just not on the radar screen for time compressed and highly competitive students; nor are they needed for medical or nursing school admission, or the many related allied health professionals schools.

In fact, William C. Roberts, MD, originally from Emory University in Atlanta, and former editor for the *Baylor University Medical Center Proceedings* and *The American Journal of Cardiology*, opined just a decade ago: "Of the 125 medical schools in the USA, only one of them to my knowledge offers a class related to saving or investing money." And so, it is important to review some basic principles of economics, finance, and accounting as they relate to financial planning in the first section of this book.

Section I is not intended as a replacement for such courses, but it will serve as a place to start the discussion, enhance independent life-long learning, or perhaps even ignite the path forward to a more formal educational journey. After all, many of our contributors are dual degreed business, legal, financial, and medical professionals of all stripes, degrees, specialties, and financial industry designations. It is good to learn from them by example, and harvest their insatiable curiosity and experiences. Such enhancement may be cumbersome and challenging, but it is always worthwhile.

1 Unifying the Physiologic and Psychologic Financial Planning Divide

Holistic Life Planning, Behavioral Economics, Trading Addiction, and the Art of Money

Bradley Klontz, Ted Klontz, Eugene Schmuckler, Kenneth Shubin-Stein, and David Edward Marcinko

CONTENTS

In any textbook of *gravitas* on financial planning, a short chapter on money psychology is typically placed at the end of the book, almost as an afterthought, if included at all. Moreover, it is rarely written by a surgeon (MBA and Certified Medical Planner™), a Certified Trauma Specialist and behavioral psychologist, two practicing financial psychologists (one a Certified Financial Planner®), and a board certified psychiatrist practicing as a Chartered Financial Analyst®. Usually, it is written by a lay-hobbyist, self-styled guru, or financial-mentalist, and included by fiat in guise of the popular sales rubric of *life* or *holistic planning*. This current marketing theory *de rigor*, also known as the *next big sales thing,* is akin to the variable annuity and limited partnership initiatives promoted by product hucksters of the past. However, we have elected to prominently place this topic at its rightful place as the premier chapter of our book.

Why? In the end, much of the success in any financial planning engagement ultimately comes down to changing human behavior—helping a client alter whatever she/he was doing toward something that will better allow them to achieve their goals. And, there is still remarkably little education or training for financial advisors focused directly on motivation or change theory. Instead, advisors are increasingly turning to health professionals to find ideas and best practices about how to help clients actually make the behavioral changes necessary to achieve their goals.

INTRODUCTION

It is no wonder why the concept of life planning has emerged within the industry, from a dedicated core group of advocates, but using the more established academic discipline of behavioral economics and finance as its pragmatic root core. Shifting the emphasis of the planning relationship to assisting clients in formulating their "life of choice" first, and then related reasons for them, physicians can strategize the financial decisions that will support the unfolding goals and objectives of their life plan and financial requirements.

THE ANATOMIC BASIS OF HUMAN PHYSIOLOGY AND BEHAVIOR

It is well-known that emotional and behavioral change involves the human nervous system. But, there are two parts of the nervous system that are especially significant for holistic financial advisor; the first is the limbic system and the second is the autonomic nervous system. And, according to Dr. C. George Boerre of Shippensburg University of Pennsylvania, this is known as the *emotional nervous system*.

THE LIMBIC SYSTEM

The limbic system is a set of structures that lies on both sides of the thalamus, just under the cerebrum. It includes the hypothalamus, the hippocampus, the amygdala, and nearby areas. It is primarily responsible for emotions, memories, and recollection.

Hypothalamus

The small hypothalamus is located just below the thalamus on both sides of the third ventricle (areas within the cerebrum filled with cerebrospinal fluid that connect to spinal fluid). It sits inside both tracts of the optic nerve, and just above the pituitary gland.

The hypothalamus is mainly concerned with *homeostasis* or the process of returning to some "set point." It works like a thermostat: When the room gets too cold, the thermostat conveys that information to the furnace and turns it on. As the room warms up and the temperature rises, it turns off the furnace. The hypothalamus is responsible for regulating hunger, thirst, response to pain, levels of pleasure, sexual satisfaction, anger and aggressive behavior, and more. It also regulates the functioning of the *autonomic nervous system*, which means it regulates functions such as pulse, blood pressure, breathing, and arousal in response to emotional circumstances. In a recent discovery, the protein leptin is released by fat cells with overeating. The hypothalamus senses leptin levels in the bloodstream and responds by decreasing appetite. So, it seems that some people might have a gene mutation that produces leptin, and can't tell the hypothalamus that it is satiated. The hypothalamus sends instructions to the rest of the body in two ways. The first is to the *autonomic nervous system*. This allows the hypothalamus to have ultimate control of things such as blood pressure, heart rate, breathing, digestion, sweating, and all the sympathetic and parasympathetic functions.

The second way the hypothalamus controls things is via the *pituitary gland*. It is neurally and chemically connected to the pituitary, which in turn pumps hormones called releasing factors into the bloodstream. The pituitary is the so-called "master gland" as these hormones are vitally important in regulating growth and metabolism.

Hippocampus

The hippocampus consists of two "horns" that curve back from the amygdala. It is important in converting things "in your mind" at the moment (short-term memory) into things that are remembered for the long run (long-term memory). If the hippocampus is damaged, a patient cannot build new memories and lives in a strange world where everything they experience just fades away; even while older memories from the time before the damage are untouched! Most patients who suffer from this kind of brain damage are eventually institutionalized.

Amygdala

The amygdalas are two almond-shaped masses of neurons on either side of the thalamus at the lower end of the hippocampus. When it is stimulated electrically, animals respond with aggression. And, if the amygdala is removed, animals get very tame and no longer respond to anger that would have caused rage before. The animals also become indifferent to stimuli that would have otherwise have caused fear and sexual responses.

Related Anatomic Areas

Besides the hypothalamus, hippocampus, and amygdala, there are other areas in the structures near to the limbic system that are intimately connected to it:

- The *cingulate gyrus* is the part of the cerebrum that lies closest to the limbic system, just above the corpus callosum. It provides a pathway from the thalamus to the hippocampus, is responsible for focusing attention on emotionally significant events, and for associating memories to smells and to pain.
- The *ventral tegmental area* of the brain stem (just below the thalamus) consists of dopamine pathways responsible for pleasure. People with damage here tend to have difficulty getting pleasure in life, and often turn to alcohol, drugs, sweets, and gambling.
- The *basal ganglia* (including the caudate nucleus, the putamen, the globus pallidus, and the substantia nigra) lie over to the sides of the limbic system, and are connected with the cortex above them. They are responsible for repetitive behaviors, reward experiences, and focusing attention.
- The *prefrontal cortex*, which is the part of the frontal lobe that lies in front of the motor area, is also closely linked to the limbic system. Besides apparently being involved in thinking about the future, making plans, and taking action, it also appears to be involved in the same dopamine pathways as the ventral tegmental area, and plays a part in pleasure and addiction.

The Autonomic Nervous System

The second part of the nervous system to have a particularly powerful part to play in our emotional life is the autonomic nervous system.

The autonomic nervous system is composed of two parts, which function primarily in opposition to each other. The first is the *sympathetic nervous system*, which starts in the spinal cord and travels to a variety of areas of the body. Its function appears to be preparing the body for the kinds of vigorous activities associated with "fight or flight," that is, with running from danger or with preparing for violence. Activation of the sympathetic nervous system has the following effects:

- Dilates the pupils and opens the eyelids
- Stimulates the sweat glands and dilates the blood vessels in large muscles
- Constricts the blood vessels in the rest of the body
- Increases the heart rate and opens up the bronchial tubes of the lungs
- Inhibits the secretions in the digestive system

One of its most important effects is causing the adrenal glands (which sit on top of the kidneys) to release *epinephrine* (adrenalin) into the blood stream. Epinephrine is a powerful hormone that causes various parts of the body to respond in much the same way as the sympathetic nervous system. Being in the blood stream, it takes a bit longer to stop its effects, and may take some time to calm down again.

The sympathetic nervous system also takes in information, mostly concerning pain from internal organs. Because the nerves that carry information about organ pain often travel along the same paths that carry information about pain from more surface areas of the body, the information sometimes get confused. This is called *referred pain,* and the best-known example is the pain in the left shoulder and arm when having a heart attack.

The other part of the autonomic nervous system is called the *parasympathetic nervous* system. It has its roots in the brainstem and in the spinal cord of the lower back. Its function is to bring the body back from the emergency status that the sympathetic nervous system puts it into.

Some of the details of parasympathetic arousal include some of the following:

- Pupil constriction and activation of the salivary glands
- Stimulating the secretions of the stomach and activity of the intestines
- Stimulating secretions in the lungs and constricting the bronchial tubes
- Decreases heart rate

The parasympathetic nervous system also has some sensory abilities: It receives information about blood pressure, levels of carbon dioxide in the blood, and so on.

There is actually another part of the autonomic nervous system that is not mentioned too often: the *enteric nervous system*. It is a complex of nerves that regulate the activity of the stomach. For example, if you get sick to your stomach with a new financial advisory client—or feel nervous butterflies with your first patient encounter as a doctor—you can blame the enteric nervous system.

The Triune Brain Model

In the 1950s the neurologist Paul McCleanin corporated the anatomic basis of human behavior reviewed above, and developed the triune theory of the brain. While simplistic and full of anatomical and evolutionary inaccuracies, the triune brain is a useful metaphor for explaining brain structure and function in terms of financial behaviors. In the book *Mind over Money: Overcoming the Money Disorders That Threaten Our Financial Health,* Klontz and Klontz use the triune brain theory as a metaphor to help understand and change self-destructive financial behaviors. That triune brain model describes the human brain as divided into three parts.

Sitting at the lowest portion of the anatomical structure is the reptilian brain. It is fully functional shortly after birth and controls basic bodily functions. Behaviorally, it takes in sensory information and determines whether or not there are signs that indicate danger. The reptilian brain tends to see everything through the lens of potential threat to its existence and as if everything and everyone, until proven otherwise, cannot be trusted. Its default state is that of anxiety. To the degree that a person's experience in childhood was one in which he or she experienced abuse or neglect, the individual's level of ambient anxiety increases. It is the first part of the brain to be fully developed and it will be the last part of the brain to cease functioning at death.

Sitting atop the reptilian brain is the mammalian brain, made up of the limbic system. It is fully developed in early childhood. Functionally, one of its tasks is to help calm the anxiety of the reptilian brain. As such, it experiments with a variety of behavioral strategies that serve to relieve stress and develops hard-wired shortcuts or automatic reactions in times of stress. These reactions are some variation of the familiar fight, flight, or freeze response. During childhood, immature and underdeveloped associations with money and beliefs about money (aka *money scripts*) are developed at an unconscious level. Beliefs about what money means, what it can do, and what it can't do are formed during early childhood and are often locked in place by emotional triggers in the mammalian brain. This part of the brain experiences the threat of not belonging or losing its standing or place in one's primary socialization groups (e.g., family, socioeconomic group, etc.) as one of the biggest potential threat to its survival. Being kicked out of one's group or "tribe" in early human history meant certain death and this fear of being excluded from one's group helps explain why individual's who come into money quickly; through inheritance, lottery wins, and so on, are often prone to self-sabotage, because the change in socioeconomic status is typically accompanied by relationship stress and threatens the basic need for attachment and affiliation in one's social group.

Together, these two parts of the brain, what is referred to as the *animal brain*, make up unconscious. It is hypothesized by many that the unconscious makes 90–99% of our day-to-day decisions. The animal brain has difficulty grasping abstract concepts, such as "retirement," or "financial security." As such, motivation is often not stimulated by abstract concepts. This helps explain why the average American "knows" they should save for the future and not spend more than they make;

however, most do the exact opposite. The only language the animal brain understands is emotional and sensory. The animal brain is self-centered and self-serving. When animal brain dominates—particularly in times of stress, elation, or fear—promises, commitments, resolutions, delaying gratification, and consideration of future consequences are all sacrificed for the expediency of relieving the stress of the moment.

Choices made by the animal brain can be self-destructive. For example, a person dying of thirst is likely to drink salt water if no other liquid is available, even though this is self-destructive. Likewise, the animal brain compels a person trapped underwater to eventually attempt to draw breath. It is estimated that the animal brain processes information at 4 billion bits per second. When emotions are mixed with high levels of stress, irrational, illogical financial choices are often made.

Human beings are posited to have six primary needs: belonging, autonomy, safety, self-expression, purpose, and connection. Every financial behavior is a strategy that attempts to meet one or more of these needs.

Positioned above the animal brain is the neocortex, or new brain. The neocortex to the animal brain is like a person sitting on an elephant, attempting to override some of the more egregious, outrageous, and impulsive choices emerging from the much larger and stronger beast. The neocortex does not become fully developed until our early to mid-20s. When fully engaged in service of our financial well being, all is well. The neocortex serves as a moderating influence, overriding immature thoughts and impulses. In fact, there is nothing quite like it that we know of in the universe. This part of the brain loves information, loves the abstract and contemplation of things as they might be. This part of the brain processes information at approximately 2 million bits of information per second and goes off-line when we sleep, over indulge in alcohol, or ingest other sedative effect drugs.

If the stress and anxiety level of the animal reaches a critical point, emotional flooding occurs, and the neocortex's moderating influence is stymied. It's in those moments that the strategies the animal brain has developed over the years to stay safe or to feel better in the moment, become the prominent behaviors.

For example, stock purchases we wish we wouldn't have bought or sold, purchases we wish we wouldn't not have made, words spoken we wish we could take back, promises broken, and behaviors we feel embarrassed about later are all evidence of this dynamic. Using the human riding the elephant metaphor, when the elephant is excited or terrified, the human is just along for the ride as the emotionally flooded elephant stampedes. On a macroeconomic level, this explains the cycle of bubbles and busts that have occurred since the beginning of recorded history and will continue to plague every area of the market as long as human beings are in existence. The challenge, of course, is to recognize when financial decisions are at risk of being hijacked by the animal brain and to engage the neocortex to make appropriate financial decisions.

Money Scripts

Money scripts are unconscious beliefs about money that are typically only partially true, are developed in childhood, and drive adult financial behaviors. Money scripts may be the result of "financial flashpoints," which are salient early experiences around money that have a lasting impact in adulthood. Money scripts are often passed down through the generations and social groups often share similar money scripts. As mentioned above, the animal brain stores associations around money based on early experiences, which can result in rigid and often problematic money attitudes. And so, we argue that money scripts are at the root of all illogical, ill-advised, self-destructive, or self-limiting financial behaviors.

In research at Kansas State University (KSU), researchers identified four distinct money script patterns, which are associated with financial health and predict financial behaviors. These include: (a) money avoidance, (b) money worship, (c) money status, and (d) money vigilance (Bradley Klontz, PsyD, CFP® and Sonya Britt, PhD, CFP®, personal communication). A summary of their findings follow:

Money Avoidance

Money avoidance scripts are illustrated by beliefs such as "Rich people are greedy," "It is not okay to have more than you need," and "I do not deserve a lot of money when others have less than me." Money avoiders believe that money is bad or that they do not deserve money. They believe that wealthy people are corrupt and there is virtue in living with less money. They may sabotage their financial success or give money away even though they cannot afford to do so. Money avoidance scripts may be associated with lower income and lower net worth and predict financial behaviors including ignoring bank statements, overspending, financial dependence on others, financial enabling of others, and having trouble sticking to a budget.

Money Worship

Money worship is typified by beliefs such as "More money will make you happier," "You can never have enough money," and "Money would solve all my problems." Money worshipers are convinced that money is the key to happiness. At the same time, they believe that one can never have enough. Money worships have lower income, lower net worth, and higher credit card debt. They are more likely to be hoarders, spend compulsively, and put work ahead of family.

Money Status

Money status scripts include "I will not buy something unless it is new," "Your self-worth equals you net worth," and "If something isn't considered the 'best' it is not worth buying." Money status seekers see net worth and self-worth as being synonymous. They pretend to have more money than they do and tend to overspend as a result. They often grew up in poorer families and believe that the universe should take care of their financial needs if they live a virtuous life. Money status scripts are associated with compulsive gambling, overspending, being financially dependent on others, and lying to one's spouse about spending.

Money Vigilance

Money vigilant beliefs include "It is important to save for a rainy day," "You should always look for the best deal, even if it takes more time," and "I would be a nervous wreck if I did not have an emergency fund." The money vigilants are alert, watchful, and concerned about their financial welfare. They are more likely to save and less likely to buy on credit. As a result, they tend to have higher income and higher net worth. They also have a tendency to be anxious about money and are secretive about their financial status outside of their household. While money vigilance is associated with frugality and saving, excessive anxiety can keep someone from enjoying the benefits that money can provide.

When money scripts are identified, it is helpful to examine where they came from. A simple technique involves reflecting on the following questions:

What three lessons did you learn about money from your mother?
What three lessons did you learn about money from your father?
What is your first memory around money?
What is your most painful money memory?
What is your most joyful money memory?
What money scripts emerged for you from this experience?
How have they helped you?
How have they hurt you?
What money scripts do you need to change?

Historical Review of Behavioral Finance and Economics

James O. Prochaska, PhD, Professor of Psychology and Director of the Cancer Prevention Research Center at the University of Rhode Island, developed the Trans-Theoretic Model of Behavior Change

(TTM) that has been evolving since 1977. Nominated as one of the five most influential authors in Psychology by the Institute for Scientific Information and the American Psychological Society, Dr. Prochaska is author of more than 300 papers on behavior change for health promotion and disease prevention.

TTM Stages of Change

In his Trans-Theoretical Model, behavior change is a process involving progress through a series of these stages:

- Precontemplation (not ready)—"People are not intending to take action in the foreseeable future, and can be unaware that their behavior is problematic."
- Contemplation (getting ready)—"People are beginning to recognize that their behavior is problematic, and start to look at the pros and cons of their continued actions."
- Preparation (ready)—"People are intending to take action in the immediate future, and may begin taking small steps toward behavior change."
- Action—"People have made specific overt modifications in changing their problem behavior or in acquiring new healthy behaviors."
- Maintenance—"People have been able to sustain action for a while and are working to prevent relapse."
- Termination—"Individuals have zero temptation and they are sure they will not return to their old unhealthy habit as a way of coping."

In addition, researchers conceptualized "relapse" (recycling) which is not a stage in itself but rather the "return from Action or Maintenance to an earlier stage." In medical care, these stages of behavior change have applicability to antihypertension and lipid-lowering medication use, as well as depression prevention, weight control, and smoking cessation.

More recently, validating the emerging alliance between psychology (human behavior) and finance (economics) are two Americans who won the Royal Swedish Academy of Science's 2002 Nobel Memorial Prize in Economic Science. Their research was nothing short of an explanation for the idiosyncrasies incumbent in human financial decision-making outcomes.

Daniel Kahneman, PhD, professor of psychology at Princeton University, and Vernon L. Smith, PhD, professor of economics at George Mason University in Fairfax, VA, shared the prize for work that provided insight on everything from stock market bubbles, to regulating utilities, and countless other economic activities. In several cases, the winners tried to explain apparent financial paradoxes.

For example, Professor Kahneman made the economically puzzling discovery that most of his subjects would make a 20-minute trip to buy a calculator for $10 instead of $15, but would not make the same trip to buy a jacket for $120 instead of $125, saving the same $5.

Initially, in the 1960s, Smith set out to demonstrate how economic theory worked in the laboratory (*in vitro*), while Kahneman was more interested in the ways economic theory mispredicted people in real life (*in vivo*). He tested the limits of standard economic *choice theory* in predicting the actions of real people, and his work formalized laboratory techniques for studying economic decision making, with a focus on trading and bargaining.

Later, Smith and Kahneman together were among the first economists to make experimental data a cornerstone of academic output. Their studies included people playing games of cooperation and trust, and simulating different types of markets in a laboratory setting. Their theories assumed that individuals make decisions systematically, based on preferences and available information, in a way that changes little over time, or in different contexts.

By the late 1970s, Richard H. Thaler, PhD, an economist at the University of Chicago, also began to perform behavioral experiments further suggesting irrational wrinkles in standard financial theory and behavior, enhancing the still embryonic but increasingly popular theories of Kahneman and Smith.

Other economists' laboratory experiments used ideas about competitive interactions pioneered by game theorists like John Forbes Nash Jr., PhD, who shared the Nobel Memorial Prize in Economic Sciences in 1994, as points of reference. But, Kahneman and Smith often concentrated on cases where people's actions departed from the systematic, rational strategies that Nash envisioned. Psychologically, this was all a precursor to the informal concept of life or holistic financial planning. Kahneman was awarded the Medal of Freedom, by President Barack Obama, on November 20, 2013.

FINANCIAL LIFE PLANNING DEFINED

Of course, comprehensive financial planners (not financial advisors, insurance agents, or stock brokers) have always consulted with their clients regarding their goals and objectives, hopes, and dreams, but typically from the point of view of money goals, rather than life ideals or business goals. The absence or presence of biological and/or psychological reasons for them was seldom considered, nor discussed. But, quantifying future subjective and objective goals, and doing a technical analysis of factors such as risk tolerance, age, insurance, tax, investing, retirement and succession planning, asset protection, and estate planning needs, has certainly been the norm for some. But, such quantifications were taken to another level by the informed advisors and enlightened authors of this book.

ENTER THE FINANCIAL PLANNERS

Life planning and behavioral finance then, as proposed for physicians and integrated by the Institute of Medical Business Advisors Inc., is somewhat similar. Its uniqueness emanates from a holistic union of personal financial planning, human physiology, and medical practice management, solely for the healthcare space. Unlike pure life planning, pure financial planning, or pure management theory, it is both a quantitative and qualitative "hard and soft" science, with an ambitious economic, psychological, and managerial niche value proposition never before proposed and codified, while still representing an evolving philosophy. Its first-mover practitioners are called Certified Medical Planners™.

Life planning, in general, has many detractors and defenders. Formally, it has been defined by Mitch Anthony, Gene R. Lawrence, AAMS, CFP® and Roy T. Diliberto, ChFC, CFP® of the Financial Life Institute, in the following Trinitarian way.

> Financial Life Planning is an approach to financial planning that places the history, transitions, goals, and principles of the client at the center of the planning process. For the financial advisor or planner, the life of the client becomes the axis around which financial planning develops and evolves.
> Financial Life Planning is about coming to the right answers by asking the right questions. This involves broadening the conversation beyond investment selection and asset management to exploring life issues as they relate to money.
> Financial Life Planning is a process that helps advisors move their practice from financial transaction thinking, to life transition thinking. The first step is aimed to help clients "see" the connection between their financial lives and the challenges and opportunities inherent in each life transition.

But, for informed physicians, life planning's quasi-professional and informal approach to the largely isolate disciplines of financial planning and medical practice management is inadequate. Today's practice environment is incredibly complex, as compressed economic stress from HMOs managed care, financial insecurity from insurance companies, Washington, DC, and Wall Street; liability fears from attorneys, criminal scrutiny from government agencies, and IT mischief from malicious electronic medical record (eMRs) hackers; economic benchmarking from hospital employers; lost confidence from patients; and most recently the Patient Protection and Affordable Care Act (PP-ACA); all promote "burnout" and converge to inspire a robust new financial planning approach for physicians and most all medical professionals.

The iMBA Inc. approach to financial planning, as championed by the Certified Medical Planner™ professional certification designation program, integrates the traditional concepts of financial life planning, with the increasing complex business concepts of medical practice management. The former topics are presented in this book, the later in our recent companion book: *The Business of Medical Practice: Transformational Health 2.0 Skills for Doctors.*

For example, views of medical practice, personal lifestyle, investing, and retirement, both what they are and how they may look in the future, are rapidly changing as the retail mentality of medicine is replaced with a wholesale and governmental philosophy. Or, how views on maximizing current practice income might be more profitably sacrificed for the potential of greater wealth upon eventual practice sale and disposition. Or, how the ultimate fear represented by Yale University economist Robert J. Shiller, in *The New Financial Order: Risk in the 21st Century,* warns that the risk for choosing the wrong profession or specialty might render physicians obsolete by technological changes, managed care systems, or fiscally unsound demographics. Or, if a medical degree is even needed for future physicians? *Say what?*

Dr. Shirley Svorny, chair of the economics department at California State University, Northridge, holds a PhD in economics from UCLA. She is an expert on the regulation of healthcare professionals who participated in health policy summits organized by Cato and the Texas Public Policy Foundation. She argues that medical licensure not only fails to protect patients from incompetent physicians, but, by raising barriers to entry, makes health care more expensive and less accessible. Institutional oversight and a sophisticated network of private accrediting and certification organizations, all motivated by the need to protect reputations and avoid legal liability, offer whatever consumer protections exist today.

Yet, the opportunity to revise the future at any age through personal re-engineering exists for all of us, and allows a joint exploration of the meaning and purpose in life. To allow this deeper and more realistic approach, the informed transformation advisor and the doctor client must build relationships based on trust, greater self-knowledge, and true medical business management and personal financial planning acumen.

The iMBA Philosophy

As you read this book, you will embrace the opportunity to receive the focused and best thinking of some very smart people. Hopefully, along the way you will self-saturate with concrete information that proves valuable in your own medical practice and personal money journey. Maybe you will even learn something that is so valuable and so powerful that future reflection will reveal it to be of critical importance to your life. The contributing authors certainly hope so.

At the Institute of Medical Business Advisors, and through the Certified Medical Planner™ program, we suggest that such an epiphany can be realized only if you have extraordinary clarity regarding your personal, economic, and (financial advisory or medical) practice goals, your money, and your relationship with it. Money is, after only, no more or less than what we make of it. Ultimately, your relationship with it, and to others, is the most important component of how well it will serve you.

This primal chapter then is about the perspectives that are appropriate to attaining a solid and grounded relationship with money, medical practice, and life. Our goal is to facilitate balance and vision within that relationship.

BEHAVIORAL FINANCE DEFINED

Behavioral finance is an evolving area within the field of finance that incorporates economics, psychology, and neurophysiology in an effort to explain human economic behavior and decision-making. Even gender differences are studied. For example, a report in *Research Magazine* (2005) a decade ago suggested that men and women may invest differently. Yet, the difference has been narrowing, recently.

Cash Allocation	Average Account Balance
Men: 26%	Men: $104,000
Women: 40%	Women: $48,000
Mutual Fund Allocation	**Trades per Quarter**
Men: 44%	Men: 2.1
Women: 38%	Women: 1.4
Self-Directed Brokerage Accounts Owned	**Equity Allocation**
Men: 45,000	Men 22%
Women: 14,000	Women 17%

Traditional finance and economic theory is based on the notion that individuals are capable of change, and will make decisions that are in their best economic interest and that are based on a rational analysis of available information. It has become apparent that these are flawed assumptions—not only will individuals often make irrational choices and cognitive errors, but these flaws in decision making are often predictable, and will be repeated by the same individual even after the error has been recognized.

The field of behavioral finance has evolved to try to better understand how emotions affect decision-making, and what seemingly "hard-wired" mistakes in decision-making are innate to human beings. As science advances, the field is drawing in economists, psychologists, physicians, and neuroscientists who are working together to explain how we make decisions and how our decision-making process changes over time due to the experiences we have. There is even an emerging theory in health-law that would allow physicians to apologize to patients for their mistakes.

Integrating Biology, Human Psychology, and Financial Planning

As we have seen, the human brain evolved to work optimally in a hunter–gatherer environment. At that time in human development it was very important to be able to recognize short-term patterns in order to find food, and to have the ability to generate quick emotional and physiologic responses, such as the fight or flight reflex, in response to certain stimuli.

Those who were good at reacting quickly and running fast toward food or away from danger prospered. There was very little downside to overreacting, while there was a tremendous risk to being a contrarian and waiting to consider whether or not one was really in danger. So, hyperreactive, crowd followers were fruitful and multiplied (thus passing on their genes), while analytical contrarians either starved or became lunch for one of the other members of the animal kingdom.

Human evolution has not kept pace with the cognitive demands of modern civilization. Long-term, independent thinkers did not reproduce at a higher rate than others, so there was no Darwinian pressure for their genes to become a predominant trait of our species.

Since successful decision-making is predicated on the ability to rationally analyze data and make decisions that optimize the chance of having a desired outcome, it is important to understand the many ways that this process goes awry. Successful financial planning requires both the doctor–client and the consulting professional to set goals, develop a plan, and have a process to reach those goals. And, very importantly, success is predicated on having the discipline to stay with the plan even when there are predictable, but painful or exciting short-term stimuli (like the stock market having a terrible or a great year).

Psychological Biases Affecting Financial Planning and Investing

The following are some of the most common psychological biases. Some are learned while others are genetically determined (and often socially reinforced). While this essay focuses on the financial implications of these biases, they are prevalent in most areas in life.

Incentives

It is broadly accepted that incenting someone to do something is effective, whether it be paying office staff a commissions to sell more healthcare products, or giving bonuses to office employees if they work efficiently to see more HMO patients. What is not well understood is that the incentives cause a subconscious distortion of decision-making ability in the incented person. This distortion causes the affected person—whether it is yourself or someone else—to truly believe in a certain decision, even if it is the wrong choice when viewed objectively. Service professionals, including financial advisors and lawyers, are affected by this bias, and it causes them to honestly offer recommendations that may be inappropriate, and that they would recognize as being inappropriate if they did not have this bias. The existence of this bias makes it important for each one of us to examine our incentive biases and take extra care when advising physician clients, or to make sure we are appropriately considering nonincented alternatives.

Denial

Denial is a well-known, but underappreciated, psychological force. Physicians, clients, and professionals (like everyone else) are prone to the mistake of ignoring a painful reality, like putting off an unpleasant call (thus prolonging a problematic situation and potentially making it worse) or not opening account statements because of the desire not to see quantitative proof of losses. Denial also manifests itself by causing human beings to ignore evidence that a mistake has been made. If you think of yourself as a smart person (and what professional doesn't?), then evidence pointing to the conclusion that a mistake has been made will call into question that belief, causing cognitive dissonance. Our brains function to either avoid cognitive dissonance or to resolve it quickly, usually by discounting or rationalizing the disconfirming evidence. Not surprisingly, colleagues at Kansas State University and elsewhere found that financial denial, including attempts to avoid thinking about or dealing with money, is associated with lower income, lower net worth, and higher levels of revolving credit.

Consistency and Commitment Tendency

Human beings have evolved—probably both genetically and socially—to be consistent. It is easier and safer to deal with others if they honor their commitments and if they behave in a consistent and predictable manner over time. This allows people to work together and build trust that is needed for repeat dealings and to accomplish complex tasks. In the jungle, this trust was necessary for humans to successfully work as a team to catch animals for dinner, or fight common threats. In business and life it is preferable to work with others who exhibit these tendencies. Unfortunately, the downside of these traits is that people make errors in judgment because of the strong desire not to change, or be different ("lemming effect" or "group-think"). So the result is that most people will seek out data that supports a prior stated belief or decision and ignore negative data, by not "thinking outside the box." Additionally, future decisions will be unduly influenced by the desire to appear consistent with prior decisions, thus decreasing the ability to be rational and objective. The more people state their beliefs or decisions, the less likely they are to change even in the face of strong evidence that they should do so. This bias results in a strong force in most people causing them to avoid or quickly resolve the cognitive dissonance that occurs when a person who thinks of themselves as being consistent and committed to prior statements and actions encounters evidence that indicates that prior actions may have been a mistake. It is particularly important therefore for advisors to be aware that their communications with clients and the press clouds the advisor's ability to seek out and process information that may prove current beliefs incorrect. Since this is obviously irrational, one must actively seek out negative information, and be very careful about what is said and written, being aware that *the more you shout it out, the more you pound it in.*

Pattern Recognition

On a biological level, the human brain has evolved to seek out patterns and to work on stimuli– response patterns, both native and learned. What this means is that we all react to something based on our prior experiences that had shared characteristics with the current stimuli. Many situations have so many possible inputs that our brains need to take mental short cuts using pattern recognition we would not gain the benefit from having faced a certain type of problem in the past. This often-helpful mechanism of decision-making fails us when past correlations or patterns do not accurately represent the current reality, and thus the mental shortcuts impair our ability to analyze a new situation. This biologic and social need to seek out patterns that can be used to program stimuli–response mechanisms is especially harmful to rational decision-making when the pattern is not a good predictor of the desired outcome (like short-term moves in the stock market not being predictive of long-term equity portfolio performance), or when past correlations do not apply anymore.

Social Proof

It is a subtle but powerful reality that having others agree with a decision one makes gives that person more conviction in the decision, and having others disagree decreases one's confidence in that decision. This bias is even more exaggerated when the other parties providing the validating/questioning opinions are perceived to be experts in a relevant field, or are authority figures, like people on television. In many ways, the short-term moves in the stock market are the ultimate expression of social proof—the price of a stock one owns going up is proof that a lot of other people agree with the decision to buy, and a dropping stock price means a stock should be sold. When these stressors become extreme, it is of paramount importance that all participants in the financial planning process have a clear understanding of what the long-term goals are, and what processes are in place to monitor the progress toward these goals. Without these mechanisms, it is very hard to resist the enormous pressure to follow the crowd; think social media.

Contrast

Sensation, emotion, and cognition work by contrast. Perception is not only on an absolute scale, it also functions relative to prior stimuli. This is why room temperature water feels hot when experienced after being exposed to the cold. It is also why the cessation of negative emotions "feels" so good. Cognitive functioning also works on this principle. So one's ability to analyze information and draw conclusions is very much related to the context with in which the analysis takes place, and to what information was originally available. This is why it is so important to manage one's own expectations as well as those of clients. A client is much more likely to be satisfied with a 10% portfolio return if they were expecting 7% than if they were hoping for 15%.

Scarcity

Things that are scarce have more impact and perceived value than things present in abundance. Biologically, this bias is demonstrated by the decreasing response to constant stimuli (contrast bias) and socially it is widely believed that scarcity equals value. People who feel an opportunity may "pass them by" and thus be unavailable are much more likely to make a hasty, poorly reasoned decision than they otherwise would. Investment fads and rising security prices elicit this bias (along with social proof and others) and need to be resisted. Understanding that analysis in the face of perceived scarcity is often inadequate and biased may help professionals make more rational choices, and keep clients from chasing fads.

Envy/Jealousy

This bias also relates to the contrast and social proof biases. Prudent financial and business planning and related decision-making are based on real needs followed by desires. People's happiness and satisfaction is often based more on one's position relative to perceived peers rather than an ability to meet absolute needs. The strong desire to "keep up with the Jones" can lead people to risk what they have and need for what they want. These actions can have a disastrous impact on important long-term financial goals. Clear communication and vivid examples of risks are often needed to keep people focused on important financial goals rather than spurious ones, or simply money alone, for its own sake.

Fear

Financial fear is probably the most common emotion among physicians and all clients. The fear of being wrong—as well as the fear of being correct! It can be debilitating, as in the corollary expression on fear: the *paralysis of analysis.*

According to Paul Karasik, there are four common investor and physician fears, which can be addressed by financial advisors in the following manner:

- Fear of making the wrong decision: ameliorated by being a teacher and educator
- Fear of change: ameliorated by providing an agenda, outline and/or plan
- Fear of giving up control: ameliorated by asking for permission and agreement
- Fear of losing self-esteem: ameliorated by serving the client first and communicating that sentiment in a positive manner

Psychological Traps

Now, as human beings, our brains are booby-trapped with psychological barriers that stand between making smart financial decisions and making dumb ones. The good news is that once you realize your own mental weaknesses, it's not impossible to overcome them.

In fact, Mandi Woodruff, a financial reporter whose work has appeared in Yahoo! Finance, Daily Finance, *The Wall Street Journal, The Fiscal Times* and the *Financial Times* among others, related the following mind-traps in a September 2013 essay for the finance vertical *Business Insider;* as these impediments are now entering the lay-public zeitgeist:

- *Anchoring* happens when we place too much emphasis on the first piece of information we receive regarding a given subject. For instance, when shopping for a wedding ring a salesman might tell us to spend 3-month salary. After hearing this, we may feel like we are doing something wrong if we stray from this advice, even though the guideline provided may cause us to spend more than we can afford.
- *Myopia* makes it hard for us to imagine what our lives might be like in the future. For example, because we are young, healthy, and in our prime earning years now, it may be hard for us to picture what life will be like when our health depletes and we no longer have the earnings necessary to support our standard of living. This shortsightedness makes it hard to save adequately when we are young, when saving does the most good.
- *Gambler's fallacy* occurs when we subconsciously believe we can use past events to predict the future. It is common for the hottest sector during one calendar year to attract the most investors the following year. Of course, just because an investment did well last year doesn't mean it will continue to do well this year. In fact, it is more likely to lag the market.
- *Avoidance* is simply procrastination. Even though you may only have the opportunity to adjust your healthcare plan through your employer once per year, researching alternative health plans is too much work and too boring for us to get around to it. Consequently, we stick with a plan that may not be best for us.
- *Loss aversion* affected many investors during the stock market crash of 2008. During the crash, many people decided they couldn't afford to lose more and sold their investments. Of course, this caused the investors to sell at market troughs and miss the quick, dramatic recovery.
- *Overconfident investing* happens when we believe we can out-smart other investors via market timing or through quick, frequent trading. Data convincingly shows that people who trade most often underperform the market by a significant margin over time.

- *Mental accounting* takes place when we assign different values to money depending on where we get it from. For instance, even though we may have an aggressive saving goal for the year, it is likely easier for us to save money that we worked for than money that was given to us as a gift.
- *Herd mentality* makes it very hard for humans to not take action when everyone around us does. For example, we may hear stories of people making significant profits buying, fixing up, and flipping homes and have the desire to get in on the action, even though we have no experience in real estate.

THE ADDICTIVE INVESTING/TRADING PERSONALITY

Dr. Deana J. Mandell, a pediatrician, always needs to leave the office 15 minutes ahead of schedule. The reason is because it takes that long to make the necessary number of trips to ensure the front door is truly locked.

Dr. Kamela A. Shaw, a general surgeon, is constantly rushing to the bathroom so that she can wash her hands. As far as she is concerned, it is not possible to get one's hands clean enough considering a recent influenza outbreak.

Although the behaviors displayed by these two doctors are different, they are consistent in that each, to some degree, display behavior that might be called obsessive–compulsive.

WHEN INVESTING OR TRADING IS NO LONGER FUN

An *obsession* is a persistent, recurring preoccupation with an idea or thought. A *compulsion* is an impulse that is experienced as irresistible. *Obsessive–compulsive* individuals feel compelled to think thoughts that they say they do not want to think or to carry out actions that they say are against their will. These individuals usually realize that their behavior is irrational, but it is beyond their control. In general, these individuals are preoccupied with orderliness, perfectionism, and mental and interpersonal control, at the expense of flexibility, openness, and efficiency. Specifically, behaviors such as the following may be seen:

- Preoccupation with details
- Perfectionism that interferes with task completion
- Excessive devotion to work and office productivity
- Scrupulous and inflexible about morality (not accounted for by cultural or religious identification)
- Inability to discard worn-out or worthless objects without sentimental value
- Reluctance to delegate tasks or to work with others
- Adopts a miserly spending style toward both self and others
- Demonstrates a rigid, inflexible, and stubborn nature

Most people resort to some minor obsessive–compulsive patterns under severe pressure or when trying to achieve goals that they consider critically important. In fact, many individuals refer to this as *superstitious behavior*. The study habits required for medical students entail a good deal of compulsive behavior.

As the above examples suggest, there are a variety of addictions possible. Recent news accounts have pointed out that even high-level governmental officials can experience *sex addiction*. The advent of social media has led to what is referred to as *Internet addiction* where an individual is transfixed to a computer, tablet PC, or smart-phone, "working" for hours on end without a specific project in mind. The simple act of "surfing," "tweeting," "texting" or merely posting opinions offers the person afflicted with the addiction some degree of satisfaction.

Still another form of addictive behavior is that of the individual with a *gambling disorder (GD)*. *GD* is recognized as a mental disorder in the American Psychiatric Association's Diagnostic and

Statistical Manual of Mental Disorders-V. This is the behavior of an individual who is unable to resist the impulse to gamble. Many reasons have been posited for this type of behavior including the death instinct; a need to lose; a history of trauma; a wish to repeat a big win; identification with adults that the "gambler" knew as an adolescent; and a desire for action and excitement. There are other explanations offered for this form of compulsive behavior. The act of betting allows the individual to express an immature bravery, courage, manliness, and persistence against unfavorable odds. By actually using money and challenging reality, he puts himself into "action" and intense emotion. By means of gambling, the addicted individual is able to pretend that he is favored by "lady luck," specially chosen, successful, able to beat the system and escape from feelings of discontent.

Greed can also have addictive qualities. In fact, a poll conducted by the *Chicago Tribune* revealed that folks who earned less than $30,000 a year said that $50,000 would fulfill their dreams, whereas those with yearly incomes of over $100,000 said they would need $250,000 to be satisfied. More recent studies confirm that goals keep getting pushed upward as soon as a lower level is reached.

Question: So how much money is enough?
Answer: Just a little bit more.

Edward Looney, executive director of the Trenton, New Jersey based *Council on Compulsive Gambling (CCG)* reports that the number of individuals calling with trading-associated problems is doubling annually. In the mid-1980s, when the council was formed, the number of people calling the council's hotline (1–800 Gambler) with stock-market gambling problems was approximately 1.5% of all calls received. In 1998 that number grew to 3%, and rose to 8% by 2012. Today, that number is largely unknown because of its pervasiveness, but Dr. Robert Custer, an expert on compulsive gambling, reported that stock market gamblers represent over 20% of the gamblers that he has diagnosed. It is evident that online trading presents a tremendous risk to the speculator. The CCG describes some of the consequences:

- Dr. Fred B. is a 43-year-old Asian male physician with a salary above $100,000 and in debt for more than $100,000. He is married with two children. He was a day trader.
- Michael Q. is a 28-year-old Hispanic male registered nurse. He is married and the father of one (7 month old) child. He earns $65,000 and lost $40,000 savings in day trading and is in debt for $25,000. He has suicidal ideation.

A QUESTION OF SUITABILITY

Since online traders are in it for many reasons, investment suitability rarely enters the picture, according to Stuart Kaswell, general counsel of the *Securities Industry Association,* in Washington, DC. The kind of question that has yet to be confronted, by day or online trading firms, is a statement, such as: "Equities look good this year. We favor technology stocks. We have a research report on our Web page that looks at the social media industry." Those kinds of things are seldom considered because they do not involve a specific recommendation of a specific stock, such as Apple, Google, Groupon, Facebook, or Twitter. However, if a firm makes a specific recommendation to an investor, whether over the cell-phone, iPad®, fax machine, face-to-face, or over the Internet, suitability rules should apply. Opining similarly on the "know your customer" requirements is Steven Caruso, of Maddox, Koeller, Harget & Caruso of New York City. "The on-line firms obviously claim that they do not have a suitability responsibility because they do not want the liability for making a mistake as far as determining whether the investor was suitable for buying any security. I think that ultimately more firms are going to be required to make a suitability, (or eventually fiduciary) determination on every trade."

ONLINE TRADERS AND STOCK MARKET GAMBLERS

Some of the preferred areas of stock market gambling that attract the interest of compulsive gamblers include options, commodities, penny stocks and bit-coins, index investing, new stock offerings, certain types of CAT bonds, crowd-sourcing initiatives, and some contracts for government securities. These online traders and investment gamblers think of themselves as cautious long-term investors who prefer blue chip or dividend paying varieties. What they fail to take into consideration is that even seemingly blue chips can both rise and precipitously drop in value again, as seen in the summer of 2003, the "crash" of 2008, or the "flash crash" of May 6, 2010. On this day, the DJIA plunged 1000 points (about 9%) only to recover those losses within minutes. It was the second largest point swing 1,010.14 points, and the biggest one-day point decline, 998.5 points, on an intraday basis in Dow Jones Industrial Average history.

Regardless of investment choice, the compulsive investment gambler enjoys the anticipation of following the daily activity surrounding these investments. Newspaper, hourly radio and television reports, streaming computer, tablet and smart phone banners, and hundreds of periodicals and magazines add excitement in seeking the investment edge. The name of the game is action. Investment goals are unclear, with many participating simply for the feeling it affords them as they experience the highs and lows and struggles surrounding the play. And, as documented by the *North American Securities Administrators Association's* president, and Indiana Securities Commissioner, Bradley Skolnik, most day or online traders lose money. "On-line brokerage was new and cutting edge and we enjoyed the best stock market in generations, until the crashes. The message of most advertisements was 'just do it,' and you'll do well. The fact is that research and common sense suggest the more you trade, the less well you'll do."

Most day or online traders are young males, some who quit their day jobs before the just mentioned debacles; or more recently with the dismal economy. Many ceased these risky activities but there is some anecdotal evidence that is resurging again with 2013–14 technology boom and market rise. Most of them start every day not owning any stock, then buy and sell all day long and end the trading day again without any stock—just a lot of cash. Dr. Patricia Farrell, a licensed clinical psychologist states that day traders are especially susceptible to compulsive behaviors and addictive personalities. Mark Brando, registered principal for *Milestone Financial,* a day trading firm in Glendale, California states, "People that get addicted to trading employ the same destructive habits as a gambler. Often, it's impossible to tell if a particular trade comes from a problem gambler or a legitimate trader."

Arthur Levitt, former Chairman of the *Securities and Exchange Commission* (SEC) is discussing the risks and misconceptions of investing are only amplified by online trading. In a speech before the *National Press Club* a few years ago, he attempted to impress individuals as to the risks and difficulties involved with day trading. Levitt cited four common misconceptions that knowledgeable medical professionals, and all investors, should know:

- Personal computers, tablets, mobile devices, and smart-phones are not directly linked to the markets—thanks to *Level II* computer software, day traders can have access to the same up-to-the-second information available to market makers on Wall Street. "Although the Internet makes it seem as if you have a direct connection to the securities market, you don't. Lines may clog; systems may break; orders may back-up."
- The virtue of *limit orders*—"Price quotes are only for a limited number of shares; so only the first few investors will receive the currently quoted price. By the time you get to the front of the line, the price of the stock could be very different."
- *Canceling an order*—"Another misconception is that an order is canceled when you hit 'cancel' on your computer. But, the fact is it is canceled only when the market gets the cancelation. You may receive an electronic confirmation, but that only mean your request to cancel was received—not that your order was actually canceled."

- *Buying on margin*—"if you plan to borrow money to buy a stock, you also need to know the terms of the loan your broker gave you. This is margin. In volatile markets, investors who put up an initial margin payment for a stock may find themselves required to provide additional cash if the price of the stock falls."

How then, can the medical professional or financial advisor tell if he or she is a compulsive gambler? A diagnostic may be obtained from *Gamblers Anonymous*. It is designed to screen for the identification of problem and compulsive gambling.

But, it is also necessary to provide a tool to be used by online traders. This questionnaire is as follows:

1. Are you trading in the stock market with money you may need during the next year?
2. Are you risking more money than you intended to?
3. Have you ever lied to someone regarding your online trading?
4. Are you risking retirement savings to try to get back your losses?
5. Has anyone ever told you that you spend too much time online?
6. Is investing affecting other life areas (relationships, vocational pursuits, etc.)?
7. If you lost money trading in the market, would it materially change your life?
8. Are you investing frequently for the excitement, and the way it makes you feel?
9. Have you become secretive about your online trading?
10. Do you feel sad or depressed when you are not trading in the market?

Note: If you answer "yes" to any of these questions, you may be moving from investing to gambling.

The cost of compulsive gambling and day trading is high for the individual medical or lay professional, the family and society at large. Compulsive gamblers, in the desperation phase of their gambling, exhibit high suicide ideation, as in the case of Mark O. Barton, the murderous day-trader in Atlanta who killed 12 people and injured 13 more in July 29th, 1999. His idea actually became a final act of desperation.

Less dramatically, for doctors, is a marked increase in subtle illegal activity. These acts include fraud, embezzlement, CPT® upcoding, medical overutilization, excessive full risk HMO contracting, Stark Law aberrations and other "white collar crimes." Higher healthcare and social costs in police, judiciary (civil and criminal) and corrections result because of compulsive gambling. The impact on family members is devastating. Compulsive gamblers cause havoc and pain to all family members. The spouses and other family members also go through progressive deterioration in their lives.

In this desperation phase, dysfunctional families are left with a legacy of anger, resentment, isolation, and in many instances, outright hate.

DAY TRADING ASSESSMENT

Internet day trading, like the Internet and telecommunications sectors, became something of a investment bubble a few years ago, suggesting that something lighter than air can pop and disappear in an instant. History is filled with examples: from the tulip mania of 1630 Holland and the British South Sea Bubble of the 1700s; to the Florida land boom of the roaring twenties and the Great Crash of 1929; to the collapse of Japans stock and real estate market in early 1990s; and to an all-time high of $1,926 for an ounce of commodity gold a few years ago. To this list, one might again include smart-phone or mobile day trading.

WHAT IS MONEY?

So, what is money? Money is elusive. It seems to demand so much from us. Not only does it seem utterly convoluted and alien, it is also bafflingly personal. In between, we find complex monetary systems, multinational legalisms; a whole host of political and cultural mythologies, our most profound personal issues and another zillion nuances that go into generating "the money forces." Then, as if to heap insult upon injury, the art of money demands competency with your own personal intangibles.

Money has strong spiritual and religious components. Indeed, our relationship with money goes straight to our souls. Getting it, keeping it, and spending it all precisely reflect our values, morals, and motivations. Some believe money has its origins in religious rituals. Others believe that the love of money is at the root of all evil. Either way, it is no accident that the money issue is the second most frequently addressed topic in the Christian Bible and is clearly a part of most major religious traditions. It has that kind of power in our lives.

What's more, money itself has much else in common with religion. Despite pretentious banalities decrying money as either secular creed or an unworthy recipient of thoughtful attention by right thinking people, and in spite of trite condemnations of its hold on our value systems, the baseline fact is that money is a belief system with all the qualities and characteristics that generally attend belief systems. It has only the values, functions, and meanings we collectively give it. No more. No less. It is myth at its best.

It also grounds humanity's best attempts to take care of its individuals while rationally allocating goods and services. Perfection? Hardly. Yet still the best system we know for delivering life's necessities to the broadest possible group of living souls.

One may suggest the following to be financial axioms of our age:

- Money is the most powerful secular force on the planet.
- Money skills are quite literally twenty-first century survival skills.
- Money skills do not come with our DNA.

Therefore, this may lead to multiple conclusions that heads directly to core realities. If these observations are true and can be taken together as working presuppositions for life in the twenty-first century, well, you know, money is just plain powerful. Our lives will go better if we have a grip on it.

Money skills come in many forms and are much more than mere technical proficiency. In fact, some money skills are simple coping mechanisms such as balancing creditors and cash flow, understanding insurance needs, or grasping the rudiments of our legal system.

Others include an ability to deal with the array of money systems that have evolved in response to complex economies including relevant bureaucracies. Also, an appreciation for history and social evolution is useful. At the very least, such an appreciation will enhance your coping skills. Much about our economic systems does not make much sense if taken in isolation.

Money has been evolving for the thousands of years. It has been an integral part of civilization. It enables the marketplace. It is easy to become cynical about money, but without it, our systems grind to a halt. This includes our healthcare systems.

Money underscores the purpose of this chapter. Its work is grounded in these beliefs and the attendant exploration of their ramifications for individual lives. In doing this work, our discussion will range from the philosophical to the intensely personal. Be forewarned, this chapter will not teach you how to get rich so much as it might, hopefully, help you live richly. To derive maximum benefit, it is imperative that you bring a willingness to look into yourself as well as the world around you.

We are too easily daunted by money. Some of our fears are justified but there are whole ranges of skill that are resolved by simply understanding some basics. For all the mysteries and myths woven around money, truly crucial money skills are easily accessible to individuals. At the level required for twenty-first century survival, money skills are not particularly complex. If you don't have them, you can generally rent them or associate with them.

The simple fact is that if you have read the entirety of this book, you have been exposed to just about all there is to know about financial planning fundamentals, and some practice management benchmarks. If you have not found it between these covers, most of what is left is just a phone call, or couple of browser clicks away.

Don't misunderstand. There are certain financial and managerial issues that are incredibly complex, that deserve years of schooling, should only be used in the hands of the most skillful, and truly merit our awe and admiration. This is comparable to those times when sophisticated surgical invasion is required. Sometimes it does the trick perfectly. But you don't do heart surgery to cure a cold and you do not necessarily need complex solutions to your financial problems. Be careful out there.

This will undoubtedly get us into some philosophical trouble, but we plead with you to understand the simple realities of the financial services and medical consulting industry. There are some great people in it. Nonetheless, in the wonderful world of personal finance and practice management, what others make complex often simply covers sales motives, crude politics, or some other form of pocketbook invasion. Or, it may be an attempt to make someone appear sophisticated. Or, it might possibly be simply an intellectual version of the old shell game, betting neither you nor a team of auditors could find the pea that has been so magnificently shuffled. Reducing gimmicks to essential components is a worthy skill. Never investing in something you do not understand is simply fundamental intelligence. If you don't "get it," please accept the possibility that it may not be you. Hold off. Even if you "get it," it is still a good idea to "get" the seller's motives. There is a difference between paranoid and prudent, but even paranoids reduce their odds of getting mugged if their fear helps them stick to safer paths.

Yet, these and other basics are pure financial muscle. Whole industries are built around them and getting around them.

True sophistication comes with tailoring your money and practice to you. Imagine what you would know if you had completely absorbed the information contained herein. You could have learned to build, staff, and plan for your medical business. You might have received an overview of various taxation systems and miscellaneous methods for best working with their demands. You could now be comfortably crunching numbers, multiplying, adding, subtracting, and dividing with the best of them. In the meantime, you have been exposed to investments, estate planning, insurance, "retirement" planning, and so forth. You could have been absorbing details, possibilities, likelihoods, and the prospective repercussions for guessing wrong. Imagine.

AND SO WHAT?

At the end of the day, the real trick is to understand this information as it applies to you, personally. Without knowledge of your own life dreams and goals, the utility of any of this knowledge is of the most dubious value.

Now step back a minute. How do these thoughts feel? Are you energized or daunted? Empowered or bewildered? Thrilled or bored? Be honest in your answers. Money has huge emotional and personal spiritual aspects to it. Overestimating either your aptitudes or your knowledge can be both expensive and time consuming. It can most certainly be intellectually daunting and spiritually depleting.

MONEY: "MINUTES TO LEARN—A LIFETIME TO MASTER"

Assuming your goals ultimately has more to do with home, heart, health, patients, and happiness than extra numbers from your practice on your bank and brokerage statements, all of this ultimately needs to be about perspective, money and you. It is about wisdom of the sort that will enable you to aspire realistically toward your visions while maintaining personal balance. Without these, money craft is fundamentally worthless.

Here we are trying to put money insights into context. We are looking at practicalities. We are also attempting to look at money from the standpoints of various modern social and economic systems. As we continue along this course, a couple of suggestions: you will be well-served by a sense of irony, a tolerance of paradox, and the well-founded belief that "everybody is weird about money." Trust me. Everybody. You. Me. Everybody.

Allow us to suggest that financial health reflects attitudes more than aptitudes. The art of money demands good judgment more than gimmicks. Greed is not only one of the seven deadly sins; it is quite clearly dangerous to your wealth. So are the other six: pride, envy, gluttony, lust, anger, and sloth. An individual's fiscal health, as with her physical well being, is more likely to respond favorably to great habits than technical mastery.

There can be no doubt that financial and managerial issues can get complicated. Yet, it is equally obvious that money fundamentals are not so difficult to grasp that folks of reasonable intelligence should be intimidated. An abiding truth is that one need not be an "expert" to function effectively and efficiently around it and within the money forces.

The relevant personal financial rules can be summarized in eight short words.

- Rule One: Save more.
- Rule Two: Spend less.
- Rule Three: Don't do anything stupid.

The relevant personal financial planning process corollaries can also be summarized briefly:

- Financial planning first, asset allocation second, your portfolio third.
- The financial planning process is insensitive to the economy and market outlook. For example, you do not buy equities because you think the market is going up. You own them because their historical returns (absolute/compared to debt) are sufficient to meet the goals and objectives of your plan.
- Diversification at all times.
- A good long-term definition for the commodity money is purchasing power. The best test of income potential overtime is total return, not current yield.
- Do not micromanage your plan, your portfolio, yourself, or your advisors.

That's it. Nothing daunting or inherently intimidating, here. Just control your spending. At the very least, spend less than you make and do it for a long time. Save regularly. Your savings are raw power. They enable you to make choices that suit you. Understand your personal issues, particularly your vulnerabilities and most particularly the essentials of your obligations as a citizen of your family and your various communities. Then, make a plan, allocate your assets, get professional help to monitor your portfolio, and don't do anything stupid.

Other relevant fundamentals include living modestly and beneath your economic means. Stay married to your spouse. Grasp basic risk management (i.e., insurance and general prudence) and investment fundamentals, most particularly notions of cycles, greed, and time. Pay your taxes on time. Master your medical specialty, tele-health, m-health, medical records documentation, and the nuances of CPT® billing codes! Adhere to the tenants of NPI numbers, HIPAA, CLIA, EMTALA, OSHA, electronic record keeping, Comparative Effective Research (CER), medical homes, value-based care, P4P initiatives, and the PP-ACA, and so on. Become skillful in financial ratio-analysis and business interpretation. Buy enough insurance to keep your promises and avoid catastrophe. Protect your assets. Be skeptical of sales pitches yet generous with others. Save and invest for growth your entire life. Have faith in any god you wish. Worry less about your appearances than your realities. Be flexible and market responsive in your medical practice specialty and future life. Develop a hobby and plan a passionate-retirement. Have faith in yourself and in your future. And, never-ever lose sight of the fact that, *above all else*, medical care should be delivered in a personal and humane manner, with patient interest, rather than self interest, as a guiding standard. *Omnia pro aegroto,* or "all for the patient."

Finally, live your life with pride and joy but don't confuse good fortune with skill. Adherence to these simple rules will generally assure a rewarding relationship with money. Truly.

Our purpose here is not to denigrate technical financial knowledge so much as to suggest that attention to the technical at the expense of one's human priorities and personal values can lead to ruined lives—which sort of misses the point of developing financial and business skills.

Assuming the above, there is substantial craft to technical financial proficiency. As with all crafts, genuine mastery requires time, experience, skill, knowledge, and discipline. The details may be easily accessible but truly appropriate use of the details takes time and the sort of experience that comes with making mistakes or seeing them made by others. Yet even then, craft is of considerably less importance than understanding and judgment.

Money tends to reward those who treat it with respect and wisdom.

Full development of the money craft takes years of education and experience. Wisdom takes longer. Wisdom is not subject to rules and regulations. Wisdom requires the integration of financial issues with your own sense of life, its purpose, and its possibilities. Wisdom includes an ability to anticipate consequences of all sorts. The craftsman will help you to maximize your estates to benefit your family. A wise advisor will ask you if your family is emotionally or spiritually prepared for receiving it. If not, they will help you to avert a train wreck for those you love. Your practice may respond well to 80-hour work weeks. Will your mental and physical health? How about your soul? Will your marriage, friends, and relationships respond as well? Or your children? All are part of behavior finance and the art of money.

As a doctor, you may hate practicing medicine, or your current work environment as an employed hospitalist, or because of managed care or the PP-ACA. You may even feel helpless and burned-out. What are the possibilities for personal re-education and changing it? What is the cost of continued misery or sense of meaninglessness? What are the intangibles for lives lived without inherent worth? Can you re-engineer and retool your life for a new career?

What may be obvious to many may be dead wrong for you. Do you want to allocate your precious life energies to deals and heels? You may choose not to play the maximization game. "Enough" may really be enough. You may make choices for reasons other than money. You can practice until you drop. You may choose to live simply. You can smell some roses. Truly, it is up to you.

Money is here to serve humans. Humans are not here to serve money. Humans are not money machines. More is not better. Enough *is* enough. Money is a terrific servant but a terrible master. Remember: You can't take it with you.

Is this heresy in a secular culture that allegedly reveres money at the expense of all else? Perhaps! Nonetheless, your relationship with money is uniquely yours. How you regard it, relate to it, use it, work with it, or play with it is entirely up to you. As ancient wisdom tells us, "Where your heart is, so shall your treasure be." Your relationship with your money will reflect both your personality and your value systems. You are revealed through money more profoundly than through your handwriting. Neither your fingerprints nor your blood work are as individuated as your relationship with this ultimate intangible.

Yet, money is inescapable. At base, we must understand that the money forces rage around us. We can no more escape money than we can escape water, nourishment, or oxygen. Money impacts everything about our lives every hour of every day. It is very strange, unique in its every aspect. It gets into the cracks of our personal, communal, regional, national and international lives in manners unlike any other part of human existence. And we need it to survive.

So, what is it, this money? First, as noted above, it is a belief system. It has value only insofar as we impart value to it. If humans ceased believing in money, money would immediately cease to be important.

Second, it is a social lubricant and intellectual fertilizer. In the immortal words of Ben Franklin "Money is like muck—Useless unless spread around." When money is used as nourishment, deserts bloom. When money serves as lubricant; social machinery functions smoothly.

Using money, we build families, communities, schools, hospitals, libraries and cultural facilities, stadiums, highways, utilities, and transportation systems.

We generate: Food, clothing, shelter, books
We create: Art, literature, science, exploration
We educate: We care, we tend, we live

Without money, we are simply an agglomeration of individuals. With it, we can be interdependent communities. Look at the bad economies of the world. Would you want to live in them? Imagine the prospect of feeding the planet's 6 billion souls without money. Not even close.

Third, money stores value. It enables trade and, in so doing, facilitates the development of resources and proficiencies with unparalleled efficiency. Imagine creating all that you consume. Inconceivable! Yet, through the miracle of money, much is enabled. The simplest act of consumption generally reflects the labors and/or mental genius of hundreds to thousands or millions, all performed in the name of money.

Fourth, it provides incentives and helps us keep score. It frequently reflects excellence and reveals mediocrity. Successful medical practices serve humanity in miscellaneous ways and are rewarded with money. Unsuccessful ones move those associated to something more "productive." Money abuses tend to bring down the incompetent and the dishonest. Inefficiencies, dishonesty, poor quality, and so on tend to contain within themselves the seeds of their own destruction.

Similarly, it often serves as palpable recognition for discipline, thoughtfulness, creativity, deferred gratification, hard work, and/or vision. "Show me the money" has become a cultural icon for the very best of reasons.

Yet it is obviously silly to accumulate money for its own sake, out of context for your life requirements. You can't eat it, wear it, or cure yourself with it. Without the hard work of others, there is no food, shelter or, indeed, much else carrying with it even a scintilla of value. It is certainly no substitute for love, self-esteem, prudence, knowledge, or professional integrity. The Disney character Scrooge McDuck may swim in it but even such a nominal utility is denied the rest of us. For all the energy we throw at it, it is remarkably insubstantial.

Indeed, money has, in fact, become the most powerful secular force on earth. Nothing of consequence in our twenty-first century world takes place without it lurking somewhere nearby. Moreover, money is simply amazing in its ability to do "good," to spread power, and counter brute force as a method of imposing will. It is my heartfelt belief that more acts of peace, love, and brotherhood occur in our daily pursuits of money than through any other aspect of our collective human existence. Nothing else induces enemies to cooperate with each other like the power of money. Lions lay down with lambs and swords are beat into plowshares in the contexts of markets and money forces. Nothing else can mobilize humans in their pursuits of knowledge, mutual benefit, and sharing. Imagine a healthcare system without money. Not likely.

The metaphors abound. It is like water in the sense that it is the giver of life to healthy human enterprises. Yet, like water, it carries the taints and poisons of its origins. "Dirty money" is no joke. Stay away from it.

It is also like water in the sense that floods of it contain the power to destroy. An old joke runs "Cocaine is God's way of telling you that you make too much money." One of many. Money without values is horrifying. It destroys ecosystems and communities along with individuals, families, and businesses. Markets may be efficient but they are not compassionate. Unfortunately, neither do they deal well with true off-balance sheet costs. Ostrich accounting often ignores the intangible or the immeasurable. However, these problems are not flaws in money so much as shortcomings in our methods of working with it.

Money issues find their way into our most intimate relationships. The family itself is a fundamental economic unit. Cities are strategically located to achieve certain economic advantages.

Money issues lurk ominously around and about most forms of human conflict. These are just more good reasons for money's prominence within morality literature. Fairy tales, myths, and fables frequently focus on money and its ramifications.

Read the Brothers Grimm, the Wizard of Oz or other world mythologies as money allegories. Fascinating! Indeed the book, *The Seven Stages of Money Maturity* finds parallels throughout history and the world's religions, literature, and wisdom (SevenStages.com). Authored by yoga-devotee, George D. Kinder, CPA, CFP®, a Harvard graduate, Bronze Medal winner in the National Uniform Certified Public Accountant examination in Massachusetts, and Buddhist teacher, the Seven Stages are outlined below.

INNOCENCE

"Innocence represents the beliefs, thoughts, stories, attitudes, and assumptions about money we hold onto for dear life no matter how fiercely the world works to remind us of their untruth. The process of entrapment in beliefs begins early in childhood, when parents pass on their own often—unstated attitudes about money. We seize upon these beliefs, sometimes burying them so deeply within that we don't even know they're there-yet they still influence every money decision we make. The desperate, often unconscious way we cling to our beliefs around money reflects the urgency of our basic needs."

PAIN

"Where Innocence consists of our belief systems, thoughts, and stories, Pain represents the wild, unbearable, chaotic feelings hooked to these systems, thoughts, and stories—emotions such as envy, greed, desire, frustration, anger, despair, fear, humiliation, boredom, and sadness—the great mass of unpleasant feeling we would just as soon avoid. Attaching these feelings to stories gives us a way of tolerating and explaining them. Because we don't like these troubling emotions and try to push them away, they attach themselves, seemingly permanently and often unconsciously, to our belief systems, thoughts, and stories. Then, we go round and round with them, inventing endless variations of the old themes as new money circumstances present themselves."

KNOWLEDGE

"The stage of knowledge, while filled with practical things like budgets and taxes and investments, is actually rooted in virtue and integrity. Without integrity economic systems and relationships fall apart. Our determination to act always with integrity in the day-to-day world forms the only healthy basis from which we can approach the universe of information and knowledge about money."

UNDERSTANDING

"Understanding is the most revolutionary teaching of all the Seven Stages. Because of its life-transforming nature, Understanding often takes us in directions and over distances we have never imagined possible. In Understanding we go back to the beginning, to contemplate Innocence and Pain again and resolve the cycle of suffering once and for all. Understanding stands at the center of the Seven Stages, the place where the transforming action of the heart takes hold. In Understanding we resolve the dilemma of childhood by unraveling the knot of suffering, letting stories and identifications go, turning suffering into wisdom and truth. Such transformation is possible because understanding gives us the capacity to enter, with grace and acceptance, the darkest areas of suffering."

Vigor

"Vigor centers on discovering purpose in life and putting one's energy into accomplishing that purpose. Vigor is centered in the throat, the place from which we speak with authority. Vigor concerns authority in the sense of 'authoring' our own lives. In the world of money, Vigor represents the energy to accomplish financial goals and completes the work of adulthood on the path to Money Maturity."

Vision

"Vision is all about seeing. It entails coming to each moment of life with the focused awareness of someone who is vital and alive. Vision directs our sense of life purpose beyond ourselves, toward the health and welfare of communities. What propels us through life is no longer the deadening, blinding suffering caused by the dance of Pain and Innocence, but the full consciousness of every moment supported by the skills of adulthood and a calling toward what needs to be done."

Aloha

"The last stage is a place of wisdom and generosity. Given or received, Aloha is unmistakable. It is humility, kindness, and blessing that pass from one person to another. Aloha lacks economic distinction; it can be given by a poor person to rich one, as well as the other way around. Aloha arises from the interior place where we have emptied ourselves of attachments to objects and stories and can give ourselves spontaneously, genuinely, and lovingly to another."

We need these stages or moral instructions about money because it is so easy to get out of whack in our relationships with it. The consequences can be huge. Indeed, individual and collective failures to attain balance and vision in our personal money relationships lead to egregious consequences in virtually every area of our lives.

Which is to say that money is serious stuff! Which is *not* to say that life, financial advice, or medical practice is all about money or that you should sacrifice beyond measure to maximize either your competencies with it, medical specialty, or your particular pile of it. It is just to say that money is serious stuff and that your life will be better if you understand it and your relationship with it.

It is also to say that it impacts everybody and that everybody has to come to terms with its role in our lives. Indeed, if you are having trouble in your own relationship with money, it might comfort you to know that you are the best of company. Remember, "Everybody is weird about money."

KNOW THYSELF

Money is personal and intimate. We are all uniquely wired in our relationship with it and our attitudes toward it. No one else is like you. You are like no one else. No one has your medical or secular experiences. No one else comes from your family, with your ears, with your traumas or joys. No one else has your prospects or your timetable.

Your own hard wiring may help or hurt you in achieving significant net worth but without understanding it, it will be difficult for you to achieve balance or vision in your personal relationship with money. This is where the cold realities of financial health meet self-awareness and the mental health disciplines. No self-help book has the capacity to explain you to you, but your personal work toward self-understanding will go a long way toward easing the trials of your own money journey.

However, there is no substitute for working with mental health professionals and skilled financial advisors. The interface of money and mental health can pose tricky ethical and practical dilemmas. We recommend working with professional advisors who have both understanding of and respect for the skills of related professions.

The exercises that follow are examples. They are designed to help with your self-awareness. While they can be useful all by themselves, it is our experience that it is difficult for humans to work them as hard as is generally necessary to receive full value. Also there may be other exercises or techniques that would be more particularly useful for you. Without some sort of coach who is in touch with you, your progress, and your responses, it would be hard to tell. Accordingly, we recommend working on these exercises in conjunction with a skilled advisor or advisory team. Licenses are not as important as skill sets. You want somebody who listens, understands what is going on, and has your best interests at heart and in mind. Financial planners, coaches, psychologists, psychiatrists, lawyers, accountants, or even Uncle Joe may all be excellent facilitators. Many with the same licenses will be terrible. It is worth the effort to find someone with whom you are comfortable, and who understands money and who also has a minimal or nonexistent sales agenda.

Every aspect of your life will be improved with a healthy relationship with money. The exercises that follow are designed to help you on your way. They will reward your efforts.

EXERCISE A

MONEY AUTOBIOGRAPHY QUESTIONNAIRE

For understanding your relationship with money, it is important to be aware of yourself in the contexts of culture, family, value systems, and experience. These questions will help you. This is a process of self-discovery. To fully benefit from this exploration, please address them in writing. You will simply not get the full value from it if you just breeze through and give mental answers. While it is recommended that you first answer these questions by yourself, many people relate that they have enjoyed the experience of sharing them with others who are important to them.

As you answer these questions, be conscious of your feelings, actually describing them in writing as part of your process.

CHILDHOOD
- What is your first memory of money?
- What is your happiest moment with money? Your most unhappy?
- Name the miscellaneous money messages you received as a child.
- How were you confronted with the knowledge of differing economic circumstances among people, that there were people "richer" than you and people "poorer" than you?

CULTURAL HERITAGE
- What is your cultural heritage and how has it interfaced with money?
- To the best of your knowledge, how has it been impacted by the money forces? Be specific.
- To the best of your knowledge, does this circumstance have any motive related to money?
- Speculate about the manners in which your forebears' money decisions continue to affect you today?

FAMILY
- How is/was the subject of money addressed by your church or the religious traditions of your forebears?
- What happened to your parents or grandparents during the Depression?
- How did your family communicate about money? Be as specific as you can be, but remember that we are more concerned about impacts upon you than historical veracity.
- When did your family migrate to America (or its current location)?
- What else do you know about your family's economic circumstances historically?

YOUR PARENTS
- How did your mother and father address money?
- How did they differ in their money attitudes?

- How did they address money in their relationship?
- Did they argue or maintain strict silence?
- How do you feel about that today?

Please do your best to answer the same questions regarding your life or business partner(s) and their parents.

CHILDHOOD: REVISITED

- How did you relate to money as a child? Did you feel "poor" or "rich"? Relatively? Or, absolutely? Why?
- Were you anxious about money?
- Did you receive an allowance? If so, describe amounts and responsibilities.
- Did you have household responsibilities?
- Did you get paid regardless of performance?
- Did you work for money?

If not, please describe your thoughts and feelings about that.
Same questions, as a teenager, young adult, older adult.

CREDIT

- When did you first acquire something on credit?
- When did you first acquire a credit card?
- What did it represent to you when you first held it in your hands?
- Describe your feelings about credit.
- Do you have trouble living within your means?
- Do you have debt?

ADULTHOOD

- Have your attitudes shifted during your adult life? Describe.
- Why did you choose your personal path? Would you do it again?
- Describe your feelings about credit.

ADULT ATTITUDES

- Are you money motivated? If so, please explain why? If not, why not?
- How do you feel about your present financial situation?
- Are you financially fearful or resentful? How do you feel about that?
- Will you inherit money? How does that make you feel?
- If you are well off today, how do you feel about the money situations of others?
- If you feel poor, the same question as above.
- How do you feel about begging? Welfare?
- If you are well off today, why are you working?
- Do you worry about your financial future?
- Are you generous or stingy? Do you treat? Do you tip?
- Do you give more than you receive or the reverse? Would others agree?
- Could you ask a close relative for a business loan? For rent/grocery money?
- Could you subsidize a nonrelated friend? How would you feel if that friend bought something you deemed frivolous?
- Do you judge others by how you perceive they deal with their money?
- Do you feel guilty about your prosperity?
- Are your siblings prosperous?
- What part does money play in your spiritual life?
- Do you "live" your money values?

There may be other questions that would be useful to you. Others may occur to you as you progress in your life's journey. The point is to know your personal money issues and their ramifications for your life, work, and personal mission. This will be a "work-in-process" with answers both complex and incomplete. Don't worry. Just incorporate fine-tuning into your life's process.

EXERCISE B

REALITY CHECK

This is where you match resources with goals. Does it work?

RESOURCES

Your so-called net worth statement does not accurately reflect the full extent of your financial resources. If your assets are those tangible and intangible pieces of your life that stand between you and financial disaster, you need to look at all aspects of your life. These include your earning power together with your knowledge and experience. Brains count. Medical acumen counts. Muscles count. Talents count. Write them down.

Resources also include your productive assets, like your medical practice, that may be worth much more to you than could conceivably be reflected on a balance sheet. Or not! Inheritances also count. While caution is appropriate against over reliance upon such anticipations, if you know that substantial resources are likely to come your way, this should be factored into your thinking. Finally, look at your family, community, patients, and other relationships that can provide trustworthy security in your various possibilities for personal disaster. They also do more for your quality of life than pieces of paper.

GOAL SETTING

Goals are the essence of financial planning. Why do you have money? Why do you want more? What do you expect it to do for you? What would you like it to do for you?

Genuine goal setting is among the most intimate and personal of undertakings. Going about it requires self-knowledge and self-honesty. There is insufficient space to enumerate all the possibilities for goal-setting tools. The following are the best we have encountered. Taken from the *Seven Stages of Money Maturity*, they are reprinted with the permission of its author, George D. Kinder, CPA, CFP®.

FIRST QUESTION

This exercise is a set of three scenarios to be worked through in order. The first one, called "plenty of money," is playful and fun as well as revealing. Here's the question to consider: You may not be as wealthy as Bill Gates or the Sultan of Brunei, but you do have all the money you need, now and in the future. What will you do with it? From this moment forward, how will you live your life?

As you write your answer, let yourself dream. This part of the exercise has nothing to do with realism. Run loose, without tether or rein. Give yourself the right to have, do, or be anything that comes to mind. Only when you have completed this part of the exercise should you go on to part two.

SECOND QUESTION

The second segment is called "just a few years left." You've just come back from a visit to a doctor who has discovered from your lab reports that you have only five to ten years to live. In a way you're lucky. This particular disease has no manifestations, so you won't feel sick. The bad part is that you will have no warning about the moment of your death. I will simply come upon you in an unpredictable instant, sudden and final.

Let the emotional import of the situation sink in, then address yourself to this interwoven question: "Knowing death is waiting for you sooner than you expected, how will you change your life? And what will you do in the uncertain but substantial period you have remaining?" Again, spend time with this question and let the full answer emerge from you. And don't go to the next part until you've finished here.

THIRD QUESTION

Now you are ready for the last step, named "Twenty-four hours to live." Again you've gone to the doctor, but this time you learn you'll be dead within twenty-four hours. The question isn't what you would to with the little time you have. Instead, ask yourself, "What feelings am I experiencing? What regrets, what longings, what deep and now-unfulfilled dreams? What do I wish I had completed, been, had, done in this life that is just about to end?" As with the other two parts of this exercise, write your answers with the greatest honesty and candor you can summon.

Goals can be linearly defined. The chart below is a tool for putting goals into a chronological context. Practicalities demand that we make it small. Obviously, you can make it as big as you choose. Pretend each blank rectangle is its own legal pad if you choose. The point is to begin conceptualizing your most important goals in terms of the different, competing arenas of your life and then to attach to each the perspective of time.

	One Week	One Month	Six Months	One Year	Three Years	Five Years	Ten Years	Twenty Years	Lifetime
Family									
Relationship									
Health									
Career									
Community									
Creativity									
Spirit									
Your category									
Your category									
Your category									
Your category									

The next exercise involves a sort of "tic tac toe" chart.

	Got to	Should	Like to
Have			
Do			
Be			

"The next step is to fill in the cells." Into the 'got to' column, put all the things that, from the level of your heart or soul, you simply must do lest your life lack or lose meaning. 'Have' refers to possessions; 'do' covers accomplishments and activities, and 'be' covers states of existence.

"The same distinctions apply to the 'should' column, which covers areas where you feel an obligation to do, have, or be." In the 'like to' column, put the fluff and extras.

"Now that you've completed the exercise, what does it reveal? Typically, issues of career, family, and home appear in the 'got-to' column. Travel, special vacations, and second homes in resort locales usually occupy the 'like-to' column. The 'should' column fills up with practical issues as well as obligations, often toward parents and sometimes toward children. It is not unusual for many issues to appear in the 'should' column."

OVERHEARD IN THE DOCTOR'S LOUNGE: PROSPECT THEORY IN CLIENT EMPOWERMENT FOR FINANCIAL DECISION MAKING

Amanda, an RN client, was just informed by her financial advisor that she needed to relaunch her 403(b) retirement plan. Since she was leery about investing, she quietly wondered why she couldn't DIY. Little does her FA know that she doesn't intend to follow his advice, anyway! *So, what went wrong?*

The answer may be that her advisor didn't deploy a behavioral economics framework to support her decision-making. One such framework is the "prospect theory" model that boils client decision-making into a "three step heuristic."

Prospect theory makes the unspoken biases that we all have more explicit. By identifying all the background assumptions and preferences that clients (patients) bring to the office, decision-making can be crafted so that everyone (family, doctor, and patient) or (FA, client, and spouse) is on the same page. Briefly, the three steps are

1. Simplify choices by focusing on the key differences between investment (treatment) options such as stock, bonds, cash, and index funds.
2. Understanding that clients (patients) prefer greater *certainty* when it comes to pursuing financial (health) *gains* and are willing to accept *uncertainty* when trying to avoid a *loss* (illness).
3. Cognitive processes lead clients and patients to overestimate the value of their choices thanks to survivor bias, cognitive dissonance, appeals to authority, and hindsight biases.

Much like in healthcare today, the current mass-customized approaches to the financial services industry fall short of recognizing more personalized advisory approaches like prospect theory and assisted client-centered investment decision-making.

Jaan E. Sidorov, MD
(Harrisburg, PA)

TELE-PSYCHOLOGY AND PSYCHIATRY

Tele-psychiatry and tele-psychology help patients and clients through online video conferencing, making access to quality mental healthcare easier and personalized. Research has shown that tele-health may be as clinically effective with counseling session results similar to on-ground patient satisfaction and clinical outcomes.

For example, the mission of 1DocWay is to serve the 80 million Americans living in rural communities with the highest quality tele-health services, quickly and easily linking them to those psychiatric and psychological professionals able to provide the proper care (www.1DocWay.com).

ASSESSMENT

Life planning is becoming a highly visibility notion to financial planning practitioners, FAs, and Certified Medical Planners™. Experimental methods are becoming hot topics for graduate and doctoral students in some top behavioral economics, statistics, and mathematics departments in the United States, Europe, Israel, and Japan.

For example, Nobel Laureate Maurice Allais, PhD, demonstrated how economic theory breaks down when used to predict people's choices between different sets of lotteries. And, human beings' limited capacity to digest information needed to make complex decisions was a prime concern of Herbert A. Simon, PhD. More recently, David I. Laibson, PhD, of Harvard University credits the rapidly rising interest in the subject to the strength of its science.

Though the 2002 Nobel Prize of Smith and Kahneman was the first to reward such work, the Nobel committee has long shown an interest in the nexus of economics, physiology, and psychology.

CONCLUSION

The obsession to gain material wealth is sad. Mihaly Csikszentmihalyi, writing in the October 1999 edition of *The American Psychologist,* suggests that material advantages do not readily translate into emotional and social benefits. Friendship, art, literature, natural beauty, religion, and philosophy become less and less interesting. The physician, mental health professional or financial advisor who only responds to material rewards becomes blind, to any other kind, and loses the ability to derive happiness from other sources.

If you are a doctor, nurse, accountant, or financial planner, as you read the remaining chapters of this book you will undoubtedly learn and reinforce information that will prove invaluable in your economic, personal consulting, and practice life.

More importantly however, as you work with other professional advisors and physicians-clients, it will help define your relationship with them, and assist in the never-ending balance between vision, finance, self-awareness, practice, risk, and reward.

COLLABORATE

Discuss this chapter online with others at www.MedicalExecutivePost.com.

ACKNOWLEDGMENTS

To Richard Wagner, JD, CFP®, WorthLiving LLC of The Nazrudin Project and George Kinder of the Kinder Institute of Life Planning, Littleton, Massachusetts.

FURTHER READING

Altman, D: A Nobel that bridges economics and psychology. *New York Times*, October 10, 2002.

Anderson, TJ: *The Value of Debt*. Wiley, New York, 2013.

Baker, HK: *Investor Behavior: The Psychology of Financial Planning and Investing*. Wiley, New York, 2014.

Baker, HK and Nofsinger, JR: *Behavioral Finance (Investors, Corporations, and Markets)*. Wiley, New York, 2010.

Benton, L: *Behavioral Finance Psychology (Bias, Emotion, & Overconfidence)*. e Pub Wealth.com, Cedar City, UT, Kindle edition, 2013.

Boerre, GC: *Shippensburg University of Pennsylvania*, webspaceship.edu, 2009.

Burton, E and Shah, S: *Behavioral Finance (Understanding the Social, Cognitive, and Economic Debates)*. Wiley Finance, New York, 2013.

Field, A: Reading a Client's Tell. *Wealth Management*, p.17, March 2014.

Gladwell, M: *David and Goliath: Underdogs, Misfits and the Art of Battling Giants*. Little Brown, New York, 2013.

Haidt, J: *The Happiness Hypothesis: Finding Modern Truth in Ancient Wisdom*. Basic Books, New York, 2006.

Health Dan and Health Chip: *SWITCH: How to Change Things When Change Is Hard*. Crown Publishing Group, New York, 2010.

Jolles, R: *How to Change Minds; The Art of Influence without Manipulation*. Berrett-Koehler, New York, 2013.

Karasik, P: The four fears. *On the Street*; August, 2003.

Kinder, G: *The Seven Stages of Money Maturity: Understanding the Spirit and Value of Money in Your Life*. Delacorte Press (Dell), New York, 2000.

Kinder, G and Galvan, S: *Lighting the Torch: The Kinder Method™ of Life Planning*. FPA Press, Denver, CO, 2006.

Kinder, G and Rowland, M: *Life Planning—A Banking Manifesto*. Serenity Point Press, Littleton, MA, 2013.

Kitces, ML: Persuading clients to do the right thing. *Financial Planning*, March, 1, 2014.

Klontz, B and Britt, S: How client's money scripts predict their financial behaviors. *Journal of Financial Planning*, 25(11), 33–43, 2013.

Klontz, B, Britt, SL, Archuleta, KL, and Klontz, T: Disordered money behaviors: Development of the Klontz money behavior inventory. *Journal of Financial Therapy*, 3(1), 17–42, 2012.

Klontz, B and Klontz, T: *Mind Over Money: Overcoming the Money Disorders That Threaten Our Financial Health*. Broadway Business, New York, 2009.

Knutson, T: When investing becomes a gambling disease. *Financial Advisor*, p. 17, March 2014.

Marcinko, DE (Ed): *Business of Medical Practice (Transformation Healthcare 2.0 Skills for Doctors)*, 3rd edition. Springer Publishers, New York, 2010.

Oechsli, M: A high-touch practice-literally. *Wealth Management*, p. 24, April 2014.

Paikert, C: High net-worth psychology: What advisors need to know? *Financial Planning*, March 25, 2014.

Pompian, M: *Behavioral Finance and Wealth Management (How to Build Optimal Portfolios that Account for Investor Biases)*. Wiley, New York, 2012.

Post, R: Why "Adviser as Therapist" is good for investors. *Wealth Management*, March 27, 2014.

Prochaska, J and Norcross, J: *Systems of Psychotherapy: A Transtheoretical Analysis*. Cengage Learning Systems; Independence, KY, 2013.

Research Magazine: Staff Writer on Gender Focus, New York, October 1, 2005.

Riekert, KA, Ockene, JK, and Pbert, L: *The Handbook of Health Behavior Changes*. Springer Publishing Company, New York, 2014.

Rosenbaum, J and Pearl, J: *Investment Banking*. John Wiley, New York, 2013.

Schmuckler, E: The addictive investing personality. In Marcinko, DE (Ed): *Financial Planner's Library on CD-ROM*. Aspen Publishing, New York, 2001.

Shubin-Stein, KH: Psychological issues for financial advisors and their clients. In Marcinko, DE (Ed): *Financial Planner's Library on CD-ROM*. Aspen Publishers, New York, 2003.

Snyder, S: *Leadership and the Art of Struggle*. Berrett-Koehler, New York, 2013.

Tversky, A and Kahneman, D: Prospect theory; an analysis of a decision under risk. *Econometrica*, 47(2), 263–291, March 1979.

Wagner, R: The art of money. In Marcinko, DE (Ed): *Financial Planning for Physicians and Healthcare Professionals*. Aspen Publishing, New York, 2003.

Zweig, J: Is your investing personality in your DNA? *WSJ*, April 4th, 2009.

2 Physician Recruitment and Reimbursement Models of the Future

Migrating from Quantity of Care ... to Outcomes from Care

Hope Rachel Hetico and Brian J. Knabe

CONTENTS

Emerging medical provider reimbursement contracts are underappreciated by some doctors, as well as their financial advisors. The mathematical methodology for evaluating the potential impact of these contracts on practice viability and personal physician income may also be vague. Nevertheless, the proto-typical solo family practice reimbursement and related models used in this chapter are applicable to most any medical specialty or for small to large group practices.

INTRODUCTION

"Are financial incentives the proper way to compensate physicians?" asked Jeffrey V. Winston, MD, an ophthalmologist, in a KevinMD.com essay on November 9, 2013; and, "How can we motivate physicians to provide preventive, cost effective, and quality care without incentive programs?", asked Alfie Kohn two decades earlier in his 1994 treatise "Incentive Plans Cannot Work" (EDO-PS-94-14) www.AlfieKohn.org.

To date, doctors and all stakeholders are still struggling with answers to these vital concerns. Clearly, even poorly devised compensation plans are detrimental. Incentive plans do not work because they are poor motivators, can be punitive, discourage risk taking, and inhibit teamwork. Furthermore, Dr. Winston said:

> Once wage earners receive adequate compensation to meet their physical needs, money is not the major motivator. There are much better motivators than money as elucidated in "Drive" by Daniel Pink. People are self-motivated by pride and accomplishment. Workers thrive on recognition by respected leaders and coworkers. Most employees want to achieve the goals of their employer and produce value for their services. Employees lose motivation when treated as automatons, chastised for outcomes that are beyond their control and denied adequate tools to succeed. A manager who provides education, tools and efficient systems will achieve far more than devising a compensation system that rewards a specific behavior.
>
> Bonuses for accomplishing goals can temporarily improve productivity and improve employee satisfaction, but when goals are not met the initial incentive when taken away becomes punitive. Effective incentive systems must reward for doing the right thing, using resources efficiently and producing quality outcomes. Glasziou in 2012 developed a checklist of 9 items that must be reviewed before implementing a financial incentive system. Designing and implementing an incentive system that meets the checklist is nearly impossible.
>
> Physicians motivated by rewards concentrate on their incentive system, avoiding innovation and risk taking. They are also distracted from achieving the overall goals of the organization or the welfare of their patients. Any time taken to improve quality and improve efficiency could threaten their current incentive bonus.
>
> Often compensation systems create additional competition between providers, which inhibits cooperation. Instead of competing based on patient satisfaction and quality care, providers may compete through contracting. If referrals are based on perceived quality, then providers will be less likely to share best practices with others in the community. Engendering teamwork to devise more efficient systems that achieve the mission and goals of the community will accomplish much more than a complex reward system.
>
> Helping many satisfied patients achieving optimal outcomes with the least resources should be enough to motivate physicians. The trick is not to pay for a behavior but to measure the desired activity or outcome. The science of quality improvement has taught us that one must measure to improve. Physicians can be encouraged to change their behavior by measuring performance and providing positive feedback. Recognition by their peers and community leaders for high practice standards can be worth more than money.

PHYSICIAN RECRUITMENT

Recruitment has become a refined art in recent years as practices and physicians themselves grow increasingly savvy about the finer points of marketing positions and securing employment. It's more competitive than ever, too. Many organizations are going after the same physicians. Add to that a shortage of doctors in key specialties in certain geographical areas and the pressure becomes that much more intense. Moreover, the aging of the physician workforce, their increased dissatisfaction with managed care, and changes in doctors' work expectations (they want more free time) have affected the demand and supply.

Additionally, both practicing physicians and residents fresh out of training have become more discerning and skillful in managing the search process. Candidates have learned to be selective based on how they're treated on the phone, how they're treated in person during site visits, or how smoothly the negotiations go. One small bump in the road and they could choose to go elsewhere. In truth, they look to rule organizations out, not in.

Even the smallest of practices must have an effective recruitment plan because they compete directly with the big guys—larger practices and hospitals that have polished their efforts and perfected their processes.

FACTS ABOUT PHYSICIAN RECRUITERS AND EXECUTIVE SEARCH FIRMS

If You Are Job Hunting, You Should Send Your Resume to Recruiters

Different recruiters know about different positions. They do not usually know about the same ones. This is particularly true with retained firms. By sending your resume out widely, you will be placed in many different confidential databases and be alerted of many different positions. If you send your resume to only a few, it may be that none you send to will be working toward positions which are suited for you. Throw your net widely.

If you change jobs, it is also wise to send follow-up letters to the recruiters and alert them of your new career move. Many search firms follow people throughout their careers and enjoy being kept up-to-date. It is a good idea to have your resume formatted in plain text so you can copy and paste it into email messages when requested to do so. Then, follow up with a nicely formatted copy on paper by postal mail.

Some estimate that only 1–3% of all resumes sent will result in actual job interviews. So, if you only send 50 resumes, you may only have less than two interviews, if that many. Send your resume to as many recruiters as you can. It is worth the postage or email time. Generally, recruiters will not share your resume with any employer or give your name to anyone else without obtaining your specific permission to do so. The recruiter will call first, talk to you about a particular position, and then ask your permission to share your resume with that employer.

Your Resume Will Be Kept Strictly Confidential by the Executive Search Firm

It is safe to submit your resume to a search firm and not worry that the search firm will let it leak out that you are job hunting. Recruiters will call you each and every time they wish to present you to an employer in order to gain your permission. Only after they have gained your permission will they submit your name or resume to the identified employer. The wonderful aspect of working with search firms is that you can manage your career and your job search in confidence and privacy.

Fees Are Always Paid by the Employer, Not the Job Candidate

Recruiters and search firms work for the employer or hiring entity. The employer pays them a fee for locating the right physician for the job opening. This is important to remember, in that when you interact with executive recruiters, you are essentially interacting with an agent or representative of the employer. Recruiters are more loyal to employers than they are to job candidates because they work for the employer. This should not present a problem, but, should cause you to develop your relationship with the recruiter with the same integrity and professionalism that you would with the employer.

Recruiters are paid fees in one of two ways—*retainer fees* or *contingency fees*. This is an important distinction and will affect your process with both the employer and the recruiter. Some employers prefer working with contingency firms and some with retained firms. Both are respected by employers and useful in your job search, but, the two types of firms will not be handling the same positions with the same employers simultaneously.

A "retained" recruiter has entered an exclusive contract with an employer to fill a particular position. The retained recruiter, then, is likely to advertise a position, sharing the specifics of the position, location, and employer openly. The retained firm feels a great obligation to fulfill the contract by finding the best person for the job.

A "contingency recruiter" on the other hand, usually does not have an exclusive relationship with the employer, and is only paid a fee if the job search is successful. Often, if the employer uses contingency firms, there will be more than one contingency firm competing to fill a certain position. As a job hunter, if you are sent to an interview by a contingency firm, you may find that you are competing with a larger number of applicants for a position. Generally, retained firms only send in from three to five candidates for a position.

Recruiters will be paid fees equal to about 25–35% of the resulting salary of the successful candidate plus expenses. This does not come out of the job candidate's salary. This is paid to the recruiter through a separate relationship between the employer and the search firm. This may seem like a large fee, but, keep in mind that recruiters incur a great many expenses when searching for successful job candidates. They spend enormous amounts of money on computer systems, long distance calls, mail-outs, travel, and interviews. Recruiters work very hard for these fees. Employers recognize the value of using recruiters and are more than willing to pay recruiters the fees. All you have to do is contact the recruiter to get the process moving.

Not All Medical Recruiters Work Only with Physicians

Some search firms work exclusively with physicians or in healthcare, while others may work in several fields at once. Some of the larger generalist firms will have one or more search consultants that specialize in healthcare. It is important for you, as a job hunter, to assess the recruiters' knowledge of your field. If you use industry or medical specialty buzz words in describing your skills, experience or career aspirations, you may or may not be talking a language the recruiter understands fully. It is wise to explore fully with the recruiter his understanding of your field and area of specialization.

Recruiters and Search Consultants Move Around

Recruiters, like many professionals, move to new firms during their careers. Often you will find that recruiters will work at several firms during their careers. Since it is much more effective to address your letters to a person rather than "to whom it may concern," it is smart for job hunters to have accurate and up-to-date information about who is who and where, since this can change frequently. Search firms also move their offices, sometimes to another suite, street, or state. If you have a list of recruiters that is over one year old, you will certainly waste some postage in mailing your resumes and cover letters. Many of your mail-outs will be returned to you stamped "nondeliverable," unless you obtain an up-to-date list. A resource, like the *Directory of Healthcare Recruiters* is updated very frequently, usually monthly (www.pohly.com/dir3.html).

Most Search Firms Work with Positions all over the Country

If you are from a particular state, and want to remain in that state, don't make the mistake of only sending your resume to recruiters in your state. Often the recruiters in your state are working on positions in other states, and recruiters in other states are working on positions in your state. This is usually the case. Very few recruiters work only in their local area, most work all around the U.S. and some internationally. Regardless of your geographic preference, you should still send your resume to all the healthcare recruiters. If you really only want to remain in your area, you can specify that preference in your cover letter.

Recruiters Primarily Work with Hard to Fill Positions or Executive Positions

Some recruiters specialize in clinical positions for physicians, managed care executive positions, healthcare financial positions, or health administration positions. Others may specialize in finding doctors, nurses, or physical therapists. Generally, an employer does not engage a recruiter's assistance in filling a position unless it is hard to fill. Sometimes employers will engage search firms to save them the valuable time of advertising or combing through dozens of resumes.

Contingency recruiters tend to work with more midlevel management and professional positions, but this is not always the case. Retained firms generally work with the higher level clinical or administrative positions.

One thing you will be assured of is that if a recruiter is working on a position that means the employer is willing to pay a fee. This usually means the position is a valued one and worth closer inspection on your part. Even in healthcare, with certain exceptions, our economy is an "employer's market." This means that employers receive a deluge of resumes for their open positions. Increasingly, employers are using recruitment firms to handle their openings and schedule the interviews because employers simply do not have the manpower or time to handle the many resumes they receive. Therefore, if a job hunter is submitted by a recruiter, that job hunter has a great advantage over all other applicants.

EMPLOYED PHYSICIAN COMPENSATION MODELS

As profit generators, physicians such as pathologists, invasive radiologists, anesthesiologists, emergency department doctors, and hospitalists demand and receive higher salaries.

According to corporate medical recruiter Kris Barlow, employed physicians can select from various employment models that may include fringe benefit packages (life, health, dental, disability insurance; medical society and hospital dues, journals, vacations, auto, and CEUs, etc.) equal to 25–40% of salary (personal communication).

INDEPENDENT CONTRACTOR OR EMPLOYEE

A payer has the right to control or direct the result of the work done by an independent contractor, and not the mean or method of accomplishing the result. By contrast, anyone who performs services for another is an employee if he or she cannot control what will be done and how it will be done. Thus, employed physicians are usually not compensated as independent contractors. Hiring authorities and medical professionals should be careful overusing this technique, in the office or other business. Why? The IRS has successfully attacked many companies that tried to classify their workers as independent contractors rather than employees. The back taxes and penalties can be fierce. However, many tasks may be successfully delegated to independent contractors or consultants without fear of such characterization.

For example, a company does not have to withhold payroll taxes for an independent contractor, but must file a 1099-MISC form whenever payments exceed $600 a year. Moreover, IRS form 1099-MISC is also required for payments greater than at least $10 in royalties or broker payments in lieu of dividends or tax-exempt interest; at least $600 in rents, services (including parts and materials), prizes and awards, other income payments, medical and healthcare payments, crop insurance proceeds, cash payments for fish (or other aquatic life) purchased from anyone engaged in the trade or business of catching fish, or, generally, the cash paid from a notional principal contract to an individual, partnership, or estate; any fishing boat proceeds; or gross proceeds of $600 or more paid to an attorney. In addition, Form 1099-MISC is used to report that you made direct sales of at least $5000 of consumer products to a buyer for resale anywhere other than a permanent retail establishment.

To distinguish between the two, there are several factors to consider. In general, the more you have control over a worker, the more the worker looks like an employee. Two brief tables below note a few of the differences:

Employee:

- Works at the medical office site of employer
- Use practice instruments or equipment
- Cannot delegate or hire others for job
- Method/timing/hours of job specified/controlled
- Expenses reimbursed
- Little invested by worker
- Payment weekly, biweekly, or monthly
- Only works for one employer
- No risk of nonpayment if poor job
- Profit/bonus limited
- No advertising
- Contract states employee relationship
- Position seems permanent
- Work done is essential to practice

Independent Contractor:

- Works off-site
- Uses own instruments and equipment
- Can hire others or delegate (outsource)
- Method/timing of job uncontrolled
- Expenses borne by worker
- More invested by worker
- Payment by the job, procedure, or flat fee
- Works for several clients
- Opportunity for profit
- Advertising to general public
- Contract says independent contractor
- Position temporary
- Work done is noncore function of practice

No single one of these factors determines status. The IRS has a 20-factor test outlined in Revenue Ruling 87–41 and discussed in Publication 1976, "Independent Contractor or Employee." When you have a relationship that is unclear, you should consult with the IRS guidelines and publications. If your intent is to hire an independent contractor physician, try to make sure the relationship has more of the factors indicative of that status, checking the latest IRS publication for all relevant factors. Because of the large amounts at stake, you should err on the side of employee status, if uncertain. You may wish to consult a tax attorney or accountant as well, especially if you have multiple workers in a gray area. In addition, you can request that the IRS make a determination of worker classification by submitting Form SS-8, "Determination of Employee Work Status for Purposes of Federal Employment Taxes and Income Tax Withholding." The IRS guidelines on this topic are rather lengthy.

SELF-EMPLOYED PHYSICIAN COMPENSATION MODELS

According to medical benefits consultant Eric Galtress, CMP™ (Hon), physicians can still seek self-employment compensation models (personal communication).

- *Independent Physicians*: A self-employed physician has great freedom but less security, because relationships with an employer are defined in return for a set compensation. Typically, this option is ideal for those who desire control, don't work well in structured environments, and are committed to maximizing personal compensation.
- *Same-Specialty Group Partnerships*: A same-specialty partnership is more restrictive than independent practice, and must balance control with the security that comes from working with colleagues along a continuum-of-care. Internal competition may be fierce, but partners maintain some autonomy while reaping rewards from economies of scale. More personal time is available too, but compensation is based on individual and group performance.

OVERHEARD IN THE DOCTOR'S LOUNGE: ON HARDWORKING PHYSICIANS

One of my favorite patients told me this anecdote as he recalled the story of the old man who spent a day watching his physician son treating HMO patients in the office.

> The doctor had been working at his usual feverish pace all morning, and although he was working hard, bitterly complained to his dad that he was not making as much money as he used to.
> Finally, the old man interrupted him and said, "Son, why don't you just treat the sick patients?"
> The doctor-son looked annoyed at his father, and responded, "Dad, can't you see, I don't have time to treat just the sick ones."

Dr. David E. Marcinko, FACFAS, MBA, CMP™
(iMBA Inc., Atlanta, GA)

NEWER COMPENSATION MODELS

Today, whether independent or employed, physicians can pursue several creative compensation models, other than fee-for service reimbursement based on Current Procedural Terminology (CPT®) codes, not popular a decade ago:

- *Pay-for-Performance Initiatives (P4P)*: According to Mark Fendrick, MD, and Michael E. Chernew, PhD, instead of the one size fits all approach of traditional health insurance, a "clinically sensitive" cost-sharing system that supports copayments related to evidence-based value for targeted patients is emerging. In 2014, for example, there were a number of changes to Medicare's pay-for-performance programs (personal communication). These value-based payment modifiers will show up in physicians' paychecks in few years, and will be expanded to practices with 10 or more eligible professionals. The program, mandated by the Affordable Care Act, assesses a provider's quality of care and costs, and increases Medicare payments for good performers and decreases them for bad ones. And, doctor performance will be reflected in adjustments to 2016 payments. As much as 2% of Medicare payments will be at risk in 2016 based on physician performance in 2014. It was only 1% for 2015, which was based on doctors' 2013 performance.
- *Physician Quality Reporting Initiative Model*: The Centers for Medicare and Medicaid Services (CMS) paid out more than $40 million in monetary incentives to medical providers who reported data on quality of care delivered between July 2010 and December 2010; as part of its PQRI. Under the PQRI, healthcare providers who participated received bonuses of 1.5% of their total CMS payments during the reporting period.

- *Direct Reimbursement Payment Model*: A Health Reimbursement Arrangement (HRA) is a tool that is used to provide direct reimbursement by an employer for qualified medical expenses. The HRA is an employer-established benefit plan and contributions to the plan may only be made by the employer. The HRA can be used in conjunction with any insurance plan, including a high-deductible plan. Qualified reimbursements made under the HRA are tax-deductible for the employer, and the payments are not counted as income for the employee. Any balance in an HRA can generally be carried over to the next year. This plan allows for flexibility and tailored to meet the particular needs of both employers and employees in a tax-advantaged manner. From the physician's perspective, increasing use of HRAs poses new challenges. Payment for services in the medical office may be required of the patient/employee before reimbursement from the employer occurs. These extra steps can easily result in delayed payment or nonpayment to medical providers who are not prepared to work with this model of reimbursement. The provisions for this model are outlined in IRS publication 969, http://www.irs.gov/pub/irs-pdf/p969.pdf.
- *Concierge Practice Model*: The concept of concierge medicine (CM), also known as retainer medicine, first emerged in Seattle, Washington, in the 1990s. With CM, the physician charges an annual retainer fee to patients. The fee usually ranges from $1000 to $20,000 per year, and the number of patients in a practice is usually limited to a few hundred. In return, patients receive increased levels of access and personalized care. This often includes same day appointments, extended visit times, house calls, and 24/7 access to the physician by pager and cell phone. An annual executive physical is often included, as well as an increased emphasis on preventive care. Many physicians choosing this type of practice model do so for lifestyle and control reasons, although the average income for a successful CM primary care physician is higher than that of a typical primary care physician.
- *Global Healthcare Model*: American businesses are extending their cost-cutting initiatives to include offshore employee medical benefits, and facilities like the Bumrungrad Hospital in Bangkok, Thailand (cosmetic surgery), the Apollo Hospital in New Delhi, India (cardiac and orthopedic surgery) are premier examples for surgical care. Both are internationally recognized institutions that resemble five-star hotels equipped with the latest medical technology. Countries such as Finland, England, and Canada are also catering to the English-speaking crowd, while dentistry is especially popular in Mexico and Costa Rica. Although this is still considered "medical tourism," Mercer Health and Benefits was recently retained by three Fortune 500 companies interested in contracting with offshore hospitals and The Joint Commission (TJC) has accredited 88 foreign hospitals through a joint international commission. To be sure, when India can discount costs up to 80%, the effects on domestic hospital reimbursement and physician compensation may be assumed to increase downward compensation pressures.
- *Locum Tenens Practitioner Model*: Locum Tenens (LT) as an alternative to full-time employment is enjoying a comeback for most specialties. Some younger physicians enjoy the travel, while mature physicians like to practice at their leisure. Employment factors to consider include: firm reputation, malpractice insurance, credentialing, travel, and relocation expenses (which are negotiable). However, an LT firm typically will not cover taxes (NALTO.org and http://www.studentdoc.com/locum-tenens.html)

Locum Tenens Specialty Compensation per 8 Hour Shift

CRNA	$750–$900
Family Practice	$425–$475
Internal Medicine	$425–$475
Pediatrics	$420–$440

OB/GYN	$625–$825
Hospitalist	$525–$775
General Surgeon	$675–$750
Orthopedic Surgeon	$825–$925
Neurosurgeon	$1350–$1450
Anesthesiologist	$1000–$1500
Psychiatrist	$500–$600
Radiologist	$1250–$1500
Cardiologist	$625–$750

Source: www.LocumTenens.com

THE CAPITATION REIMBURSEMENT MODEL

According to the *Dictionary of Health Economics and Finance*, capitation reimbursement represents a health insurance company contract with a medical provider. It is a fixed, prearranged monthly payment received by a physician, clinic, or hospital per patient (pp) enrolled in the plan. Payment per month (pm) is calculated one year in advance and remains fixed for that year, regardless of how often the patient needs services (pp/pm). Counter-intuitively, a full waiting room becomes less desirable than an empty one.

Such shifts in payer mix can cause dramatic impacts to the financial performance of a medical practice. While it is important for the MD and FA to try to evaluate the impact before taking on capitated business, similar principles apply as physician practices shift back to fee for service business from capitation. Before accepting capitation contracts, participants should answer three questions:

1. How much capitation should I accept as a percent of my total business?
2. How will the shift to capitation affect my practice financially?
3. How much will I need to reduce operating expenses in order to break even or profit from capitation?

As physicians' practices shift back to fee for service from capitation, two additional considerations must be addressed:

1. How much capitation is too little?
2. How will another shift in payer mix impact my practice cost structure?

THE SHIFT TO CAPITATION

In the traditional fee for service practices, there are three key financial measures:

1. Net revenue and net revenue per patient visit
2. Office expenses including fixed expenses such as rent, and those that vary with patient volume such as medical supplies
3. Net income, the amount remaining to be paid as physician compensation or reinvested in the practice

By adding capitation to the practice, a physician must consider two additional factors:

- The capitation rate per member/per month (PM/PM)
- The estimated number of visits for each capitated patient

It is often difficult to isolate the financial performance related to one specific payer contract because the same resources are used to care for all the practice's patients. One way to evaluate the impact of a new contract is to determine what the practice's breakeven volume level is before and after the shift to capitation. Breakeven can be described as the level of patient volume required to cover all practice expenses. It is an important measure because once a practice achieves breakeven volume each additional visit contributes to practice net income. Two variables that impact breakeven are revenue per visit and variable cost per visit. Breakeven volume equals:

Total Fixed Expenses

(Net Revenue per Visit—Variable Expenses per Visit)

In some cases, the impact of a shift in payer mix on breakeven volume can be dramatic. This is illustrated in the following examples.

BASELINE EXAMPLE

The baseline example is an internal medicine physician in solo practice. Currently, payment for services is from traditional fee-for-service sources including indemnity insurance, some discounted rate plans, self-pay patients, and Medicare. To analyze the potential financial impact of a shift in payer mix to or from capitation, it is necessary to establish a few key statistics from the practice's most recent 12-month period. Total net patient revenue and total operating expenses can be easily identified. Next, identify fixed operating expenses, which are those costs that generally do not change with volume within a defined range of capacity, such as space, most staffing, and utilities. Subtracting fixed expenses from total operating expenses provides total variable expenses, or those costs that are directly related to patient volume, such as medical supplies. Average variable expense per visit is calculated by dividing total variable expenses by the number of patient visits. The baseline practice profile is shown in Table 2.1.

In the baseline example, the practice needs 2028 annual visits to break even. Any additional visits contribute $81.38, or the difference between net revenue and variable expenses, to net income.

PAYER MIX SCENARIOS

We can now develop scenarios to help evaluate the impact of changes in payer mix. Computerized spreadsheets are idea for analyzing these "what-if" scenarios. In each scenario, assume that the practice is at capacity with 4800 visits, so new capitated patients represent a shift from fee for service business, and are not incremental business to the practice.

SCENARIO 1

Let's assume that 333 of the practice's patients shift to a capitated plan, and that on average, a capitated patient has three visits per year, for 1000 total visits. The physician receives a capitation

TABLE 2.1
Baseline Practice Profile

	Total Annual	Average per Visit
Patient visits FFS	4800	
Total net revenue	$480,000	$100.00
Fixed expenses	$165,000	$34.38
Variable expenses	$89,400	$18.62
Total practice expenses	$254,400	$53.00
Net income	$225,600	$47.00
Breakeven visits	2028	
Contribution to net income after breakeven		$81.38

TABLE 2.2
Payer Mix Scenario 1: Shift to Capitation

	Total Annual w/No Expense Reductions	Avg per Visit w/No Expense Reductions	Total Annual w/Expense Reductions	Avg per Visit w/Expense Reductions
Patient visits—FFS	3800		3800	
Patient visits—capitation	1000		1000	
Total net revenue	$428,000	$89.17	$428,000	$89.17
Fixed expenses	$165,000	$34.38	$148,500	$30.94
Variable expenses	$89,400	$18.62	$80,440	$16.76
Total practice expenses	$254,400	$53.00	$228,940	$47.70
Net income	$173,600	$36.17	$199,060	$41.47
Breakeven visits	2339		2051	
Contribution to net income after breakeven		$70.55		$72.41

payment of $12 per member per month. The average revenue per visit under the capitated agreement is $48 ($12 per month times 12 months, divided by 3 visits), a substantial reduction from the fee for service average of $100. Therefore, the breakeven number of visits for the practice increases to 2339 as the overall average net revenue per visit decreases to $89.17. In order to maintain the fee for service breakeven level of 2028, the practice would need to reduce total costs significantly.

However, even modest reductions in operating expenses can help to compensate for the downward pressure of capitated contract rates on net revenue. In Scenario 1, total expenses are reduced by 10% through a combination of fixed and variable cost reductions. Scenario 1 is shown in Table 2.2.

As a medical practice shifts back from capitation to better paying fee for service business, it is important to remember two things:

1. Increasing revenue per visit does not mean costs should increase.
2. Be careful to maintain enough capitated business to average out the effect of a few high utilizers, or get out of capitation entirely.

Maintain Practice Cost Savings

Let's assume that the practice was able to decrease operating expenses by 10%. With the shift to capitated business, the practice's net income is $199,060. What happens if the practice's business shifts back to fee for service? If the costs revert back to the levels before cost savings were implemented, the practice's net income and breakeven volume are the same as they were originally under the baseline scenario.

But, if the practice is able to maintain the cost savings it experienced, net income increases by $25,460, breakeven volume decreases by 244 visits, and each visit above breakeven contributes $83.24 to the bottom line. This is shown in Table 2.3.

Manage the Level of Capitated Business

Physicians are paid a fixed amount per member per month to care for capitated patients. Capitation rates paid to the practice are determined actuarially based on demographics of the patient population covered, including their anticipated utilization of resources. When a practice has a significant number of capitated patients, the effects of a few high utilizers are usually offset by the utilization patterns of the rest of the population.

TABLE 2.3
Shift from Capitation to Fee for Service

	With Old Cost Structure	With New Cost Structure
Total visits	4800	4800
Net revenue	$480,000	$480,000
Total expenses	$254,400	$228,940
Net income	$225,600	$251,060
Breakeven visits	2028	1784
Contribution to net income after breakeven	$81.38	$83.24

TABLE 2.4
Shift from Capitation to Fee for Service

	333 Capitated Patients	50 Capitated Patients	15 Capitated Patients
Capitated patient visits	1000	220	115
Average visits per capitated patient	3.00	4.40	7.67
Annual capitation revenue	$48,000	$7200	$2160
Capitation revenue per visit	$48.00	$32.73	$18.78
Variable expense per visit	$16.76	$16.76	$16.76
Contribution to net income after breakeven	$31.24	$15.97	$2.02

For example, if the average number of visits per year for a capitated patient is three, it is likely that a few patients will have more visits, but that most patients will visit the physician less frequently. In a practice with a large capitated population, those patients offset the additional use of resources (cost) required to care for the higher utilizers.

Assume the practice's capitated enrollment shifts mostly back to fee for service, so that only 50 capitated patients remain. Ten of those fifty are high utilizers, requiring ten visits per year. The contribution to net income drops by nearly half, from $31.24 to $15.97. As an extreme example, assume that only 15 capitated patients remain and that 10 of them are high utilizers. The contribution drops to only $2.02 per visit, barely enough to cover variable costs. The impact of this is shown in Table 2.4.

NURSING CAPITATION

Capitated reimbursement is predominantly, but not exclusively, within the realm of physician providers. But a recent Community Nursing Organization project examined an innovative approach to community nursing and ambulatory care services for Medicare beneficiaries. The hypothesis was that provision of such services would promote the timely and appropriate use of healthcare and to reduce the use of costly acute care services.

Organizations participating in the CNO demonstration were paid a fixed per-member-per-month capitated rate for covered services. But, the participating CNOs were only at risk under capitation for a subset of Medicare benefits (partial-capitation or carve-out). The financial incentive was to minimize utilization covered under the capitated payment, but not necessarily to minimize utilization of services not covered because traditional Medicare, not the CNO, would be at risk.

Final results indicated that the CNO model under partial capitation led to increased Medicare costs based on findings consistent across several analytic approaches. The cost differences between treatment and control or reference groups persisted after the application of increasingly complex risk-adjustment methods. Moreover, the differences increased over time and were robust to changes in the way CNO participation was defined. Finally, there was no statistically significant evidence of

TABLE 2.5

Sample Allocation Formula for Comprehensive Payment System

25% Primary Care Physician Reimbursement: $250,000 before Bonus/Fringe Benefits

60% Staff, fringe, rent, office expense (assumes hiring of multidisciplinary office team charged with timely delivery of personalized comprehensive care): $600,000

- Nurse practitioner $100,000
- Nurse $90,000
- 0.5 FTE nutritionist $35,000
- 0.5 FTE social worker $35,000
- Receptionist $60,000
- Medical assistant $50,000
- Rent $40,000
- Office expenses $50,000
- Insurance $50,000
- Physician FBs $75,000–$90,000

10% Information technology/patient safety/quality monitoring: $100,000

Purchase/lease/setup of electronic health record and quality monitoring system $35,000, data manager $35,000

5% Performance bonus, annual meeting mutually established goals: $50,000

Source: A. H. Goroll, R. A. Berenson, S. C. Schoenbaum et al., Fundamental Reform of Payment of Adult Primary Care: Comprehensive Payment for Comprehensive Care, *Journal of General Internal Medicine,* March 2007 22 (3) 410–15; Voluntary Partial Capitation: The CNO Medicare Demonstration Project, Austin Frakt, Steve Pizer, Robert Schmitz, and Soeren Mattke—Health Care Financing Review 2005.

Note: Example assumes an average comprehensive payment of $800/year/patient, an average panel size of 1250 patients/ full time primary care physician and team, 30% fringe benefit unless otherwise specified, and gross revenue of $1 million/full time equivalent primary care physician and team.

increase in physical or social functioning of the treatment group, as compared with the control group. CNOs cost more without providing any health benefits along dimensions measured (see Table 2.5).

EMERGING HYBRID PAYMENT MODELS

Current reimbursement structures involve the submission and payment of medical CPT® coded claims. But, some doctors feel they need to "up-code" to maximize revenue or "down-code" for fear of having a claim denied. Contradictory business goals bastardize the system into a payer *versus* provider tug-of-war, with patient care as a potential bargaining chip. Instituting quality metrics should be included in this equation and, a hybrid reimbursement model may be a viable option while integrating quality care metrics and reducing costs for all stakeholders.

This hybrid reimbursement system might use a two-payment structure. For the first payment, claims would be paid at hypothetical rate of 60% within one week of submission. The second payment, consisting of the remaining zero to 40% of some total maximum allowable fee, is paid quarterly. It would be based on scores like patient satisfaction and stewardship of healthcare resources by analyzing a statistically valid sample of patient encounters taken from the electronic health record.

Such a hybrid system would remove unnecessary steps, like resubmitting claims, and would lower the operational and administrative costs of claims processing. These changes would decrease operational cost and drive quality stewardship of the healthcare dollar.

ASSESSMENT

Changes in payer mix, to and from the various medical reimbursement models described above, will have significant impacts on physician income and ought to be considered by all physician focused financial advisors. And, it is important that physicians understand the financial, service responsibility, and administrative terms of payer contracts themselves.

CONCLUSION

And so, by understanding the accounting fundamentals of this chapter, physicians and their advisors can anticipate and prepare for the emerging changes that are likely to occur in the near future; especially as the PP-ACA of 2010 is fully implemented in 2014 through 2016.

COLLABORATE

Discuss this chapter online with others at www.MedicalExecutivePost.com.

ACKNOWLEDGMENTS

To Angela Herron, CPA, and Allan Gordon of Executive Healthcare Consulting, LLC, of Phoenix, Arizona.

FURTHER READING

Barlow, K and Merriman, C: Establishing healthy medical partner relations. In, Marcinko, DE [editor]. *Business of Medical Practice*. Springer Publishing, New York, 2005.

Baum, N: *Hiring a New Associate: Tips to Find Dr. Right*. HCPro/Opus Communications, New York, 2006.

Baum, N: *Marketing Your Clinical Practice: Ethically, Effectively, Economically*. Jones and Bartlett Publishers, Sudbury, MA, 2010.

Chien, AT, Wroblewski, K, Damberg, C, Williams, TR, Yanagihara, D, Yakunina, Y and Casalino, LP: Do physician organizations located in lower socio economic status areas score lower on P4P measures. *Journal of General Internal Medicine* 27(5), 2012: 548–54.

Coker Group: *Physician Recruitment and Employment: A Complete Reference Guide*, 2nd Edition, Jones and Bartlett, Sudbury, 2009.

Felt-Lisk, S, Gilbert, G and Stephanie, P: Maliong P4P Woek in Medicaid. *Health Affairs* 26(4), 2007: w516–27.

Freeman, CK: *Physician Recruitment, Retention and Separation*. AMA Press, Chicago, IL, 2002.

Glasziou, PP, Buchan, H, Del Mar, C, Doust, J, Harris, M, Knight, R, Scott, A, Scott, IA and Stockwell, A: When financial incentives do more good than harm: A checklist. *BMJ* 345, August 13, 2012: e5047–e5047.

Kearns, M: Employers of doctors changing pay models. *Health Care Finance News*, March 11, 2014.

Marcinko, DE and Hetico, HR: Analyzing and negotiating cost-volume profit medical contracts. In, Marcinko, DE [editor]: *Healthcare Organizations [Journal of Financial Management Strategies]*. iMBA Inc Publishing, Atlanta, GA, 2010.

Marcinko, DE and Hetico, HR: *Dictionary of Health Economics and Finance*. Springer Publishing Company, New York, 2007.

Marcinko, DE and Hetico, HR: Physician compensation trends, models and approaches. In, Nash, David, B [editor]: *Practicing Medicine in the 21st Century*. American College of Physician Executives, Tampa, Florida, 2006.

Mullen, KJ, Richard, GF and Meredith, BR: Can you get what you pay for [P4]. National Bureau of Economic Research, Working Paper 14886, April 2009.

Pink, DH: Drive: *The Surprising Truth about What Motivates Us*. Riverhead Books, Penguin Books Groups, New York, 2011.

Pohly, P: *The Directory of Healthcare Recruiters*, 9th Edition, Hays, KS, 2009.

Stewart, J: *The Story of Dr. Sidney R. Garfield: The Visionary Who Turned Sick Care into Health Care*. The Permanente Press, San Francisco, CA, 2009.

Theuns, S: New-wave physician recruitment and retention. In, Marcinko, DE [editor]: *The Business of Medical Practice*. Springing Publishing, New York, 2010.

Tinsley, R: *Medical Practice Management Handbook*. Aspen Publishers, NY, 2000.

Werner, R and Dudley, RA: Medicare's new hospital value based purchasing program likely to have only a small impact on hospital payments. *Health Affairs* 31(9), 2012: 1932–40.

Werner, R, Kolstad, JT, Stuart, EA and Polsky, D: The effect of P4P in hospitals. *Health Affairs* 30(4), 2011: 690–8.

White, C: Employers of doctors changing pay models. *National Institute for Health Care Reform; Bulletin* 2, February 2014.

HOSPITAL/CLINIC RECRUITMENT AGREEMENT CHECKLIST

- Does the agreement provide the following incentives to the physician?

Income guarantee	YES	NO
Recruitment bonus	YES	NO
Relocation assistance	YES	NO
Marketing allowance	YES	NO
Expense subsidy	YES	NO
Loan guarantee	YES	NO
Practice start-up assistance	YES	NO
Other: _____	YES	NO
Other: _____	YES	NO

- If the agreement provides the physician with an income guarantee, determine if incentive is a gross income guarantee or a net income guarantee.
- Determine if the physician can obtain a net income guarantee, since this type of arrangement removes risk from the physician.
- Under the income guarantee arrangement, determine who will be responsible for the payment of any debt service.
- If the agreement provides for a gross income guarantee, assess the following:
  Must physician pay for his or her own debt service out of gross income guarantee? YES   NO
  Is amount of guarantee reasonable? YES   NO
  After paying expenses and debt service, is the net amount remaining enough to pay physician compensation? YES   NO
- If the agreement provides for a net income guarantee, assess the following:
  Must the physician pay for debt service out of the net amount? YES   NO
  Are there any limitations on practice expenses? YES   NO
  Is amount of net guarantee reasonable for the physician's medical specialty? YES   NO
- Determine when advances will be needed by the physician under the income guarantee arrangement. Make sure that the contract provides for such advances. For example, if the physician starts practice on the first of the month, he or she will need money to make payroll on the 15 of the same month. Thus, make sure that the hospital will make a necessary advance in this and possibly other situations.
- Determine how incentives will be repaid (cash, service, or forgiveness).
  (Attempt to secure repayment in the following order: (1) forgiveness, (2) service, (3) combination of forgiveness and service, (4) combination of forgiveness and cash, (5) combination of service and cash, and (6) cash.)
- Assess tax consequences, both immediate and in the future, related to the repayment option in the agreement. Pay strict attention to immediate tax consequences related to any repayment in service.
- Determine when Form 1099s will be issued by the hospital and for how much.
- Based on an assessment of tax consequences, determine if the practice should incorporate.
- If the hospital is not providing certain incentives because it is a not-for-profit hospital, have the hospital answer the following questions:
  Is there a documented community needed for the physician?
  Are the incentives reasonable?
  Were incentives negotiated at arm's length?
  Are state benefits going to the hospital by securing the physician's services?
  (If the hospital can favorably answer the above questions, it should not be limited in the number and amount of incentives it can provide to the physician.)
- Does the agreement restrict the physician's ability to obtain privileges at other hospitals? If so, would this restrict his or her ability to open a satellite office or take emergency calls

at other hospitals at some time in the future? Attempt to negotiate the physician's right to obtain other hospital privileges.

- Determine if the agreement violates any Medicare fraud and abuse statutes.
- Other issue: _____
- Other issue: _____

3 Debt and Salary Review for Medical Professionals

Considerations for the Next Generation of Providers

Hope Rachel Hetico and Brian J. Knabe

CONTENTS

Almost a decade ago, *Fortune* magazine carried the headline "When Six Figured Incomes Aren't Enough. Now Doctors Want a Union." To the man in the street, it was just a matter of the rich getting richer. The sentiment was more precisely quantified, according to health economist and financial advisor Dr. David E. Marcinko, MBA, CMP™, in the March 31, 2005 issue of *Physician's Money Digest*, who with Editor Gregory Kelly reported that a 47-year-old doctor with $184,000 in annual income would need about $5.5 million dollars for retirement at age 65.[1]

Of course, physicians were not complaining back then under the traditional fee-for-service system; the imbroglio only began when managed care adversely impacted income, or when the stock market crashed in 2008; or with passage of the Patient Protection and Affordable Care Act (PP-ACA) in 2010 or its full implementation in 2014 through 2016.

INTRODUCTION

A decade later, the situation is vastly different as medical professionals struggle to maintain adequate income levels. Rightly or wrongly, the public has little sympathy for affluent doctors following healthcare reform. While a few specialties flourish, others, such as primary care, barely move. In the words of Atul Gawande, MD, a surgeon and author from Brigham and Women's Hospital in Boston, "Doctors quickly learn that how much they make has little to do with how good they are. It largely depends on how they handle the business side of practice." So, it is critical to understand contemporary thoughts on physician compensation and related trends.

And, private banker Jorge Russe, MBA, CMP™ *candidate*, whose wife is an employed emergency room physician, stated: "I've seen physician salaries, compensation structures and third-party reimbursement models change more in the past five years, than in the prior three decades" (personal communication).

MEDICAL STUDENT ESTIMATES OF SUPPLY AND DEMAND

Projecting future clinician supply and demand informs stakeholders and policy makers about the healthcare workforce implications of expected changes in the healthcare environment, including demographic shifts in the population and changing public policies. The National Center for Health Workforce Analysis is charged with estimating supply and demand of the U.S. healthcare workforce and works to overcome the inherent challenges projecting the future by improving available data, integrating projection systems, and enhancing scenario modeling, including building nurse workforce microsimulation models that facilitate localization, improve accuracy and factor in other types of clinicians. But, in essence, there is a projected shortage of 45,000–60,000 allopathic physicians for the next decade (average 7 years pipeline, postbaccalaureate degree). These forecasts do not account for changes in how primary care is delivered, however.

In the face of this projected doctor shortages and debate about the future of medicine, a record number of students applied to, and started, allopathic medical school for the academic 2014 year. About 20,000 students enrolled in 2013, about 2.8% more than the year before, according to the data distributed by the Association of American Medical Colleges (AAMC). First-time applicants—an important indicator of interest in medicine—increased by 5.8% to 35,727.

Meanwhile, osteopathic medical schools saw a continued surge in their new student pool, with an 11.1% growth in enrollment, according to the Association of American Colleges of Osteopathic Medicine (AACOM).

And, the American Association of Colleges of Podiatric Medicine (AACPM) reported that there are now nine (up from the original five) schools of podiatric medicine in the country (Arizona, Florida, Iowa, Ohio, New York, Illinois, Pennsylvania, and California [Pamona and Oakland]) with increasing enrollment levels.[2]

UNBALANCED SPENDING ON PHYSICIAN TRAINING

There is an imbalance in how Medicare distributes its $10 billion a year for graduate medical education. For example, New York State received 20% of all Medicare's graduate medical education funding while 29 states, including places struggling with a severe shortage of physicians, got less than 1%. Other states at the top in funding are Massachusetts, Rhode Island, Pennsylvania, Michigan, and Connecticut. Each gets more than $71 in funding per each resident compared to $14 for Florida and $11.50 for Texas. At the bottom is Montana, which gets $1.94 per resident. The distribution is important because while some medical residents move elsewhere after training, most practice near where they train.

REGISTERED NURSE VIEWS ON HEALTHCARE REFORM

Nurses (ages 19–39) are confident about their ability to supply the demands of healthcare reform, despite today's shortages. Approximately 45% of young nurses believe that the shortage has improved during the last 5 years, while older nurses were less optimistic. The generational differences are even more apparent when asked whether healthcare reform will ensure an adequate supply of quality nurses, with 38% of younger nurses citing confidence compared to 29% and 27% of older nurses ages 40–54 and 55+, respectively.[3]

ON HEALTH EDUCATION ASSISTANCE LOANS

Federal Health Education Assistance Loans (HEALs) to student borrowers were discontinued as of September 30, 1998. From fiscal year 1978 through 1998 the Federal HEAL Program insured loans made by participating lenders to eligible graduate students in schools of medicine, osteopathy, podiatric medicine, dentistry, veterinary medicine, optometry, public health, pharmacy, chiropractic, or in programs in health administration, and clinical psychology. HEAL refinancing occurred from fiscal year 1994 through fiscal year 2004. Now, they are administered privately under the following deferral guidelines.

INTEREST RATES

The maximum interest which may be charged to the borrower on the unpaid balance of a HEAL loan may not exceed the average bond-equivalent rate during the prior calendar quarter for 91-day Treasury bills sold at auction, plus 3%, rounded to the next higher 1/8 of 1%. Payment of principal and interest may be deferred during specific eligible periods of deferment. The HEAL program does not provide a subsidy payment for interest. Accrued interest may be compounded once annually by adding it to the principal amount of the loan.

Repayment

Repayment begins the first day of the 10th month after the month the borrower ceases to be a full-time student at a HEAL school. The 9-month period before the repayment period begins is called the "grace period." However, if the borrower becomes an intern or resident in an accredited program within 9 full months after leaving school, repayment will begin the first day of the 10th month after the borrower ceases to be an intern or a resident. A borrower has from 10 to 25 years to repay the loan after the repayment period starts, even when the borrower participates in an authorized deferment program. There is no penalty for prepayment. Overdue accounts will be aggressively pursued and referred to collection agencies and credit bureaus or for legal action when borrowers fail to meet the terms of their loans.

Repayment schedule provisions may vary and affect the total amount to be repaid.

- Lenders *must* offer a graduated repayment option that requires smaller payments early in the repayment period.
- Lenders *must* offer an income contingent loan repayment schedule that, during the first 5 years of repayment is based on borrower income.

Forebearance

Forbearance is an extension of time for making loan payments or the acceptance of smaller payments than previously scheduled to prevent a borrower from defaulting. Lenders have the authority to grant forbearance in 6-month increments up to a maximum of 3 years. Periods of forbearance may be extended beyond 3 years with the approval of the secretary. Any such period would be in addition to the 3-year period that lenders/holders can grant. Any period of forbearance granted to a HEAL borrower shall not be included in the 25-year loan repayment period for loans made on or after 10/13/1992. Lenders must notify each borrower of the right to request forbearance; however, if the lender determines that the default of the borrower is inevitable and that forbearance would be ineffective in preventing default, the lender is not required to grant forbearance.

Deferment

Repayment of principal and interest can be deferred, but interest continues to accrue during periods of

- Full-time study at a HEAL school or at an institution of higher education participating in the Federal Family Education Loan Program
- Up to 3 years for full time active duty in the Armed Forces
- Up to 3 years each in the Peace Corps, VISTA, or National Health Service Corps
- Up to 2 years for certain fellowship and educational training programs
- Up to 4 years for internship and residency training
- Up to 1 year for graduates of schools of chiropractic
- Up to 3 years for completion of an internship or residency training program in osteopathic general practice, family medicine, general internal medicine, preventive medicine, or general pediatrics and is practicing primary care
- Up to 3 years for providing healthcare services (beginning 02/01/1999) to Indians through any health program or facility funded in whole or part by the Indian Health Service for the benefit of Indians

Total and Permanent Disability

To be totally and permanently disabled the borrower must be unable to engage in any substantially gainful activity because of a medically determinable impairment that is expected to continue for a long and indefinite period of time or to result in death.

Due Diligence (Lenders Must)

- Contact the borrower every 6 months to notify him/her of the amount of the debt
- Contact the borrower in writing 30–60 days before the commencement of the repayment period to establish the repayment terms
- Contact both the borrower and any endorser at least 4 times at regular intervals during the first 120 days of any delinquency period
- Notify national consumer credit reporting agencies regarding accounts overdue by more than 60 days
- Request preclaim assistance from the HEAL program when the borrower is 90 days delinquent

Litigation

Lenders and holders are required to litigate defaulted loans and obtain a judgment against the borrower in most cases. Litigation is not required when the loan involved was made in an amount of less than $5000 prior to 11/04/1988 or the loan was made in an amount of less than $2500 on or after 11/04/1988 or if the defaulted claim is less than $1000. Schools may assist in the collection of delinquent HEAL loans. HEAL loans are exempted from any State or Federal Statute of Limitations provisions which limit the period within which a loan may be collected.

Postdefault Activities

Defaulted borrowers are subject to the following:

- Account referred to a collection agency
- Referral to the Inspector General, DHHS, and the Department of Justice (DOJ)
- DOJ registers the judgment in Federal court for enforced collection
- Exclusion from Medicare; IRS offset
- Publish names of defaulters (who have not entered into a settlement agreement) in the Federal Register and on the website at www.defaulteddocs.dhhs.gov[4]

Medical Student Debt Burden and Loan Defaults

Medical student debt burdens (averaging $100,000–$250,000) must now be factored into personal financial planning endeavors since they may be economically devastating. Since inception, for example, the federal HEAL program has squeezed significant repayment settlements from its top deadbeat doctor debtors, and excluded more than a thousand practitioners from Medicare and other federal/state programs. Historically, student loans are difficult to discharge through bankruptcy. Alterations to the Bankruptcy Code in late 1998 made student loans almost nondischargeable, unless the borrower can establish substantial hardship and the "nondischarge of such debt would be unconscionable" (42 U.S.C. sec. 292f[g]). Changes in 2005 made even private student loans nondischargeable, subject to state modifications in 2014.

StudentLoanJustice.org, a website propelled by the current credit squeeze and economic malaise was launched by Alan Collinge of University Place, Washington, who runs the site.

The Next Generation of Antimillionaire Doctors

CBS *Moneywatch* published an article entitled "$1 Million Mistake: Becoming a Doctor" Aside from the possibility that devoting one's life to helping others might be considered a mistake, medical student Dan Coleman was struck by the "$1 million" figure. Before medical school, he worked in the pharmaceutical industry and even turned down a hefty promotion to his education as soon as possible, rather than defer for a year or two. But, his financial calculations made it fairly obvious that, including benefits, bonuses, and potential promotions, his medical decision was not a $1 million mistake, but was more like a $1.3 million dollar disaster. Still; he opined:

Yet, even today, as we stare down the barrel of the Affordable Care Act, being a doctor is a very desirable job. We may not be famous, but we will be well-respected. We may not be rich, but we will certainly live comfortably. We may work a lot, but we will never be out of work. To future doctors, the young and impecunious, the anti-millionaires, tuition is a mere afterthought. All that matters is the MD.[5]

OVERHEARD IN THE MEDICAL STUDENT'S LOUNGE: ODE TO THE ANTIMILLIONAIRES

We are medical students.
We are young, proud, and righteous.
We have made the hard choice (medicine), but we have cleared the high hurdle (getting into school).
We know healthcare is a difficult, imperfect art, but we are devoted.
We arm ourselves with the weapons of knowledge and compassion, prepared to defend against the onslaught of trauma, disease, and time.
We are here to the bitter end, for our patients and ourselves.
And above all, we know the cost of our choice.
And if we're lucky, it will stay under 6% interest through graduation.

Daniel Coleman
(First-year student, Georgetown University School of Medicine)

PHYSICIAN COMPENSATION DATA SOURCES

A growing number of surveys measure physician compensation, encompassing a varying depth of analysis. Physician compensation data, divided by specialty and subspecialty, is central to a range of consulting activities including practice assessments and valuations of healthcare enterprises. The AMA maintains the most comprehensive database of information on physicians in the United States, with information on over 940,000 physicians and residents, and 77,000 medical students. Started in 1906, the AMA *Physician Masterfile*, which contains information on physician education, training, and professional certification information, is updated annually through the Physicians' Professional Activities questionnaire and the collection and validation efforts of AMA's Division of Survey and Data Resources (SDR). A selection of other sources of healthcare-related compensation and cost data is set forth below.

Physician Characteristics and Distribution in the United States is an annual survey based on a variety of demographic information from the *Physician Masterfile* dating back to 1963. It includes detailed information regarding trends, distribution, and professional and individual characteristics of the physician workforce.

Physician Socioeconomic Statistics, published from 2000 to 2003, was a result of the merger between two prior AMA annuals: (1) *Socioeconomic Characteristics of Medical Practice;* and, (2) *Physician Marketplace Statistics.* Data has been compiled from a random sampling of physicians from the *Physician Masterfile* into what is known as the *Socioeconomic Monitoring System*, which includes physician age profiles, practice statistics, utilization, physician fees, professional expenses, physician compensation, revenue distribution by payor, and managed care contracts, among other categories.

The American Medical Group Association (AMGA), formerly known as the American Group Practice Association, has conducted the *Medical Group Compensation and Financial*

Survey (known as the "Medical Group Compensation and Productivity Survey" until 2004) for 22 years. This annual survey is cosponsored by RSM McGladrey, Inc., who is responsible for the independent collection and compilation of survey data. Compensation and production data are provided for medical specialties by size of group, geographic region, and whether the group is single or multispecialty.

The Medical Group Management Association's (MGMA) *Physician Compensation and Production Survey* is one of the largest in the United States with approximately 2000 group practices responding as of the 2009 edition publication. Data is provided on compensation and production for 125 specialties. The survey data are also published on CD by John Wiley & Sons ValueSource; the additional details available in this media provide better benchmarking capabilities.

The MGMA's *Cost Survey* is one of the best known surveys of group practice income and expense data, having been published in some form since 1955, and obtaining over 1600 respondents, combined, for the 2008 surveys: *Cost Survey for Single Specialty Practices* and *Cost Survey for Multispecialty Practices*. Data is provided for a detailed listing of expense categories and is also calculated as a percentage of revenue and per FTE physician, FTE provider, patient, square foot, and relative value unit (RVU). The survey provides information on multispecialty practices by performance ranking, geographic region, legal organization, size of practice, and percent of capitated revenue. Detailed income and expense data is provided for single specialty practice in over 50 different specialties and subspecialties.

The *Medical Group Financial Operations Survey* was created through a partnership between RSM McGladrey and the American Medical Group Association (AMGA), and provides benchmark data on support staff and physician salaries, physician salaries, staffing profiles and benefits, and other financial indicators. Data is reported as a percentage of managed care revenues, per full-time physician and per square foot, and is subdivided by specialty mix, capitation level, and geographic region with detailed summaries of single specialty practices in several specialties.

Statistics: Medical and Dental Income and Expense Averages is an annual survey produced by the National Society of Certified Healthcare Business Consultants (NSCHBC), formerly known as the National Association of Healthcare Consultants (NAHC), and the Academy of Dental CPAs. It has been published annually for a number of years and the *2008 Report Based on 2007 Data* included detailed income and expense data from over 2200 practices and 4600 physicians in 60 specialties.

MEDICAL SPECIALTY TRENDS

The characteristics of both the practice and the profitability of different physician specialties vary greatly. Information on trends affecting specific specialties should further refine the types of industry information gathered including changes in treatment, technology, competition, reimbursement, and the regulatory environment. For many of the subspecialties, oversupply and undersupply issues and the corresponding demand and compensation trends are central to the analysis of potential future earnings and the value of established medical entities. Information that is available and that may be gathered can range from broad practice overviews to, for example, specific procedural utilization demand and forecasts for a precise local geographic area.

A large number of national and state medical associations and organizations gather and produce information on these various aspects of the practice of different individual physician specialties and subspecialties. Information may be found in trade press articles, medical specialty associations and their publications, national surveys, specialty accreditation bodies, governmental reports and studies, and elsewhere. The American Medical Association's (AMA) as well as the MGMA both publish comprehensive physician practice survey information.

Twelve Best Jobs in Healthcare, 2014–2015

(Profession, Annual Media Salary, and Projected Growth)

1. Biomedical Engineer $86,960–62%
2. Dental Hygienist $70,210–38%
3. Occupational Therapist $75,400–33%
4. Optometrist $97,820–33%
5. Physical Therapist $79,860–39%
6. Chiropractor $66,160–28%
7. Speech Pathologist $69,870–23%
8. Pharmacist $116,670–25%
9. Podiatrist $116,440–20%
10. Respiratory Therapist $55,870–28%
11. Medical Records Technician $34,610–21%
12. Physician Assistant $90,930–30%[6]

Sample Salary Offered to Recruited Medical Specialties[a,b,c]

	Low	Average	High	
Family Practice				
2013/14				$180,000
2008/09	$120,000	$173,000	$245,000	
2007/08	$120,000	$172,000	$275,000	
2006/07	$120,000	$161,000	$250,000	
2005/06	$115,000	$145,000	$220,000	
Family Practice with Obstetrics				
2013/14				$200,000
2008/09	$140,000	$184,000	$275,000	
2007/08	$140,000	$184,000	$275,000	
2006/07	$145,000	$159,000	$200,000	
2005/06	$140,000	$158,000	$180,000	
Internal Medicine				
2013/14				$210,000
2008/09	$140,000	$186,000	$300,000	
2007/08	$125,000	$176,000	$330,000	
2006/07	$135,000	$174,000	$275,000	
2005/06	$130,000	$162,000	$250,000	
Hospitalist				
2013/14				$220,000
2008/09	$160,000	$201,000	$300,000	
2007/08	$150,000	$181,000	$300,000	
2006/07	$145,000	$180,000	$250,000	
2005/06	$140,000	$175,000	$190,000	
General Surgery				
2013/14				$370,000
2008/09	$175,000	$321,000	$616,000	
2007/08	$240,000	$321,000	$450,000	
2006/07	$225,000	$301,000	$350,000	
2005/06	$150,000	$272,000	$350,000	
Orthopedic Surgery				
2013/14				$590,000
2008/09	$300,000	$481,000	$990,000	
2007/08	$250,000	$439,000	$750,000	

continued

Sample Salary Offered to Recruited Medical Specialties (continued)

	Low	Average	High	
2006/07	$250,000	$413,000	$650,000	
2005/06	$250,000	$370,000	$515,000	
OB/GYN				
2013/14				$360,000
2008/09	$150,000	$266,000	$655,000	
2007/08	$160,000	$255,000	$405,000	
2006/07	$200,000	$247,000	$345,000	
2005/06	$175,000	$234,000	$450,000	
Psychiatry				
2013/14				$220,000
2008/09	$160,000	$200,000	$300,000	
2007/08	$120,000	$189,000	$230,000	
2006/07	$160,000	$186,000	$230,000	
2005/06	$130,000	$174,000	$230,000	
Cardiology				
2013/14				$490,000
2008/09	$180,000	$419,000	$990,000	
2007/08	$250,000	$392,000	$999,000	
2006/07	$250,000	$391,000	$500,000	
2005/06	$175,000	$342,000	$500,000	
Pediatrics				
2013/14				$200,000
2008/09	$120,000	$171,000	$350,000	
2007/08	$120,000	$159,000	$265,000	
2006/07	$115,000	$159,000	$200,000	
2005/06	$115,000	$151,000	$180,000	
Neurology				
2013/14				$270,000
2008/09	$180,000	$258,000	$375,000	
2007/08	$150,000	$230,000	$325,000	
2006/07	$170,000	$234,000	$275,000	
2005/06	$150,000	$210,000	$250,000	
Emergency Medicine				
2013/14				
2008/09	$185,000	$244,000	$302,000	
2007/08	$190,000	$240,000	$258,000	
2006/07	$150,000	$239,000	$300,000	
2005/06	$130,000	$210,000	$270,000	
Pulmonology				
2013/14				$245,000
2008/09	$215,000	$293,000	$400,000	
2007/08	$200,000	$283,000	$525,000	
2006/07	$225,000	$266,000	$350,000	
2005/06	N/A	N/A	N/A	
Urology				
2013/14				
2008/09	$230,000	$401,000	$550,000	
2007/08	$300,000	$387,000	$550,000	
2006/07	$275,000	$400,000	$500,000	
2005/06	$250,000	$320,000	$375,000	
Gastroenterology				
2013/14				$395,000

continued

Sample Salary Offered to Recruited Medical Specialties (continued)

	Low	Average	High	
2008/09	$250,000	$393,000	$600,000	
2007/08	$250,000	$379,000	$475,000	
2006/07	$200,000	$365,000	$450,000	
2005/06	$175,000	$315,000	$500,000	
Radiology				
2013/14				
2008/09	$300,000	$391,000	$500,000	
2007/08	$230,000	$401,000	$750,000	
2006/07	$250,000	$380,000	$500,000	
2005/06	$240,000	$351,000	$500,000	
Hematology/Oncology				
Today:				$400,000
2008/09	$250,000	$335,000	$450,000	
2007/08	$225,000	$365,000	$500,000	
2006/07	$300,000	$339,000	$500,000	
2005/06	N/A	N/A	N/A	
Otolaryngology				
2013/14				
2008/09	$280,000	$377,000	$450,000	
2007/08	$275,000	$362,000	$600,000	
2006/07	$200,000	$312,000	$400,000	
2005/06	$175,000	$272,000	$350,000	
CRNA				
2013/14				$370,000
2008/09	$125,000	$189,000	$250,000	
2007/08	$155,000	$185,000	$230,000	
2006/07	$130,000	$164,000	$200,000	
2005/06	$87,000	$156,000	$210,000	
Anesthesiology				
2013/14				
2008/09	$250,000	$344,000	$500,000	
2007/08	$250,000	$336,000	$480,000	
2006/07	$220,000	$300,000	$425,000	
2005/06	$275,000	$306,000	$375,000	
Dermatology				
2013/14				$365,000
2008/09	$200,000	$297,000	$400,000	
2007/08	$250,000	$315,000	$400,000	
2006/07	$200,000	$318,000	$400,000	
2005/06	N/A	N/A	N/A	
Phlebology[c]				
2013/14	$195,000			
2008/09	$175,000			
Podiatry[b]				
2013/14	$120,000			
2008/09	$125,000			

Source: http://blogs.wsj.com/health/2009/06/17/how-much-do-rookie-doctors-make-the-latest-scorecard/.

Note: Base salary or income guarantee only; does not include production bonus or benefits.

[a] Merritt Hawkins and Associates.

[b] Podiatry Management Compensation Report 2014.

[c] iMBA Inc, Proprietary Compensation Statistics 2014.

Most recently, a "top five" medical specialty list was developed for primary care specialties by the National Physicians Alliance (http://npalliance.org/). This initiative was funded through the American Board of Internal Medicine (ABIM) Foundation's "Putting the Charter into Practice" grants, which fund organizations to develop initiatives to advance physician professionalism, including management of finite resources. What follows are the median (50% earn more, 50% earn less) salaries for the six highest-paying and six lowest-paying medical specialties in 2010:

- Six Highest
  - Orthopedic surgeons: $580-k to $640-k
  - Cardiac and thoracic surgeons: $507,143
  - Radiologists: $438,115 to $478,000
  - Radiation therapy: $413,518
  - Gynecological oncology: $406,000
  - Cardiology: $398,034
- Six Lowest
  - Family medicine: $197,655
  - Pediatrics: $202,832
  - Internal medicine: $205,441
  - Psychiatry: $208,462
  - Geriatrics: $211,425
  - Hospitalists: $211,835

These specialties enjoyed the biggest jumps from a year earlier: neurology, noninvasive cardiology, anesthesiology, emergency medicine, and internal medicine.[7]

THE PHYSICIAN SALARY GENDER GAP

Facebook (FB) chief operating officer Sheryl Sandberg is an expert on this general topic noting that a smaller percentage of women than men reach the top of their respective professions. Here are the health financial facts according to the 2011 U.S. Census Bureau:

- Women physicians earn $0.62/dollar compared to men.
- Women physicians start careers with a $17,000 pay gap.
- Midcareer women physician researchers are paid $12,000 less than males.

A 2013 study by *Health Affairs* suggested the following but did not point to discrimination as a reason for wage gaps.

1. The gender gap in physician salaries is not related to specialty choice or work hours.
2. The gender gap has grown nearly five times from 1999 to 2008 and from a $3600 difference in 2008 to a $16,819 difference in 2012.
3. Women choosing lower-paying primary care specialties have nothing to do with this trend because women have increasingly not been going into primary care specialties.

So how can female doctors increase their compensation, and how can a physician-focused financial advisor assist them? Be sure to suggest and do the following:

1. *Negotiate*: Start out realizing that whatever is offered, it is probably 15–40% less than a man. So, look at the first offer as only a place to commence negotiations.
2. *Know specialty worth*: Know that some self-reporting mechanisms underestimate worth due to the variations and complexities of salary determination methods.

3. *Leverage the doctor shortage*: Medical services are more valuable if there are few who can provide them. But remember, the medical market-place is not really free and transparent.
4. *Know geography*: Consider geographic locations that need doctors (i.e., Central US).[9]

THE EFFECT OF HEALTHCARE REFORM LEGISLATION ON PHYSICIAN COMPENSATION

With the passage of healthcare reform legislation, officially known as the Patient Protection and Affordable Care Act of 2010, many questions remain regarding its effect upon physicians' livelihood as it is fully rolled-out in 2014–16. Undoubtedly, this bill moves the healthcare system several steps closer to a socialized model, but the effects on physicians' salaries and compensation models are far from clear. We suggest that a way to estimate the effect this shift may have on future compensation is to look to other countries, many of which already have a more socialized system in place.

For example, according to the CRS Report for Congress, US Health Care Spending in comparison with other OECD countries (http://assets.opencrs.com/rpts/RL34175_20070917.pdf): the US specialists rank near the top in compensation compared to the other countries, trailing the Netherlands and Australia. In this survey the average specialist in the United States made $230,000. The comparable salary in Canada is $161,000, $150,000 in the United Kingdom, and $253,000 in the Netherlands. Generalists in the United States are at the top in terms of compensation with an average of $161,000. This compares to $107,000 in Canada, $118,000 in the United Kingdom, and $117,000 in the Netherlands.

Another indicator of physician salary trends is the change in compensation adjusted for inflation. According to the American Medical Association (AMA), the inflation-adjusted income for the average patient care physician declined from $180,930 to $168,122 from 1995 to 2005, a 7% decrease. And, the inflation adjusted decrease is more substantial given the low interest rate environment through 2010 and going forward.

	Average Net Income		
	1995	**2005**	**Decrease (%)**
All patient care physicians	$180,930	$168,122	7
Primary care physicians	$135,036	$121,262	10
Medical specialists	$178,840	$175,011	2
Surgical specialists	$245,162	$224,998	8

Source: http://www.ama-assn.org/amednews/site/free/prsc0724.htm.

Given these trends, as well as the fact that an increasing percentage of healthcare payments are coming from dwindling government sources, it is likely that physician salaries will decline as "healthcare reform" legislation is implemented. In fact, it is likely that this trend will accelerate. A 15% to 25% inflation-adjusted decline in salaries over the next decade is a reasonable prediction.

It is also important to note that the level of student debt in the United States continues to rise, while college and medical education are usually subsidized in other countries. Many foreign physicians graduate with no student loan debt. The ratio of debt level to salary in the United States continues to become more onerous for new physicians.

DOCTOR COMPLAINTS ABOUT ACA's HEALTH INSURANCE EXCHANGES PAY

Despite the trends, opinions, and anecdotes, doctors fear they will be paid less to care for the millions of patients projected to buy coverage through the health law's new health insurance exchanges

(HIEs). Some have complained to medical associations, including those in New York, California, Connecticut, Texas, and Georgia, saying discounted rates could lead to a two-tiered system in which fewer doctors participate, potentially making it harder for consumers to get the care they need.

And, insurance companies are acknowledging they have reduced rates in some plans, under enormous political pressure to keep premiums affordable. Physicians will make up for lower pay by seeing more patients, since the plans tend to have smaller networks of doctors. But many primary care doctors, family practice providers, and internists barely have time to take care of the patients they have now.

The conflict sheds light on the often murky world of insurance contracts in which physicians don't always know which plans they're listed in or how much they're being paid to treat patients in a particular plan. As a result, some doctors are just learning about the lower pay rates in some plans sold in the online markets or exchanges. And, they are fearful of diminishing compensation.

PHYSICIAN EXECUTIVE PAY

The median total compensation of physician executives increased 7% to $325,000 in 2013 from $305,000 two years ago, keeping pace with the salary growth rate in 2011, according to Paul Esselman and Cejka Executive Search conducted with the American College of Physician Executives (personal communication).

The payment of chief quality/patient safety officers had the most significant growth at 22%, along with a category referred to as other C-suite officers, at 25%. These include new titles that have emerged with healthcare reform, such as chief operations officer, chief integration/implementation officer, and chief strategy/innovation/transformation officer. The growth rate of physician CEO compensation lagged behind other clinical department chairs and division chiefs. Physician CEOs reported median compensation rose 4% since 2011 to $410,000, while payment for chief medical officers was 6% higher to $365,000 (personal communication).

OTHER MEDICAL PROFESSIONAL SALARIES

DOCTORS OF PODIATRIC MEDICINE

The salary range for a podiatrist, or Doctor of Podiatric Medicine (DPM), in 2006 was $128,000–$292,000 according to Allied-Physicians.com (http://www.allied-physicians.com/salary_surveys/physician-salaries.htm).

This robust growth was likely due to expanded education, training, and general allopathic and osteopathic acceptance by the medical community, as well as by insurance companies, employers, patients and various governmental agencies and third-party payers. Increased surgical subspecialization, in-patient hospital and ambulatory out-patient surgical center activity were also positive compensation factors.

Doctors in solo and self-employed practice (34%) reported a median net income decrease of 9%. In 2012, the cumulative gross income per solo practitioner was $251,000. In 2011 it was $247,725 and in 2010 it was $225,000. Overhead expenses averaged 50%. However, by 2014 the annual Podiatry Management 31st annual survey entitled "Working Smarter" revealed that patient numbers and net income dropped for doctors in group practice; while DPMs cut costs and invested in the long term with more spending on equipment such as digital x-rays, staff, eHRs, and related computer technology. Net income solo practice compensation in 2012 was $117,750, but the average a podiatrist takes home rose to $177,000 by 2014, according to Paul Michael, *Wisebread* (2/20/14).

Seventy-five percent of podiatrists are male, while 25% are female. Eighty-one percent are in the American Podiatric Medical Association (APMA), and two-thirds are board certified in at least one subspecialty. Over 90% of all podiatrists accept Medicare assignment and 10% have been audited.

Doctors of Dental Surgery/Doctors of Dental Medicine

In 2002, the average practitioner's net income was $174,350. The average dental specialist's net was $291,250. These figures represent a 0.7% and a 5.8% increase over 2001, respectively. Net income rose steadily since 1986, when general dentists made an average of $69,920 and specialists an average of $97,920. A 2003 Survey of Dental Practices reported net income from dentistry-related sources. Dentists differ from physicians in that 90% are in private practice. By 2011, according to PayScale.com, the average general dentist earned $98,276–$157,437; a decreasing trend allocated as follows.

Salary	$93,750–$148,000
Bonus	$2000–$20,000
Profit sharing	$1100–$28,500
Commissions	$485.74–$33,000

Source: http://www.ada.org/prof/resources/pubs/dbguide/newdent/income.asp#private; http://www.payscale. com/research/US/Job=Dentist/Salary.

By 2013 the average dental salary became $125,982, with an expanded range of $79,242–$242,000. And, the American Dental Association (ADA) Health Policy Resources just reported on an "environmental scan" of the dental care sector titled "A Profession in Transition: Key Forces Reshaping the Dental Landscape."

Using various modeling scenarios, the results indicate that dental spending will remain fairly flat in the coming decades—a departure from the decades of historically robust growth in the dental economy. Clearly, the economic recovery, when it does finally kick into gear, may not bring back the dental spending growth many are anticipating, and practitioner earnings.

Among other findings:

- Dental benefits are likely to continue to erode for adults and potentially further influence dental care utilization. But benefits will expand for children, mostly because of the Affordable Care Act. Up to 8.7 million additional children will gain dental benefits by 2018 as a result of the law.
- There will be pressure to increase value and reduce costs from all payers—governments, employers, and individual consumers. This will be driven by a shift toward value-or outcome-based payment within both public and private plans and a new wave of healthcare consumerism among the population.
- Commercial dental plans will increasingly use more selective networks and demand more accountability through data and performance measures.
- The trend toward larger, consolidated multisite practices will continue, driven by changes in the practice patterns of new dentists, a drive for efficiency and increased competition for patients.

Nevertheless, many dentists are struggling to get by—hoping for a business turn around that may not come for years. Unresponsive and ineffective dental leadership may be blamed for dentists' current business weakness. It is no accident that dentists have been led to believe that criticizing dental care stakeholders such as EDR vendors, discount dentistry brokers and even the ADA is somehow unprofessional. Even though it is a somewhat morbid task for the professional organization to perform, some think the ADA should take the next step and report the level of dental practice bankruptcies in the nation. Those considering dentistry, as a profession, have a right to be warned. Without transparency, dental patients who stand to lose the most are always left out of the loop. (D. Kellus Pruitt, DDS; Fort Worth, TX, personal communication).

DOCTORS OF CHIROPRACTIC

According to Salary.com, the median salary for strictly office-based chiropractors was $78,994 in 2005; while Collegegrad.com reported the median annual earnings of a salaried chiropractor as $65,330 in 2002; with the middle 50% earning between $44,140 and $102,400.

The U.S. Bureau of Labor Statistics estimated chiropractors earned an average salary of $84,020 in 2004. A Chiropractic Economics survey in 2005 suggested mean salary at $104,363. But, bankruptcies and HEAL loan defaults are high in this segment. Another survey for 2007 in *Chiropractic Economics* is available here: http://www.chiroeco.com/article/2007/Issue8/images/CES&ESurvey2007.pdf

A range of $44,511–$82,826 was reported in 2010 by PayScale.com, allocated as follows:

Salary	$42,106–$78,129
Bonus	$1008–$10,205
Profit sharing	$973–$8139
Commission	$750–$10,113
Total pay	$44,511–$82,826

XTotal Pay combines base annual salary or hourly wage, bonuses, profit sharing, tips, commissions, overtime pay, and other forms of cash earnings, as applicable for this job. It does not include equity (stock) compensation, cash value of retirement benefits, or the value of other noncash benefits (e.g., healthcare).

Source: http://www.payscale.com/research/US/Job=Chiropractor/Salary.

ALLIED HEALTHCARE PROVIDER SALARIES

CERTIFIED REGISTERED NURSE ANESTHETIST

Some nurses land higher salaries than primary care doctors, and in 2008 anesthetists recruited through the staffing firm Merritt Hawkins & Associates, landed salaries that averaged $185,000; compared to the pay for family practice doctors hired through the firm, who averaged $172,000; and internists, who averaged $176,000; according to a *Wall Street Journal* report, on June 18, 2008.

The Merritt Hawkins figures for the nurses are higher than some other sources, like the Medical Group Management Association. The MGMA also tracks healthcare salaries and puts nurse anesthetists' median compensation at $140,000 per year. The discrepancy may be because fewer employers go through recruiters to hire the nurses, and those who do are willing to pay top dollar.

And, according to a January 2009 Salary.com report, a certified registered nurse anesthetist (CRNA) received an average annual base salary of $175,319.00. And, that's just 76% of total income. The other benefits include the following:

1. Bonuses: $50.00
2. Social Security: $9164.00
3. 401(k)/403(b): $6313.00
4. Disability: $1754.00
5. Healthcare: $5722.00
6. Pension: $8067.00
7. Time Off: $22,933.00

So, this is a total package, benefits, and salary, amounting to about $229,334.00. Of course, the Salary.com figures are not statistically correct. Nevertheless, this should be compared to an average general practitioner (MD/DO) salary of less than $150,000.

PHYSICIAN ASSISTANT

The salary range for a physician's assistant (PA) is $69,626–$119,179 with a Median of $88,737 as reported by PayScale.com in 2013. According to Salary.com, the median expected salary for a typical PA was $92,208.

I'M A DOCTOR: WHAT, ME WORRY?

Most doctors love their work, but are frustrated about flat and declining income and other increasing challenges. A *Medical Economics 2013 Physician Earnings Survey* took a look at compensation trends, secondary incomes, malpractice, technology frustrations, work/life balance, and attitudes about the future of healthcare.

Here are the most frequently cited concerns:

- Fees and reimbursement (68%)
- Burden of paperwork (56%)
- Healthcare reform (54%)
- Value of primary care versus specialty care and use of midlevels (43%)
- Third-party interference (43%)
- Malpractice/tort reform (39%)
- Doctor shortage (29%)
- EHRs (28%)
- Accountable care organizations (17%)[12]

MEDICARE PAYMENT TRANSPARENCY

In 2014, Medicare announced that it would tell the public how much individual (not aggregate) doctors are paid to treat patients. And, *MedPage Today/New York Times* reported that in 2012 Medicare paid $69.6 billion dollars to 800,000 providers (2013 and 2014 results not available from centers for medicare and medicaid services (CMS)). This was only 12% of Medicare's overall fee-for-service spending. A tiny fraction of the 880,000 doctors and other healthcare providers who accept Medicare payments accounted for nearly a quarter of the roughly $77 billion paid out to them under the federal program, in some cases receiving millions of dollars each in a single year, according to the most detailed data ever released in Medicare's nearly 50-year history.[13]

THE BEST-PAID 2% OF DOCTORS

Among doctors who billed Medicare, the highest-paid 2% accounted for almost one-quarter of total Medicare payments.

Highest-paid 2% of doctors, by specialty, paid by Medicare for 2012

1. Ophthalmology
2. Hematology/Oncology
3. Cardiology
4. Radiation Oncology
5. Internal Medicine
6. Dermatology
7. Rheumatology
8. Medical Oncology
9. Diagnostic Radiology
10. Nephrology

11. Pathology
12. Family Practice
13. Orthopedic Surgery
14. Urology
15. Pulmonary Disease
16. Vascular Surgery
17. Neurology
18. Physical Medicine and Rehabilitation
19. Interventional Pain Management
20. Hematology
21. General Surgery
22. Infectious Disease
23. Gastroenterology
24. Interventional Radiology
25. Anesthesiology
26. Podiatry
27. Pain Management
28. General Practice
29. Physical Therapist
30. Endocrinology[14]

Medicare Payments: Breakdown of Top 15 Medical Specialties Ranked by Average Paid to Individual Billers

Provider Type	Number of Providers	Total Paid in Millions	Average Amount Paid per Provider
Hematology/oncology	7374	$2703.9	$366,677.0
Radiation oncology	4135	$1499.6	$362,566.0
Ophthamology	17,067	$5585.0	$327,239.0
Medical oncology	2613	$806.6	$308,702.0
Portable x-ray	7	$2.0	$288,020.0
Rheumatology	4053	$1044.5	$257,701.0
Nephrology	7503	$1685.6	$224,657.0
Cardiology	22,241	$4965.3	$223,248.0
Dermatology	10,507	$2235.3	$212,745.0
Interventional pain management	1856	$366.1	$197,229.0
Peripheral vascular disease	74	$14.3	$193,441.0
Hematology	687	$127.6	$185,757.0
Cardiac electrophysiology	1117	$204.0	$182,641.0
Vascular surgery	2696	$485.3	$180,019.0
Urology	8791	$1385.4	$157,589.0

Data Source: Centers for Medicare and Medicaid Services.

Publication Source: Medicare Spending Tied to Sliver of Providers, April 9, 2014, *Wall Street Journal*.

FIND OUT HOW MUCH YOUR DOCTOR RECEIVED FROM MEDICARE

Use the interactive link below to find a doctor or other medical professional among the more than 800,000 healthcare providers that received payments in 2012 from Medicare Part B, which covers doctor visits, tests, and other treatments. You will need to input the physicians' name and/or zip code.

Link: http://www.nytimes.com/interactive/2014/04/09/health/medicare-doctor-database.html.[15]

THE COMPENSATION VERSUS VALUE PARADOX

Regardless of specialty, degree designation, or delivery model, the private practice physician salary is traditionally inversely related to independent medical practice business values. In other words, the more a doctor takes home in compensation from his practice, the less ownership in a private practice is worth, and *vice versa*. This is the difference between a short-term and long-term compensation strategy.

OVERHEARD IN THE DOCTOR'S LOUNGE: BEWARE STATISTICS

Reading statistical income information can be full of pitfalls. One needs to look at the mean and median. Both give useful information. By comparing the two, one can ascertain if there are outliers that affect the results.

For example, if a sample of 10 physicians has one earning $1,000,000 and the other nine earning $100,000, the average (mean) income is $190,000; but the median income is $100,000.

Just using this information alone, one can tell there are some outliers that could affect the results.

Dr. Edmond F. Mertzenich, DPM, MBA
(Rockford, IL)
PNews, March 4, 2014

ASSESSMENT

Money, received as salary in the present, can earn money over a period of time (making the amount ultimately larger than if the same initial sum were received later). Therefore, both the amount of investment return and the length of time it takes to receive that return affect the rate of return (i.e., the value of the return). This financial planning principle, known as the time-value of money (TVM), is a vital compensation issue regarding ultimate wealth accumulation.

CONCLUSION

This TVM concept, along with the Marcinko/Kelly retirement report, should serve as a wake-up call that physicians may need to cut personal consumption and professional expenses, and to save more aggressively to harvest the eventual lifestyle and retirement dream all are working toward.

COPYRIGHT NOTICE

The sections entitled *Physician Compensation Data Sources* and *Medical Specialty Trends* are owned and copyrighted by Health Capital Consultants LLC, St. Louis, Missouri. They are reprinted with permission (HCC President Robert James Cimasi—MHA, ASA, FRICS, MCBA, CVA, CM&AA, Certified Medical Planner™). Health Capital Consultants, LLC specializes in healthcare valuation, merger & acquisition, litigation support & expert testimony, financial analysis, and related health industry economics and capital evaluation research services (www.HealthCapital.com).

COLLABORATE

Discuss this chapter online with others at www.MedicalExecutivePost.com.

ACKNOWLEDGMENT

To David B. Nash, MD, MBA, FACP, The Raymond C and Doris N. Professor and Chair of the Department of Health Policy Director, Office of Policy and Clinical Outcomes, Jefferson Medical College, Thomas Jefferson University, Philadelphia, Pennsylvania.

REFERENCES

1. http://www.physiciansmoneydigest.net/issues/2005/92/3951.
2. Physician News Digest, October 25, 2013.
3. AMN Healthcare.
4. HEAL website: www.bhpr.hrsa.gov/dsa/healsite; Defaulted Docs website: www.defaulteddocs.dhhs.gov.
5. http://in-training.org/medical-students-the-anti-millionaires-4361.
6. Career Cast.
7. http://www.abimfoundation.org/Professionalism/Professionalism%20in%20Practice.aspx.
8. http://blogs.wsj.com/health/2009/06/17/how-much-do-rookie-doctors-make-the-latest-scorecard/.
9. Linda Brodsky, a pediatric surgeon at The Brodsky Blog. She founded Women MD Resources (personal communication).
10. http://www.ada.org/prof/resources/pubs/dbguide/newdent/income.asp#private; http://www.payscale.com/research/US/Job=Dentist/Salary.
11. http://www.payscale.com/research/US/Job=Chiropractor/Salary.
12. November 25, 2013: http://medicaleconomics.modernmedicine.com/medical-economics/news/flat-declining-salaries-inflate-physician-worries-over-payments-red-tape.
13. The information presented here is from a database released by the Centers for Medicare and Medicaid Services.
14. Centers for Medicare and Medicaid Services. Includes only services billed by an individual, not a company; excludes ambulances, laboratories, and other facilities.
15. The database excluded, for privacy reasons, any procedures that a doctor performed on 11 or fewer patients. The total reimbursement for each doctor does not include those procedures either. Results shown include only the individuals such as doctors, nurses, or technicians but not organizations like *Walgreens*. While some providers could have multiple offices, the address shown is the main address indicated in the database. Descriptions of the procedures are from the American Medical Association (AMA).

FURTHER READING

Abelson, R: Sliver of Medicare Doctors Get Big Share of Payouts. *New York Times*, April 9, 2014.
Barlow, K: Establishing Healthy Medical Partner Relations. In, Marcinko, DE (Ed): *The Advanced Business of Medical Practice* (second edition). Springer Publishing, New York, 2005.
Black's Law Dictionary, 7th West Publishing, Co; St. Paul, Minnesota, 2009.
Cimasi, RJ and Alexander, T: Industry Benchmarking for Emerging Healthcare Organizations. In, Marcinko, DE (Ed): *Healthcare Organizations (Journal of Financial Management Strategies)*. iMBA Inc Atlanta, GA, 2010.
Galtress, E: Human Resource Options for the Harried Physician. In, Marcinko, DE (Ed): *Business of Medical Practice*. Springer Publishing, New York, 2005.
Gawande, A: *Complications*. Profile Books Ltd; New Ed edition (July 3, 2003)
Kelly, G.J: Are Your on Your Way to $5.5 Million? *Physicians Money Digest*, March 31, 2005.
Marcinko, DE: *Financial Planning CD-ROM*. JB Publishing, Sudbury, MA, 2006.
Marcinko, DE and Hetico, HR: *Dictionary of Health Economics and Finance*. Springer Publishers, New York, 2007.
Marcinko, DE and Hetico, HR: Physician Compensation Trends, Models and Approaches. In, Nash, David, B (Ed): *Practicing Medicine in the 21st Century*. American College of Physician Executives, Tampa, Florida, 2006.
Marcinko, DE, Hetico, HR, and Knabe, BJ: In, Marcinko, DE (Ed): *Business of Medical Practice* (third edition). Springer Publishing Company, New York, 2010.
Nash, DB: *Practicing Medicine in the 21st Century*. ACPE, Tampa, FL, 2008.
Prince, RA: *Wealth Preservation for Physicians*. Primedia, New York, 2006.
Ritchie, A and Marbury, D: Shifting Reimbursement Models: The risks and rewards for primary care. *Medical Economics*, April 8, 2014.

US Dept. Health and Human Services (HRSA Bureau of Health Professions), Washington, DC, 2010.
Will the Last Physician in America Please Turn Off the Lights? A Look at America's Looming Physician Shortage, Fourth Edition © 2008 Merritt Hawkins & Associates Merritt Hawkins & Associates Guide.

PHYSICIAN EMPLOYMENT AGREEMENT OUTLINE

1. DURATION OF THE CONTRACT
   a. Length of the contract
      i. Option: Annual with automatic renewal
   b. Effective date of the contract
2. CONDITIONS UNDER WHICH CONTRACT CAN BE TERMINATED
   a. Voluntary termination by employee or employer with thirty (30) days' written notice
   b. Death of employee
   c. Suspension, revocation, or cancelation of employee's right to practice medicine in the State of (State)
   d. Employee loses privileges to any hospital at which practice regularly maintains admission privileges
   e. Employee fails or refuses to follow reasonable policies or directives established by the practice
   f. Employee commits acts amounting to gross negligence or willful misconduct to the detriment of the practice or its patients
   g. Employee is convicted of a crime involving moral turpitude, including fraud, theft, or embezzlement
   h. Employee breaches terms of the employment contract
   i. Employee becomes and remains disabled in excess of three (3) consecutive months
3. COMPENSATION
   a. Amount of annual salary
   b. Incentive bonus, calculated as follows: (formula)
   c. Determine how long physician will be paid during period of disability and how much
4. BENEFITS
   a. Health insurance
   b. Retirement plan contribution
   c. Malpractice insurance
      i. Malpractice tail-end premium?
   d. Dues, books, and periodicals
   e. Licenses
   f. CME expenses
      i. Annual allowance of $ (dollar amount)
   g. Entertainment
   h. Automobile
   i. Relocation
   j. Vacation leave
   k. Sick leave
   l. Life and disability insurance
   m. Cellular phone
   n. Pager
   o. Other
5. OUTSIDE INCOME
   a. Decide on the type of outside income the physician can retain and the type of outside income earned by the physician that the practice will be entitled to retain.
   b. At the same time as (A), discuss the physician's restrictions on outside employment.

6. PHYSICIAN'S DUTIES
   a. Required work hours
   b. Required on-call schedule
   c. Discuss any restrictions on the acceptance of new patients by the physician.
   d. Discuss any provision if the physician is called to jury duty or related duty.
7. TERMINATION COMPENSATION
   a. Determine how much the physician will be paid if employment is terminated.
8. OPPORTUNITY TO BUY INTO PRACTICE OWNERSHIP
   a. How long after joining the practice?
   b. What exactly will the physician be allowed to buy into?
      i. Accounts receivable
      ii. Hard assets of the practice
      iii. Goodwill
   c. How will the assets be valued?
      i. By independent appraiser
      ii. By fixed formula
   d. If applicable, how will accounts receivable be valued?
   e. How will fixed assets be valued?
   f. How will the buy-in price be paid for?
9. REASONABLENESS OF COVENANT NOT TO COMPETE
10. OTHER ISSUES

4 Hospital Fringe Benefits Plans and Stock Options

Understanding Employer and Employee Perspectives

David Edward Marcinko and Perry D'Alessio

CONTENTS

This chapter examines hospital employee benefits and equity participation, both from the healthcare organization employer and employee perspectives. Employee benefits include employer payment of personal expenses on behalf of employees, as well as methods for deferring taxation of compensation earned by employees. If a public healthcare entity or hospital, stock options allow employees to benefit from the appreciation in the value of employer securities without having to deplete cash resources to purchase shares at the time appreciation begins.

INTRODUCTION

When selecting an employer, understanding the value of the benefits offered is critical. Just because one employer may offer a higher salary doesn't mean they are offering more total compensation than other options.

CASE MODEL EXAMPLE

So, let's explore the value of benefits received by a hypothetical 60-year-old hospital-based respiratory therapist (RT) employee who is married and has two children (ages 18 and 15). We'll assume this individual earns $51,017, which was the median average household income in 2012–2013.

HOW MUCH ARE EMPLOYER BENEFITS WORTH?

PAYROLL TAXES

The value of some benefits is easier to calculate than others. For instance, regardless of your income, your employer is required to pay half your FICA—Federal Insurance Contributions Act—taxes (which covers Social Security and Medicare). The combined FICA tax is 15.3% of your income; so you pay 7.65% and your employer pays 7.65% (6.2% for the Social Security portion and 1.45% for Medicare).

Note: This had been reduced by 2–4.2% over the past few years as part of a payroll tax holiday to help with the economic recovery. All the fiscal cliff discussions did not address this and the rate has reverted back to what it was 2 years ago.

SOCIAL SECURITY

The first $113,700 of wages is taxed at 6.2% for Social Security. Anything above this amount is not taxed.

MEDICARE TAX

This is taxed at 1.45% of wages and there is no wage base limit.

NEW IN 2013

Employers must withhold a 0.9% additional Medicare from wages paid to an employee in excess of $200,000 in a calendar year if single and $250,000 if married. Employers are required to begin withholding additional Medicare Tax in the pay period in which wages in excess of $200,000 are paid to an employee and continue to withhold it in each pay period until the end of the calendar year.

Now, assuming a salary of $51,017, your employer's FICA contribution is **$3903**.

It should be noted that any employer you affiliate with will be required to contribute their 7.65% portion of the payroll tax. Of course, the actual dollar amount they contribute will increase as your salary rises. Alternatively, self-employed individuals are required to pay almost the full 15.3% payroll tax themselves (less a modest reduction, and a deduction for half the self-employment tax as an adjustment to income.) In comparison, a halving of the payroll tax is a significant benefit to non-self-employed workers.

RETIREMENT PLAN CONTRIBUTIONS

Of course, not all employers offer a 401(k) match, and the amount of the match offered varies. However, let's assume a fairly common matching policy where the employer will match 50% of the first 6% of your salary that you contribute. Assuming you take full advantage of the match, your employer will contribute 3% of your salary to your retirement plan, or **$1530**.

PAID TIME OFF

Most employers offer a mixture of vacation, holidays, and sick days. Assuming you get 10 days for vacation, five paid sick days, and seven paid holidays, you get a total of 22 paid days off per year. If you make $51,017 per year and work 260 days, your daily pay rate is $196 ($51,017/260). Multiplying the daily rate by 22 paid days off, you actually make **$4312** for days you don't work.

HEALTHCARE

Notwithstanding the Patient Protection and Affordable Care Act (PP-ACA), some benefits, such as healthcare, are much less predictable. Of course, not all employers offer healthcare, and it is difficult to determine the value of any benefits offered. However, according to ehealthinsurance.com, our 60-year-old married individual with two kids could purchase a healthcare plan from Select Health with a $1000 deductible per individual and $2500 deductible per family for $1243 per month or $14,916 per year. Many employers won't cover this entire cost, but let's assume the employer covers 60% of this cost, leading to a total healthcare benefit of **$8949** contributed by the employer.

LIFE INSURANCE

Life insurance, when provided by an employer, is typically term insurance and fairly cost-effective. Assuming the employer provides life insurance equal to two times your salary, they would provide $102,034 of coverage. On intelliquote.com, we found a company willing to provide this level of coverage for $41 per month, or **$492** per year.

LONG-TERM DISABILITY

When offered, employers usually provide long-term disability coverage amounting to approximately 50% of your salary. On Mutual of Omaha's website, we found that a long-term disability policy providing a $2000 per month benefit (47% of salary) after a 60-day elimination policy would cost our 60-year-old employee $175 per month, or **$2100** per year.

ADDING IT UP

So, how much are the benefits for our hypothetical employee worth?

- FICA contributions: **$3903**
- Retirement plan contributions: **$1530**
- Paid time off: **$4312**
- Healthcare: **$8949**
- Life insurance: **$492**
- Long-term disability: **$2100**

Total employer-paid benefits based on a $51,017 income: **$21,290**

Consequently, although salary may be $51,017, total compensation is $72,307, and the benefits provided by the employer represent approximately 30% of compensation. This example is typical—the U.S. Department of Labor reports that benefits are worth 30% of an average employee's total compensation.

Clearly, benefits can amount to a significant portion of compensation and should be closely analyzed when choosing an employer. Even if not currently considering changing employers, knowing how much an employer pays for benefits might help you appreciate your job at least a little bit more (Lon Jefferies MBA, CFP®, www.NetWorthAdvice.com, personal communication).

HOSPITAL EMPLOYEE BENEFITS

Now, let's drill down a bit deeper. There are three categories of benefits that hospital employers typically provide to their employees:

- Those that are totally income-tax free. Some of these are still taxable for FICA (Social Security and Medicare).
- Those that are not taxed at their full economic value, or are taxed at a special preferential rate.
- Those in which a tax liability is not incurred until sometime after the employee receives the benefit.

Tax-Free Benefits

The following are the benefits typically provided by hospitals that are tax free to employees:

- Group term life insurance
- Accident and health benefits
- Moving expense reimbursement
- Dependent-care expenses
- Meals and lodging
- Adoption expense assistance
- Use of athletic facilities
- Employee awards
- Educational assistance
- Qualified employee discounts
- No additional-cost services
- Retirement-planning service
- De minimus benefits
- Qualified transportation benefits
- Working-condition benefits
- General fringe benefits and miscellaneous specialized provisions

All tax-free benefits have varying conditions, which can include

- What constitutes a benefit to qualify (as defined by the Indian Revenue Service [IRS])
- What constitutes an employee to qualify? The most commonly restricted employee types are S Corporation employees who owned >2% of the corporation's stock in the taxable year, highly compensated employees, and key employees
- Which employees are excluded
- Monetary caps
- IRS reporting requirements
- Exclusion from what type of taxes (income, FICA, and federal unemployment tax [FUTA])

ACCIDENT AND HEALTH BENEFITS

These are the most common types of tax-free benefits provided to employees. They include payments for healthcare insurance, payment to a fund that provides accident and health benefits directly to the employee, company-direct reimbursements for employee medical expenses, and contributions to an Archer MSA (medical savings account).

The IRS definition of an employee, for healthcare benefit purposes, is very broad.

Health benefits are exempt from income, FICA, and FUTA. This saves the employer 7.65% that would otherwise be the "matching" 6.2% Social Security tax and the 1.45% Medicare Tax components due if these were true wages. The employer also saves the 0.8% FUTA tax, but since FUTA taxes only the first $7000 of calendar year wages, per employee, this usually doesn't factor in.

CALCULATION

If you pay the full state unemployment tax, then your FUTA tax = gross salary * .08%—The maximum amount is $56 per employee:

$50,000 Salary = ($7000) * (.8%) = $56.00
$5000 Salary = ($5000) * (.8%) = $40.00

The hospital employee saves federal income taxes on health benefits received, at their marginal tax rate, and, their components of FICA taxes. Depending on the coverage provided, these plans, when fully funded by the employer, can save the employee thousands of dollars in taxes each year.

IRS restrictions include

- Certain payments to S Corporation employees who are 2% shareholders are subject to FICA taxes
- Certain long-term care benefits
- Certain payments for highly compensated employees

EXAMPLE 4.1

Let's say the annual cost of providing medical coverage for an employee, age 50, with a spouse and two minor children is $7500. An employee in the 30% tax bracket who received this amount in cash each year and then paid for his or her own medical coverage would be liable for as much as $2250 in income taxes. In addition, FICA taxes save another 7.65% or $574, for a total savings to the employee of $2824. The employer saves $574 in FICA taxes.

GROUP TERM LIFE INSURANCE

A hospital employee usually must include in gross income the amount of life insurance premiums paid by the employer on the employee's life if the policy proceeds are payable to a beneficiary named by the employee. However, the cost of providing group term life insurance on an employee's life up to $50,000 is excluded from the employee's gross income. The cost of any amount over $50,000 provided by the employer is included in the employee's income. The amount excludable under this provision for an employee who is 60 years of age is approximately $500 per year.

MOVING EXPENSE REIMBURSEMENTS

A company may pay the qualified moving expenses of an employee, except meals, directly or indirectly, and exclude them from the employee's gross wages for income-tax calculations.

DEPENDENT-CARE EXPENSES

The first $5000 of annual dependent-care expenses (for married-filing jointly employees, $2500 for married filing separately) paid by an employer is exempt from the employee's gross income. This is limited by the IRS-defined earned income for either the employee or spouse. The expenses must be made for a qualifying person, and, their care must allow an employee to work. The amount must be expended by the employee to a qualified day care with a federal identification number described on the employee's income-tax return or the pretax amounts will be added back to income on the income-tax return level. This can be for a current employee, a sole proprietor, a leased employee, and a partner who performs services for a partnership. It excludes highly paid employees defined as any employee paid more than $115,000 in the preceding year.

These benefits are reported in Box 10 of the employee's W-2.[1]

MEALS AND LODGING

Under very limited circumstances, meals and lodging provided to an employee, by the employer on the business premises of the employer, may be excludable from the gross income of the employee. Usually, lodging is a condition of employment where the employee must live on the premises to properly perform their duties. S Corporation employees who are at least 2% shareholders are excluded.

ADOPTION ASSISTANCE

If you're thinking of adopting a child in 2014, you should know about the tax credit. In 2014, the maximum credit for adopting a child with special needs is $12,970. The special needs adoption credit, which typically applies to harder-to-place children, including children in foster care, can be claimed regardless of your actual adoption expenses. The maximum credit for other adoptions is your qualified adoption expenses (including attorney's fees, agency fees, travel fees, etc.) up to $12,970. The adoption credit, as of 2013, is not refundable. It'll reduce your tax liability, but you won't get a check in the mail for any leftover credits. Also, this credit begins to phase out with a modified adjusted gross income of $194,580.[2]

USE OF ATHLETIC FACILITIES

A company may provide employee access to on-site athletic facilities, and exclude the value of such a benefit from gross wages, if all employees and their families have equal access to it.

EMPLOYEE AWARDS

Awards to employees, such as for safety or length of service, are excludable from the employee's gross income up to the amount of the cost to the employer, or $1600, or, $400 for nonqualified plan awards. The type of award that qualifies for exemption from gross income is limited. Specifically, cash and its equivalents and intangible property such as vacations are excluded. S Corporation employees who are 2% shareholders are excluded.

EDUCATIONAL ASSISTANCE

Up to $5250 of employer-paid, qualifying educational assistance can be excluded from the employee's gross pay. Since 2002, qualifying expenses include graduate courses.

Assistance over $5250: If you do not have an educational assistance plan, or you provide an employee with assistance exceeding $5250, you can exclude the value of these benefits from wages if they are working-condition benefits. Property or a service provided is a working-condition benefit to the extent that if the employee paid for it, the amount paid would have been deductible as a business or depreciation expense.

QUALIFIED EMPLOYEE DISCOUNTS

Companies can provide discounts on goods and services to employees and exclude the value of these from gross income. This is limited to 20% of nonemployee charges for the same services and the gross profit margin on merchandise. Stocks and bonds are excluded.

RETIREMENT PLANNING

If the hospital has a qualified retirement plan, an employer may provide retirement-planning services to the employee and his/her spouse. Advice may include nonemployer retirement issues but cannot provide tax preparation, legal, accounting, or brokerage services.

WORKING-CONDITION BENEFITS

Examples of working-condition fringes are employer-paid business travel, use of company cars, job-related education, and business-related security devices.

DE MINIMUS FRINGE BENEFITS

De minimus fringes include items such as occasional parties or picnics for employees, traditional holiday gifts of property with a small fair market value (FMV), or occasional theater or sporting-event tickets. Cash is never allowed except for occasional meal money or transportation fare. Examples are holiday gifts of low value, limited use of a copying machine, parties, picnics, occasional movie or sports tickets, transportation fare, and so on.

QUALIFIED TRANSPORTATION BENEFITS

A qualified transportation fringe is any of the following provided by the employer to an employee: (1) transportation in a commuter highway vehicle if such transportation is in connection with travel between the employee's residence and place of employment, (2) a transit pass, or (3) qualified parking.

MISCELLANEOUS SPECIALIZED PROVISIONS

There are other narrowly focused statutory provisions, such as personage allowances and certain military benefits that allow for exclusion of income. Because of their very limited application, these specialized benefits are not addressed in this portfolio.

BENEFITS THAT ARE NOT TAXED AT FULL ECONOMIC VALUE

When a benefit does not qualify for exclusion under a specific statute or regulation, the benefit is considered taxable to the recipient. It is included in wages for withholding and employment-tax purposes, at the excess of its FMV over any amount paid by the employee for the benefit.

For example, hospitals often provide automobiles for use by employees. Treasury regulations exclude from income the value of the following types of vehicles' use by an employee:

- Vehicles not available for the personal use of an employee by reason of a written policy statement of the employer

- Vehicles not available to an employee for personal use other than commuting (although in this case commuting is includable)
- Vehicles used in connection with the business of farming [in which case the exclusion is equal to the value of an arbitrary 75% of the total availability for use, and the value of the balance may be includable or excludable, depending upon the facts (Treas. Regs. § 1.132-5(g) involved)]
- Certain vehicles identified in the regulations as "qualified non-personal-use vehicles," which by reason of their design do not lend themselves to more than a de minimus amount of personal use by an employee (examples are ambulances and hearses)
- Vehicles provided for qualified automobile demonstration use
- Vehicles provided for product testing and evaluation by an employee outside the employer's workplace

If the employer-provided vehicle does not fall into one of the excluded categories, then the employee is required to report his personal use as a taxable benefit. The value of the availability for personal use may be determined under one of the several approaches. Under any of the approaches, the after-tax cost to the employee is substantially less than if the employee used his or her own dollars to purchase the automobile and then deducted a portion of the cost as a business expense.

COST COMPARISON: EMPLOYER-PROVIDED TRANSPORTATION

EXAMPLE 4.2

Kurt purchases an automobile for $15,000.

His hospital business use is 80% and he drives 20,000 total miles per year. Operating costs for the year, including gasoline, oil, insurance, maintenance, repairs, and license fees, are $4000. If Kurt owns the car for 5 years, ownership will cost $35,000 ($4000 × 5 = $20,000, $20,000 + $15,000 = $35,000), or $7000 per year. For, each personal use mile costs $1.75 (100%−80% = 20%, 20% × 20,000 miles = 4000 miles, and $7000/4000 miles = $1.75). Kurt's employer reimburses him 34.5 cents per mile for the business-related miles. As a result, the business use of the car is only partially reimbursed (16,000 business miles × 34.5 cents = $5520).

However, the business usage costs Kurt $5600 (80% of $7000). Kurt subsidizes the employer 9.25 cents per mile ($7000 − $5520 = $1480, $1480/16,000 = 9.25 cents). Kurt's total cost of ownership is $1.84 per mile, or $36,850 ($1.88 × 20,000 personal miles over the 5-year life).

EXAMPLE 4.3

Ben uses a hospital employer-provided vehicle 4000 miles per year in 2003.

He reimburses the employer 34.5 cents per mile. His cost for 5 years is $6900 (5y × 4000 = 20,000 miles, 20,000 miles × 34.5 = $6900).

Beginning on January 1st 2013, the standard mileage rates for the use of a car (also vans, pickups, or panel trucks) were:

- 56.5 cents per mile for business miles driven
- 24 cents per mile driven for medical or moving purposes
- 14 cents per mile driven in service of charitable organizations

Note the dramatic contrast, from the employee's perspective, between the above two examples, of the company reimbursing the employee for business use of his personal car, versus the employee reimbursing the company for personal use of the vehicle.

The business, medical, and moving expense rates decrease one-half cent from the 2013 rates. The charitable rate is based on statute.[3]

TAX-DEFERRED BENEFITS

There are several types of arrangements, listed below, which allow employees to receive economic benefits currently without having to pay taxes until a later taxable year. Furthermore, some of these arrangements may even provide for a lower taxation rate at that time. These types of benefits are not totally excludable from income forever, as are those listed in the first two sections. Rather, they primarily provide deferral of taxable income.

The classic example is a retirement plan. Employers may establish pension, profit sharing, stock bonus, or annuity plans, as well as 401(k) and 403(b) plans. The tax consequences and most of the formal requirements of these plans are similar. These plans are often referred to as "qualified retirement plans."

The hospital employer makes contributions on behalf of participating employees. The contributions are placed in a trust fund, custodial account, or annuity contract. The funds are held and accumulated for the benefit of plan participants. The distribution of the funds to a participant normally occurs no sooner than the participant's termination of service with the employer, and, no later than attainment of normal retirement age, as defined in the plan. The method of distribution may be a lump-sum payment of all of the employee's benefits, an installment payment over a number of years (usually 10–15), and an annuity that provides payments over the employee's and/or spouse's lifetime.

The extremely favorable tax consequences of qualified retirement plans are the reason for their popularity. When the hospital makes a contribution on the employee's behalf to the qualified plan, the employer receives a deduction for the amount contributed; however, the employee will not have to report the contribution as income until the funds are finally distributed. Contributions to the trust or other qualified fund are accumulated tax free. Distributions are taxable, but the recipient is generally in a lower marginal tax bracket during retirement than when contributions to the retirement plan were made. This treatment is a truly startling departure from the normal practice under the Internal Revenue Code (IRC).

The following examples demonstrate how the tax-free accumulation of income (contributions and interest) offers the employee great advantages, *even* if his or her tax rates are the same at the time of deferral as at the time of distribution.

EXAMPLE 4.4

Tony, a hospital employee in the 30% tax bracket, decides to place a portion of his $150,000 annual salary for the next 5 years in a qualified retirement plan that pays an 8% return. He decides to let that deferred income compound for 10 years. Depending on the percentage he decides to apply to the plan each year, the following table shows the total economic benefit of the deferral he can expect after 10 years:

Tax-Free Compounding

Years of deferral	5		
Annual investment return	8%		
Years of compounding	10		
Tax rate	30%		
% of salary deferred	5%	10%	15%
Amount of deferral per year	$7500	$15,000	$22,500
Total deferred	$37,500	$75,000	$112,500
Value at the end of 10 years	$64,650	$129,299	$193,949
Income tax due on receipt	$19,390	$38,790	$58,185
Value remaining	$45,255	$90,509	$135,764
Value remaining, if $ not deferred (tax paid on receipt and on investment earnings)	$38,554	$77,107	$115,661
Economic benefit of deferral	$6701	$13,402	$20,103

The moral here is twin benefits of the time value of money and deferred taxation, at least with a stable investment.

Deferral arrangements (retirement plans) using employees' salaries to supplement employer-funded qualified plans have become increasingly popular. Such plans are commonly called 401(k) plans, after the section of the Code that defines them. Under these plans, an enrolled employee is permitted to make an elective deferral of a portion of their compensation, or part or all of a year-end bonus, and have the employer contribute such amounts to the plan, rather than receiving them directly. If made within the statutory limits, the amounts are not included in the employee's income and the earnings from investment of such contributions accumulate tax free until distributed to the employee. Thus, in addition to employer contributions, the employee can get all the qualified benefits on a portion of his or her own salary. These salary deferral arrangements are obviously voluntary and are subject to severe restrictions.

TAX-FREE BENEFIT RECEIPTS

Many of the special tax-free benefits discussed above only apply to hospital employees, and not to owners of medical clinics, and so on. Thus, S Corporation employee/shareholders, and sole proprietors, cannot take full advantage of all the nontaxable benefits outlined above.

There is some tax relief available to those who do not receive tax-free benefits as employees. 100% of healthcare insurance premiums may be deducted as itemized deductions in the medical expense section of federal Schedule A, along with other unreimbursed medical costs. However, only qualified medical expenses over 7.5% of the taxpayer's AGI are allowed. Thus, the total medical expenses, including the 70% allowable for healthcare insurance premiums, falling beneath the 7.5% AGI threshold produce no tax benefits. Additionally, the total allowable itemized deductions must exceed the IRS standard deduction to produce tax benefits. Third, allowable itemized deductions on Schedule A phase out with higher AGI and S Corporation employees who own at least 2% of the corporations stock.

Special rules apply to certain employees of S corporations who are also substantial shareholders. Any 2% shareholder of an S corporation is treated as a partner in a partnership for purposes of taxing certain fringe benefits. Regular rules apply to holders of smaller ownership interests, as well as to all common-law employees. The following fringe benefits provided by an S corporation are taxable under these special rules, and the affected shareholder must pay for them with after-tax dollars:

- Accident and health-plan benefits
- Group term life insurance
- Meals and lodging furnished for the convenience of an employer

The nontaxable benefits providing dependent-care assistance programs and certain general fringe benefits, such as no-additional-cost services or qualified employee discounts, are not subject to any special rules for self-employed individuals and, therefore, are not subject to any special rules with respect to the shareholder employees of an S corporation, regardless of the amount of stock they own.

KEY HOSPITAL EMPLOYEES

Effective January 1, 2014, the limitation on the annual benefit under a defined benefit plan under Section 415(b)(1)(A) is increased from $205,000 to $210,000. For a participant who separated from service before January 1, 2014, the limitation for defined benefit plans under Section 415(b)(1)(B) is computed by multiplying the participant's compensation limitation, as adjusted through 2013, by 1.0155.

The limitation for defined contribution plans under Section 415(c)(1)(A) is increased in 2014 from $51,000 to $52,000.

The Code provides that various other dollar amounts are to be adjusted at the same time and in the same manner as the dollar limitation of Section 415(b)(1)(A). These dollar amounts and the adjusted amounts are as follows:

- The limitation under Section 402(g)(1) on the exclusion for elective deferrals described in Section 402(g)(3) is increased to $17,500.
- The annual compensation limit under Sections 401(a)(17), 404(1), 408(k)(3)(C), and 408(k) (6)(D)(ii) is increased from $255,000 to $260,000.
- The dollar limitation under Section 416(i)(1)(A)(i) concerning the definition of a key employee in a top-heavy plan is increased from $165,000 to $170,000.
- The dollar amount under Section 409(o)(1)(C)(ii) for determining the maximum account balance in an employee stock ownership plan (ESOP) subject to a 5-year distribution period is increased from $1,035,000 to $1,050,000, while the dollar amount used to determine the lengthening of the 5-year distribution period is increased from $205,000 to $210,000.
- The limitation used in the definition of a highly compensated employee under Section 414(q)(1)(B) is increased from to $115,000.
- The dollar limitation under Section 414(v)(2)(B)(i) for catch-up contributions to an applicable employer plan other than a plan described in Section 401(k)(11) or Section 408(p) for individuals aged 50 or over is increased from $5000 to $5500. The dollar limitation under Section 414(v)(2)(B)(ii) for catch-up contributions to an applicable employer plan described in Section 401(k)(11) or Section 408(p) for individuals aged 50 or over remains unchanged at $2500.
- The annual compensation limitation under Section 401(a)(17) for eligible participants in certain governmental plans that, under the plan in effect on July 1, 1993, allowed cost-of-living adjustments to the compensation limitation under the plan under Section 401(a)(17) to be taken into account, is increased from $380,000 to $385,000.
- The compensation amount under Section 408(k)(2)(C) regarding simplified employee pensions (SEPs) is increased from $500 to $550.
- The limitation under Section 408(p)(2)(E) regarding SIMPLE retirement accounts is increased from $12,000.
- The limitation on deferrals under Section 457(e)(15) concerning deferred compensation plans of state and local governments and tax-exempt organizations is increased to $17,500.
- The compensation amounts under Section 1.6-21(f)(5)(i) of the Income Tax Regulations concerning the definition of "control employee" for fringe benefit valuation purposes is increased from $100,000 to $105,000. The compensation amount under Section 1.61-21(f) (5)(iii) is increased from $205,000 to $210,000.

The Code also provides that several pension-related amounts are to be adjusted using the cost-of-living adjustment under Section 1(f)(3). These dollar amounts and the adjustments are as follows:

- The adjusted gross income limitation under Section 25B(b)(1)(A) for determining the retirement savings contribution credit for married taxpayers filing a joint return is increased from $35,500 to $36,000; the limitation under Section 25B(b)(1)(B) is increased from $38,500 to $39,000; and the limitation under Sections 25B(b)(1)(C) and 25B(b)(1)(D), is increased from $59,000 to $60,000.
- The adjusted gross income limitation under Section 25B(b)(1)(A) for determining the retirement savings contribution credit for taxpayers filing as the head of the household is increased from $26,6250 to $27,000; the limitation under Section 25B(b)(1)(B) is increased from $28,875 to $29,250; and the limitation under Sections 25B(b)(1)(C) and 25B(b)(1)(D), is increased from $44,250 to $45,000.
- The adjusted gross income limitation under Section 25B(b)(1)(A) for determining the retirement savings contribution credit for all other taxpayers is increased from $17,750 to

$18,000; the limitation under Section 25B(b)(1)(B) is increased from $19,250 to $19,500; and the limitation under Sections 25B(b)(1)(C) and 25B(b)(1)(D), is increased from $29,500 to $30,000.

- The applicable dollar amount under Section 219(g)(3)(B)(i) for determining the deductible amount of an individual retirement account (IRA) contribution for taxpayers who are active participants filing a joint return or as a qualifying widow(er) is increased from $95,000 to $96,000. The applicable dollar amount under Section 219(g)(3)(B)(ii) for all other taxpayers (other than married taxpayers filing separate returns) is increased from $59,000 to $60,000. The applicable dollar amount under Section 219(g)(7)(A) for a taxpayer who is not an active participant but whose spouse is an active participant is increased from $178,000 to $181,000.

- The adjusted gross income limitation under Section 408A(c)(3)(C)(ii)(I) for determining the maximum Roth IRA contribution for married taxpayers filing a joint return or for taxpayers filing as a qualifying widow(er) is increased from $178,000 to $181,000. The adjusted gross income limitation under Section 408A(c)(3)(C)(ii)(II) for all other taxpayers (other than married taxpayers filing separate returns) is increased from $112,000 to $114,000.

- Administrators of defined benefit or defined contribution plans that have received favorable determination letters should not request new determination letters solely because of yearly amendments to adjust maximum limitations in the plans.[4]

WHAT IS A HOSPITAL CAFETERIA PLAN?

Under cafeteria plans, each eligible employee may choose to receive cash or taxable benefits, or, an equivalent of qualified, nontaxable, fringe benefits. The amounts contributed by the employer are not taxable to the employee. In effect, the employee pays for the benefits with before-tax dollars. They remain nontaxable even though the employee could have elected to receive those amounts in cash. An additional benefit for both the employee and employer is that nontaxable cafeteria plan benefits are not subject to FICA taxes, thus saving 7.65% on amounts that would otherwise be under the Social Security wage base. However, if the employee does not use all the monies that are diverted into the cafeteria plan, the unused amounts are forfeited.

The essence of a hospital cafeteria plan is that it permits each participating employee to choose among two or more benefits. In particular, the employee may "purchase" nontaxable benefits by foregoing taxable cash compensation.

This ability of participating employees, on an individual basis, to select benefits fitting their own needs, and to convert taxable compensation into nontaxable benefits, makes the cafeteria plan an attractive means of offering benefits to employees. Other qualified employee benefits, described above, are excluded from cafeteria plans.

Cafeteria plans may include the following nontaxable benefits:

- 401(k) retirement plan
- Health and accident insurance
- Adoption assistance
- Dependent-care assistance
- Group term life insurance including premiums for coverage over $50,000

CAFETERIA PLANS AND HEALTH CARE

It is always to the tax advantage of an employee to receive employer-provided health and accident benefits in a tax-free form, rather than paying them with after-tax money. Note that there is the potential draw back of employees thinking of healthcare benefits as an implicit condition of employment instead of true noncash compensation.

Because of increases in healthcare costs, employers are not always willing or able to provide coverage for all of an employee's medical expenses. This means many employees must often pay for a portion of their medical costs under a co-pay provision. If an employee is fortunate, the employer may establish a cafeteria plan to allow the employee to fund the co-pay healthcare costs with before-tax dollars.

For example, if an employee must spend $3000 annually to provide healthcare coverage for his or her dependents, then the income-tax savings to the employee could be as much as $1129.50 annually, if the employee is in the 30% tax bracket ($900 in income taxes and $229.50 of FICA taxes). The employer saves $229.50, the 7.65% of gross pay "matching" FICA taxes.

CAFETERIA PLANS AND OTHER NONTAXABLE BENEFITS

A cafeteria plan may be expanded to cover more than just medical benefits. It may offer participants a choice between one or more nontaxable benefits, and cash resulting from the employer's contributions to the plan or the employee's voluntary salary reduction. Participants in cafeteria plans are sometimes given a choice of using vacation days, selling them to the employer and then getting cash for them, or buying additional vacation days. Some cafeteria plans also include one or more reimbursement accounts, often referred to as "flexible spending accounts" or "benefit banks." Under these plans, cash that is foregone by an employee by means of a salary-reduction agreement or other agreement, is credited to an account and drawn upon to reimburse the employee for uninsured medical or dental expenses, or for dependent-care expenses. Many cafeteria plans include both insurance coverage options and reimbursement accounts.

ELECTIONS REGARDING BENEFITS UNDER A CAFETERIA PLAN

A hospital employee given the opportunity to participate in a cafeteria plan should consider the following.

HEALTHCARE

If the employee is married and has a spouse who also works, and, the employer-provided health benefits are better under the spouse's plan, then the employee should elect to be covered by the spouse's plan and choose another nontaxable benefit or a cash benefit that would be taxable under his or her own cafeteria plan, such as dependent-care coverage or group term insurance coverage. Switching health insurance requires planning and eliminating potential gaps in coverage created by insurance enrollment criteria. If the employee does not need the salary or cafeteria-plan benefits to meet the current expenses, he or she should consider contributing the cash to a 401(k) plan and defer the tax liability.

If the employee has no working spouse and the employee's plan is the only source for certain health benefits, the employee should consider what type of benefits he or she really needs for his or her family. In other words, can the employee get the necessary benefits under the company plan cheaper than he or she could individually, after taking into account that individual coverage will be paid with after-tax dollars, whereas under a cafeteria plan, such benefits can be paid with before-tax dollars? For example, if an employee who is in the 30% tax bracket is provided a $6000 plan by her employer. He or she would have to be able to get a comparable plan independently for only $3741 to be in the same position on an after-tax basis ($6000 minus income taxes of $1800 = $4200, or, $4200 minus $459 of avoided FICA).

DEPENDENT-CARE COSTS

An employee who has a choice of including dependent-care costs may be entitled to an income-tax credit for such expenses if, the employer does not reimburse them. Thus, if a credit is worth the same or more than the payment under the cafeteria plan, the employee may choose to contribute those dollars toward additional health or life insurance.

SHOULD AN EMPLOYEE USE A TAX CREDIT OR EMPLOYER-SPONSORED BENEFITS TO OFFSET DEPENDENT-CARE COSTS?

A tax credit is available to qualified individuals to help offset expenses, such as child and dependent-care costs, which enable them to be gainfully employed. The question then arises whether it is to the employee's advantage to opt out of any employer-sponsored dependent-care benefit program and take the tax credit, or vice versa.

As shown above, an employer-sponsored reimbursement plan is usually more advantageous than the tax credit, but, employees whose marginal tax rate is 15% may be better off taking the credit. As a taxpayer has increasing amounts of income in the 25% bracket, however, the exclusion under an employer-provided program will be more attractive than the credit.

EMPLOYEE ELECTIONS REGARDING DEFERRALS UNDER A HOSPITAL 403(b) PLAN

Code § 403(b) authorizes a special type of funded deferred compensation arrangement that is generally available to employees of tax-exempt hospital organizations. This also includes entities organized and operated exclusively for religious, charitable, scientific, public safety testing, literary, or educational purposes, or to foster national or international amateur sports competitions, or for prevention of cruelty to children or animals, subject to certain restrictions prohibiting political action. These arrangements are called 403(b) plans.

Much like a 401(k) plan for profit-making organizations, these plans provide for salary-reduction (deferral) contributions to be made by employees. If made within the statutory limits, the amounts are not included in the employees' income and the earnings from investment of such contributions accumulate tax free until distributed to the employee. Although there are technical differences between 403(b) plans and 401(k) plans, and the limits on the amount that may be deferred may be different, the effect on the employee is the same. Thus, the same analysis used by an employee under a 401(k) plan should also be applied to an employee who participates in a 403(b) plan.

INCOME-TAX REDUCTIONS ON RETIREMENT PLAN DISTRIBUTIONS

A hospital employee has alternatives to consider when attempting to reduce income taxes on distributions from qualified retirement plans. To help understand the choices, an advisor must understand not only the income-tax implications but also the federal estate-tax implications of each alternative and the distribution requirements imposed by law.

Generally, all payments received from a qualified retirement plan that are payable over more than 1 year are taxed at ordinary income rates. IRS Publication 575, *Pension and Annuity Income*, defines the allowed methods for structuring distributions. The 5-year averaging option was repealed in 2002. Distributions are reported to the IRS and the taxpayer via a Form 1099-R.

An additional 10% penalty is applied to withdrawals from a qualified plan before death, disability, or attainment of age 59½. SIMPLE plans may incur a 25% penalty. Insufficient withdrawal, per IRS guidelines, can incur a 25% excise tax penalty.

However, the additional tax does not apply to distributions in the form of an annuity payable over the life or life expectancy of the participant (or the lives or joint life and last-survivor expectancy of the participant and the participant's beneficiary), or to distributions made after the participant has attained the age of 55, separated from service, and satisfied the conditions for early retirement under the plan.

Lump-sum distributions from a qualified retirement plan, such as when an employee leaves the sponsoring company, may be rolled over, tax free, by the employee or surviving spouse of the employee to an IRA or another qualified retirement plan. This must occur within 60 days, and as always, there are exceptions. In 2002, the definition of a qualified plan was expanded to include 403(b) and Section 457 deferred compensation plans. This applies to direct rollovers, where the recipient has no physical control of the funds. Twenty percent withholding is required on distributions made to employees pending rollover.

Note that for some clients, this may allow a 60-day loan of 80% of their retirement funds. In addition, distributions of less than the balance to the credit of an employee, as well as distribution of the entire balance, under a qualified retirement annuity may now be rolled over, tax free, by the employee (or surviving spouse of the employee) to an IRA, as long as they are not one of the several installment payments.

ROLLOVERS

In many cases, it may be more financially beneficial to defer receipt of benefits as long as possible, assuming the client's cash flow is sufficient. Under the Economic Growth and Tax Relief Reconciliation Act of 2001 (EGTRRA), marginal tax brackets dropped. Income taxes are payable only when the benefits are received; so, deferring the receipt of benefits means that the payment of tax is deferred. If the recipient's income tax liability is deferred, there may be a greater amount left to invest during the period over which distributions are being made. Benefits retained in a qualified plan or IRA, pending distribution, continue to earn income on a tax-deferred basis. Payment in installments also results in a natural averaging effect, and may push some income into retirement years of the beneficiary, when his or her tax bracket may be lower.

There are still several potential income-tax benefits that are available on rollovers of distributions to a traditional IRA or Keogh (HR 10) plan because of special rules. Lump-sum distributions that are rolled over are excluded from gross income for the year in which they are made. This can avoid imposition of the special 10% penalty on early distribution.

Amounts rolled over are also exempted from the requirement that lump-sum treatment may be elected and that only one such election may be made. As a result of the election exemption, a rollover can be used in certain situations to avoid having to include the value of an annuity in a special 10-year averaging calculation when two dissimilar plans are involved, one of which would ordinarily distribute an annuity. For example, an employee who desires an annuity from her pension plan, and a lump-sum distribution from her profit-sharing plan, could avoid the tax-rate increase that comes from having to include the value of an annuity in the special 10-year averaging calculation by taking a lump-sum distribution from the pension plan and rolling it over into an IRA annuity.

In situations involving multiple lump-sum distributions in the same year from dissimilar plans, or distributions that might involve a look-back calculation, the election exemption may result in lower overall taxation by rolling over one or the other distribution, thus deferring the tax on the aggregated lump-sum distribution to subsequent years, when the comparative effective rate might be lower.

The relative value of a rollover as compared to a lump sum first depends on what the individual wants to do with the money. If he has an immediate need for consumption and not investment, the rollover option is generally not appropriate. But if he or she does not need to consume all the funds in a short period of time, and will invest it in the same type of assets whether it is rolled over or taken in a lump sum, then it is appropriate to compare the financial differences between the two strategies. The table below compares the results of rolling over a distribution to a traditional IRA compared to taking it as a lump-sum distribution. The figures are based on a 30% income-tax rate and an 8% annual return on all invested amounts.

A retiree can roll over his or her distribution into as many traditional IRAs as desired, if diversification of the funds is an objective.

It is sometimes advantageous to roll over distributions to a Keogh plan rather than to a traditional IRA because a subsequent lump-sum distribution from a Keogh plan may qualify for favorable 10-year income-tax averaging. Unlike traditional IRAs, Keogh plans are available only to the self-employed. However, an employer–participant might have outside self-employment income (e.g., director's fees or freelance activities) or an employee may be expecting to receive self-employment income in the form of consulting fees from the employer following retirement. Where an employee's distribution is imminent, and the employee has self-employment income, a Keogh plan rollover may be the best alternative.

In deciding whether a tax-free rollover to a traditional IRA is preferable to the various taxable options discussed above, retirees should understand that later distributions out of the traditional IRA do not qualify for either the capital gains or 10-year averaging rules that apply to lump-sum distributions from the qualified retirement plans.

IRA ROLLOVER VERSUS PAYING THE LUMP-SUM TAX

EXAMPLE 4.5

Ron, an RN, receives a lump-sum distribution qualifying for 10-year averaging treatment. The amount of distribution is $1,500,000. Since Ron will not need to use the funds for the next 20 years, he should elect a rollover that will yield annual cash flow of $106,945, instead of 10-year averaging, which will yield annual cash flow of $72,737.

Distribution amount	$1,500,000
Death benefit exclusion	0
Form 1099-R Box 2 (capital-gain portion)	0
Form 1099-R Box 9 (current actuarial value)	0
Marginal income-tax rate	30.0%
Expected investment return (before taxes)	8.0%
How many years will you need income?	20
Risk tolerance	Low
IRA Rollover	
Required annual withdrawals	$152,778
Less income tax	45,833
Net annual cash flow	$106,945
10-Year Averaging	
Invested funds after paying income tax	$867,790
Net annual cash flow	$72,737

ROLLOVER TO ROTH IRA

Another option is to transfer the lump-sum distribution to a Roth IRA. The advantage of such a conversion is that future earnings on the Roth IRA will be tax free, possibly for future generations as well. Unfortunately, however, current taxes would be paid on the lump sum when the transfer takes place. These taxes would reduce the amount of funds available for reinvestment. Allowable Roth IRA annual contributions are $5500 if under the age of 50 or $6500 for those who are of age 50 or over.

ROTH CONVERSIONS ALLOWED FOR HIGH-INCOME INDIVIDUALS AFTER 2009

A taxpayer ordinarily may not convert any part of an IRA to a Roth IRA if (1) the taxpayer's modified "adjusted gross income" for the tax year exceeds $100,000 or (2) the taxpayer is married filing a separate return. However, after 2009, a taxpayer will be able to convert an IRA to a Roth IRA regardless of the level of his or her income—and regardless of a separately filed return.

Extension of Roth Conversions into Eligible Retirement Plans

Taxpayers have long been able to convert their regular IRAs into Roth IRAs. However, to convert funds in an employer retirement plan into a Roth IRA, taxpayers have generally had to roll the funds over first to a regular IRA and then convert the regular IRA into a Roth IRA. In contrast, after 2007, a taxpayer may directly convert all or part of an "eligible plan" into a Roth IRA without using a regular IRA as an intermediary. For this purpose, an eligible plan is a qualified retirement plan, a Section 403(b) tax-sheltered annuity (TSA), or an eligible state and local government plan.

Conversions of eligible plans into Roth IRAs will be subject to the same conditions that apply to regular IRA conversions. That is, before 2010, a taxpayer may generally make the conversion only if (1) the taxpayer's modified "adjusted gross income" for the tax year does not exceed $100,000 and (2) the taxpayer is not a married individual filing a separate return. After 2009, a taxpayer will be able to make the conversion regardless of the level of his or her income—and regardless of a separately filed return. Of course, conversions into Roth IRAs are taxable (exclusive of return of investment) whether the converted funds come from a regular IRA or an eligible plan (Tax Increase Prevention and Reconciliation Act of 2005, Pub. L. No: 109-455, § 512—Pension Protection Act of 2006, Pub. L; No. 109-280, § 824(a), (b), (c); I.R.C. § 408A).

HOSPITAL ESOPS

The growth over the past few decades of plans that give employees a stake in the ownership of their company has been a significant development in the area of employee compensation and corporate finance. Although there are many forms of employee ownership, the ESOP has achieved widespread application. The rapid growth in the number of ESOPs being created has important ramifications for employees, corporations, and the economy at large.

An ESOP is a special kind of qualified retirement plan in which the sponsoring employer establishes a trust to receive the contributions by the employer on behalf of participating employees. The trust then primarily invests in the stock of the sponsoring employer. The plan's fiduciaries are responsible for setting up individual accounts within the trust for each employee who participates, and the company's contributions to the plan are allocated according to an established formula among the individual participants' accounts, thus making the employees beneficial owners of the company where they work.

Like all qualified retirement plans, ESOPs must be defined in writing. Furthermore, in addition to the usual rules for qualified deferred compensation plans, ESOPs must meet certain requirements of the Internal Revenue Code with respect to voting rights on employer securities. In general, employers that have "registration class securities" (publicly traded companies) must allow plan participants to direct the manner in which employer securities allocated to their respective accounts are to be voted on all matters. Companies that do not have registration class securities are required to pass through voting rights to participants only on "major corporate issues." These issues are defined as merger or consolidation, recapitalization, reclassification, liquidation, dissolution, sale of substantially all the assets of a trade or business of the corporation; and under treasury regulations there are similar issues. On other matters, such as the election of the Board of Directors, the shares may be voted by the designated fiduciary unless the plan otherwise provides. In regard to unallocated shares held in the trust, the designated fiduciary may exercise its own discretion in voting such shares.

As owners, hospital employees may be more motivated to improve corporate performance because they can benefit directly from company profitability. A growing company showing significant increases in the value of its stock can mean significant financial benefits for participating employees. However, because the assets of the ESOP trust are primarily invested in the stock of one company, there is a higher degree of risk for the employee.

An ESOP is the only employee-benefit plan that may also be used as a technique of corporate finance. Thus, in addition to the usual tax benefits of qualified retirement plans, studies have shown that ESOPs provide employers with significant amounts of capital, which often result in financial benefits far superior to other employee-benefit plans, while employees can share in the benefits realized through corporate financial transactions. Until January 1, 2003, the employee did not incur FICA tax on exercised stock options.

ESOPs, like all qualified deferred compensation plans, must meet certain minimum requirements spelled out in Code § 401(a) in order for the contributions to be tax deductible to the sponsoring employer. Many employers who set up ESOPs do so not to take advantage of the very substantial tax incentives they can receive, but rather to provide their employees with a special kind of employee benefit—one with many implications for the way a company does business.

HOW DO ESOPs BENEFIT EMPLOYEES AND THEIR EMPLOYERS?

When participants in an ESOP terminate their employment, they are entitled to receive the shares previously allocated to their account. The employee may then hold or sell them, but for tax purposes, these shares are treated like any other distribution from a qualified deferred compensation plan; that is, upon distribution of employer stock, the employee is not taxed on an unrealized appreciation until the shares are sold.

However, to ensure that there is a market for the stock distributed by closely held companies, these companies are required to provide a "put option" to the recipient. For lump-sum distributions from an ESOP that are then put to the employer, the employer (or the ESOP) must pay the FMV of such shares to the terminated participant, in substantially equal payments over a period not exceeding 5 years. The following table shows how the gain on stock from an ESOP distribution is taxable when the stock is later sold.

Value of stock when purchased by ESOP	$2500	100 shares × $25/share	
Value of stock when distributed	$5000	100 shares × $50/share	
Years held after distribution, until sale	3	5	10
Value in the later year of sale	$6613	$8745	$17,589
Gain on sale	4113	6245	15,089
Tax on sale (20%)	−823	−1249	−3018
Value remaining	$5790	$7496	$14,571

For the purpose of broadening the ownership of capital and providing employees with access to capital credit, Congress has granted a number of specific incentives meant to promote increased use of the ESOP concept. These ESOP incentives provide numerous advantages to the sponsoring employer and can significantly improve corporate financial transactions. Chief among these incentives is the leveraged ESOP, which provides for a more-accelerated transfer of stock to employees. The sponsoring employer of a leveraged ESOP can deduct contributions to repay the principal as well as interest on the debt. This allows the employer to reduce the costs of borrowing and enhance cash flow and debt financing. The contribution limits are increased for employers to allow them to repay any ESOP debt.

Employers are also permitted a tax deduction for dividends paid on ESOP stock to the extent that the dividends are paid to employee participants or are used to reduce the principal or pay interest on an ESOP loan. Certain lenders may exclude from this taxable income 50% of the interest earned on loans made to ESOPs for the purpose of acquiring shares.

UNDER WHAT CIRCUMSTANCES CAN A SHAREHOLDER DEFER INCOME TAXES ON THE SALE OF EMPLOYEE SECURITIES TO AN ESOP?

An additional ESOP incentive, provided by the 1984 Tax Reform Act, allows shareholders of a closely held company to sell their stock to the company's ESOP and defer all taxes on the gain from the sale.

For shareholders to qualify for this so-called ESOP rollover, the ESOP must own at least 30% of the company's stock immediately after the sale, and the shareholder must reinvest the proceeds from the sale in "qualified replacement property"—generally, the stocks and bonds of domestic operating corporations; government securities do not qualify—within a 15-month period beginning 3 months before the date of the sale. The seller, certain relatives of the seller, and 25% shareholders in the company are prohibited from receiving allocations of stock acquired through an ESOP rollover, and the ESOP generally may not sell the stock acquired through a rollover transaction for 3 years.

An ESOP rollover may be attractive to a selling shareholder for a number of reasons. Normally, the owner of the stock in a closely held company may either sell his or her shares back to the company, if such a transaction is feasible; sell to another company or individual, if a willing buyer can be found; or exchange a controlling block of stock with another company. Rolling over the same stock to the company's ESOP, on the other hand, allows the stockholder to sell all or only a part of his or her stock and defer taxes on the gain. In addition to the favorable tax treatment, selling to an ESOP also preserves the company's independent identity, whereas other selling options may require transferring control of the company to outside interests. A sale to an ESOP also provides a significant financial benefit to valued employees and can assure the continuation of their jobs. In the case of owners retiring or withdrawing from a business, an ESOP allows them to sell all or just part of the company, and withdraw from involvement with the business as gradually or suddenly as they like.

Employer securities that can be sold to an ESOP for purposes of the tax-free rollover are common stock with the greatest voting and dividend rights, issued by a domestic corporation with no stock outstanding, and readily tradable on an established securities market. In addition, the securities must have been held by the seller for 6 months and must not have been received by the seller in a distribution from a qualified employee-benefit plan or a transfer under an option or other compensatory right to acquire stock granted by or on behalf of the employer corporation.

The seller's gain on a sale of stock to an ESOP will be retained by adjusting the seller's basis in the qualified replacement property. If the replacement securities are held until death, however, a stepped-up basis for the securities is allowed. The tax-free rollover must be elected in writing on the seller's tax return for the taxable year of the sale.

Careful documentation of ESOP rollover transactions is required, and the transactions must conform to regulations developed by the IRS, but if constructed properly, an ESOP rollover can provide significant benefits to the selling shareholder, the employees, and the company itself.

HOW MAY A HOSPITAL EMPLOYEE RECEIVE EMPLOYER SECURITIES?

There are a number of different methods, other than qualified retirement plans, by which stock may be transferred to hospital employees.

The first and simplest method is a *stock bonus,* whereby the employer makes an outright grant of shares to the employee. In this case, the employee immediately owns his or her shares and has full voting and dividend rights. The employee is taxed at ordinary income rates on the full value of the stock when it is received. This sort of arrangement is very beneficial to the employee, since he or she is able to acquire stock for a cost of the income tax payable on receipt of the stock. Of course, cash flow may not be sufficient to support increased income taxes due for noncash compensation. Thus, if the employee receives $10,000 worth of stock, he or she has essentially acquired the stock for $3000, if he or she is in the 30% marginal tax bracket.

The employer may insist that when the shares are granted, the employee satisfies certain conditions either relating to continued employment for a period of time or attainment of certain performance goals. Until the restrictions are met, the shares cannot be sold and remain subject to forfeiture. Using restriction periods ensures that employees will hold their shares and helps to support employee retention. Moreover, because grants can be made contingent on meeting specific goals, employers can create a stronger performance linkage than stock price alone.

As soon as the rights to the stock are not subject to a substantial risk of forfeiture, the employee is subject to ordinary income taxation. The amount to be included in income is the excess of the FMV of the stock at the time it is no longer subject to the risk of forfeiture.

EMPLOYEE-OWNED STOCK WITH RESTRICTIONS

EXAMPLE 4.6

The Olympia Hospital granted stock to one of its executives on July 1, 1998, when the stock is trading at $10 per share. The stock is not freely transferable and must be forfeited if the executive ceases to be employed prior to July 1, 2001. In 2001, the stock is worth $20 per share and the executive is still with the company. The executive ultimately sells the stock in 2015 for $30 per share. The executive is not subject to taxation in 1998, since the stock is subject to a substantial risk of forfeiture and is not freely transferable. In 2001, when the restriction lapsed, the executive recognizes ordinary income of $20 per share. When the executive ultimately sells the stock in 2015 for $30, he recognizes a capital gain of $10.

If the stock had been sold to the executive for $5 per share rather than given as a bonus, the basic analysis would not change. The executive would simply reduce any total gain by the amount paid, and the gain would be $15. This represents the excess of the FMV of the stock at the time of the transfer minus the amount paid.

The following table demonstrates the tremendous economic benefit an employee can realize through such a program.

Advantages of a Straightforward Stock Bonus Plan

Value of shares granted	$50,000		
Years until restrictions lapse	3	5	10
Value (assume 10% growth rate)	$66,125	$87,450	$175,894
Income tax due (assuming 30%)	−19,837	−26,235	−52,768
Economic benefit remaining	$46,288	$61,215	$123,126

A program allowing stock to be purchased at a discount can also provide great advantages to the employee.

Value of shares purchased	$50,000		
Years until exercised	3	5	10
Value (assume 10% growth rate)	$66,125	$87,450	$175,894
Cost of shares = 75%	37,500	37,500	37,500
Taxable portion	28,625	49,950	138,394
Income tax due on compensation (assume 30% rate)	−8588	−14,985	−41,518
Economic benefit remaining	$20,037	$34,965	$96,876

WHAT IS A SECTION 83(b) ELECTION, AND HOW IS IT BENEFICIAL TO AN EMPLOYEE?

Code § 83(b) allows a hospital employee who receives employer stock on a tax-deferred basis to be taxed immediately in the year the stock is transferred, regardless of the presence of a substantial risk of forfeiture. If the employee makes such an election, any subsequent appreciation is not taxable as compensation. Once made, the IRS must approve any change you may want to make. There are several reasons why a taxpayer might want to make such an election.

First, absent a Section 83(b) election, any appreciation in the value of the stock that occurs after transfer will then be subject to ordinary income taxation at the time of vesting for the full amount by which the then-appreciated FMV exceeds the amount paid, if any. If a Section 83(b) election is made, any post-transfer appreciation will not be taxed until the stock is sold and will only be subject to capital-gain taxation on its ultimate sale.

If one expects the restricted property to appreciate substantially before vesting and one plans to hold the property for a long time after it vests, such delay in taxation of the appreciated amount may be a significant benefit. If the taxpayer holds the property until death, any post-transfer appreciation will escape income taxation entirely.

The main disadvantage of the Section 83(b) election is the triggering of current taxation for the excess of FMV (without regard to any restrictions or risk of forfeiture) over the amount paid. In addition, the Code provides that, if a Section 83(b) election is made before the lapse of the restrictions and such property is subsequently forfeited due to the failure to meet the conditions, no deduction can be made.

Furthermore, if a Section 83(b) election is made and the property later declines in value; only a capital loss is allowed. Finally, the employer receives no deduction for any later appreciation before vesting, nor will the company be able to take a deduction in the case of transferred stock on any dividends after the transfer that are paid to the employee. The following example shows the benefit of electing Section 83(b) in certain circumstances.

EXAMPLE 4.7

In 2005, Horizon Hospital Corp., a newly founded and highly promising hospital network, grants restricted stock worth $10,000 to Anne, a senior executive, conditioned upon her remaining with Horizon for the next 5 years. In 2012, when the stock vests, its value is $100,000. Anne has no immediate intention of selling the stock. If she makes a Section 83(b) election on transfer, she will recognize $10,000 of ordinary income for that year, and the subsequent $90,000 of appreciation will be subject to the lower capital-gains rate only if and when she sells the stock. If she does not elect to use Section 83(b), she would not recognize any income for 2005, but, in 2011, she would have recognized ordinary income in the full amount of $100,000.

The election consists of a written statement, mailed to an IRS center where you file your return, within 30 days of the triggering transaction. It must include everything about the transaction.

HOW MAY AN EMPLOYEE ACQUIRE HOSPITAL SECURITIES WITHOUT ANY CURRENT CASH ACTIVITY?

To alleviate cash-flow problems of their employees, hospitals that want their employees to take part in a discounted stock-purchase program may lend the money to the employees to pay any taxes due and any purchase price for the stock.

However, it is important that any such loan be subject to a full recourse liability; if the loan is secured by the stock on a nonrecourse basis, the transaction may be treated as if it was a grant of an option, and thus, there would be no transfer of property until the loan is paid.

The rationale for treatment as an option is that if the property drops in value below the amount of the debt, the employee will not pay the debt and walk away from the property, as he would if he had an option. Thus, until the note is paid, no transfer has occurred. This could negate the effect of a Section 83(b) election.

The following example demonstrates how the use of employer loans, in connection with a Section 83(b) election, can be used to a great advantage to an employee. The employer in the example on Section 83(b) election (above) lends the employee the cash necessary to meet the income-tax liability of the $10,000 grant at 30%, or $3000. The employee gives the employer a promissory note for $3000, bearing interest at 8%. Thus, the employee acquires $100,000 worth of employer stock ownership after 5 years with no out-of-pocket cost at the date of the grant and an interest cost of approximately $1300, payable over 5 years.

Of course, in lieu of making a loan to the employee, the employer can simply agree to give the employee, as a bonus, sufficient cash to cover the tax liability. This is obviously more costly to the employer, as it results in the employee acquiring stock at no out-of-pocket cost.

HOW MAY AN EMPLOYEE PARTICIPATE IN THE EQUITY OF A HOSPITAL WITHOUT OWNING VOTING STOCK?

Many closely held hospitals or healthcare organizations may not wish to transfer actual shares of stock but may wish to give their employees an interest that parallels actual equity ownership. There are two ways to do this: phantom stock plans and stock appreciation rights (SARs).

Phantom Stock Plans

As an alternative to granting an interest in stock or awarding stock options, an employer may establish the so-called phantom stock or shadow stock plan. Under these arrangements, the employee is treated as if he or she had received a certain number of shares of the company stock, but instead of actually issuing shares, the employer establishes an account for the employee. The employer then issues "units" to the employee's account. The number of units that the employee receives under such a contractual arrangement is pegged to the price or value of the company's stock. Once the units have been credited to the employee, the equivalent of dividends on these units are generally paid to the employee and are reinvested to purchase additional units or deferred with interest. The plan normally provides for appropriate adjustment in the value of units if changes are made in the capitalization of the stock with respect to which the units are priced. Benefits under such a plan are usually deferred for a specific period of time or an event such as death or retirement. When benefits are payable, they may be paid in cash, either in a lump sum or installments, or in the form of stock.

Since a phantom stock plan does not require the actual issuance of shares of the employer's stock, it may enable the employer to offer much of the practical benefit of stock ownership without causing dilution of equity, securities law problems as to stock that would otherwise have been issued, or other problems such as risking the loss of S corporation status.

The phantom stock is taxed like any other nonqualified deferred compensation plan. The granting of the phantom stock units is not taxable to the employee. When the cash or stock is distributed to the employee, it is taxed as ordinary income, equal to the amount of cash received or the value of the stock. If the stock distributed is subject to a substantial risk of forfeiture, it will be subject to taxation when such risk lapses in accordance with Code § 83(b).

Hospital SARs

Another alternative to the actual transfer of shares to an employee is the issuance of the so-called SARs. This is a contractual arrangement that, when exercised, entitles an employee to receive, in stock, cash, or a combination of the two, an amount equal to the appreciation in the employer's stock subsequent to the date the SARs were granted (or related to such appreciation, if the SARs are valued higher than the FMV of the stock when the SARs were granted). The grant of SARs does not constitute the constructive receipt of income even though the option is immediately exercisable, because the exercise of the option means that the grantee will not get the benefit of additional appreciation of the stock on which the value of the SARs is based.

Any declarable income with SARs occurs at the sale, not acquisition. Income received from the exercise of SARs is ordinary, and is equal to the amount of cash received or the value of the appreciated stock received. This amount will generally be reportable in the income of the employee in the year of receipt; however, if the SARs are exercised for stock and the stock is subject to a substantial risk of forfeiture, it will be subject to tax when the substantial risk of forfeiture lapses pursuant to Code § 83, as discussed above.

When the SARs are exercised, a deduction is available to the employer.

The income from the SARs is also subject to withholding and employment taxes on the employer and employee. As a practical matter, if the individual is an employee at the time the tax is determined, there will often be very little additional payroll taxes to pay because he or she will already have exceeded the Social Security taxable wage base.

WHAT ARE HOSPITAL STOCK OPTIONS, AND WHY ARE THEY SO POPULAR?

Hospital stock options require a special contractual arrangement that gives employees the right, for a designated period, to purchase stock in their hospital at a set price.

For example, a hospital employer grants to an employee the right, at any time over the next 10 years, to purchase stock of the employer at a price of $10 a share. Thus, if the stock value increases to $20 a share and the employee exercises the option, he will pay $10 for an asset worth $20. On the other hand, if the stock value decreases to $5, the employee simply does not exercise the option and the option lapses. This arrangement allows the employee in effect to enjoy the risk-free benefits of an increase in value without any economic cost.

Stock options are so popular because they offer advantages to both employees and employers. Employees can share in the growth of a company's equity just like a shareholder, but without any immediate cash outlay. They can acquire stock at less than FMV, and, under certain conditions, obtain the economic benefit of the excess of the stock's FMV over the option price without an immediate tax gain (which will be reported only on the subsequent sale of the stock).

Options have simultaneous advantages to employers. First, they can provide incentives to employees without a cash outlay. In fact, the employer receives cash when the employee exercises the option. Also, if properly structured under the current accounting rules, there is no change to the employer's earnings for financial reporting purposes, either on the grant or the exercise of the option.

HOW DO ISOs WORK, AND HOW DO THEY BENEFIT HOSPITAL EMPLOYEES?

There are two basic types of stock options: the nonqualified stock option (NQSO) and statutory stock options. Statutory stock options include incentive stock options (ISOs) and employee stock-purchase plans (ESPPs). ESPPs are discussed below.

An ISO is similar in operation to other compensatory options. However, there are restrictions on how the option may be structured and when the option may be transferred, and there is special income-tax treatment given to both the employee and the employer.

An ISO must satisfy the following statutory requirements:

- The option is granted pursuant to a plan that states the aggregate number of shares that may be issued under options and the employees (or class of employees) eligible to receive options, which are approved by the stockholders of the granting corporation within 12 months before or after the date the plan is adopted.
- The option is granted within 10 years from the date the plan is adopted, or the date the plan was approved by the shareholders, whichever is earlier.
- The option by its terms is not exercisable after the expiration of 10 years from the date it is granted.
- The option price is not less than the FMV of the stock at the time the option is granted.
- The option by its terms is not transferable by the employee (except upon death pursuant to a will or the laws of descent and distribution) and is exercisable only by the employee during his or her lifetime.
- The employee, at the time the option is granted, does not own more than 10% of the total combined voting power of all classes of stock of the corporation, its parent, or its subsidiary.
- The aggregate FMV of the stock for which options may be granted to an employee in the calendar year in which the options are first exercisable may not exceed $100,000, determined as on the date the option is granted. This limitation automatically applies to ISOs

in the order of their grant dates. This does not mean the ISO must be limited to $100,000; rather, to the extent the value of the stock exceeds $100,000 in the year in which it first becomes exercisable, the excess will not be considered as an ISO.
- If an option specifies that it is not an ISO, it will not be treated as one even though it satisfies all of the above requirements.

Under special stock ownership attribution rules, for purposes of the percentage limitations, the employee will be considered as owning the stock owned, directly or indirectly, by or for his or her brothers and sisters (whether by the whole or half-blood), spouse, ancestors, and lineal descendants. Stock owned, directly or indirectly, by or for a corporation, partnership, estate, or trust shall be considered as being owned proportionately by or for its shareholders, partners, or beneficiaries.

Under an ISO, no gain is recognized when the option is granted; nor is any income recognized when it is exercised. Gain is recognized by the employee only upon disposition of the stock, provided the IRS holding period requirement is met. The gain recognized on the disposition is taxed at long-term capital-gains rates. The gain may be taxed as ordinary income if the holding period requirement is not met. The employer is not entitled to any deduction at any time. The difference between the option price and the FMV of the stock at the exercise date is a tax preference and could cause imposition of the alternative minimum tax (AMT).

ECONOMIC BENEFIT OF ISO

EXAMPLE 4.8

Nurse Joyce is granted an option to purchase $50,000 of her hospital employer's stock at a price equal to the FMV of the stock at the date of grant. The economic benefit is shown in the following table:

FMV of the stock when the option is granted	$50,000		
Years until the option is exercised	2	4	9
Value when exercised	$57,500	$76,044	$152,951
Cost of exercising the option	–50,000	–50,000	–50,000
Remaining value of the option	$7500	$26,044	$102,951
Years until the stock is sold	3	5	10
Value when sold (assumed)	$66,125	$87,450	$175,894
Capital gain on sale	16,125	37,450	125,894
Income tax due on capital gain (18-month hold)	–3225	–7490	–25,197
Economic benefit of the option remaining[a]	$12,900	$29,960	$100,697

[a] Value when sold—Income tax due on capital gain.

The favorable income-tax treatment of an ISO is available to the employee only if he or she does not dispose of the shares within 2 years of the date of the grant of the option, or within 1 year after the exercise of the option. This is the IRS-required holding period.

Further, the grantee must be an employee of the granting corporation or its parent or subsidiaries, or of a corporation issuing or assuming a stock option continuously during the period from the day of the granting of the option until 3 months before the option is exercised. Termination of employment may occur up to 1 year before exercised if the grantee of the option is disabled. If the option is exercised after the death of the employee by the decedent's estate or by a person who acquired the right to exercise such option by bequest or inheritance or by operation of law, the holding and employment requirements listed in this paragraph do not apply.

If the employee disposes of the stock received in <2 years from the date the option was granted, or <12 months after the option is exercised and the stock is received, any gain must be reported as ordinary income.

In such a case, however, the employer may be able to claim a deduction equal to the amount of ordinary income reported, whereas ordinarily, the employer would be able to claim no deduction at all.

If an individual who has acquired stock through an ISO disposes of it at a loss (i.e., a price less than the exercise price) within 2 years from the date of the granting of the option, or 1 year from the date of the exercise of the option, the amount includable in the gross income of the individual, and the amount that is deductible from the income of the employer [pursuant to Code § 83(h)] as compensation attributable to the exercise of the option, will not exceed the excess (normally zero) of the amount realized on the disposition over the adjusted basis of the stock.

HOW DO NQSOs WORK, AND HOW DO THEY BENEFIT HOSPITAL EMPLOYEES?

NQSOs are options that do not satisfy the requirements for an ISO or options not granted under a qualified ESPP. Most hospital employee options fit into this category.

When an NQSO is granted to an employee, there is no tax effect at the time of the grant, assuming the option does not have a readily ascertainable FMV. When an NQSO has a readily discernable FMV, the employee must include it as income for the year received. Almost all employee options are nontransferable and therefore, they are not considered to have a readily ascertainable value. Upon exercise of the option, the employee will usually recognize income to the extent of the difference between the FMV of the stock and the option price. However, if the stock received on exercise of the option is subject to a substantial risk of forfeiture, no gain is recognized until the risk lapses. Any future appreciation realized on the stock will be taxed as capital gain at the time the stock is sold. The hospital receives a tax deduction equal to the amount of the gain recognized by the employee on option exercise.

ECONOMIC BENEFIT OF NQSO

EXAMPLE 4.9

Dr. Hilary is granted an option to purchase $50,000 of her hospital employer's stock at a price equal to the FMV of the stock at the date of grant. The economic benefit of the NQSO is shown in the following table:

FMV of the stock when the option is granted	$50,000		
Years until the option exercised	3	5	10
Value when exercised (assume a 10% increase per annum)	$66,125	$87,450	$175,894
Cost of shares	–50,000	–50,000	–50,000
Compensation element	$16,125	$37,450	$125,894
Income tax due on compensation[a]	–4838	–11,235	–37768
Economic benefit remaining[b]	$11,287	$26,215	$88,126

[a] 30% marginal tax bracket.
[b] Value when exercised—Cost of shares—Income tax due on compensation.

Greater flexibility in the pricing, permissible time of exercise, employment status, and other matters are possible with an NQSO than with an ISO or an option granted under a qualified ESPP.

For example, an NQSO could be offered that would permit the grantee to purchase stock at a price of $5 per share even though the stock was worth $10 a share at the date of the grant of the option. The option could be granted to a consultant who was not an employee, and the option could be exercisable for a period in excess of 10 years. None of these terms would be possible with an ISO.

Some companies will grant a "discounted stock option," under which the exercise price is intended to be substantially below the value of the stock at the time of grant. When used, this form of option is typically offered to officers or directors in lieu of bonuses or directors' fees.

For example, suppose the directors' fee for a company was $10,000 per year and the company's stock was selling at $100 per share. At the beginning of the year, the director might be offered the choice of the customary $10,000 directors' fee, or an option to purchase 100 shares of company stock at $5 per share. The advantage to the director of the option is that, assuming no constructive receipt, there will be a deferral of recognition of income until the option is exercised.

IS A HOSPITAL ISO MORE ADVANTAGEOUS THAN AN NQSO?

The difference in tax treatment between an ISO and an NQSO can be crucial in determining which stock option is more advantageous to an employee.

For a designated amount of shares, an ISO is usually more beneficial to a hospital employee than an NQSO. The employee can defer recognition of all gains until he or she sells the shares and can report all of his or her gains at long-term capital-gains rates. The following table shows how an ISO usually provides a greater advantage than an NQSO to an employee exercising the option:

FMV of stock when the option is granted	$50,000		
Years until the option exercised	2	4	9
Value when exercised	$57,500	$76,044	$152,951
Economic benefit remaining[a]			
ISO	$12,900	$29,960	$100,697
NQSO	$11,126	$25,841	$86,867
Difference	$1774	$4119	$13,830

[a] Value when exercised—Exercise cost—Income tax due on sale.

Note that in the above example, the ISO had an option price equal to the FMV at the date of grant.

If the employer is willing to set the option price substantially below the FMV at the date of the grant of the option, the NQSO may be more beneficial, notwithstanding the less-favorable tax treatment.

The following table shows how an NQSO involving a deep discount in the price of the stock may be to the employee's advantage:

FMV of stock when the option is granted	$50,000		
Years until the option exercised	2	4	9
Value when exercised	$57,500	$76,044	$152,951
Cost of exercising the option	−25,000	−25,000	−25,000
Compensation element	$32,500	$51,044	$127,951
Income tax due on compensation	−10,075	−15,824	−39,665
Economic benefit remaining	$22,425	$35,220	$88,286

Since corporate tax rates are currently higher in general than individual tax rates, there may be a net-tax advantage to the corporation and the employee to using an NQSO over an ISO. Since an employer gets no tax deduction for the ISO, the employer may be willing to grant NQSOs consisting of more shares after considering the after-tax cost of the program.

EXAMPLE 4.10

Healthorama Corporation, (a C corporation), grants an NQSO to its employee, Alex, entitling him to purchase 1000 shares of stock at $10 per share, the current price of the stock.

Healthorama simultaneously grants an ISO to another employee, Beth, entitling her also to buy 1000 shares of Healthorama stock at $10 per share. A year later, the stock rises to $20 per share and both Alex and Beth exercise their options in full, receiving $20,000 of stock (not subject to a risk of forfeiture) for $10,000. Alex will recognize $10,000 of ordinary income at that time (taxable at 27%), and Healthorama will be entitled to a $10,000 deduction (at its 34% rate). Thus, there is a net-aggregate tax savings of $700 (Alex's tax of $2700 minus Healthorama's tax of $3400).

If Healthorama was to give $3857 to Alex as a bonus (enough to pay Alex's $2700 tax costs and the additional tax cost to Alex of the bonus), Healthorama would have a total net-tax savings of $4711 (34% of 3857 = 1311, 3400 + 1311 = 4711). Alex would have no net loss (except for the issuance of the stock), and he would pay no net taxes. In contrast, Beth will not recognize any income at the time of exercise, and Healthorama will have no deduction. Subsequent appreciation in Healthorama's stock will be treated as a capital gain to either Alex or Beth on disposition of the stock, assuming that Beth holds the stock for at least a full additional year and meets the other requirements for an ISO.

However, Alex's basis will be $20,000 (the $10,000 paid and the $10,000 recognized as ordinary income when the option was exercised), and Beth's basis will be $10,000 (the $10,000 paid). Thus, if the stock acquired through exercise of NQSO is sold at $20,000, no further gain will be recognized.

HOW ARE EXERCISES OF HOSPITAL STOCK OPTIONS FUNDED?

The holder of a stock option may encounter financial difficulty in exercising the option and holding the stock. Unless the exercise price is nominal, the employee will need funds to purchase the stock, and, if the option is an NQSO, there will be a need for cash to pay the tax on the taxable income in the year of exercise.

The optionee could sell the stock immediately following the exercise of the option under the so-called cashless exercise and sell program. Using this method, an optionee finances the exercise of an option and sells the underlying shares on the same day. By using the optionee's exercise notice as collateral, a brokerage firm can finance the exercise of the option, plus any applicable withholding taxes. As an alternative, the optionee may sell only the number of shares required to cover the costs of the exercise (including withholding taxes and brokerage fees).

The immediate sale of the stock acquired by exercising the option is normally undesirable from the employer's viewpoint, since the employer wants the employee to continue to have the equity interest. Instead, the company might permit the employee to pay the option exercise price with stock already owned, but then grant the employee additional options equal to the number of shares tendered and at an exercise price equal to the value of the stock at the time of such tender.

Suppose an employee owned 1000 shares of the company and had been granted an option to purchase 500 more shares at $10 per share. When the price is $30 per share, the employee exercises the option. The exercise price is paid by transferring 334 shares to the employer. The employer issues the 500 shares resulting from the option and grants an additional 334 shares to the employee, exercisable at $30 per share. This takes the cash bite out of exercising the option (assuming the employee already owns shares), but permits the employee effectively to retain the same equity interest as before. However, it also reduces the potential for the employee to gain on the stock, since the employee will end up with fewer shares than if he or she had used cash to exercise the option.

If an optionee does not have other employer stock available to use in exercising the option, an employer could simply allow the employee to surrender a portion of the option grant as consideration for exercising the remaining shares. This option reduces the potential gains on the stock by reducing the total number of shares held by the employee. An alternative to this method, which is conceptually the same, is the use of SARs issued in tandem with options.

SARs can be granted in connection with stock options. If the SARs are granted in connection with a stock option, cash received on the exercise of the SARs will help the employee pay for the stock when he or she exercises the options.

For example, a key hospital employee might be granted an NQSO to buy 1000 shares of stock and SARs on another 1000. The SARs would entitle the employee to be paid by the company the difference between the FMV of those shares at the time of exercise of the SARs, over the FMV of the stock at the time the SARs were granted, or, to receive that amount in shares of company stock. Thus, if both the stock option and SARs were granted when the stock is $10 per share, and the NQSO is exercised when the FMV is $25 per share, the key employee will have to provide $10,000 to purchase the stock and then must pay tax on ordinary income of $15,000. By exercising the SARs and electing to take $15,000 cash (which will also be taxable), the employee will be better able to afford the cash-flow problems caused by purchase of the stock and the payment of taxes and will, therefore, be more likely to hold the stock.

Sometimes, when a stock option and SARs are issued together, the exercise of the SARs is automatic on the exercise of the stock option, and vice versa. The SARs and the stock option may be issued in tandem so that the exercise of the SARs for cash reduces the amount of stock options that may be exercised. For example, if SARs for 1000 units were issued, and the recipient exercised 750, that recipient could purchase only 250 shares of stock through the stock option. In this case, the SARs can be written to be exercisable in stock, in cash, or in a combination of the two.

The SARs can be issued in conjunction with an ISO (as well as an NQSO) as long as the ISO is not thereby made subject to conditions or granted other rights inconsistent with an ISO.

In some instances, the optionee can finance the exercise of an option and hold the underlying shares through the use of a margin account with a broker.

Again, the hospital may lend the employee the funds necessary to finance the exercise price and any income-tax withholding requirements. It is important to reiterate that the debt must be of full recourse and must bear interest.

Finally, a hospital employer can simply give enough cash to the optionee as a bonus to cover the costs of exercising the option.

WHEN SHOULD HOSPITAL EMPLOYEE OPTIONS BE EXERCISED?

The decision of when to exercise an option depends on whether the employee is going to hold the stock following the exercise, or is going to sell the stock immediately. If the employee intends to sell the stock, then he or she should try to time the exercise so that the stock is at its highest value. If the employee is going to hold the acquired stock for future investment, then he or she should exercise the option as late as possible. The employee thus enjoys all upside potential without any investment and has nothing at risk.

There are two exceptions to the general rule. First, if the rate of dividends is sufficient to cover the financing cost, or is at least equal to other investment returns, then exercise of the options makes sense.

How Dividends Can Affect Decisions about Exercising Stock Options

	NQSO	ISO
Value of stock	$87,450	$87,450
Cost of the option	50,000	50,000
Income tax due on exercise	11,610	0
Total cash cost of exercise	$61,610	$50,000
Annual cost of borrowing at 8%	$4929	$4000
Dividend rate necessary to exceed costs of borrowing	5.6%	4.6%

Second, if the option is an ISO, the potential application of the AMT rules may force the employee to stagger the exercise, as shown in the following table.

How AMT Can Affect Stock Options

	Regular Tax without Exercise	AMT: Exercise 1000 Shares in Year 7	AMT: Exercise 500 Shares in Year 7	AMT: Exercise 500 Shares in Year 8
Adjusted gross income	$175,000	$175,000	$175,000	$175,000
Itemized deductions	−28,000	−23,000	−23,000	−23,000
Exemptions (4)	−10,000	n/a	n/a	n/a
Tax preference[a]	n/a	65,653	32,827	41,500
AMT exemption amount	n/a	−28,087	−36,293	−34,125
Taxable amount	$137,000	$189,566	$148,533	$159,376
Tax	$41,324	$49,579	$38,089	$41,125
AMT due	n/a	8255	None	None
Total tax paid	$41,324	$49,579	$41,324	$41,324

[a] Difference between FMV and option price at the date of exercise [IRC § 56(b)(3)].

HOW DO HOSPITAL ESPPs WORK, AND HOW DO THEY BENEFIT EMPLOYEES AND THEIR HOSPITAL EMPLOYERS?

An ESPP qualified under Code § 423 allows eligible employees to purchase stock of an employer under special tax rules and favorable prices.

An ESPP is intended to benefit virtually all employees, not just exceptional ones or limited groups. Since the granting of options to purchase employer stock under an ESPP cannot discriminate in favor of key employees, usually, the plan will appeal only to an employer who simply wants to provide, as a general benefit of employment, the right to buy employer stock, or believes that owning employer stock will act as an incentive to employees to perform well. A hospital ESPP must meet the following requirements:

- Options may be granted only to employees of the employer corporation, or its parent or subsidiary corporations, to purchase stock in the employer, parent, or subsidiary.
- The stockholders must approve the plan within 12 months before or after the date the plan is adopted.
- The plan must provide that an employee cannot be granted an option if the employee, immediately after the option is granted, owns 5% or more of the total voting power or value of all classes of stock of the employer corporation, or its parent or subsidiary, computed using special attribution rules.
- The plan must require that the options must be granted to all employees on a nondiscriminatory basis. However, the options granted to different employees may bear a uniform relationship to the total compensation or the basic or regular rate of compensation of employees. The plan may also provide for a ceiling on the amount of stock to be purchased by any employee.
- The exercise price must be at least 85% of the FMV of the stock on the date the option is granted.

The broad participation requirements of ESPPs mean that the stock is likely to be widely owned. Problems of marketing the employer stock and the securities problems inherent in issuing shares of stock to a number of employees will probably discourage employers who do not have an established market for their stock, and who do not want to face the securities problems related to public trading in their stock. Both NQSOs and the direct transfer of stock are available to the employer as potentially less cumbersome means of obtaining the results of an ESPP. Since a nonqualified plan is not subject to the restrictions of the qualified plan, normally, the main reason for the employer choosing to implement an ESPP is to gain for the employees the favorable tax consequences of such a plan and thereby create a widespread base of company stock ownership among employees.

On receipt of an option to purchase stock under an ESPP, the employee does not report any income, even though the exercise price of the stock may be less than the FMV at the time; nor will the employee recognize income on the exercise of the option and acquisition of the stock at a subsequent date. Only on disposition of the stock will the employee recognize taxable income. As long as the disposition occurs 2 years or more after the date the option is granted to the employee, and the employee has held the stock at least 12 months after exercising the option, any profit will be treated as capital gains.

There is a minor exception to this favorable tax treatment. Upon disposition of stock purchased under the plan, a portion of the gain will be treated as ordinary income equal to the discount of 0–15%.

HOW CAN "RABBI" AND SECULAR TRUSTS BE USED TO PROVIDE SECURITY AND TO DEFER INCOME TAX ON NONQUALIFIED DEFERRED COMPENSATION CONTRACTS AND PLANS?

An employer may establish a nonqualified deferred compensation contract, which can provide the needed tax and retirement advantages, and in some cases, enable the employer to offer much of the practical benefit of stock ownership. Although they lack the tax advantages of tax-qualified plans, nonqualified deferred compensation arrangements are used today to retain key employees while often permitting the employer greater flexibility than do qualified plans, which are subject to participation, vesting, and funding requirements under the Code and Title I of the Employee Retirement Income and Security Act (ERISA). Since they are not necessarily subject to the funding requirements that apply to qualified plans, nonqualified deferred compensation arrangements may be an attractive option for new businesses with potential but which have limited cash resources.

A traditional reason for establishing a nonqualified deferred compensation plan has been to permit an employee to reduce his or her taxes by deferring payments for service rendered until such time as he or she is in a lower tax bracket.

Nonqualified plans can be found in a variety of forms. They may offer hospital employees an opportunity to elect to defer the current compensation or provide for additional deferred compensation contingent upon the employee's remaining with the employer for a certain length of time, and perhaps on meeting certain performance goals. Benefits under such agreements may, for example, be expressed in specific dollar amounts, correlated with other compensation, or related to the value of the employer's stock. Nonqualified deferred compensation plans may provide for retirement payments that supplement retirement income provided by a qualified retirement plan—which is particularly important with the increasing cutbacks in such tax-favored plans in benefits for the highly compensated.

Thus, the trade-off for deferral for the employee is that the amounts due from the employer remain subject to some risk.

RABBI TRUSTS

To help provide some additional security for the hospital employee, and at the same time defer taxation, an employer may establish the so-called Rabbi trust to hold the assets set aside to meet its obligations under a deferred compensation arrangement. Such a trust simply restricts the use of the funds solely to meeting its obligations to the employee, and rights to benefits under the trust cannot be sold, transferred, assigned, or otherwise alienated. However, if the employer should be bankrupt or insolvent, the trust assets will be subject to the claims of the employer's creditor.

To provide additional security for an employee will result in the arrangement being considered "funded" for tax purposes and therefore taxable to the employee when set aside.

SECULAR TRUSTS

A secular trust is typically an irrevocable trust designed so that creditors of the hospital employer, including bankruptcy creditors, cannot attach its funds. Consequently, the employer's contributions to an irrevocable trust, often means the trust's earnings are taxable income to the employee. Benefits are normally payable to the employee upon the occurrence of specific events, such as the passage of a certain number of years, retirement, disability, or death. Since they protect against a loss of benefits if the employer becomes insolvent, secular trusts may be preferred to Rabbi trusts by executives.

If corporate tax rates exceed an individual's tax rate, and if the employee is regarded as the grantor of the trust, secular trusts can produce a tax savings in comparison to Rabbi trusts.

For example, if a corporation's marginal tax rate is 34% and an individual's marginal tax rate is 30%, then for each $1000 of income that the corporation contributes to the trust, the corporation receives a deduction of $340 while the individual pays tax of $300. An employer may also pay an additional bonus to cover the taxes owed by the individual. The net effect on the corporation is about the same as if it had received no deduction and was in the 34% tax bracket.

In contrast, if a Rabbi trust is used, the corporation does not get a current deduction, but rather pays tax of $340 on each $1000 of income. Once the taxpayer includes the contribution in his or her income, the corporation gets a deduction—but until that occurs—the earnings on past contributions are taxed at a rate of 34%. If the employee is not treated as the grantor of the trust, the tax results are much less clear. In such cases, it is possible that a secular trust will result in a greater total tax burden than a Rabbi trust.

SECULAR ANNUITIES

A secular annuity is an alternative to a secular trust. One approach that is sometimes used is for the hospital to purchase single-premium deferred annuities to fund executive benefits that accrue during the year. The executive receives ownership of the annuity, and income earned on amounts contributed to secular annuities is postponed until such amounts are distributed.

A hospital employee is taxed on the value of the annuity contract when his rights under the contract are no longer subject to a substantial risk of forfeiture [IRC § 403(c)]. Although the employee is taxed on the amount of premium payments made by the employer, the employer can make supplemental cash payment to cover the tax. If the rights of an employee become substantially vested, the value of the annuity contract on the date of the change is included in the employee's gross income.

EMPLOYEE BENEFITS LIABILITY INSURANCE

As we have seen, virtually, each medical practice, hospital, or healthcare facility has employee non-cash benefits in addition to their payroll. These benefits usually include group insurance and some form of retirement plan (e.g., 403(b)).

However, each of these benefit packages exposes the employer to liabilities under state and federal statutes. Employee benefits liability insurance covers an employer, or if so stipulated by some policies, the employees who act on behalf of the employer, against liability claims involving alleged errors or omissions, or improper advice or administration of the employee fringe benefit plans.

For example, an employer may be liable for not enrolling an employee on a timely manner resulting in no medical coverage. Frequent litigation also arises out of violations of the ERISA of 1974. Since 1974, the provisions and reach of this act has become massive and errors can occur.

Assessment

Voluntary health benefits market by the seller:

- Benefits brokers 55%
- Career agents 21%
- Traditional worksite brokers 14%
- Enrollment companies 8%
- Occasional producer 2%[5]

CONCLUSION

This chapter examined hospital employee benefits from the perspective of all stakeholders. If available, from a public hospital, stock options allow employees to benefit from appreciation without having to expend cash to purchase shares upon receipt.

COLLABORATE

Discuss this chapter online with others at www.MedicalExecutivePost.com.

ACKNOWLEDGMENTS

To the late LaVerne L. Dotson, JD, CPA; Thomas P. McGuiness, CPA, CVA of Reimer, McGuinness & Associates, PC in Houston, Texas; and Thomas Bucek, CPA, CVA in Houston, Texas.

SAMPLE NEW PHYSICIAN LETTER OF EMPLOYMENT INTENT

Dear Dr. *(Name of Physician)*

On behalf of [Name of medical practice or clinic] (hereinafter called the "practice"), this letter sets out a proposed agreement for your initial employment in Dr. [Name of physician]'s medical practice. After both you and Dr. [Name of physician] have agreed upon all issues related to your employment, a formal physician employment agreement will be prepared for your review and signature.

1. *Term:* You will be an employee of the practice for an initial [Duration]-month period starting [Month, Date, and Year]. Should you and the practice want to proceed past this initial employment period, an offer of co-ownership may be made to you as described in item 9 below.

    Your employment with the practice will essentially be "at will," since you or the practice may voluntarily terminate it at any time upon 30 days' written notice to the other. However, the following are the conditions under which the practice may terminate your employment immediately: (a) upon your death or disability for three (3) consecutive months; (b) upon the suspension, revocation, or cancelation of your right to practice medicine in the State of [State]; (c) if you should lose privileges at any hospital at which the practice regularly maintains admission privileges; (d) should you fail or refuse to follow reasonable policies and directives established by the practice; (e) should you commit an act amounting to gross negligence or willful misconduct to the detriment of the practice or its patients; (f) if you are convicted of a crime involving moral turpitude, including fraud, theft, or embezzlement; and (g) if you breach any of the terms of your employment contract.

2. *Compensation:* Your salary for the initial 12-month period will be $[dollar value] and $[dollar value] in the second 12-month period, each year payable in monthly installments. You will also be entitled to an incentive bonus calculated as follows: [Percentage]% of your collected production when such collections exceed $[dollar value] in the first year and $[dollar value] in the second year. The bonus each year will be calculated and paid on a semiannual basis. You will also be entitled to receive a one-time signing bonus of $[dollar value] if you sign your employment contract before [Month, Date, and Year].

    A portion of your compensation may be paid for by proceeds received from [Name of hospital] under the terms and conditions of a hospital recruitment agreement. The parties to this agreement will be the hospital and the practice only. However, forgiveness of any advances made by the hospital will be directly contingent upon the length of time you remain with the practice. Therefore, should your employment terminate for any reason, the practice will require you to repay to it any amounts the practice repays the hospital, in no matter what form, as per the terms and conditions in the hospital recruitment agreement. (Note: Use this if the practice signs a hospital recruitment agreement with the hospital.)

3. *Benefits:* In addition to your base compensation and incentive bonus, the practice will pay for the following: (a) health insurance, (b) malpractice insurance, (c) continuing medical education (CME) costs, (d) medical license fee, (e) board certification exam fee, (f) reasonable cellular phone costs, and (g) a pager. You will also be entitled to a moving-cost allowance for relocating to [Location]. You will be entitled to 2 weeks of paid vacation, 10 working days as paid sick leave, and 4 days paid time off for CME or the board certification exam.

4. *Disability leave:* In case of absence because of your illness or injury, your base salary will continue for a period not exceeding 30 days per calendar year, plus any unused vacation time and sick leave. You will be entitled to any incentive bonus payments that may be due to you as collections are received on your prior production. Absence in excess of 30 days would be without pay. Unused sick leave cannot be carried over to succeeding years, nor will it be paid for at any time.

5. *Exclusive employment:* As an employee, you will be involved full time in the practice and you may not take any outside employment during the term of your employment agreement without the practice's written approval. However, you will be entitled to keep compensation from honorariums, royalties, and copyrights if approved by the practice in writing. If the practice does not give approval, then the income from such activities shall remain the property of the practice.

6. *Termination compensation:* Should your employment terminate for any reason, you will be entitled to accrued but unpaid base compensation, earned but unpaid incentive bonus, and unused vacation leave.

7. *Nonsolicitation:* During the course of your employment, the practice will introduce and make available to you its contacts and referring physician relationships, ongoing patient flow, general hospital sources, business and professional relationships, and the like. Since you have not been in private practice in the area previously, you acknowledge that you currently have no established patients following you. If there should be a termination, the practice will not restrict your ability to practice medicine in the area; however, it will require you to enter into a nonsolicitation agreement in which you agree not to solicit the employees of the practice nor its patients to follow you into your new medical practice. (Note: Insert covenant not to compete here, if applicable.)

8. *Employee-only status:* During the term of your employment, you will not be required to contribute any money toward the practice's equipment or operations, but likewise, your work will give you no financial interest in the assets of the practice. However, the practice intends to offer you the opportunity to buy into the ownership of the practice as set forth in item 9 below.

9. *Ownership opportunity:* At the end of your employment period, the practice will evaluate your relationship and may offer you the opportunity to become a co-owner in the practice (or enter into an office-sharing relationship). This offer is not mandatory and is at the total discretion of the practice. Should an offer not be tendered for some reason, the practice will wait until the end of your next 12-month employment period to decide whether to tender an offer of co-ownership. If an offer of co-ownership is made, Dr. [Name of physician] will discuss with you the following: (a) what percentage of the practice you will be allowed to acquire, (b) how best to value such interest, and (c) how you will pay for the acquisition of such interest. The practice hopes to achieve mutually agreeable solutions to these ownership issues.

We hope this offer meets with your approval. If so, please contact Dr. [Name of physician] as soon as possible. This letter is not intended to be a legally binding agreement; it is, rather, a tool to be used to prepare your formal physician employment agreement. If you should have any questions, please do not hesitate to contact myself or Dr. [Name of physician] at your convenience.

Sincerely,
Atlantic Physicians Group
Medical Group Practice, LLC
Lantana, Florida

REFERENCES

1. http://www.irs.gov/publications/p503/index.html.
2. http://www.irs.gov/instructions/i8839/ch02.html.
3. http://www.irs.gov/newsroom/article/0,id=200505,00.html.
4. http://www.irs.gov/newsroom/article/0,id=187833,00.html.
5. Employee benefit advisor, March 2013.

5 Basic Concepts of Personal Financial Planning
Revising Economic Principles for the New Normal

David Edward Marcinko and Hope Rachel Hetico

CONTENTS

In 1972, Nobel Laureate Kenneth J. Arrow, PhD, shocked academe by identifying health economics as a separate and distinct field. Yet, the seemingly disparate insurance, tax, risk management, and financial planning principles that he also studied are just now becoming transparent to some medical professionals and their financial advisors, despite the fact that a basic, but hardly promoted, premise of this new wave financial planning era is imprecision.

Nevertheless, to informed cognoscenti like Certified Medical Planners™, the principles served as predecessors to the modern physician-focused financial advisory niche sector. In 2004, Arrow was selected as one of eight recipients of the National Medal of Science for his innovative views.

And now, as a three-decade-long bull market in bonds and equities is over, and if the current "new-normal" prevails—meaning a 4.5% real annualized rate of return on equities and a 1.5% real rate on bonds—wealth accumulation for all may be reduced.

AN IMPRECISE SCIENCE

There is a major variable, dominant in any marketplace, that pushes an economy in a forward direction. It is called *consumerism*. This became apparent while waiting in a doctor's office one recent afternoon.

SCENARIO

The front office receptionist, who appeared to be about 21 years old, was breaking for lunch and her replacement, and who appeared not much older, came over to assist. Realizing the propensity for a long wait, one was taken by the size of the waiting room and the number of patients coming in and going out of the office. (Americans consume healthcare and a lot of it.) There was another notable peculiarity. The sample prescription bags being carried out of the door were no match for the bags under everyone's eyes, including the doctor's. The office staff was probably working overtime, if not two jobs, and the doctor was working harder and faster in a managed care system.

Why? So that they all could afford to buy and voraciously consume for their children and themselves. Americans indeed work longer hours than any other industrialized nation.

Additionally, female medical professionals entered the workforce in unprecedented numbers, and the stock markets reached an all-time high in 2014, even as money was spent at a feverish pace as the Federal Reserve pumped out money in inflammatory fashion.

INTRODUCTION

In the medical space, a study by the Kaiser Permanente Foundation in California reported that doctors there chose to work 4 h longer each week rather than take a 10% pay cut. Consumerism is what keeps economies alive and well. What a perfect way to describe medical and healthcare professionals, sans most basic economic fundamentals of modern financial planning.

WHY DOCTORS DON'T GET RICH

> Physicians have a significantly low propensity to accumulate substantial wealth.
>
> **Thomas Stanley—Author,** *The Millionaire Next Door*
> (*New York Times*)

How come doctors fail to get rich? Re-read the above!

The Institute of Medical Business Advisors Inc. identified several reasons based on observations working with medical professionals and physician clients over the years.

A LATE START

By the time doctors finish medical school and residency they're typically in their mid- or late thirties. Many have families to feed, and substantial student loans to pay off. It will be years before they can even start accumulating wealth. Consider that physicians typically enter careers at later ages, often with larger debts from training. Some specialties may not lead a medical case until gaining 10 years of practice, and many specialties have limited longevity. Peak earning years may also be shorter for healthcare providers than other professionals. Financial survival skills are paramount for converting the limited earnings time period into personal financial security.

Challenging Sociopolitical Environment

It is increasingly challenging to practice medicine. With the Medicare Trust Fund slated to go bust in 2019, the Center for Medicare and Medicare Service (CMS) is increasingly resorting to cutting physician reimbursements and implementing capitation and bundled value-based medical payments models. The medical reimbursement effects of the Patient Protection-Affordable Care Act (PP-ACA) are not yet fully discerned, but appear to continue the decline in compensation. And to illustrate this potential governmental control, in what other industry can participants debate the simple question "Who is the customer?"

Lifestyle Expectations

Society expects a doctor to live like a doctor, dress like a doctor, and drive like a doctor. Meeting social expectations can be quite expensive.

Time and Energy

A doctor can't be just a doctor any more. S/he also has to deal with ever-increasing regulatory mandates, paperwork requirements by state and federal agencies, and capricious insurance companies. It is estimated that for every hour spent on patient care, an additional half-hour is spent on paperwork. To date, the use of electronic medical records has exacerbated, not ameliorated this problem. The demand on their time is mind-boggling. A typical doctor works a 10–12 h a day. After work and family, they simply don't have time and energy left to do comprehensive financial planning.

Financially Naive

Doctors are smart. They're highly trained in their area of expertise. But that doesn't translate into understanding about finance or economics. Because they are smart, it's easy for them to think they can easily master and execute concepts of personal financial planning, as well. Often, they don't.

Lack of Trust and Delegation

Many doctors don't trust financial advisors working for major Wall Street banks. They have the good instinct to realize that their interests are not aligned. Not knowing there are independent advisors out there who observe a strict fiduciary standard, they tend to do everything by themselves.

In fact, Paul Larson, CFP®, president-CEO of the firm Larson Financial Group LLC, noted a disquieting trend among physician clients in his firm (personal communication). Almost 90% of them fail to take care of their own family finances in a comprehensive manner, while only 10% are succeeding at it. The strategies in this chapter and book are common to their success.

Too Trusting

Another aspect of naivety is that many physicians do not realize that the financial advisory industry lacks the same discipline and regulation that the average physician operates in. A primary care doctor would never even attempt a complicated surgery on a patient, but is trained to refer such patients to a specialist in the field with the proper training and experience. Financial advisors often come from a sales background and are trained to keep a client in house even if the advisor is lacking in expertise. Also, many physicians are not trained to discern a qualified financial advisor from a sales person dressed up like a financial advisor. It is illegal to call yourself a physician in the United States unless you have the credentials to back it up, yet, anyone in the United States can legally call themselves a financial advisor or a financial planner.

BASIC MACROECONOMIC CONCEPTS

Money lending, or extending credit, is probably one of the oldest professions. It precedes the creation of currency. It wasn't long ago that the term "usury" was used to describe the charging of interest on borrowed money. Today it is associated with an unlawful rate of interest. The usury rate is the maximum rate that may be charged for loans made by nonregulated lenders. That rate is measured by the average coupon on Treasury Bills maturing within 6 months. The rate is calculated and disclosed on the last day of each month by the Treasury commissioner.

FEDERAL RESERVE ACTIVITIES

The price of the commodity "money" is its interest rate. There are two types of short-term interest rates: the *discount rate* is what the Federal Reserve System (Janet L. Yellen, PhD, Chair of the Board of Governors the Federal Reserve) charges member banks, and the Federal Funds rate is what the member banks charge each other. A third rate, known as the prime rate, is what banks charge to their most creditworthy clients. Be aware, however, that the law of supply and demand determines long-term interest rates, not the Federal Reserve banking stem.

Perhaps the most vital functions of the Federal Reserve itself includes keeping member banks afloat; providing a system of check collecting and clearance; supplying member banks with paper currency reserve balances; supervising and regulating member banks; and regulating the supply of money and credit. The Federal Open Market Committee (FOMC) achieves these short-term goals in the following two ways:

1. By decreasing the overall money supply, the Federal Reserve sells government securities, forcing member banks to pay for them with dollars. This shrinks free reserves and the capability of banks to supply funds to personal and business owners, such as medical professionals. The borrowed money ultimately leaves the money supply. This is called a tight or contractionary monetary policy.
2. By increasing the overall money supply, the Federal Reserve buys government securities, paying banks with dollars. This expands free reserves and the capability of banks to supply funds to personal and business borrowers, such as medical professionals. The money ultimately enters the money supply. This is the easy or expansionary money policy that exists today.

Of course, the ability to make new loans and increase the money supply is controlled by FOMC reserve requirements. For example, an increase in the reserve requirement lowers free reserves, reduces the ability to borrow, and is contractionary. On the other hand, a decrease in the reserve requirements raises free reserves and is the environment that now exists.

EXAMPLE 5.1

Total of all bank reserves	$50,000 MM
Required reserves	49,400 MM
Excess reserves	600 MM
Reserves borrowed from FOMC	300 MM
"Free" reserves	300 MM

1. Reserves = percentage of deposits banks must keep on hand
2. An increase in reserves multiplies the money banks can lend
3. A 20% reserve requirement means $5 to loan for every $1
4. Bank loans create new deposits and increase the money supply
5. Banks borrow from the FOMC to meet reserve requirements
6. But only "free" reserves are available to create new loans

Therefore, reserves drive deposits, as indicated by the various money supply measures. If the FOMC removes additional reserves, this extraction could begin a painful contraction process as interest rates rise, potentially causing stock market prices to fall.

MONEY SUPPLY MEASURES

M1 = demand deposits (checking accounts) + money in circulation (cash and coins), plus NOW (negotiated order of withdrawal) accounts.

M2 = is the most reliable measure of money supply. It equals M1 plus savings accounts + money market accounts (4 × M1). Of course, since equity investors have decided that holding cash is unwise in a bull market, valuations may rise but not much purchasing power is leftover for consumption.

M3 = M2 + other large financial institutions and large time deposits.

VELOCITY OF MONEY

The velocity of money is the rate of circulation in the money supply. The more often money changes hands, the greater the level of commerce. The velocity of money is determined by money supply, interest rates, inflation, commerce, and the Federal Reserve. Medical professionals, like most consumers, tend to hold less money as interest rates and inflation increase, and therefore, the velocity of money increases. Velocity is reduced when people increase their money holdings. This occurs in periods of low interest rates and low inflation; the opposite occurs when rates and inflation are high.

MONETARY AND FISCAL POLICIES

Government intervention attempts to bring a social and economic justice to a system that tends to distribute its resources efficiently, in the manner which supply and demand naturally creates. Democracy and capitalism work as countermeasures within our economic system. Economic policies can have a dramatic effect on financial planning results for the medical professional, and it is important to understand them in order to position investments accordingly.

By controlling interest rates and the money supply, the Federal Reserve Board tries to entice or suppress the consumption spending in the economy. In some cases, monetary policy is designed to stimulate the economy, thereby avoiding a recession. In other cases, it is designed to suppress economic growth and slow down or lower inflationary pressures.

Congress, on the other hand, controls taxes and government spending. Congress and the president are not always in agreement with the Federal Reserve Board. For example, after the Great Depression of the 1930s, Congress believed that deficit spending would revitalize the depressed economy. In 1936, John Maynard Keynes introduced the concept of demand-side economic policy. The government would become the ultimate consumer and therefore push up the systems capability for production. This would increase employment and wages, and push the economy forward. This pump-priming policy was used to solve a demand-side problem. When inflation occurred, the government would enact policies to retard the economic system, thereby suppressing inflation. This did not work in the 1970s when monetary manipulation, combined with government's fiscal stimulus, actually caused inflation to increase.

Tax policies were also used to achieve economic justice. Congress could stimulate the economy by striving for certain social initiatives. Hence, the marginal income tax rates (MITR), which became progressively higher with higher incomes, allowed tax payers to only keep the percentage of income that was left over, and above, their tax rate (1–MITR), or $(1 - 28\% = 0.72)$, for example. This redistribution of wealth was seen as fair and a way to stimulate growth. With the 1970s only a memory, Congress adopted a new fiscal strategy that later became known as supply-side economics. Congress needed to boost productivity capacity and proceeded to cut income taxes. The idea was that the prevailing high tax rates were creating a disincentive to invest, save, and produce. It was later found that although tax rates were lower, tax revenues increased. Because after-tax revenue was now higher, this created an incentive to work harder and longer. Lower taxes were levied on greater revenue, thereby increasing tax receipts.

The tax acts of 1993, 2001, and 2013–2014 put a damper on supply-side economics by increasing/decreasing the marginal tax rates on income and the capital gains rates. Going forward today, rates seem poised to rise as medical professional and physician financial wellness may yet be determined by actions taken in response to upcoming monetary and fiscal policies, by political fiat.

Major Economic Theories

The above policies led to the development of the two dominant economic theories today.

Monetarists

Monetarists believe the FOMC reserve should not be used to influence the business cycle or economy. Money supply is believed to be the prime mover of the U.S. economy. Monetarists control demand and money becomes more or less expensive, in relation to domestic or foreign markets via the International Monetary Fund (IMF).

INTERNATIONAL TRANSACTIONS VIA INTERNATIONAL MONETARY FUND

Money leaving the United States	Money coming into the United States
The United States purchases foreign currency	Foreign purchases of U.S. currency
Current account payments by the United States	Current account payments to the United States
Goods and services imports	Goods and services exports
Merchandise trade imports	Merchandise trade exports
Service payments	Service fees
Foreign aid payments	Foreign aid receipts
Capital account outflows	Capital account inflows
U.S. private investments abroad	Foreign investments in the United States
Central bank debt	Central bank credit

STRONGER U.S. $ DOLLARS = MORE EXPENSIVE GOODS/SERVICES

Example #1: To illustrate how foreign currency exchange rate fluctuations may affect consumer purchasing power, consider the example of auto aficionado, Dr. M. Rappaport, whose auto dealer contracted to import 20 BMWs, each at a price of 40,000 German marks. If the current exchange rate was 2 marks per U.S. dollar, upon placement of an order, the dealer told Dr. Rappaport to expect to pay about $20,000 for a car. Dr. Rappaport agreed to pay upon delivery, 3 months later. However, the exchange rate fell to 1.5 marks per dollar, and the BMW now costs Dr. R. about $26,666. Of course, if the price of a dollar, in terms of the mark were to rise, the cost in dollars would fall. Fortunately, currency risk may be mitigated somewhat by forward transactions in which traders purchase marks at a fixed price for delivery 1–3 months in the future.

Example #2: Another illustration of currency fluctuations occurs when dealing with American Depository Receipts. An ADR represents individual foreign shares of a company that are held by a custodian bank. They are available from the NYSE, AMX, or NASDAQ, and may be either sponsored or unsponsored. The former provide American style financial information, while the latter do not.

KEYNESIANS

Keynesians believe the FOMC should be used to influence the business cycle or economy. Supply and demand is the prime mover of the U.S. domestic economy. Fiscal policy uses spending and taxes to control supply.

GROSS DOMESTIC AND NATIONAL PRODUCTS

Gross domestic product (GDP) and gross national product (GNP) are measures of the total amount of money changing hands. GDP is the dollar value of all goods and services produced during 1 year. GDP is a measure of a country's productivity when shown on a per capita basis. To get this number, divide GDP by the number of productive workers in the country. It does not include income earned by workers overseas.

In December 1991, the Bureau of Economic Analysis began using GDP instead of GNP, as the primary measure of U.S. production. The GNP measures output of all multinational companies that are U.S.-owned, where the profits are expected to return. In GDP, the profits are attributed to the country where the product is produced or located, even though profits would eventually wind up in the country that owns the factory. It includes the manufacture of tangible personal property such as vehicles, durable medical equipment, furniture, bread, and services used in daily living such as education, healthcare, and auto repair. The accounting shift facilitates comparisons between the United States and other countries, which is the standard used in international commerce accounting. Other important definitions, for medical professionals, include

Current (medical) dollar GNP (nominal GNP) is slightly different and uses medical service values. It measures changes in actual physician production.

Constant (medical) dollar GNP (real GNP) is adjusted for medical inflation and uses an implicit price deflator (index) to arrive at a realistic inflationary adjustment.

CONSUMER PRICE INDEX AND PRODUCER PRICE INDEX

There are various indices to track economic growth. The consumer price index (CPI) is a measure of the average change, over time, in the prices paid by urban consumers for a predetermined market basket of consumer goods and services from A to Z. It is the most commonly used economic indicator of inflation. However, it is not to be confused with the cost-of-living index (CLI). The CPI is an index of price changes only. For example, the CPI would exclude income taxes and social security taxes. The Bureau of Labor Statistics (BLS) chooses over 200 specific items within selected business establishments. One of the items measured is the average fee to visit a doctor's office.

The BLS set the base average index level for the CPI using the 36-month period from 1982 to 1984. That period is said to have a base of 100. Changes are measured in relation to this base figure. The index level for March 2000, for example, was 168.2. This means that there was a sixty-eight and one fifth-percent increase in average price since the base period.

Chained CPI

An alternative for the CPI was recently introduced to remove the biases associated with new products, changes in quality, and discounted prices. The chain-weighted CPI incorporates the average changes in the quantity of goods purchased along with standard pricing effects. This allows the chain-weighted CPI to reflect situations where customers shift the weight of their purchases from one area of spending to another. The chain-weighted CPI incorporates changes in both the quantities and prices of products.

For example, let's examine clothing purchases between 2 years. Last year, you bought a sweater for $40 and two t-shirts at $35 each. This year, two sweaters were purchased at $35 each and one t-shirt for $45.

Standard CPI calculations would produce an inflation level of 13.64%.

$$((1 \times 35 + 2 \times 45)/(1 \times 40 + 2 \times 35)) = 1.1364$$

The chain-weighted approach estimates inflation to be 4.55%.

$$((2 \times 35 + 1 \times 45)/(1 \times 40 + 2 \times 35)) = 1.0455$$

Using the chain-weighted approach reveals the impact of a customer purchasing more sweaters than t-shirts.

BLS began publishing the chained CPI for all urban consumers effective with the release of July 2002 CPI data. Designated the C-CPI-U, the index supplements the existing indexes already produced by the BLS: the *CPI for All Urban Consumers (CPI-U)* and the *CPI for Urban Wage Earners and Clerical Workers (CPI-W)*.

The C-CPI-U employs a formula that reflects the effect of substitution that consumers make. Traditionally, the CPI was considered an upper bound on a CLI in that the CPI did not reflect the changes in consumption patterns that consumers make in response to changes in relative prices. Since January 1999, a geometric mean formula has been used to calculate most basic indexes within the CPI; this formula allows for a modest amount of substitution within item categories as relative price changes.

The geometric mean formula, though, does not account for consumer substitution taking place between CPI item categories.

For example, pork and beef are two separate CPI item categories. If the price of pork increases while the price of beef does not, consumers might shift away from pork to beef. The C-CPI-U is designed to account for this type of consumer substitution between CPI item categories. In this example, the C-CPI-U would rise but not by as much as an index that was based on fixed purchase patterns.

With the geometric mean formula in place to account for consumer substitution within item categories, and the C-CPI-U designed to account for consumer substitution between item categories, any remaining substitution bias would be quite small.

Many policymakers and economists believe that C-CPI-U is a more accurate index than CPI for calculating the changes in the cost of living from inflation. However, a backlash by federal entitlement recipients and other benefits tied to CPI fear that that C-CPI-U will produce smaller benefit checks and protest the adoption to the new standard.

Producer Price Index

The PPI is a group of indexes that measure the change, over time, in the prices received by domestic producers of goods and services. It measures price changes from the perspective of the seller rather than the consumer, as with the CPI. The CPI would include imported goods, while the PPI is relevant to U.S. producers, and therefore would not include imports. The PPI measures over 10,000 products and services. It reports the price changes prior to the retail level. This information is useful to the government in formulating fiscal and monetary policies. The data gathered from the PPI is often used in escalating purchase and sales contracts. That is the dollar amount to be paid at some time in the future. Long-term managed medical care contracts of the future will seek escalation clauses for increases in prices.

THE BUSINESS CYCLE

The business cycle is also known as the economic cycle and reflects the expansion or contraction in economic activity. Understanding the business cycle and the indicators used to determine its phases may influence investment or economic business decisions and financial or medical planning expectations. Although often depicted as the regular rising and falling of an episodic curve, the business cycle is very irregular in terms of amplitude and duration. Moreover, many elements move together during the cycle and individual elements seldom carry enough momentum to cause the cycle to move. However, elements may have a domino effect on one another, and this ultimately drives the cycle. We can also have a large positive cycle, coincident with a smaller but still negative cycle, as seen in the current healthcare climate of today.*

1. *First phase:* Trough to recovery (production driven)
   Scenario: A depressed GNP leads to declining industrial production and capacity utilization. Decreased workloads result in improved labor productivity and reduced labor (unit) costs until actual producer (wholesale) prices decline.
2. *Second phase:* Recovery to expansion (consumer driven)
   Scenario: CPI declines (due to reduced wholesale prices) and consumer real income rises, improving consumer sentiment and actual demand for consumer goods.
3. *Third phase:* Expansion to peak (production driven)
   Scenario: GNP rises leading to increased industrial production and capacity utilization. But labor productivity declines and unit labor costs and producer (wholesale) prices rise.
4. *Fourth phase:* Peak to contraction (consumer driven)
   Scenario: CPI rises making consumer real income and sentiment erode until consumer demand, and ultimately purchases, shrink dramatically. Recessions may occur and economists have an alphabet used to describe them. For example, with a V, the drop and recovery is quick. For U, the economy moves up more sluggishly from the bottom. A W is what you would expect: repeated recoveries and declines. An L shaper recession describes a prolonged dry economic spell or even depression.

BULL AND BEAR MARKETS

A bull market is generally one of rising stock prices, while a bear market is the opposite. There are usually two bulls for every one bear market over the long term. More specifically, a bear market is defined as a drop of 20% or more in a market index from its high, and can vary in duration and severity. While a bull market has no such threshold requirement to exist other than they exist between these two periods of sharp decline.

WHITHER THE BEAR?

As a doctor, your action plan in a bear market depends on many variables, with perhaps your age being the most important.
  In your 30s

- Pay off debts, school loan or practice loan

---

* Historically, contractions have had a shorter duration than expansions.

- Invest in safe money market mutual funds, cash, or CDs
- Start retirement plan or 401(k) account

In your 40s

- Increase your pension plan or 401(k) contributions
- Stay weighted more toward equity investments
- Review your goals, risk tolerance, and portfolio

In your 50s

- Position assets for ready cash instruments
- Diversify into stock, bonds, and cash

In retirement

- Maintain 3 years of ready cash living expenses
- Reduce but still maintain your exposure to equities

ECONOMIC INDICATORS

There are 12 leading, 6 lagging, and 4 coincidental indicators for the U.S. economy. As seen in the table below, their purpose is to help evaluate which period of the business cycle is in play.

Leading Economic Indicators:
1. Average workweek for manufacturing production workers
2. Layoff rate in manufacturing
3. New orders for consumer goods
4. Vendor performance and slow/on-time deliveries
5. New business formation
6. New building permits for private housing[a]
7. Contracts and orders for plants and equipment
8. Net changes in inventories
9. Change in sensitive prices
10. Change in total liquid assets
11. Stock prices
12. Money supply

Coincidental Economic Indicators:
1. Employees on nonagricultural payrolls
2. Personal income
3. Industrial production
4. Manufacturing and trade sales

Lagging Economic Indicators:
1. Average duration of unemployment
2. Manufacturing and trade inventories
3. Labor costs per unit of output
4. Average bank prime interest rates
5. Commercial and industrial loans outstanding
6. Ration of consumer installment dent to personal income

[a] Often considered the leading economic indicator.

Other important economic indicators for medical professionals include

1. Medical labor production is a measure of medical professional output per hour, or per each unit (patient) of labor. Managed care has decreased labor production cost in medicine.
2. Unit medical labor costs represent the cost of physician labor (treatment), per unit (CPT® code) of output.
3. Capacity of medical utilization is a percentage of the maximum rate at which a medical office, clinical hospital, or surgi-center can operate under normal conditions. At the rate nears 100%, efficiency declines due to mechanical breakdowns, burnout of doctors and employees, and less experienced medical care extenders and para-professionals.

BASIC MICROECONOMIC CONCEPTS

Now that some macroeconomic concepts have been reviewed from a medical perspective, important microeconomic concepts can be reviewed.

SHORT-TERM ASSETS

Short-term goals (less than 12 months) require liquidity or short-term assets. These assets include cash, checking and saving accounts, certificates of deposit, and money market accounts. These accounts have two things in common. The principal is guaranteed from risk of loss, and pay a very low interest rate. As an investment, they are considered substandard and one would only keep what is actually needed for liquidity purposes in these accounts.

LONG-TERM ASSETS

Long-term assets (more than 12 months) include real estate, mutual funds, retirement plans, stocks, and life insurance cash value policies. Bonds may also be an appropriate long-term investment asset for a number of reasons; for example, if you are seeking a regular and reliable stream of income or if you have no immediate need for the amount of the principal invested. Bonds also can be used to diversify your portfolio and reducing the overall risk that is inherent in stock investments.

SHORT-TERM LIABILITIES

Short-term liabilities (less than 12 months) include credit card debt, utility bills, and auto loans or leasing. When a young doctor leaves residency and starts practice, the foremost concern is student debt. This is an unsecured debt that is not backed by any collateral, except a promise to pay. There are recourses that an unsecured creditor can take to recoup the bad debt. Usually, if the unsecured creditor is successful obtaining a judgment, it can force wages to be garnished, and the Department of Education can withhold up to 10% of a wages without first initiating a lawsuit, if in default.

It is also probable that young medical professionals have been holding at least one credit card since their sophomore year in college. Credit card companies consider college student the most lucrative target market and medical students hold their first card for an average of 15 years. There are several other types of unsecured debt, including department store cards, professional fees, medical and dental bills, alimony, child support, rent, utility bills, personal loans from relatives, and health club dues, to name a few.

LONG-TERM LIABILITIES

A secured debt, on the other hand, is debt that is pledged by a specific property. This is a collateralized loan. Generally, the purchased item is pledged with the proceeds of the loan. This would include long-term liabilities (more than 12 months) such as a mortgage, home equity loan, or a car loan. Although the creditor has the ability to take possession of your property in order to recover a bad debt, it is done very rarely. A creditor is more interested in recovering money. Sometimes, when borrowing money, there may be a requirement to pledge assets that are owned prior to the loan.

For example, a personal loan from a finance company requires that you pledge all personal property such as your car, furniture, and equipment. The same property may become subject to a judicial lien if you are sued and a judgment is made against you. In this case, you would not be able to sell or pledge these assets until the judgment is satisfied. A common example of a lien would be from unpaid federal, state, or local taxes. Doctors can be found personally liable for unpaid payroll taxes of employees in their professional corporations.

Be aware that some assets and liabilities defy short- or long-term definition. When this happens, simply be consistent in your comparison of financial statements, over time.

Personal Net Worth

Once the value of all personal assets and liabilities is known, net worth can be determined with the following formula: *Net worth = assets minus liabilities.* Obviously, higher is better.

In *The Millionaire Next Door,** Thomas H. Stanley, PhD, and William H. Danko give the following benchmark for net worth accumulation. Although conservative for physicians of a past generation, it may be more applicable in the future because of current managed care environment. Here is the guide: Multiple your age by your annual pre-tax income from all sources, except inheritances, and then divide by 10.

EXAMPLE 5.2

As an HMO pediatrician, Dr. Curtis earned $90,000 last year. So, if she is 35, her net worth should be at least $315,000.

How do you get to that point? In a word, consume less and save more. Stanley and Danko found that the typical millionaire set aside 15% of earned income annually and has enough invested to survive 10 years, at current income levels if he stopped working. If Dr. Curtis lost her job tomorrow, how long could she pay herself the same salary?

Common Liability Management Mistakes

A common liability management mistake is not recognizing when you are heading for trouble. If doctors are paying only the minimum payments on credit card debt, while continuing to charge purchases at a rate faster than the paydown, trouble is brewing. If you don't categorize your debt, you could find yourself paying down nonpriority debt while ignoring priority debt. A priority debt is one that is essential or subject to serious consequences, if not paid. Examples include rent, mortgage payments, utility bills, child support, car payments, unpaid taxes, and other secured debt. If in 1 month, a doctor had to choose between paying his accounting bill or his rent, it would be essential to pay the rent. A doctor cannot practice from the street.

HOME MORTGAGES

Before you apply for a home mortgage, review your credit history and then prequalify before you begin house hunting. A big car note, excessive credit card debt, medical school or residency loan burdens, are big obstacles to securing a favorable mortgage. For buyers of moderately priced homes,

---

* Longstreet Press, Oct. 1996.

Fannie Mae and Freddie Mac raised the mortgage limit for single-family homes to $417,000 in 2012. Jumbo mortgages above this amount can be privately arranged, but at a higher interest rate.

Also, consider using a buyer's agent to find your dream home, since it probably won't cost you a thing, but may require a retainer for a very large home. A buyer's agent's fee comes from splitting commission with selling agents. However, unlike a seller's agent, a buyer's agent works for you and will not disclose any information that might help the seller.

Once you have found a home, the following types of mortgages should be considered:

An adjustable-rate mortgage (ARM) is a long-term mortgage with short-term (usually annual) adjustments to the interest rate. It is common to start with an interest rate two percentage points below comparable fixed mortgage rates. If the prevailing rate on mortgages increases over time, so will the rate on the ARM. There is usually a high cap which the rate cannot exceed. An ARM is almost always cheaper than a fixed mortgage in the short run, such as the first 5 years. After that, it will have to be reevaluated to see if it is worth converting into a fixed mortgage. If lower monthly housing costs are needed in order to make ends meet, an ARM may be the correct choice. Also, if you only want to live in the house for the next 5 years or less, then an ARM is applicable. In some cases, the lender allows the ARM to be assumed by the new buyer.

A new physician just beginning practice in a new area may be wise to buy a modest home with the plan to upgrade in a few years once a comfort level with the new practice and area are established. Likewise, an ARM might be a very wise mortgage to consider, especially when considering the usual cost savings. In normal markets, the yield curve becomes gradually positive, so a 5-year ARM will have a lower interest rate than a conventional 30-year mortgage. Considering just 1% in rate difference, a physician could save $1000 in interest costs every year for each $100,000 borrowed. The biggest risk is that in 5 years (assuming a 5-year ARM), the physician is at the mercy of prevailing interest rates when negotiating a new mortgage. If terms like 7/1 ARM with a 2/6 cap are confusing, the simplicity of a locked rate for 30 years might provide some peace of mind regarding the incremental cost.

If on the other hand, you feel comfortable with the current mortgage rate and monthly payment, you may want to lock in the rate with a fixed-rate mortgage. If the idea of increasing rates and payments is distasteful, a fixed mortgage might be appropriate. As your income rises, you can allocate more toward retirement and other goals, or perhaps pay down the principal faster. There is a preferable way to accomplish this. What many doctors do is send to their lender an extra $100 or $200 each month, in addition to the scheduled payment. This requires the lender to recalculate your amortization schedule every time you make a payment. Some lenders are more equipped to do this than others. Still, others will only do this once per year on your anniversary date. You should never have to pay for such mortgage accelerator programs. A better way to keep track of your outstanding balance would be to pay down the exact principal amount due in the next or several monthly payments. You can do this easily by requesting an amortization schedule from the lender right from the beginning. If you have a 30-year fixed mortgage, for example, you will have a schedule with payments numbered from 1 to 360. You could then submit your regular payment (let's say #1) and the principal amounts from payments numbers 2, 3, and 4. In this way, you will be advancing yourself in the amortization schedule and you can at any time figure out your outstanding balance, remaining term, and interest saved. You also make it easier for the lender as well.

There are other types of mortgages; hybrids, multistep, interest-only, balloons, and so on. Other more sophisticated mortgage types include biweekly mortgages, growing equity mortgages (GEMs), graduated payment mortgages (GPMs), FHA, and veteran's loans. Avoid them all, if possible, and omit mortgage insurance with a traditional down payment of 20%.

Tip: Before the passage of the Mortgage Relief Act of 2007, any home mortgage debt discharged was treated as taxable income. The act allowed taxpayers to exclude any such relief of mortgage debt through foreclosure, as well as any debt reduced by mortgage restructuring, for as much as $2 million. But this provision expired on December 31, 2013, which means any cancelation of debt income is now taxable. This tax break was designed to help those with underwater mortgages, as it allowed them to not pay taxes on any debt they had been forgiven.

REFINANCING

Recently, fixed mortgages were near their lowest rates in almost 30 years. If your mortgage was taken out within the past 5 years, it may be worthwhile to refinance if you can get financing that is at least one to two points lower than your current interest rate. You should plan on staying in the house long enough to pay off the loan transaction charges (points, title insurance, attorney's fees, etc.). Generally, points and origination fees can be deducted in the first year on original mortgages, but not on refinancing. For refinancing, the deduction must be spread over the life of the mortgage. Real estate commissions on a home sale are not tax deductible.

EXAMPLE 5.3

A 30-year, $100,000 refinancing loan with 1% origination fee and one point. Total points are the equivalent of 2%, or $2000. So, you may deduct $2000/30 years = $66.67 each year as pre-paid interest. Often, points and fees can be added to the loan, but if you refinance again, you may deduct rather than amortize the remainder of the points you paid on the refinance. If you have refinanced twice, but did not deduct the points from the first refinancing, you may file an amended tax return to recapture the deduction.

EXAMPLE 5.4

If you took out a $150,000 30-year fixed-rate mortgage at 7.5% (including transaction charges), your monthly payment is now $1049. Refinance at 6% with a 30-year fixed-rate mortgage of $150,000 (including transaction fees), and your payment will be $899 per month. That's a savings of $150 per month, which you can then use to invest, add to your retirement fund, pay off medical school debt or do whatever you wish.

Private mortgage insurance (PMI) premiums range from about 0.5% of a home mortgage to about 1%. PMI can be avoided with a down payment of at least 20%. The insurance protects the lender, not you, should a default occur. When rising home values boost your equity, PMI can be dropped upon request. Similarly, most mortgages can be prepaid without penalty. If a penalty does exist, it is treated as interest and may be deducted in the year paid.

Tip: If you're not behind on your mortgage payments but have been unable to get traditional refinancing because the value of your home has declined, you may be eligible to refinance through the Home Affordable Refinance Program (HARP). It is designed to help achieve a new, more affordable, more stable mortgage. HARP refinance loans require a loan application and underwriting process, and refinance fees apply. You may be eligible for HARP if you meet all of the following criteria:

- The mortgage must be owned or guaranteed by Freddie Mac or Fannie Mae.
- The mortgage must have been sold to Fannie Mae or Freddie Mac on or before May 31, 2009.
- The mortgage cannot have been refinanced under HARP previously unless it is a Fannie Mae loan that was refinanced under HARP from March to May 2009.
- The current loan-to-value (LTV) ratio must be greater than 80%.
- The borrower must be current on the mortgage at the time of the refinance, with a good payment history in the past 12 months.

Source: Fannie Mae: www.KnowYourOptions.com, (800)7Fannie, OR FreddieMac.com, (800)Freddie, OR 888-995-HOPE (4673).

Reverse Mortgages

A reverse mortgage gives medical professionals several options for withdrawing equity from their homes.

1. Line of credit option allows you to decide the timing and amount of withdrawals.
2. Tenure option involves equal monthly payments for as long as the home is occupied as a principal residence.
3. Modified tenure option is a mixture of loan payments and an available line of credit. Reverse mortgages may be ideal for medical professionals who own their own homes "free and clear," since payments are considered a "return of principle" and not taxable income. They can be prepaid at any time. Moreover, you do not give up any of the benefits or responsibilities of home ownership with a reverse mortgage, but upon death, your heirs must pay the balance of the mortgage, normally with proceeds from sale of the house. But they are not a panacea as fees are expensive.

Tip: While the housing market is still recovering, 30–60% of properties are assessed at higher than their current value, and fewer than 5% of taxpayers appeal assessments, according to the National Taxpayers Union. Yet, many people are still paying real estate tax on values that date back to 2006 and 2007, despite the fact that 20–30% of appeals generally have some success. For example, a $2.4 million home in Westchester County, New York, reassessed at $2.1 million, yields about $6000 in savings on a property-tax bill. This translates into about $82,000 in savings over 10 years, assuming the tax rate increases at historical levels.

Tip: Homebuyers looking at properties with Home Owner Associations in place should ask about associations' financial situation. This report suggests 70% of them are short on cash. *Source*: http://realestate.msn.com/blogs/post-report-70-percent-of-homeowners-associations-are-short-on-cash.

Renting

Most medical professionals should probably not spend more than 30% of take-home pay for rent on a personal apartment. Advantages of renting include freedom and flexibility, more square footage for the money, less concern about property values, and more liquidity for other financial needs or desires. Be sure to get replacement cost coverage renter's insurance rather than the older cash value-type insurance policy. The current environment however, does not favor renters in many geographic locations.

For example, a 2014 analysis of home prices and rents by RealtyTrac® found that in more than 90% of the counties it looked at, the average rent is higher than the cost of buying a median-priced home. The exceptions was a handful of highest-priced housing markets in the country—places like San Francisco, New York, and Arlington, Virginia. The list also includes some out-of-the-way housing hot spots like Teton County, Wyoming, and Gallatin County, Montana.

On the other extreme, renters come out way behind in places like Baltimore, where the average renter pays $1600 a month—roughly 3.6 times the cost of buying a median-price home. Other high-rent counties include Clayton, Georgia (where rents are 4.5 times the cost of buying), and Wayne, Michigan (4.8 times the cost of buying). *Source*: FIU News: https://news.fiu.edu/2011/03/second-thoughts-on-the-american-dream-of-home-ownership-study-reveals-that-renting-can-be-a-better-financial-choice/22483.

Automobiles

Generally, medical professionals should try to avoid luxury cars and prudently not spend more than 10–15% of gross income on the cost of a car, including gas, insurance, and maintenance, regardless of whether it is new or preowned. Be aware that some new cars depreciate 10–20% the moment they are driven off the lot, so resist the urge to buy new. Never finance for more than 4 years, sell your old car yourself, and make your car last at least 7 years. Some insurance companies will give you a reduced rate for cars equipped with a driver-side airbag or antilock brakes, as well as for doctor's who live less than 10 miles from the office.

Driving Costs

The Automobile Association of America (AAA) recently released its' *2013 Your Driving Costs* report, which revealed what Americans are really paying to drive. It showed an almost 2% increased cost to own and operate a vehicle in the United States.

For example, if you drive a mid-size sedan, like a Toyota Camry, Chevy Impala, or Ford Fusion, you're paying about 60.8 cents per mile, or $9122 a year. That is based on driving 15,000 miles per year, which is common for American workers. If you drive an SUV, you're paying about $11,600 per year. That's a lot of money. And, more than some medical interns, resident, fellows, and other allied healthcare providers pay for rent.

According to the AAA, here's a breakdown of the costs that drove the 2% increase in operating and owning a vehicle:

- Maintenance costs—up 11.26% between 2012 and 2013
- Fuel costs—increased 1.93%
- Tire costs—no change between 2012 and 2013
- Insurance costs—rose 2.76%
- Depreciation costs—increased by 0.78%

Source: http://newsroom.aaa.com/wp-content/uploads/2013/04/YourDrivingCosts2013.pdf.

Automobile Leases

Leasing a car may have several advantages, such as convenient maintenance, low down and monthly payments, no resale responsibility, and tax savings since you pay sales tax on the lease portion rather than the purchase price of the car. It might also be worthwhile if the after-tax borrowing cost of a home equity loan is less than the lease financing rate.

There are two major types of leases: open and closed ended. In the former type, if the car is worth more than the set price upon expiration of the lease, you are responsible for the underage or coverage. In the more advantages latter type, the responsibility of the value of the car is shifted to the leasing company. Other tips on care leasing include

- Inform the lessor how you want the auto equipped; do not accept unwanted options.
- Obtain all delivery and other charges in advance, including down payment, security deposit, registration fees, interest rates, residual value, rebates, and all taxes (sales, personal property, use and gross receipt).
- Know the capitalized cost (selling price) of the car.
- Know the annual mileage limits, usually 15,000–18,000 miles, and all excess use charges.
- Avoid maintenance and service contracts, and arrange for your own insurance.
- Understand that terms, such as money factor, or interest factor, may be used instead of the term interest rate. In this case, simply multiply the rate by 24 for an estimate of the true interest rate involved.
- Read the contract and understand all penalties, especially for premature or late termination, purchase or return terms, and consequences of theft.
- Check the lease terms through an independent company, such as First National Lease Systems.

A rough rule of thumb to determine whether to buy or lease involves multiplying all the payments required by the number of months you will have to pay, and add the down payment to yield the total amount of the purchase. Then, multiply the lease payment by the number of months, and add required upfront costs, as well as residual value (end-of-lease buyout cost), to determine the total amount to lease. Compare the two figures to determine the most economical deal. Typically, a cash deal is less expensive in the long run, providing a higher after-tax rate of return is not available, as an alternate investment, for the funds.

Perhaps the worse reason to lease a car is to drive one that you could not otherwise afford to drive. This is because most low monthly payments are only composed of two portions: interest on the note and the prorated cost of auto depreciation. No money is applied to the ownership of the vehicle. Finally, do not buy "gap" insurance to cover the difference between what your auto insurer would pay if your car was totaled, and what you would owe the leasing firm. It's usually too expensive and the risk is minimal.

Weddings for Medical Professionals

The average wedding costs about $25,525 and medical professionals often spend much more. Do you want a big wedding party for your family and friends or an earlier retirement for yourself?

Personal Financial Ratios

The economic platitude of the past, such as don't spend more than 15–20% of your net salary on food, or 5–10% on medical care, among others, have given rise to the more individualized personal financial ratio concept. Personal ratios, like business ratios, represent benchmarks to compare such parameters as debt, income growth, and net worth.

According to Edward McCarthy, MIB, CFP®, a personal financial expert from Warwick, Rhode Island, the following represents useful ratios for the medical professional (personal communication).

- Basic liquidity ratio = liquid assets/average monthly expenses. Should be 4–6 months, or even longer, in the case of a medical professional employed by a financially insecure health maintenance organization (HMO). In a low interest rate environment, iMBA Inc. offers 12–24 months for consideration.
- Debt to assets ratio = total debt/total assets. A percentage that is high initially and should decrease with age as the medical professional approaches a debt-free existence.
- Debt to gross income ratio = annual debt repayments/annual gross income. A percentage representing the adequacy of current income for existing debt repayments. Medical professionals should try to keep this below 25–30%.
- Debt service ratio = annual debt repayment/annual take-home pay. Medical professionals should try to keep this ratio below about 40%, or have difficulty paying down debt.
- Investment assets to net worth ratio = investment assets/net worth. This ratio should increase over time, as retirement for the medical professional approaches.
- Savings to income ratio = savings/annual income. This ratio should also increase over time, especially as major obligations are retired.
- Real growth ratio = (income this year − income last year)/(income last year − inflation rate). It is desirable for the medical professional to keep this ratio growing faster than the core rate of inflation.
- Growth of net-worth ratio = (net worth this year − net worth last year)/net worth last year − inflation rate. Again, this ratio should stay ahead of inflation.

By calculating these ratios, perhaps on an annual basis, the medical professional can spot problems, correct them, and continue progressing toward stated financial goals.

CURRENT RATE OF RETURN

Another important concept to understand is the current rate of return (CCR). According to this principle, the current rate of a taxable return must be evaluated in reference to a similar non-taxable rate of return. This allows you to focus on your portfolio's real (after-tax return), rather than its nominal, or stated return. Since most medical professionals own a combination of both vehicles, it is important to calculate the average rate of return (ARR), as demonstrated in the following matrix. Usually, this will result in the assumption of more risk, for the possibility of great return.

To compare after-tax yields, with taxable yields, use the following formulas:

Tax equivalent yield = yield/(1 − MTB), while taxable yield X (1 − tax rate) = tax exempt yield

EXAMPLE 5.5

If the yield on a tax exempt municipal bond was 6%, and you are in a 28% tax bracket, the equivalent taxable yield (ETY) is 8.3%, calculated in the following manner: 06/1.00 − 0.28 = 0.083, or 8.3% ETY. This means that you would need a taxable instrument paying almost 9% to equal the 6% tax exempt bond.

PERSONAL BUDGETING RULES

Budgeting is probably one of the greatest tools in building wealth. However, it is also one of the greatest weaknesses among physicians who tend to live a certain lifestyle. This includes living in an exclusive neighborhood, driving an expensive car, and wearing imported suits and a fine watch, all of which do not lend themselves to expense budgeting. Only one in 10 medical professionals has a personal budget. Fear, or a lack of knowledge, is a major cause of procrastination. The following guidelines will assist in this microeconomic endeavor.

1. Set reasonable goals and estimate annual income. Do not keep large amounts of cash at home or in the office. Deposit it in a money market account for safety and interest.
2. Do not pay bills early, do not have more taxes withheld from your salary than you owe, and develop spending estimates and budget fixed expenses first. Fixed expenses are usually contractual, and may include housing, utilities, food, telephone, social security, medical, debt repayment, homeowner's or renter's insurance, auto, life and disability insurance, maintenance, and so on.
3. Make variable expenses a priority. Variable expenses are not usually contractual, and may include clothing, education, recreational, travel, vacation, gas, entertainment, gifts, furnishings, savings, investments, and so on.
4. Trim variable expenses by 10–15%, and fixed expenses, when possible. Ultimately, all fixed expenses get paid and become variable in the long run.
5. Use carve-out or set-asides for big-ticket items and differentiate "wants from needs."
6. Know the difference between saving and investing. Savers tend to be risk adverse and investors understand risk and takes steps to mitigate it.
7. Determine shortfalls or excesses with the budget period.
8. Track actual expenses.
9. Calculate both income and expenses as a percentage of the total, and determine if there is a better way to allocate resources. Then, review the budget on a monthly basis to determine if there is a variance. Determine if the variance was avoidable, unavoidable, or a result of inaccurate assumptions, and take needed corrective action.

Verify Your Budget and Follow a Financial Plan

The process of establishing a budget relies heavily on guesswork, and the use of software or "apps," which seamlessly track expenditures and help your budget and your financial plan become more of reality. Most doctors underestimate their true expenses, so lumping and best guesses on expense usually prove very inaccurate. Personal financial software and mobile phone applications make the verification of budgets easier. Once your personal accounts are set up, free apps like MINT.com will give you a detailed report on where your money is going and the adjustments you must make. Few professions make larger contributions to the Internal Revenue Service than physicians and the medical profession. It is very important to categorize different budget categories not only to be proactive about your expenses, but also to accurately reflect the effect your different expenditures have on your real savings capability. All expense dollars are not equal. For example, a mortgage payment, which is mostly interest expense in the early years, is likewise mostly tax deductible. Spending money on your family vacation is typically not tax deductible. Itemized deductions, which are deductions that a U.S. taxpayer can claim on their tax return in order to reduce their adjustable gross income (AGI), may include such costs as property taxes, vehicle registration fees, income taxes, mortgage expense, investment interest, charitable contributions, medical expenses (to the extent the expenses exceed 10% of the taxpayers AGI), and more.

Employing qualified financial planner that utilizes a cash-flow-based financial planning software program may help the physician identify their actual after-tax projected cash flow and more accurately plan their future.

ZERO-BASED BUDGET

A zero-based budget means you start with the absolute essential expenses, and then add expenses from there until you run out of money. This is an extremely effective, yet rigorous exercise for most medical professionals and can be used personally or at the office. Guess what your first personal financial item should be? That's right, retirement plan contributions. Then your mortgage and other debt payments, and other required fixed expenses. From the office perspective, the first budget item should be salary expenses, both your own and your staff.

Operating assets and other big-ticket items come next, followed by the more significant items on your net income statement. Some doctors even review their P&L statements quarterly, line by line, in an effort to reduce expenses. Then add discretionary personal or business expenses that you have some control over. Do you run out of money before you reach the end of the month, quarter, or year? Then you better cut back on entertainment at home or that fancy new, but unproven piece of office or medical equipment. This sounds Draconian until you remind yourself that your choice is either (a) entertainment now but no money later or (b) living a simpler lifestyle now as you invest so you're able to enjoy yourself at retirement. When you were a young doctor, it may have been a difficult trade-off. But at mid-life, you're staring ultimate retirement in the face.

OVERHEARD IN THE ADVISOR'S LOUNGE: ON SALES INCENTIVES

OverTable Bay Financial recently distributed an email to its trainees offering a Maserati automobile to advisors who sell $7.5 million of annuities in 2014. Could the lure of luxury cars incentivize a financial advisor to recommend investments that aren't in a client's interest?

So, this is a great reminder that when hiring a financial planner, don't just ask him what he knows. Ask who taught him what he knows!

Lon Jefferies, MBA, CFP®
http://blogs.wsj.com/moneybeat/2014/02/14/
whos-training-your-retirement-navigator/tab/print/

USE AND ABUSE OF CREDIT

The horror stories involving debit cards and credit card debt, and credit reporting, are well known. In this age of healthcare reform, understanding the rules of the personal credit and credit card use is vital for all medical professionals.

PREAPPROVED CREDIT CARDS

The offer a new doctor gets from a credit card company, with preapproval for a low interest rate, is a classic case of reading the fine print. Many times, preapproval simply means that you are on the mailing list bought from a consumer reporting agency, based upon your current credit score. After you respond, they purchase a credit report and then decide whether or not to issue credit to you.

MEDICAL EMPLOYERS AND CREDIT REPORTS

What makes you qualify for credit? Certainly, medical professionals are no longer as desirable as they were only a decade ago, as all financial institutions now look at occupational growth potential. HMOs, hospitals, and other employers will also often run a credit report on prospective medical employees, since legal limits to the type of questions that can be asked have been curtailed. This is a valuable tool since many believe that how you manage your personal finances may say something about your ability to handle job responsibilities. For example, if you live a lifestyle you cannot afford, you may not be objective in a decision-making role over tough medical utilization reviews. This may sound harsh, but financial personality profiling is on the rise. Thus, don't be surprised if your next job application contains an authorization for credit reports and a background check.

COMPILING CREDIT REPORTS

Your credit report is a data image of your payment history. It contains personal information, such as your social security number, date of birth, current and previous real and email addresses, and financial payment information. Some credit reports also include your past or current employers. Credit bureaus are information gatherers. Banks, mortgage lenders, credit card companies, and anyone else who is considering extending credit are information hunters. Credit reporting agencies sell credit reports. The three best known are Experion (formerly TRW Information Systems Inc.), Trans Union Corporation, and Equifax.

READING CREDIT REPORTS

When you read your credit report, ensure the accuracy of information and write down any errors, or circle them on the report. Among the most common mistakes are loans and credit repair not being updated. For example, medical and professional school loans are notorious for being mishandled. This is because of ever-changing deferment rules. If your loan payments are due to start 9 months after graduation, and you entered medical school after taking a year off, look out. You will have made three payments and then be able to further withhold payments while you remain a student. The confusion arises when your payments stop. With most loans, a missed payment is a late payment. This halting of payments, perfectly legitimate for students, can be misinterpreted to mean late payments and possible default. As a medical professional, you should strongly consider obtaining your credit report and looking carefully at your loan payment history.

CREDIT RATING AND SCORING

The category in which a credit agency classifies you is based upon payment history. Recently, credit reporting agencies have shifted away from ratings to a system known as credit scoring. Your score is determined by proprietary formulas that are based on your credit history; the higher the better. The practical benefits of this scoring system are numerous. First, medical professionals do not need to be experts at deciphering credit reports since the same scoring system is used by many different companies.

CORRECTING CREDIT REPORT ERRORS

A credit bureau is not the place to get an item fixed on your credit report. Rather, you must take it up directly with the credit issuer. In any case, a late payment noted on a credit report by a durable medical equipment vendor, for example, has to be addressed directly with that merchant. The durable medical equipment (DME) merchant then has 30 days to acknowledge your complaint and respond to you. In the meantime, you do not have to pay for the disputed items. Most credit errors cannot be reported or kept on your credit report for more than 7 years. For legitimate late payments, you should contact the credit grantor and negotiate to take one of the following steps. Be tenacious, and either remove the late payment or write a letter explaining that the problem has been resolved and you now are a good credit risk again. This letter is a powerful tool and should be saved with other permanent financial records. The industry term for it is a letter of correction.

CREDIT REPAIR SERVICES

Credit repair services are oversold and their claims tend to be exaggerated. They do not have an inside track to the consumer reporting agencies. Good credit repair services are experienced in communicating with creditors and can help with legitimate repairs. They cannot restore your credit rating or your good name. However, realize that with some time and effort you can accomplish the same results yourself.

DEBT RATIOS AND CREDIT

The debt to income ratio is a formula used by most lenders and is represented as take-home pay divided by your monthly debt. For example, let's say that ABC Bank has issued you a VISA card with a $1500 limit. You use the card and one day receive a letter stating that your credit limit has been increased. The new higher limit is considered "available credit." Then, XYZ bank sends you a MasterCard. Your credit limit is $2000, and all you have to do is call their toll-free number to activate it. You wisely determine that you do not need the card and don't activate it. Unfortunately, the $2000 is still considered available credit and may be held against you. Now, when you apply for a loan, the loan issuer will run a credit report on you. It will add up your total credit card limits, whether they are active or not. This is your available credit. If your available credit is considered too high, you will not be approved for your loan, or approval will cost a higher interest rate. Taking it one step further, the potential creditor will add your total available credit and figure out the minimum monthly payment. This number is used against you.

DISPOSABLE CREDIT CARDS AND "CHIP AND PIN" TECHNOLOGY

Disposable credit cards are the newest innovation to help reduce fraud and assumed identity scams on e-commerce-based websites. As with traditional credit cards, these cards are numbered, but used only once. Then, electronically they are erased so that there is nothing left in the merchant's database for hackers to steal.

But, in 2014, Congress began looking at new ways to keep personal credit card information safe after several high-profile security breaches at some of America's top retailers. Why? Current credit cards use easy-to-hack magnetic strip technology from the 1960s. Many consumers want more secure "pin & chip" cards that have been in use in Europe for years. Even though microchip technology costs billions to implement, merchants are moving in that direction as they issue new cards to consumers. Most modern polls show nearly half of all people surveyed are extremely concerned about the safety of their personal credit card information.

CREDIT CARD MISTAKES TO AVOID

No number has as far-reaching an impact on your money as your credit scores. Here are some obstacles you should dodge on the road to financial security:

- Don't pay for a credit card repair service.
- Don't miss a payment.
- Don't max out your card.
- Don't take a cash advance.
- Don't skip using your cards.
- Don't chase interest rates.
- Don't apply for several credit cards all at once.
- Don't co-sign a loan.
- Don't spread your car or mortgage payments.

DENIED CREDIT

If you are denied a credit card, you have the right to obtain a credit report free from the agency that denied you. Your request must be made in writing and within 30–60 days. Consumer credit is governed by the Fair Credit Reporting Act (FCRA). The regulations are issued by and enforced by the Federal Trade Commission. Certain states offer consumers additional rights. Credit reporting agencies are referred to as a "consumer reporting agency."

DEBIT CARDS

Unlike credit cards, debit cards deduct the amount of purchase directly from your checking or other account. There is no grace period or "float" on them, and the safeguards against loss or theft aren't as strict as with conventional credit cards.

Reorganization and Bankruptcy

The medical professional should be familiar with the two kinds of bankruptcy: liquidation and reorganization. In the United States, the first bankruptcy laws date back to the early 1800s. Today's law is the Bankruptcy Act, which was enacted by Congress in 1978. Chapter 7 of the Act involves liquidation bankruptcy. Chapters 11 and 13 involve reorganizations, which require a repayment plan.

As a physician, if you file for a Chapter 7 bankruptcy, you are requesting that the court eliminate your debt. You must disclose all that you own and all the income you earn. The court then assigns a trustee. The trustee has the authority to take control of any nonexempt property you purchased prior to the filing. You keep control of property you claim to be exempt. What assets you claim to be exempt is scrutinized by the trustee.

Chapter 13 bankruptcy follows the same administrative procedure and paperwork. You still need to claim your assets, debts, and income. However, you also must provide a loan repayment plan that fits into your budget. You are allowed to pay your reasonable living and office expenses. If there is any surplus, that amount is surrendered to the trustee who in turn pays your creditors. If at the end of a 3-year period all debts are not fully repaid, they are usually forgiven. One type of debt that is usually not forgiven is HEAL loans and federal income taxes. The IRS will, however, stop accruing interest on the outstanding balance. Chapters 7 and 13 of the Act will also not discharge alimony or child support, debts stemming from accidental infliction of personal injury or death, DWI-related debt, and criminal fines.

Chapter 11 bankruptcy applies to healthcare professionals with unusually high debts. Typically, businesses undergoing reorganization that want to remain in business would opt for Chapter 11. It is also available to individual doctors with debt in excess of Chapter 13 limits of unsecured debt and/or secured debt, or substantial nonexempt property such as real estate. The debtor would remain in control of the assets, so in effect, the debtor becomes the trustee. Therefore, the debtor has the power to reject creditor claims with no penalty, extend the time for repayment, and even reduce the debt owed to the creditor. Chapter 11 may sound like a windfall for debtor doctors, but it does not come without great cost. It can take an extremely long time, averaging between several months and several years. There are filing fees, professional fees, legal retainers, and so on. Before the court confirms Chapter 11, the doctor debtor must provide a plan of reorganization. This requires a tremendous effort in prebankruptcy planning. Many Chapter 11 physician bankruptcies turn into Chapter 7 bankruptcies.

OVERHEARD IN THE DOCTOR'S LOUNGE: ON FINDING PHYSICIAN-FOCUSED FINANCIAL ADVICE

The financial planner is a like juggler, trying to keep a variety of balls simultaneously in the air. Each aspect of practice becomes critical, just as action is needed.

Some of the activities of operating a successful financial planning practice generally attract more attention than others, such as marketing and advertising, closing engagements, and office administration. Because product review, selection, and implementation are often related to advisor compensation, they attract a great deal of the financial juggler's concentration.

But, the heart of financial planning, niche advice, often receives little attention. Not because it is unimportant, it just doesn't seem immediately and predictably urgent. Here, that ball does not seem to be dropping so rapidly.

However, retaining clients and receiving referrals from other professionals is very dependent on the quality of the advice delivered. And, the first line of protection from practitioner liability exposure is to not deliver incorrect or incomplete advice.

But, where does the financial advisor turn for ideas and organized research in the healthcare sector?

Edwin P. Morrow, CFP™, CLU, ChFC, RFC
(Middletown, Ohio, USA)

BASIC FINANCIAL PLANNING CONCEPTS

Most principles of personal financial planning evolve from the following concepts.

MARKETABILITY AND LIQUIDITY

Marketability and liquidity are two concepts that are interrelated but often confused by the medical professional. Marketability deals with the speed at which an asset can be turned into cash. *Liquidity*, on the other hand, deals with an asset that can be turned to cash without a significant loss of value. A physician's practice may still be good investment, but it is not particularly marketable or liquid. A common stock traded on the New York Stock Exchange can be easily sold for its quoted fair market value.

TIME VALUE OF MONEY

To the young physician starting a career, the time value of money is not a primary concern. It involves spending dollars in the future compared with spending today. Paying off high student loans while earning a relatively low salary leaves barely enough for present personal consumption. In the past, the rationale to spend today, forsaking the future, was not only a function of necessity but stemmed from the probability that future income would grow appreciably higher. Today, this is no longer a given for medical professionals.

In the simplest terms, a dollar today is worth more than a dollar tomorrow. The supply and demand for a dollar today to be paid back in the future is what determines interest rates. This calls for an understanding of the concepts of present and future value.

Present value is what you have today. So, a dollar is worth a dollar. Future value is what that dollar will grow to when compounded at a given interest rate. If you started with 100 dollars and earned 10% for 5 years, you would end up with 161 dollars.

Year	Paying Amount of	Interest Factor	Ending Amount	Interest (Annual)
1	$ 100	1.10	$110.00	$10.00
2	110	1.10	121.00	11.00
3	121	1.10	133.10	12.10
4	133.10	1.10	146.41	13.31
5	146.41	1.10	161.05	14.64
				$61.05

Whenever you do not have a financial calculator, such as a Hewlett-Packard 12-C, Texas Instruments BA III plus, apps, SAAS, or computer spreadsheet handy, you can figure future value with this formula.

$$FV = PV(1 + i)^N$$

FV is future value and PV is present value. The periodic interest rate is represented by i. The number of periods being compounded is n. N means to the power of some number. In the example above, the equation would appear as follows:

$$FV = \$100(1 + 0.1)^2$$
$$FV = \$100(1.21)$$
$$FV = \$121$$

Likewise, the formula for present value is PV = amount/(1 + i).

Other concepts of money time values are easily determined with a calculator or interest table, include the future value of multiple (equal) cash flows (ordinary annuity), conversion to an annuity due, the present value of multiple (equal) cash flows (ordinary annuity), and the conversion to an annuity due.

EXAMPLE 5.6: DETERMINING A FUNDING AMOUNT

Dr. Smith has a daughter who plays the piano very well. He wishes to accumulate funds for his daughter Mackenzie's advanced music education. He estimates that she will need $6000 per year in today's dollars, and will start school at age 18. She is 10 years old now. Costs are expected to increase 6% annually. Dr. Smith and his financial advisor believe that he can earn 9% after tax on his funds. How much is required?

Step #1: Determine the future value of $6000 8 years from now. Or, what will Mackenzie's first-year piano school cost, considering inflation?

Using a financial calculator, such as the HP 12-C: @ 8n (years), 6i (interest rate), $6000 PV, the future value is $9563.

Step #2: Next, determine the lump sum necessary to provide the above amount at the start of each year (present value annuity due).

Again, using the HP12-C @ $9563 PMT, g7 (PVAD), 4N, 1.09/1.06i, the present value is $36,702.

Step #3: Compute the annual savings required at the end of each year (ordinary annuity) to provide the lump sum needed at age 18.

Finally, calculate with the HP 12-C @ g8 (ordinary annuity), $36,702FV, 8 N, 9i, and solve for PMT = $3328.

PREPARING A NET WORTH AND NET INCOME STATEMENT

The key to starting the financial planning process is determining your current financial position. A statement of net worth includes all your assets and liabilities, at a specific point in time, whether owned by you or provided by your practice. This is similar to a corporate balance sheet, except that a balance sheet shows assets at their original cost. Your net worth statement shows assets at their fair market value.

Below is a sample net worth statement for you to get started with your financial planning process. Because this part of the process is the basis of so many others, we separate the ownership of assets. This provides you with the backdrop for estate or retirement planning.

Net Worth Statement, Drs. David and Hope Smith, as of July 20, 2015			
Assets	Your Name	Spouse's Name	Joint Name
Bank Accounts:			
Checking	————	————	————
Savings	————	————	————
Savings Bonds	————	————	————
Money Market Funds	————	————	————
CDs	————	————	————
Credit Union Account	————	————	————
Stocks	————	————	————
Bonds	————	————	————
Mutual Funds	————	————	————
Life Insurance (Cash Value)	————	————	————
Residence (Current Value)	————	————	————
Other Real Estate	————	————	————
Practice Interest	————	————	————
Other Business Interest	————	————	————
Receivables	————	————	————
Trusts	————	————	————
Tax Shelters	————	————	————
Personal Property:	————	————	————
Jewelry	————	————	————
Autos	————	————	————
Furnishings	————	————	————
Collectibles:	————	————	————
Antiques	————	————	————
Fine Art	————	————	————
Precious Metals	————	————	————
Retirement Plan Accounts:	————	————	————
Pension/Profit Sharing Plan	————	————	————
Annuities	————	————	————
IRAs	————	————	————
Stock Option Plans	————	————	————

Saving & Incentive Plans	————	————	————
401(k) Plans	————	————	————
Deferred Compensation	————	————	————
Total Assets	$ ————	$ ————	$ ————
Liabilities			
Mortgages	————	————	————
Notes	————	————	————
Personal Loans	————	————	————
Business Loans	————	————	————
Credit Card Balances	————	————	————
Auto Loans/Lease	————	————	————
Total Liabilities	$ ————	$ ————	$ ————
Net Worth (Assets Less Liabilities)	$ ————	$ ————	$ ————

CASH FLOW PLANNING

Since almost all areas of financial planning are controlled by cash flow, it is important to construct a cash flow net income or profit and loss statement that is accurate and believable. The success of your plan rides on your implementation of financial strategies that arise from the foundation of your cash flow statement. If you don't believe the numbers, you will not implement the strategies, thereby allowing your plan to fail.

For example, your retirement plan may depend on your being able to save a periodic amount of your surplus income. Your surplus income is determined by your net income (income after taxes and less your expenses), which comes directly from your cash flow statement. You will not save what you do not believe exists, that is, surplus income. Also, your targeted retirement income is a function of your current standard of living, adjusted for inflation and anticipated lifestyle changes. Your standard of living is a function of your cash flow statement. Your target must be believable to be achievable.

Cash flow planning also affects how medical professionals provide for their children's college education. The added cost of saving for future education must be balanced against saving for retirement. Or, if education is to be paid out of current income, how will it affect cash flow? As another example, an accurate cash flow plan affects investment decisions, risk management programs, income tax planning, survivorship planning, and long-term care planning. Moreover, cash flow planning also relates to estate planning by determining the most efficient transfer of wealth to heirs. When planning for lifetime gifts, the medical professional must consider the potential loss of income from assets transferred. Finally, when life insurance is applicable, you must determine the added expense during life in order to provide the liquidity necessary to pay estate taxes at death.

A Lifestyle Plan

A cash flow plan covers a specific period of time, and is the most difficult financial statement to construct because many doctors perceive it to be a tool for setting up a budget. Most doctors do not live a disciplined spending lifestyle and the thought of a budget is viewed as a possible compromise to their lifestyle. It is not designed to be a budgeting tool, although it certainly can be. A cash flow plan is designed to provide comfort when there is surplus income, which can be diverted for other planning needs. If there is no surplus income, perhaps a budget is in order to generate the funds needed? For example, if retirement savings are treated as just another periodic bill, you are more likely to succeed.

A comprehensive cash flow statement, or lifestyle budget outline, begins with an analysis of your operating checkbook and a review of various source documents, such as your tax return, credit card and statements, pay stubs, and insurance policies. A typical statement will show all cash transactions that occur within 1 year. It is helpful to establish a monthly equivalent to all items of income and expense, but for the purposes of getting started, items of income and expense may be noted by the frequency you are accustomed to receiving or spending them.

Cash Flow Statement, Drs. David and Hope Smith, from 01/01/2015 to 12/31/2015

Cash Receipts or Inflows	Monthly Amount	Quarterly Amount	Annual Amount
Income from practice	$ ———	$ ———	$ ———
Income from employment			
Pensions/annuities			
Interest			
Dividends			
Net Rentals			
Equipment Leases			
Miscellaneous			
Total Inflows	$ ———	$ ———	$ ———
Cash Disbursements or Outflows			
Housing:			
Mortgage payment/rent	$ ———	$ ———	$ ———
Real estate tax			
Home improvements			
Utilities			
Maintenance/repairs			
Home Insurance			
Food (home)			
Lunches (away from home)			
Clothing			
Transportation:			
Finance/lease payment			
Gas/oil/maintenance			
Auto Replacement Fund			
License/registration			
Insurance			
Education			
Insurance:			
Disability			
Liability			
Malpractice			
Life			
Health			
Umbrella			
Long-Term Care			
Other			
Miscellaneous:			
Unreimbursed Business Expenses			
Medical Expenses			
Alimony			
Child Support/Maintenance			
Child Care			
Parental Support			
Discretionary:			
Charitable Contributions			
Vacation & Travel			
Vacation Home Expenses			
Club Dues (Golf, Tennis, Health)			

Restaurants			
Entertainment (Guests)			
Entertainment			
(Self, theater, sports, movies)			
Babysitting			
Books, Magazines, CDs			
Gifts (Holidays, Wedding,			
Birthdays)			
Personal Expenses (hair care, etc.)			
Dry Cleaning			
Hobbies			
Family Pets			
Liquor, Cigarettes, Cigars			
Other			
Wealth Accumulation:			
SEP-IRA/IRA Contributions			
Qualified Plan Contributions			
Salary deferrals			
Mutual Fund Purchases			
Systematic Savings			
Investment Real Estate			
Other Investments			
Taxes:			
FICA/Medicare			
Federal			
State			
Miscellaneous:			
Debt financing			
Student Loans			
Practice Development			
Practice Buyout			
Other			
Total Disbursements	$	$	$
Surplus (Deficit)	$	$	$

COMMON CASH FLOW MISTAKES

1. Preparing a cash flow budget is a planning tool, not a punishment. Keep the credit cards hidden until you've paid all prior credit card bills. If this means you must use some of your savings to pay off credit card debt, so be it. It is better to save the 21% finance charge than to earn 1% on your savings.
2. Don't live beyond your means. If that translates to you owning a late model American car, and not a new foreign sports car, your checkbook will thank you in the long run. But do not deny your spouse an occasional luxury, and agree on major purchases before making them. A classic physician financial blunder is "rewarding" yourself after years of medical school and residency poverty by buying the $80,000 luxury car and the $950,000 first home, especially when a very nice car and home can be obtained at half the price. The cost of this reward to the physician is limited options later on in life, such as earlier retirement or more flexible hours.
3. Do not confuse your marginal tax rate with your average tax rate. The former is the highest tax rate on your last increment of income, while the latter is your total tax due, divided by your tax base. Obviously, your marginal rate is higher than your average rate.

4. Do not confuse a tax credit with a tax deduction. A credit is a dollar for dollar deduction from your income tax liability, while a deduction is only an equivalent of your marginal tax bracket (MTB). For example, in a 28% MTB, a $1 credit still equals one dollar. But, a one dollar deduction only equals 28 cents, although it can also reduce some state income taxes.

5. Refinancing consumer debt with a home equity loan will not only save you interest, but it will also save you income taxes as well. Shop around for the lowest rate. Don't just use the bank you do business with.

6. Entertainment is a luxury, not a necessity. This is the first area to cut back on if you find yourself short at the end of a month.

7. Pay your estimated income taxes on time, and pay fourth-quarter state estimated taxes by December 31. There is nothing worse than having to come up with a huge lump sum for taxes at the same time you have to fund your practice retirement plan.

8. Find a physician-focused financial advisor, financial planner, or Certified Medical Planner™ that both you and your spouse are comfortable with, since s/he will understand the risks and benefits of most personal economic opportunities. Be sure the advisor is a fiduciary working on your behalf, and not for a brokerage firm. Get it in writing, eschew suitability rules, do not agree to arbitrate problems, or waive your right to sue. Strive for a symbiotic and trusting stewardship standard.

WHAT SHOULD A PERSONAL FINANCIAL PLAN INCLUDE?

Financial planning can be accomplished on a comprehensive or modular basis, handling one issue at a time before moving on to the next. Unfortunately, of all available careers, medicine is probably one of the busiest and precious little time is left for planning needs. Therefore, the assistance of a trusted and competent financial planner is suggested. The time devoted to the task is well worth it and has a long-term payoff.

Therefore, once you have completed the cash flow and net worth statements, you are ready to draft your financial plan.

ESTABLISHING SHORT- AND LONG-TERM GOALS AND OBJECTIVES

The success of a financial plan depends on the clear identification of all goals and objectives. Each goal should be identified and quantified. The amount should be represented in today's dollars, or, at their present value. An assumed inflation rate will determine the future value assigned to those goals.

Short-term goals may be personal or practice related. For example, a personal short-term goal might be the purchase of a summer home, a boat, college education for your 12-year-old daughter, or a major home improvement. Short-term goals involving your practice might be the purchase of a new piece of medical equipment requiring some minimum capital requirement. Another short-term goal might be to provide for insurance coverage to protect against malpractice claims.

The most common long-term goal in a financial plan is to retire comfortably. Once financial independence has been achieved, the next most common goal is estate and gift planning. Often, the financial planner provides great value by identifying, quantifying, and agreeing upon goals that previously were unconfirmed. Along with this discussion must be the agreement of certain financial assumptions. These assumptions impact upon the growth of your investment portfolio. In addition, it is also assumed that the income tax laws will change and a new analysis is required each year.

The following assessment guide serves to help quantify and rank your financial goals. It is important to assign a time frame for accomplishing these goals.

THE ABSTRACT/CONCRETE DUALITY

Any comprehensive and integrated financial plan must be both abstract and concrete regarding goals, amounts, and timelines. Vague abstractions do not work in the real world and must be quantified for more reliable results. Astute medical professionals might use the following chart to establish both abstract and concrete goals and objectives. This exercise mimics the popular style of Atul Gawande, MD, in his acclaimed work *The Checklist Manifesto.*

Example of Abstract Doctor Financial Goals: What Are Your Investment Objectives?

Liquidity (instant cash availability)

Very Important				Not Important
1	2	3	4	5

Current income (monthly cash flow from investments)

Very Important				Not Important
1	2	3	4	5

Future income (maximize income in future periods)

Very Important				Not Important
1	2	3	4	5

Inflation protection (protection against loss of purchasing power)

Very Important				Not Important
1	2	3	4	5

Capital growth (real increase in value of assets)

Very Important				Not Important
1	2	3	4	5

Safety of principal (minimal risk of losing principal)

Very Important				Not Important
1	2	3	4	5

Diversification (to minimize risk by investing in a variety of asset classes)

Very Important				Not Important
1	2	3	4	5

Marketability (investments should be convertible into cash quickly)

Very Important				Not Important
1	2	3	4	5

Ease of practice management (relief from day-to-day investment decisions)

Very Important				Not Important
1	2	3	4	5

Example of Concrete Doctor Financial Goals: What Are Your Specific Financial Goals? Within Each Time Period, Circle the Level of Importance of Each Goal. List Any Additional Financial Objectives You May Have Personally

	Short-Term (Within the Next Year)		Medium-Term (Within the Next 5 Years)		Long-Term (Within the Next 5–10 Years)		Longest-Term (10+ Years)	
Buy a house								
Estimated cost:	$ _____							
	Important	1	Important	1	Important	1	Important	1
		2		2		2		2
		3		3		3		3
		4		4		4		4
	Not Important	5	Not Important	5	Not Important	5	Not Important	5

continued

Example of Concrete Doctor Financial Goals: What Are Your Specific Financial Goals? Within Each Time Period, Circle the Level of Importance of Each Goal. List Any Additional Financial Objectives You May Have Personally (continued)

	Short-Term (Within the Next Year)		Medium-Term (Within the Next 5 Years)		Long-Term (Within the Next 5–10 Years)		Longest-Term (10+ Years)	
Education expenses (self or children)								
Estimated cost: $ _____								
	Important	1	Important	1	Important	1	Important	1
		2		2		2		2
		3		3		3		3
		4		4		4		4
	Not Important	5	Not Important	5	Not Important	5	Not Important	5
Debt reduction								
Current debt: $ _____								
	Important	1	Important	1	Important	1	Important	1
		2		2		2		2
		3		3		3		3
		4		4		4		4
	Not Important	5	Not Important	5	Not Important	5	Not Important	5
Make home improvements								
Estimated cost: $ _____								
	Important	1	Important	1	Important	1	Important	1
		2		2		2		2
		3		3		3		3
		4		4		4		4
	Not Important	5	Not Important	5	Not Important	5	Not Important	5
Buy a car								
How much: $ _____								
	Important	1	Important	1	Important	1	Important	1
		2		2		2		2
		3		3		3		3
		4		4		4		4
	Not Important	5	Not Important	5	Not Important	5	Not Important	5
Make other large purchase (boat, plane, art, jewelry)								
Estimated cost: $ _____								
	Important	1	Important	1	Important	1	Important	1
		2		2		2		2
		3		3		3		3
		4		4		4		4
	Not Important	5	Not Important	5	Not Important	5	Not Important	5
Take a vacation								
Estimated cost: $ _____								
	Important	1	Important	1	Important	1	Important	1
		2		2		2		2
		3		3		3		3
		4		4		4		4
	Not Important	5	Not Important	5	Not Important	5	Not Important	5

continued

Example of Concrete Doctor Financial Goals: What Are Your Specific Financial Goals? Within Each Time Period, Circle the Level of Importance of Each Goal. List Any Additional Financial Objectives You May Have Personally (continued)

	Short-Term (Within the Next Year)		Medium-Term (Within the Next 5 Years)		Long-Term (Within the Next 5–10 Years)		Longest-Term (10+ Years)	
Change profession or specialty								
Current salary:	$							
Potential salary:	$							
	Important	1	Important	1	Important	1	Important	1
		2		2		2		2
		3		3		3		3
		4		4		4		4
	Not Important	5	Not Important	5	Not Important	5	Not Important	5
Cover expenses with investment portfolio income								
Estimated need:	$							
	Important	1	Important	1	Important	1	Important	1
		2		2		2		2
		3		3		3		3
		4		4		4		4
	Not Important	5	Not Important	5	Not Important	5	Not Important	5
Adequate retirement income								
Estimated need:	$							
	Important	1	Important	1	Important	1	Important	1
		2		2		2		2
		3		3		3		3
		4		4		4		4
	Not Important	5	Not Important	5	Not Important	5	Not Important	5
Buy a vacation home								
Approx. cost:	$							
Maintenance:	$							
	Important	1	Important	1	Important	1	Important	1
		2		2		2		2
		3		3		3		3
		4		4		4		4
	Not Important	5	Not Important	5	Not Important	5	Not Important	5
Have children								
How many now?								
Planned:								
	Important	1	Important	1	Important	1	Important	1
		2		2		2		2
		3		3		3		3
		4		4		4		4
	Not Important	5	Not Important	5	Not Important	5	Not Important	5
Increase level of charitable giving								
Estimated current level:	$							
Estimated increase:	$							
	Important	1	Important	1	Important	1	Important	1
		2		2		2		2
		3		3		3		3

continued

Example of Concrete Doctor Financial Goals: What Are Your Specific Financial Goals? Within Each Time Period, Circle the Level of Importance of Each Goal. List Any Additional Financial Objectives You May Have Personally (continued)

	Short-Term (Within the Next Year)		Medium-Term (Within the Next 5 Years)		Long-Term (Within the Next 5–10 Years)		Longest-Term (10+ Years)	
		4		4		4		4
	Not Important	5	Not Important	5	Not Important	5	Not Important	5
Take early retirement								
	Important	1	Important	1	Important	1	Important	1
		2		2		2		2
		3		3		3		3
		4		4		4		4
	Not Important	5	Not Important	5	Not Important	5	Not Important	5
Start a non-medical business What type? _____								
	Important	1	Important	1	Important	1	Important	1
		2		2		2		2
		3		3		3		3
		4		4		4		4
	Not Important	5	Not Important	5	Not Important	5	Not Important	5
Financial independence								
	Important	1	Important	1	Important	1	Important	1
		2		2		2		2
		3		3		3		3
		4		4		4		4
	Not Important	5	Not Important	5	Not Important	5	Not Important	5
Other goals _____								
	Important	1	Important	1	Important	1	Important	1
		2		2		2		2
		3		3		3		3
		4		4		4		4
	Not Important	5	Not Important	5	Not Important	5	Not Important	5

ASSESSMENT

A decade ago, there was no way to balance a bank account, or pay bills on a PC or cell phone. So, here are some financial apps leading the way today: Manilla, Expensify, Mint, PayPal, Budgt, and Spendee, among others. And, five more financial planning apps for the iPad: CashFlow, Bloomberg, Jumsoft Money, Easy Books, and MoneyDance.

CONCLUSION

The basic concepts of financial planning have been reviewed in this chapter. An appreciation of these principles is needed for the new economic norm for medical professionals, and us all.

COLLABORATE

Discuss this chapter online with others at www.MedicalExecutivePost.com.

ACKNOWLEDGMENTS

To Brian Orol, CFP® of Strategic Wealth Management, Raleigh-Durham, North Carolina; David K. Luke, MS-PFP, MIM, CMP™ of the Net Worth Advisory Group in Sandy, Utah; and Lawrence J. DeNoia, MBA, CFP®, CPA, financial advisor, ITI Strategies, Inc., Peekskill, New York.

FURTHER READING

Corley, T: *Rich Habits*. Langdon Street Press (a division of Hillcrest Publishing Group, Inc.) March 1, 2010.

Marcinko, DE (editor): *Financial Planners*. *CD-ROM*. Aspen Publishing, New York, 2001, 2002, and 2003.

Marcinko, DE and Hetico, HR: *Business of Medical Practice* (3rd edition). Springer Publishing Company, New York, 2010.

Marcinko, DE and Hetico, RN: *Dictionary of Health Economics and Finance*. Springer Publishing Company, New York, 2007.

Marcinko, DE and Hetico, RN: *Dictionary of Health Insurance and Managed Care*. Springer Publishing Company, New York, 2006.

6 Rudimentary Financial Accounting Statement Analysis
Understanding Cash Flow Management and Financial Ratio Analysis

Gary L. Bode and David Edward Marcinko

CONTENTS

Financial statements report medical practice (any business) activity for a specific accounting period through horizontal or linear analysis. Showing changes in this fashion forms a perspective for variances that have taken place.

The three traditional statements are: (1) Income Statement (IS), also known as the *Profit & Loss Statement*, (2) Balance Sheet (BS), and (3) the Statement of Cash Flows (SCFs). A newer fourth is the Statement of Changes in Owner's Equity. Note that although exact names for these four financial statements change depending on the type of business entity they represent, the functions remains the same.

Doctors and financial advisors must have a basic understanding of financial statements for investing and valuation purposes, proactive tax, strategic and retirement planning, asset class inclusion in portfolio management, and host of other reasons.

INTRODUCTION

There are many types of asset classes used in investing (stocks, bond, mutual funds, and alternative investments like real estate, etc.). Modern portfolio analysis tells us to use many noncorrelated classes in order to achieve an optimal portfolio based on personal risk tolerance. But, asset classes are always changing and morphing; and their value rises and falls with the business cycle, scarcity, human emotions, and so on. Beyond traditional stocks and bonds, there are several distinct types of investments that have been referred to as alternative investments (AIs). While such investments (derivatives, collectibles, bit coins, CAT bonds and precious metals, etc.) often have features that differentiate them from the equity and fixed income securities that are central to modern portfolio construction approaches, AIs can be distilled down to their basic expected cash flows (usually low).

MEDICAL PRACTICE AS AN ASSET CLASS

A medical practice is much like an alternative asset class in two respects. First, it provides the work environment that generates personal income which has been considered generous, to date. Second, it has inherent appreciation and sales value that can be part of an exit (retirement) or succession planning transfer strategy. So, much like the emerging thought that offers social security payments as a surrogate for a federally insured AAA bond—a medical practice may also be considered an asset class within the ecosystem of a well-diversified modern investment portfolio.

Assigning a value to a medical practice involves a number of considerations. The future positive cash flow is dependent not just on the economic environment and competitive nature of the local healthcare market at the time of the practice sale, but also the mix of practice insurance payments, the reputation and profitability of the practice, and the value of the practice's tangible assets. Often the largest value of a practice is the intangible goodwill, the patient list, and the retention of those patients. Whether the retiring physician stays with the new owner for the transition also affects the value of the future cash flow of the practice.

Now, since cash flow is the lifeblood of any medical practice, business, or equity, it is vital to understand the three financial statements related to cash flows to maximize the value of this asset.

INCOME STATEMENT

The Net Income Statement (IS), or Profit and Loss (P&L) statement, reflects patient revenues and those medical expenses considered general overhead. The IS may report physician compensation and benefits as an expense category, during an interval period of time. Smaller practices report income and expenses on a "cash accounting" basis reflecting income actually received and expenses actually *paid*. However in these practices CPAs generally use "tax basis" which is a hybrid method of cash that adds depreciation as required by the IRS.

The accrual method of accounting records expenses when they are *incurred* and income when *earned*, not when paid or received as in the cash method. The cash method is easier, but the accrual method is more accurate and most surgical practices use this method. Accrual accounting revenue will increase because it generally records gross fees which may include contractual write offs and bad debt. Eventually, of course, write-offs bring accrual income down to match cash revenue, but the timing is different. So, accrual accounting records revenue sooner. Cash accounting records only the eventual payment which generally occurs later and is already net of write offs. Moreover, for medical groups wanting to switch from the cash to accrual method, it is best to make the change after a fiscal calendar quarter. However, accountants may be leery of the shift because they are filing taxes on a cash-modified basis.

BALANCE SHEET (STATEMENT OF FINANCIAL POSITION)

The BS reports the practice's financial position in terms of its assets, liabilities, and owner's equity in the practice, at a specified point in time.

1. Fixed assets are furniture, equipment, and property. Current assets include those that can be converted into cash within a short period of time, such as accounts receivable (AR), checking accounts, and money funds. Intangible assets include goodwill.
2. Accounts payable (AP) and current liabilities are short-term debts and notes while long-term liabilities are loans repaid over many years.
3. The last category reflects ownership in the form of retained earnings or equity and represents the difference between total assets and total unit liabilities.

STATEMENT OF CASH FLOWS

The cash flow statement is the lifeblood of a medical office because it summarizes the effects of cash on three activities.

- *Operating* activities include cash inflows (receipts, interest, and dividends) and outflows (inventory, supplies, and loans).
- *Investing* activities include the disposal or acquisition of noncurrent assets, such as equipment, loans, or marketable securities.
- *Financial* activities generally include the cash inflow or outflow effects of transactions and other events, such as issuing capital stock or notes involving creditors and physician owners.

The SCFs concern liquidity, as opposed to profitability, and may have accompanying schedules that help explain the aggregated figures in the primary document.

TABLE 6.1

Doctor's Medical Clinic (Statement of Owner's Equity) for the Year Ended December 31, 2015

	Dr. 1	Dr. 2
Partners' equity	$7000	$9000
Add: DME income (net)	$20,000	$20,000
	$27,000	$29,000
Deduct: Equipment repair	$19,000	$18,000
Partners' equity Dec. 31st	$8000	$11,000

Notes: Partnership agreement limits withdrawals as follows:

Dr. 1	$5000 per year
Dr. 2	$7000 per year

STATEMENT OF CHANGES IN OWNER'S EQUITY

This statement reconciles the amount in the Owner's Equity section of the BS which uses a time period, the same figure in the current BS (see Table 6.1).

Note: A medical corporate owners' (stockholders') equity statement shows the paid-in capital invested in the business in exchange for stock as of the beginning of the accounting period. It also shows how the income shown on the Income Statement was paid out as dividends, or plowed back into the business as retained earnings.

CASH FLOW ANALYSIS

A medical practice's bills and obligations are paid out of cash flow, not net income. So, it makes sense to look to the SCF and not the IS for liquidity. Therefore, cash flow evaluation deducts from cash revenues only those overhead operating expenses that consume cash. Under this method, each item on the IS are directly converted to cash. For example, assume that office revenues are stated at $100,000 on an accrual accounting basis. If the accounts receivable (ARs) increased by $5000, cash collections from patients and third-party insurance companies would be $95,000. All remaining items on the income statement are also converted to a cash basis.

As a general rule, an increase in a current asset (other than cash) decreases cash inflow or increases cash outflow. Thus—when ARs increase—professional service revenues on cash basis decrease. When cast materials, splints, or other DME inventories increase, the cost of goods sold on a cash basis increases (increasing cash outflow). So, when a pre-paid expense, like malpractice liability insurance increases, the related cash expense increases. The effect on cash flows is just the opposite for decreases in these other current assets (see Table 6.2).

Similarly, an increase in a current liability increases cash inflow or decreases cash outflow. Thus, when accounts payable (APs) increases, the cost of goods sold on a cash basis decrease. When an accrued liability—like salaries payable increase—the related operating expenses on a cash basis decreases. Decreases in current liabilities have just the opposite effect.

Alternately, the *indirect* (add-back) method starts with accrual net income and indirectly adjusts it for items that affect reported net income (accrual) but do not involve cash. For instance, net income is adjusted (rather than adjusting individual items in the income statement) for: (1) changes in current assets (other than cash) and current liabilities and (2) items that were included in net income but did not affect cash. The most common example of an expense that does not affect cash is depreciation.

The end result of CFA is usually a budget, or projected cash inflows and outflows expected/required by period, usually monthly. In the typical case of a smaller healthcare practice, the

TABLE 6.2
Cash Flow Model

For Changes in These Current Assets and Current Liabilities	Make These Adjustments to Convert Accrual Basis Net Income into Cash Basis Net Income	
	Add	Deduct
Accounts Receivable	Decrease	Increase
D.M.E. Inventory	Decrease	Increase
PrePaid Expenses	Decrease	Increase
Accounts Payable	Increase	Decrease
Accrued Liabilities	Increase	Decrease

preparer is the practitioner and it is paramount that the underlying practice logisitics are thoroughly understood.

Revenue is often the most difficult to project. Most cash is collected at various points after services are performed. Booked gross fees are usually reduced, if even collected, by contractual write offs. It is generally prudent to break revenue into its various streams, usually by third-party payer. Analysis of billing system reports provides past amount and timing of cash payment information. For gross analysis, knowing that 76% of insurance company X's fees will eventually be collected is enough: 52% at 45 days, 20% in 60 days, and 4% at greater than 90 days. However by the time CFA is implemented, the practice may already be experiencing cash flow problems. So investigating why that 4% takes so long to arrive is also prudent. This may show that an additional 2% of gross fees is contractually allowed by the insurance company, but never paid because it is unchallenged by the practice.

Sometimes expenses are complex too. For example, many practitioners think of payroll in terms of net pay. But workman's compensation insurance, pension contributions, payroll taxes, healthcare insurance premiums, paid childcare, unemployment taxes, and so on, all payroll related, have to be calculated and paid at various times. Such detail is not often shown in the analysis and instead requires a thorough knowledge of the practice.

The Financial Accounting Standards Board (FASB) encourages the use of the direct method, but permits use of the indirect method. Regardless of the method used, the SCF reflects the internal generation of funds available to owners, investors, and creditors to assess the following:

- The practice's ability to generate positive future net cash flows
- The practice's ability to meet its financial obligations
- The practice's ability to generate profits and dividends
- The practice's need for external financing
- Reasons for differences between net income and cash receipts/payments
- Effects on financial position for both investing and financing transactions

ACCOUNTABLE CARE ORGANIZATION EXAMPLE

Given Cash Flow Model

Suppose that in a new Accountable Care Organization (ACO) contract, a certain medical practice was awarded a new global payment or capitation styled contract that increased revenues by $100,000 for the next fiscal year. The practice had a gross margin of 35% that was not expected to change because of the new business. However, $10,000 was added to medical overhead expenses for another assistant and all Account's Receivable (AR) are paid at the *end* of the year, upon completion of the contract.

Costs of Medical Services Provided

The Costs of Medical Services Provided (COMSP) for the ACO business contract represents the amount of money needed to service the patients provided by the contract. Since gross margin is 35% of revenues, the COMSP is 65% or $65,000. Adding the extra overhead results in $75,000 of new spending money (cash flow) needed to treat the patients. Therefore, divide the $75,000 total by the number of days the contract extends (one year) and realize the new contract requires about $205.50 per day of free cash flows.

Assumptions

Financial cash flow forecasting from operating activities allows a reasonable projection of future cash needs and enables the doctor to err on the side of fiscal prudence. It is an inexact science, by definition, and entails the following assumptions:

- All income tax, salaries, and APs are paid at once.
- Durable medical equipment inventory and pre-paid advertising remain constant.
- Gains/losses on sale of equipment and depreciation expenses remain stable.
- Gross margins remain constant.
- The office is efficient so major new marginal costs will not be incurred.

Physician Reactions

Since many physicians are still not entirely comfortable with global reimbursement, fixed payments, capitation or ACO reimbursement contracts; practices may be loath to turn away short-term business in the ACA era. Physician executives must then determine other methods to generate the additional cash, which include the following general suggestions.

Extend Accounts Payable

Discuss your cash flow difficulties with vendors and emphasize their short-term nature. A doctor and her practice still has considerable cache' value, especially in local communities, and many vendors are willing to work them to retain their business.

Reduce Accounts Receivable

According to most cost surveys, about 30% of multi-specialty group's accounts receivable (ARs) are unpaid at 120 days. In addition, multi-specialty groups are able to collect on only about 69% of charges. The rest was written off as bad debt expenses or as a result of discounted payments from Medicare and other managed care companies. In a study by Wisconsin-based Zimmerman and Associates, the percentages of ARs unpaid at more than 90 days is now at an all-time high of more than 40%. Therefore, multi-specialty groups should aim to keep the percentage of ARs unpaid for more than 120 days, down to less than 20% of the total practice. The safest place to be for a single specialty physician is probably in the 30–35% range as anything over that is just not affordable.

The slowest paid specialties (ARs greater than 120 days) are: multi-specialty group practices; family practices; cardiology groups; anesthesiology groups; and gastroenterologists, respectively. So work hard to get your money, faster. Factoring, or selling the ARs to a third party for an immediate discounted amount is not usually recommended.

Borrow with Short-Term Bridge Loans

Obtain a line of credit from your local bank, credit union, or other private sources, if possible in an economically constrained environment. Beware the time value of money, personal loan guarantees, and onerous usury rates. Also, beware that lenders can reduce or eliminate credit lines to a medical practice, often at the most inopportune time.

Cut Expenses

While this is often possible, it has to be done without demoralizing the practice's staff.

Reduce Supply Inventories

If prudently possible; remember things like minimal shipping fees, loss of revenue if you run short, and so on.

Taxes

Do not stop paying withholding taxes in favor of cash flow because it is illegal.

HYPER-GROWTH MODEL

Now, let us again suppose that the practice has attracted nine more similar medical contracts. If we multiply the above example 10-fold, the serious nature of potential cash flow problem becomes apparent. In other words, the practice has increased revenues to 1 million dollars, with the same 35% margin, 65% COMSP, and $100,000 increase in operating overhead expenses. Using identical mathematical calculations, we determine that $750,000/365 days equals $2055.00 per day of needed new free cash flows! Hence, indiscriminate growth without careful contract evaluation and cash flow analysis is a prescription for potential financial disaster.

BENCHMARK A MEDICAL PRACTICE WITH FINANCIAL RATIOS

Financial ratios are figures or percentages derived from components of the financial statements described above. Even with the inherent limitations, financial ratios are the cornerstone of interpreting financial statements. They are being increasingly used by external sources to value and evaluate practices for situations like divorce, sale or practice purchase, succession planning or hospital mergers and acquisitions, and so on. Thus, it behooves doctors and advisors to understand them. Some financial ratios are valuable in the managerial report: a time series of certain practice financial ratios helps reveal its trends, strengths, and weaknesses. All practice information, including financial ratios, should be integrated into the "big picture" and undue emphasis on a single facet may skew interpretation. So, although these financial ratio values are "benchmarked" to values obtained by surveys which become "industry standard," realize that the average practice's financial statements have some inherent problems, making the derived financial ratios suspect. The government regulates, and the accounting industry strongly guides, the accounting principles used to generate publicly held company's financial statements. This makes them more uniform and accurate than the average financial statements of a private healthcare practice.

Financial ratios fall into four main classifications: (1) liquidity and solvency, (2) asset management, (3) debt management, and (4) profitability ratios.

LIQUIDITY AND SOLVENCY FINANCIAL RATIOS

The two most useful small- to mid-sized (SMB) medical practice financial ratios are: the current ratio and the current liabilities to net worth.

CURRENT RATIO

$$\frac{\text{Current Assets}}{\text{Current Liabilities}} = \text{Current Ratio}$$

The *Current Ratio* measures short-term solvency. Unfortunately, practice financial statements often do not segregate out current and long-term assets and liabilities accurately. Current assets include cash on hand, the percentage of accounts receivable you can reasonably expect to collect, and short-term investments like a 3-month CD. Current liabilities are notes payable and loans due within one year. This ratio should be at least one, preferably higher. A Certified Medical Planner™, banker, physician focused financial advisor or venture capitalist probably wants to see this be in the range of about 1.3–1.5.

Short-term solvency has an impact on the ability to pay current obligations, which dramatically affects credit, which is an essential tool to controlling practice expenses. Thus, it is an important figure to track internally over time. Establish your definitions that allow consistent calculation of the current ratio.

For example, if you enter gross fees into accounts receivable and then adjust for contractual write off and bad debt, use the last six month's figures of these adjustments to establish the true eventual cash value of accounts receivable.

CURRENT LIABILITIES TO NET WORTH

$$\frac{\text{Current Liabilities}}{\text{Net Worth}} = \text{Current Liabilities to Net Worth}$$

This should be low, probably beneath .5, but not zero. Net Worth, or owner's equity, is often distorted on the financial statements, as most practitioners take out all the money "left over" as salary or distributions. This can be especially true if the practitioner holds major assets personally, like the building (a common scenario), and "leases" them to the practice. Bankers circumvent this by evaluating the practitioner and practice simultaneously.

ASSET MANAGEMENT FINANCIAL RATIOS

The four most important are the: (1) average collection period, (2) fixed assets utilization, (3) fixed assets to net worth, and (4) total assets utilization ratio.

AVERAGE COLLECTION PERIOD

$$\frac{\text{Total Accounts Receivable}}{\substack{\text{Average Daily Charges} \\ \text{(those not collected on the day of service)}}} = \text{Average Collection Period}$$

The acceptable figure depends on the type of practice. A practice that handles a lot of personal injury cases has a higher number than one that deals mostly in cash. Note that the total accounts receivable is inherently over valued if it includes eventual contractual write off and bad debt. Average daily charges would vary on the time period sampled and can be difficult to obtain. This is a vital practice parameter however, and, it is well worth setting up the process to obtain and track the required figures. Tracked over time, it provides essential monitoring of the entire collections and billing process. For internal managerial purposes, the top dollar, third-party payer components should be tracked individually as the aggregate figure may not immediately detect a rapid change in a single insurance company.

Each extra day of this parameter means someone else is enjoying the float or interest on your money for an additional day. 10 extra days of $50,000 in accounts receivable means at least an additional expense to you of $30 a year, if you could have banked this at 2% APR. Since a practice with protracted collections usually has cash flow problems, this probably translates out to $270 if you're borrowing money at 18% APR.

FIXED ASSETS UTILIZATION

$$\frac{\text{Net Revenue}}{\text{Net Fixed Assets}} = \text{Fixed Assets Utilization}$$

This shows how productively a practice utilizes its assets. Obviously, you would like any asset you invest in to render as much as possible in additional revenue. Asset evaluation issues (like accumulated depreciation described) and true practice assets being held by the practitioner for tax purposes, make the managerial use of this figure marginal.

FIXED ASSETS TO NET WORTH

$$\frac{\text{Fixed Assets}}{\text{Net Worth (Doctor Owners Equity)}} = \text{Fixed Assets to Net Worth}$$

A higher ratio indicates a greater investment in fixed assets which, conversely, may indicate low working capital. This is a great concept in publicly held companies with strict accounting, but less useful to the average practitioner.

TOTAL ASSETS UTILIZATION

$$\frac{\text{Net Revenue}}{\text{Total Assets}} = \text{Total Assets Utilization}$$

This is similar to the fixed assets to net worth described above, but eliminates some of the asset evaluation problems. If the proper definitions are consistently employed, this is a good figure to track internally over time. An example of an appropriate definition might be any asset originally costing over $250 that is in current use, including any held "artificially" by the practitioner for tax purposes. While a "soft" figure, it has value as an indicator of productivity.

DEBT MANAGEMENT RATIOS

The two most common are (1) total debt to total assets and (2) total liabilities to net worth.

TOTAL DEBT TO TOTAL ASSETS

$$\frac{\text{Total Debt}}{\text{Total Assets}} = \text{Total Debt to Total Assets}$$

Obviously, less debt is generally preferable, so this ratio should be low. Remember debt can be a useful managerial tool if used wisely, and a total debt to total assets figure of zero might have negative implications. A consultant, advisor, or banker looks for a low figure since he is being asked to provide more debt and wants to ensure his investment.

TOTAL LIABILITIES TO NET WORTH

$$\frac{\text{Total Liabilities}}{\text{Net Worth}} = \text{Total Liabilities to Net Worth}$$

This can be a useful figure if appropriate definitions are used and some practitioners track this internally. Generally, lower is better.

PROFITABILITY RATIOS

These include (1) profit margin and (2) return on investment ratios

PROFIT MARGIN

$$\frac{\text{Net Income}}{\text{Net Revenue}} = \text{Profit Margin}$$

Generally expressed as a percentage, this figure reflects how much profit the practice makes on each dollar of revenue, usually gross fees. When the practitioner's salary encompasses "what's left over," this is zero. For internal purposes it can be considered as potential practitioner salary over gross fees. Obviously, higher is better.

RETURN ON INVESTMENT

$$\frac{\text{Net Income}}{\text{Total Assets}} = \text{Return on Investment}$$

This reflects how well assets are used to generate net income. Again, one would strive to make the most money with a given asset, making this figure as high as possible. This concept appears in a break even analysis where the expected return on investment on an individual asset is calculated before buying it. Sometimes it makes sense to refer potential gross fees to outside sources, despite inherent clinical expertise, because of the equipment cost involved. Other times, traditionally out sourced services now performed in house help the practice.

OTHER NONFINANCIAL RATIOS

Other useful financial ratios can also be correlated to help show practice efficiency. For example, staff gross salary as a ratio of gross fees and/or collections, helps monitor the amount of revenue produced by each dollar of staff salary. This is analogous to the asset utilization financial ratios explained above. And, the current ratio can generally be derived without the financial statements. Tracking it may help keep the important topic of short-term liquidity in mind.

A medical practice needs hands on management. A managerial report made of financial ratios is a good tool for managing a practice in a time efficient manner. It is a valuable exercise that can help spot both negative and positive trends earlier than they would otherwise become apparent.

OVERHEARD IN THE DOCTOR'S LOUNGE: THE *WHITE COAT* INVESTOR*

Although I think a physician is perfectly capable of doing his own financial planning and investment management, the majority of doctors want, and would benefit from hiring a competent, fiduciary, fee-only advisor who can give them good advice at a fair price. The more familiar an advisor is with the unique financial planning issues associated with physicians, such as properly managing hundreds of thousands of dollars in students loans and acquiring specialty-specific disability insurance, the better.

Unfortunately, it is surprisingly difficult for a doctor to hire such an advisor as the vast majority of those who bill themselves as financial advisors are little more than commissioned mutual fund or insurance salesmen. Many of these so-called advisors state that they "specialize in physicians," but in reality, merely specialize in marketing to physicians. To make matters worse, a doctor may assume that these advisors are trained professionals comparable to accountants, attorneys, or physicians, when in reality the advisor may only have a few days of formal training, and most of that in sales.

Obtaining high-quality, physician-specific, financial advice offered at a fair price sometimes seems like trying to find the Holy Grail.

Note: The white coat ceremony is a medical school ritual that marks the transition from the study of preclinical to clinical health sciences. WCCs typically involve a formal "robing" or "cloaking" of students in white coats, the garb doctors have traditionally worn for over a century.

James M. Dahle, MD, FACEP
(Author: The White Coat Investor: A Doctor's Guide to Personal Finance and Investing; Editor: www.whitecoatinvestor.com)

ASSESSMENT

Accounting financial statements, with an emphasis on ratio analysis and medical office cash flow management, were reviewed in order to understand their importance and the potential pitfalls of practice growth in the new environment of value-based global payments and capitated care.

If medical professionals perform this analysis, much can be ascertained about the operational efficiencies of the practice within the confines of an integrated and comprehensive financial plan, as suggested by the Institute of Medical Business Advisors Inc., and the nation's leading Certified Medical Planners™.

CONCLUSION

Having access to the analytic tools needed to determine the information in this chapter is vital to medical practice, and personal, survival. Related financial analysis will only increase business entity value to the benefit of all stakeholders.

COLLABORATE

Discuss this chapter online with others at www.MedicalExecutivePost.com.

ACKNOWLEDGMENTS

To David K. Luke, MS-PFP, MIM, CMP™ of the Net Worth Advisory Group in Sandy, Utah.

FURTHER READING

Cimasi, RJ: *Accountable Care Organizations [Value Metrics and Capital Formation]*. CRC and Productivity Press, Boca Raton, FL, 2013.

Fabozzi, FJ: *Handbook of Finance*. Wiley, New York, 2008.

Fight, A: *Cash Flow Forecasting: A Volume in the Essential Capital Markets Series*. Butterworth-Heinemann, New York, 2005.

Ittelson, TR: *Financial Statements*. Career Press, New York, 2009.

Kieso, D: *Intermediate Accounting*. Wiley, New York, 2008.

Marcinko, DE and Hetico, HR: *Financial Management Strategies for Hospitals and Healthcare Organizations*. CRC and Productivity Press, Boca Raton, FL, 2013.

Marcinko, DE and Hetico, HR: *Hospitals and Healthcare Organizations*. CRC and Productivity Press, Boca Raton, FL, 2013.

Marcinko, DE and Hetico, RH: *Business of Medical Practice*. Springer Publishing, New York, 2010.

Section II

For New Practitioners

New medical practitioners are typically in their late-twenties or early-thirties and it may be a decade, or more, before they independently lead a case. Often, they are in debt and with a new spouse and children. And, it is not unusual for them to desire nice homes, automobiles, clothes, and take vacations as a reward for their years of hard work. After all, they've earned it. In retrospect, they step back, look at their peers from college who are farther along in their careers and wonder if it was all worth it. It is about this same time that so-called "financial advisors" seek them out for gain. But is it for their benefit or advisor self-benefit?

Of course, the IRS is vicious and young doctors need an account, says the CPA. And, you must protect your business, career, life, kids, and possessions with insurance, says the insurance agent. Ditto for an investing plan and stock portfolio, says the financial advisor as they all recommend their products or hawk their services of choice. Insiders are aware that there is a truism in the financial services sector that suggests most every problem can be solved with an insurance product or financial plan. So it's no surprise that goaded physicians might prefer "investing" vehicles like the guaranteed minimum death benefit of variable annuities, or the assurance that comes with disability or long-term care insurance, or traditional cash value life insurance policies, despite their decidedly higher costs and commissions. All salesmen—as uber bloger Michael Kitecs, MSFS, MTAX, CFP®, CLU, ChFC, RHU, REBC, and CASL—opines "all financial planning is about sales, sales, and sales" (personal communication, Kitces.com, Reston, VA).

Yet, for true physician-focused financial advisors, this is an exciting time to be practicing because there is much research and creative enlightenment occurring in the academic and practitioner communities. But, one must be willing to abandon ancient thoughts and remain open to new ideas that identify and provide solutions to the contemporaneous problems of healthcare professionals. As an example of this epiphany, the economist Christian Gollier revisited the *raison d'être* of insurance, by asking: should one even buy insurance since the industry itself is so skilled at exploiting human foibles? Although this emerging work is descriptive, it is not yet time tested since some of it aspires to be normative, as developing modern models of savings and consumption hint that insurance may deserve a smaller role in personal risk management than previously believed.

So, in Section II, we review insurance plans, risk management topics, tax and asset protection fundamentals and strategies, and then introduce the various investment vehicles and platforms used in professional and self portfolio construction.

7 Establishing a Solid Foundation of Insurance Planning
The Bedrock of Life and Medical Practice

Thomas A. Muldowney, Gary A. Cook, and David Edward Marcinko

CONTENTS

Unless you are a financial advisor, Certified Medical Planner™, or insurance agent advising physicians, there will be a strong tendency to skip this chapter. The word insurance seems to have that effect on many doctors. The physician is assured, however, that each topic, while important, will not be covered in laborious detail.

The basis for much of today's insurance evolved from the seventeenth century study of probabilities and what is called the Law of Large Numbers. Actually, it's the language of science—mathematics—and more precisely, statistics. Statistically, whenever a potentially random event is to be predicted, the more events recorded or tested, the more likely the final outcome will match the predictions—the first concept of the Law of Large Numbers. Actuaries believe this instinctively. It seems that the rest of us are always trying to beat the odds.

For example, looking at all the readers of this chapter as a sample set, and assuming that they are all licensed drivers, we could predict that the reader has been involved in a minor automobile accident at sometime in his lifetime. If only one person ever reads this section, the likelihood of this prediction being wrong is fairly high. The more people that read it, however, the more likely this prediction will be right on target. Depending on the reader's age and sex, the number of miles driven in a year, his particular area of the country, and some other factors, the actuary can actually predict how often this will occur and, to an uncanny degree, even the extent of the damage. Accuracy of the predictions, then, leads to profits.

Expanding on this second concept within the Law of Large Numbers, the insurance company's marketing department is tasked with enticing enough drivers (readers), into the company's risk pool to ensure the frequency distribution (experience accuracy) of the actuarial predictions. Insurance coverage can generally be obtained for car-related accidents, tornado damage, cancer expenses, theft losses, cost of repairing tooth decay, being killed by a falling space lab, or any other statistically predictable event. The potential of finding an insurance underwriter willing to predict the event and develop rates usually depends equally on finding enough willing buyers to make the predictions accurate. It's not personal; it's just business. The business of insurance is basically that simple.

GENERAL TYPES OF INSURANCE POLICIES COVERING DOCTORS

LIFE INSURANCE OVERVIEW

Life insurance transfers the financial loss resulting from death. A myriad of different families of life insurance policies exist, but they basically have two main branches: term insurance and permanent insurance.

TERM INSURANCE

Term insurance is the simplest form of life insurance and is a sensible place to begin any discussion of life insurance. Term insurance is exactly what the name implies: it provides life insurance coverage for a specified period of time, that is, the term. At the end of the term, the policy is either canceled or continued, typically by paying higher premiums.

Annual Renewable Term

The oldest form of term insurance is that of Annual Renewable Term (ART). These polices have premiums which typically begin very low, but increase steadily each year. At the end of each year, the policy owner has the option to renew coverage at the higher premium, or cancel the coverage. By the time an insured reaches age 60, and the probability of dying becomes more pronounced, the premiums start to rise drastically. The increased premium is simply a reflection of the increased chance of dying combined with the obvious fact that there are fewer lives at that age to spread the risk over. ART insurance has lost much of its popularity recently since level-premium term products have captured more market share.

Level Term Insurance

Level term policies offer a premium which remains level for a specified period of time, usually 5, 10, 15, 20, 25, or 30 years. The most popular products have premiums that are guaranteed to remain level for the prescribed period. Beware, however, policies do exist where the insurance company has the right to change the premiums during this period. Following the selected level-premium period, the term policy is typically canceled, although the owner may keep the policy in-force by paying higher premiums. The premiums, however, may increase drastically, sometimes even to the absurd.

The affordability (during the selected term period) and simplicity of these products have made them very popular. It is easy to see why a 40-year-old physician would be attracted to a term policy that guarantees its premium for 20 years. It is entirely reasonable for many to obtain affordable coverage that would end exactly when it is anticipated that it will no longer be needed—at retirement. A seemingly very nice fit, unless justification can be made for longer coverage, like the potential for poor health and the need to renew the policy when needed most (noncancelable feature).

Decreasing Term Insurance

Decreasing (or reducing) term is another common style of term insurance that not only lasts for a specified period of time but also reduces in death benefit each year. These are often recommended by lenders to cover mortgages as the mortgage balance decreases each year. These policies have become very rare because level term insurance is so affordable that it makes little sense to buy decreasing coverage.

As currently marketed, term products generally have excellent premiums which allow a policy owner to purchase substantial coverage for a very affordable price. But it is important to keep in mind why the premium is so affordable—because the vast majority of term policies never pay a death benefit. The simple reason for this unexpected fact is that most people outlive the term period or their policies are not in-force when they die.

Triple X

Regulation XXX, also referred to as Triple X, is a model regulation from the National Association of Insurance Commissioners (NAIC) that was implemented on January 1, 2000. This regulation has substantially changed the manner in which an insurance company must set aside reserves for any term policy with a premium guarantee longer than 15 years, or a universal life policy with a secondary guarantee of more than 5 years (this will be covered soon). It basically requires higher reserves for policies with longer guarantee periods. Higher reserves generally resulted in the insurance companies increasing their premiums. As a direct result, if the physician has a current policy with a premium or death benefit guarantee longer than 5 years, the policy should probably not be replaced or lapsed without some serious thought.

PERMANENT INSURANCE

Permanent insurance differs from term insurance in two major ways. First, it is usually designed to last to age 95 or 100 (commonly referred to as the maturity date) without any future requirement to requalify for the coverage by providing proof of good health. Some newer contracts, in fact, have no maturity date at all and are being illustrated as lasting until age 115. Second, permanent policies have built in reserves, as mentioned above. It is the reserves that end up as a form of cash value accumulation.

One permanent insurance policy can cover a single life, two lives, or an entire family. Policies covering two lives can provide a death benefit either on the first death or the last death.

Generally, permanent insurance has a predefined level-premium payable until a stated maturity, but the premium-paying period can potentially be shortened in a number of ways. Regardless, the predefined premium is substantially higher in a permanent policy than for a comparable face-amount term insurance policy. This higher premium results in the aforementioned aspect of an internal accumulation of cash value.

This accumulation was originally designed by actuaries to help level the premium over longer periods of time. It has since, however, been seen by many as a convenient method of accumulating funds in a tax-deferred manner.

Common Types of Permanent Insurance

Permanent insurance comes in four standard variations: whole life, variable life, universal life, and variable universal life. Do not be fooled by the title *permanent*, however. Today's life insurance products are very complex and few policies are truly permanent. Events can occur which result in policies lapsing or paying reduced benefits, even when specified premiums have been submitted in a timely manner. The word permanent simply reflects the fact that these policies are expected to last until the insured's death no matter when that may be.

Whole Life

Whole life, also called straight life or ordinary life, is the oldest and the most classic type of permanent insurance. It typically has the highest required premium of the four standard variations, but it is also the least risky for the policy owner. Whole life remains in force until maturity and is guaranteed to pay the full death benefit if the required premiums are paid in a timely manner. The whole life family of policies also includes those referred to as Life Paid-up at 65, 83, 85, 95, and so on. The life paid up at age "X" refers to the insured's age at which the larger premiums (larger than the premium for whole life) may be stopped even though the policy death benefits will be guaranteed to remain in force until the insured person dies.

Whole life premiums are fixed, that is, they cannot be arbitrarily changed from year to year, and they must be paid in a timely manner if the entire death benefit is to be kept intact. Whole life is more rigid than universal life, but it counters by offering the highest level of guarantees. Whole life, like all permanent policies, offers growing cash values that can be borrowed by the policy owner if needed.

Because whole life is considered expensive, companies have created ways, such as term riders, to temporarily increase the death benefit but to hold the premium to more affordable levels. However, the drawback of these term riders is that more risk falls upon the policy owner. When term riders are added to a whole life policy, the premium becomes cheaper, but the entire policy is no longer guaranteed to last to maturity and/or may pay reduced death benefits under some situations.

When purchasing a whole life contract, the death benefit is fully guaranteed, as long as the premium is paid on time every year. At the maturity date, the internal cash values (to be discussed later) will equal the amount of guaranteed death benefit: this is called Endowment.

If the insurance company offers a "participating policy" and has good experiences with its business over the years, that is, fewer people die than expected, the company may illustrate that the policy "participates" and receives a refund of premiums. These refunds are called "dividends."

Because dividends are paid to participating policies and are considered a return of the policy owner's premium they are, therefore, not taxable income. A policy owner can generally take them in cash, use them to buy paid-up additions, use them to buy one-year term additions, or have them accumulate at interest, like an additional savings account. Using the dividend to buy paid-up additions or allowing them to accumulate at interest will provide the policy owner an additional source of future premiums or increased death benefit.

At some point in the policy's life, these funds may be sufficient to allow the policy owner to cease paying premiums and direct the insurance company to take its annual premium from these excess values. This is sometimes called a "vanishing" premium or a "short pay" premium or a "premium offset." The premiums are still due and still paid each year, but instead come from the excess external policy values rather than the owner's pocket.

A life insurance agent or CFP© may illustrate this discontinued premium flow as a benefit of their policy. Beware! This is only a *projection*. This means the company is not guaranteeing the ability to stop paying premiums. This may possibly occur if the company keeps doing well. It is not guaranteed!

Many whole life policies were sold this way in the past, and while some policies actually did allow the owner to stop paying premiums, many policies did not. This surprised many policy owners who were expecting to cease their premiums. The medical professional or healthcare practitioner must make sure they understand what policy aspects are guaranteed and what are merely projections.

A well-informed physician, when purchasing a whole life policy, will ask his/her insurance agent to check both the Standard and Poor's (or Moody's) company rating, and the *AM Best's*

Annual Historical Dividend Report. The first rates financial stability of the company, while the second reports how a company's actual dividends compared to their projections for each year. It is wise to be leery of illustrations from companies that consistently fail to meet their projections.

Before a whole life product is purchased, ask to see what happens to the death benefit and premiums if the company experiences a lower dividend scale (worse business conditions). This will allow the purchaser to see how sensitive the policy is to different business conditions. Beware of whole life policies that are very sensitive to reduced dividend scales.

Universal Life Insurance

Universal life was developed in the late 1970s, and has become a very popular product in a very short time. Generally, in terms of price and risk to the policy owner, it falls between term and whole life.

Universal life is similar to a bank savings account but has automatic monthly withdrawals from the account, to pay for the death benefit. Each universal life premium goes into the policy and becomes part of the cash value just as a bank savings deposit becomes part of a savings account. Some policies have a premium expense charge that generally is designed to pay the individual state premium tax. The cash value also has monthly debits to pay for the death benefit and/or any riders and most also charge a monthly administrative fee. The resulting cash value of the policy earns a competitive money market-like interest rate. Finally, policy owners receive an annual report that itemizes all relevant costs, to the penny. Universal life has often been called "whole life unbundled" because of this feature.

Clearly, the cash value of the universal life policy will depend on which is greater: the amount going into the policy (premiums and interest) or the amounts leaving the policy (the cost of the death benefit and the monthly administrative fees). Additionally, the charges for the death benefit will rise over time, as the insured doctor gets older (just like the ART rates mentioned at the beginning of this topic).

Typically, in the early policy years, the amounts flowing into the policy are greater than the internal charges and the subsequent cash value increases. If at some point the outflows exceed the inflows, the cash value will cease growing and may even decline. If the cash value falls to zero, the policy generally lapses unless more premiums are paid.

The policy owner can periodically adjust the amount and timing of the universal life premiums and even skip premiums (without incurring a loan, which is the result with whole life). Any change in premium amount or mode of payment will also change the cash value projections on a policy illustration. Skipping premiums will cause a drop in cash values and possibly cause a policy to lapse. If ample cash value has accumulated in the contract, the ability to skip premium without adverse consequences becomes more probable. This flexibility is one of the reasons for the popularity of universal life policies.

Because universal life polices are very interest rate sensitive, a policy owner needs to keep track of the policy values each year to make sure the policy is performing as expected. When a policy owner receives their "Annual Report," it is a good idea to use this as a reminder to request (from the agent or the company) a reprojection of future amounts based on the then current assumptions. This is commonly called an in-force projection or midstream proposal.

Just as with "vanishing premium" whole life projections, there have also been problems with universal life. In the 1980s, interest rates were very high and this appeared to make universal life policies appear very inexpensive, compared to whole life. Unfortunately, interests rates have declined dramatically and by now those polices have been credited far less interest than originally illustrated. As a result, the cash values were lower than expected and policy owners had to either increase their premiums or risk the policies lapsing.

If purchasing a universal life policy, the doctor should definitely ask to see illustrations reflecting declining interest rates. Typically this does not need to be to the guaranteed rate. Ask the agent,

CFP©, or broker for a history of the company's rates and gauge your request accordingly. If policy performance is drastically affected, commit to a higher premium so that coverage is not jeopardized in the event of falling interest rates.

Besides being interest rate sensitive, the insurance company can also change the internal cost of the death benefit on a universal life policy. Obviously, increasing these charges could cause the cash values to drop and the policy to lapse. Companies try to avoid doing this, but it can and does happen. A potential buyer should also inquire as to the company's history of "mortality cost" increases before purchasing any universal life policy. Avoid companies which have a history of raising their insurance costs or which fail to provide this vital information.

Variable Life Insurance

Variable life is a type of permanent insurance that comes in the same two forms discussed above: universal life and whole life.

The same general design of whole life and universal life, as just described, also apply to variable whole life and variable universal life. The only real difference is the availability of investment choices for the cash value of the policy. With whole life and universal life, the insurance companies generally invest the money in fixed income investments like bonds and mortgages. The insurance company then declares the interest rate that gets credited to the company's policies (except term, which has no cash value).

With variable policies, the company offers the policy owner a choice of investment options. These investment options are called separate accounts and resemble traditional mutual funds. Good variable life policies should offer a wide array of investment choices to include money market funds, bond funds, balanced funds, stock funds, and international funds. It is not unusual to find policies offering in excess of 30 such separate accounts.

The policy owner then chooses the account, or accounts, which match his/her investment risk. Most policy owners put a majority of their premium dollars into equity accounts because they have historically provided better returns than most other investments. Of course, the higher the actual returns of the separate accounts, the more the cash value grows.

This results because the internal policy expense costs of a variable policy are typically higher than the internal costs of a fixed interest rate policy. It therefore takes a higher return inside of a variable life to offset the effect of these higher internal costs. Generally, one should not purchase a variable policy unless he/she expects the separate accounts to earn an average of at least 8.5% per year.

Variable life policies give the policy owner more control over how their premium dollars are invested. These polices allow greater potential returns, but at greater risk, because the policy owner assumes the investment risk. Variable policies became very popular during the bull market of the 1990s. To their surprise, if they bought the policy during those periods, setting premiums based on those high equity returns, by now they must provide large amounts of additional premium or replace the policy with one that is currently more affordable. These products are most appropriate for policy owners with a moderate to high-risk tolerance, that believe in the long-term superiority of equities as investments, and who have a long-term time horizon and the ability to pay additional premiums if necessary.

The same principles that apply to investing in general also apply to variable policies. A wise variable policy owner will invest his/her premiums in several separate accounts in order to achieve diversification. Most variable policies will also allow dollar cost averaging and asset rebalancing.

Other Varieties of Life Policies

Survivorship Life Insurance

Survivorship life is commonly referred to as Second-to-Die life insurance. Unlike the typical life insurance policy that has one primary insured and pays a death benefit when that person dies, a survivorship life policy generally has two insured's and only pays a death benefit when both of the insured's are deceased.

Survivorship products have existed for about 30 years, but became very popular after passage of the unlimited marital deduction in the Economic Recovery Tax Act (ERTA) of 1981. These policies are used almost exclusively in the estate planning realm where the husband and wife have a combined net worth of more than 2 times the current unified credit, that is, 5.25 million dollars in year 2014. The amount of the unified credit will increase with inflation. Wealthy couples, with estates in excess of $10.5 million, typically between the ages of 50 and 70, purchase survivorship insurance to assist in providing adequate liquidity for estate transfer and settlement costs routinely due at the second death.

In 1996, a new feature—a secondary guarantee—was seen in universal life and, in particular, survivorship universal life policies. The primary guarantees in these policies were that of a guaranteed minimum credited interest rate and a maximum amount of monthly charges and, specifically, a maximum charge for mortality. The earlier versions of these policies illustrated poorly with regard to guaranteed cash values, unless a whole life-type premium was paid.

Secondary guarantees have also been called no-lapse guarantees. Basically, these policies are guaranteed to stay in force for a specified number of years as long as the policy owner pays a required cumulative premium as of a particular date, even if the underlying primary guarantees would allow the policy to otherwise lapse. Most importantly, the new no-lapse premiums were still considerably lower than that of a whole life policy. Unfortunately, Triple X regulations have forced most insurance companies to remove these products from sale or substantially increase their premium requirements for this benefit.

Joint First-to-Die Life Insurance

Just as with survivorship life insurance, a joint First-to-Die policy generally insures two people. Unlike survivorship insurance, however, a joint First-to-Die policy pays upon the death of the first insured.

Joint First-to-Die policies typically make sense in family insurance planning for households, who have dependent children, where both parents work, and occasionally they are used for mortgage (loan) protection. The vast majority of joint First-to-Die plans, however, are used in the business world. These policies are particularly well suited for multiple key-people or for stock redemption (entity) buy-sell plans.

It is important to remember that when the first insured dies under a joint First-to-Die policy, the death benefit is paid, and the policy is terminated: coverage no longer exists on the remaining insured(s). This problem can be solved by buying a guaranteed insurability option on the policy that allows the remaining insured to purchase a new joint policy with no underwriting immediately after the first death.

Another rider that should be considered when joint policies are purchased for business planning reasons is a substitute insured rider. This allows the policy owner to exchange an insured with a new insured. This rider comes in very handy if one of the insured's leaves the business and is replaced by someone else. Many insurance companies, unfortunately, have withdrawn this rider because of the difficulty in administering it.

Interest Sensitive Whole Life

Interest sensitive whole life, also referred to as current assumption whole life, is a hybrid of whole life and universal life. Like whole life, the premiums are fixed. Some companies fix the premium for the life of the policy, but most fix the premium only for a specified period of time. Like universal life, the current internal mortality charges are lower than for a whole life policy, but the insurance company retains the right to raise them. Also like universal life, a competitive interest rate is credited to the policy cash values each month. These polices are currently not very common.

Group Life

Group life insurance coverage is very common, and the vast majority of people have this form of coverage at work, and/or have the opportunity to purchase more group life insurance coverage through their employer or other associations to which they belong. Most group life insurance policies are group term because term is affordable and easy to understand, but group universal life and group variable universal life policies exist as well.

Many employers, especially larger ones, typically offer a minimum of group life insurance as an automatic employee benefit. Since current tax code provisions allow up to $50,000 of group coverage as a totally tax-free benefit, this is often the initial amount of coverage. Many employers also offer the employee the ability to purchase additional group life insurance with the premium being deducted from each paycheck. The main advantage of group life insurance is its convenience.

The major disadvantages concern the lack of flexibility. It may not be easy to change your coverage under a group life policy, and if you leave your company, it may not be possible to take the coverage with you. For this reason, most people prefer to purchase their own individual life insurance policy for the bulk of their life insurance protection.

Single Premium Life

Single premium life is exactly as the name implies: the owner pays one premium for lifetime coverage. Clearly, the premium will be much larger than any other type of insurance for an equivalent death benefit.

These policies have become quite rare since the Modified Endowment Contract (MEC) rules were established to discourage large premiums early in the life of a policy (see "Life Insurance Taxation" later in this section). Nonetheless, these polices still have a limited number of uses. These policies may be appropriate if tax-deferred growth is desired and the money is not needed during the insured's lifetime.

The 5–100 Rule

With any universal life insurance policy (and certainly all variable life policies), fluctuating rates of return, the actual timing of the premium payments, and potential internal policy changes by the insurance company, all contribute to results that will probably differ substantially from the original illustration. The 5–100 Rule states that as a result of accounting for these elements, all initial projections of cash value beyond 5 years, will necessarily be 100% incorrect when compared to actuality. A prudent policy owner should therefore keep on top of any changes and react accordingly. If a policy owner ignores his/her policy for even 5 years, any adverse changes could be so drastic as to make rectifying them very costly.

DEATH BENEFIT SETTLEMENT OPTIONS

Settlement options refer to the different ways a beneficiary can receive the death benefit payable upon the death of the insured. A beneficiary commonly receives the entire death benefit in a lump sum, but that is certainly not the only choice. Another possibility is the interest only option where the beneficiary leaves the death benefit with the insurer and receives the monthly interest. Another common option is the lifetime annuity option where the death benefit is paid out as a guaranteed lifetime income.

Settlement options can be left to the discretion of the beneficiary. In this way, the beneficiary, with capable advice, can hopefully make an informed choice based on their particular situation at the time. Alternatively, the policy owner can specify a particular settlement option. During the life of the insured, the policy owner can instruct the insurance company to pay the beneficiary according to a design the policy owner feels appropriate. It is the opinion of the authors, however, that a better alternative would be to establish a trust for any beneficiary unable to manage their funds, rather than use a restrictive settlement option.

A LOOK AT LEVEL LIFE INSURANCE COMMISSIONS: OF INTEREST TO ALL INSURANCE AGENTS

According to David K. Luke, MIM, MS-PFP, CMP™ (www.NetWorthAdvice.com), the current structure of the life insurance industry regarding cash-value life insurance policies with most major insurance companies is to reward the selling agent with the entire commission upfront on a newly issued policy. The criticism to this practice is that this of course reduces the needed client-agent reviews and interaction and generates more "churning" and "flipping." Unscrupulous agents are tempted to sell physician-clients another policy for another commission rather than encourage them to maintain and keep their existing policy, which most likely would have lower costs than any new policy considering the client was younger and most likely in better health with the existing contract. A model in which the insurance agent would have a financial incentive for their client's continued patronage could create a win–win for both parties. We see this "pay as you" model currently operating successfully with wealth advisors and property/casualty agents, so why not life insurance agents (personal communication)?

There are some flaws to this argument. The reality is that the captive life insurance industry and their agents prefer this form of lump compensation. The claim is that selling an individual a life insurance policy (the ultimate intangible product) is hard work, and likewise the 70–110% of the first year premium is fair compensation for the efforts. For existing agents to reduce their current income to a fraction of this commission upfront, but convert it into a trail over a multiyear period is actually quite distasteful. Therefore, this change will likewise not be initiated from the insurance agent or insurance industry side unless other forces prevail.

The drive by the consumer to change this up front lump form of compensation has not yet presented itself in full force. After all, why does the consumer care about how the agent is paid if the consumer is satisfied with the end result? One must acknowledge that the drive to reduce commissions and up front loads in the investment advisory business was driven by the consumer that insisted on lower fees and costs.

However, the relevant costs of a life insurance policy are not quite as obvious. Only by comparing a quote from different companies can a consumer compare costs, and even then it is unknown and not understood how the pricing mechanisms used by the insurance company work. The advent of nonagent sold policies however is decreasing the cost of life insurance (there is no big commission check written to the selling agent) and is hitting the radar of consumers. The consumer can notice this difference if the consumer compares the proposed agent sold policy premium with one sold directly by a financial institution such as USAA or AARP. These companies have a work force of sales people that are compensated primarily on salary. Likewise the company can structure more competitive pricing and, in effect, offers a levelized cost (in place of commission) insurance product.

For example, Mark Maurer, CFP®, of Low Load Insurance Services believes that a levelized compensation basis will not occur unless all the insurance companies were to go to such a plan all at once. If an agent can "pick and choose" he/she may use a "levelized compensation" policy when in a competitive situation, as such a policy should in theory make a policy more inexpensive. An agent would then use the higher "front-end" policy when there is a large up-front premium or in a scenario with limited competition. Mark believes the answer to the whole argument is full disclosure. Both agents and home offices would not want the purchaser to know that 100% or more of their premium is going to sales costs and then products would then get better (personal communication).

The insurance industry has a powerful lobby in Washington. Only market pressure will cause a change in this decades old insurance industry practice that has made many life insurance policies expensive and inefficient. Pricing from nonagent sold life insurance companies will be the impetus that drives the old-line insurance companies to restructure their commissions to agents.

Insurance agents also remember the days of 8% load mutual fund commissions and minimum $60 dollar commissions on stock trades in the late 1980s! That is an inflation equivalent of more than $130 per trade, minimum commission, today. The current investing world would laugh at these costs (charges) today. When the physician-consumer realizes, through full disclosure and outside competitive market pressures, that life insurance protection can be more affordable from other non-traditional channels, then s/he will insist on a better, more affordable product. Ultimately, the big agent-driven life insurance companies will have to change their commission structure. The transition is currently in process. Only time will tell now (personal communication).

TAXATION OF LIFE INSURANCE

Life insurance has a number of tax advantages that can be potentially rewarding. However, there are also some pitfalls that should be avoided.

INCOME TAX FREE DEATH BENEFIT

The simplest tax advantage of life insurance is that the death benefit is received free of any income tax by the beneficiary. When the insured dies, the named beneficiary generally receives all death proceeds free of any income taxes. The word "generally" is used because there are situations that can cause the entire death benefit; or a large part of it, to become subject to income tax.

TRANSFER FOR VALUE PROBLEM

This is a situation that can cause the death benefit of a life insurance policy to be income taxable. This can be a complicated topic and the situation may arise unexpectedly, especially when life insurance is used for business purposes.

Generally, if an existing life insurance policy is transferred to a new owner for some type of consideration (money, exchange of property, or a *quid pro quo* arrangement), then the death benefit becomes taxable to the beneficiary to the extent the proceeds exceed the tax cost basis in the policy. Basis becomes the amount of consideration paid at the time of transfer and all future premiums following the transfer, paid by the new owner. There are five exceptions to this rule:

1. Transfers by any person or company of their ownership to the person insured by the policy
2. Transfers by a business partner (in the strictest sense, i.e., not a co-shareholder) to another partner in the same business
3. Transfers to a partnership by any of the partners
4. Transfers to a corporation in which the insured is a stockholder or officer
5. Transfers between corporations (under certain conditions) in a tax-free reorganization

If a transfer for value falls under one of these exceptions, then the policy retains its tax-free death benefit status.

TAX-DEFERRED GROWTH

Another tax advantage of life insurance is its income tax-deferred cash value growth. As mentioned earlier in this section, life insurance products other than term have cash accumulation potential. The cash values will depend on the policy style, the amount of the premiums, and also the general economic environment. If there is growth in the cash value, the growth will be tax-deferred under current tax laws.

WITHDRAWALS AND LOANS

Income taxes are not generally an issue unless cash values are removed from the policy while the insured is still alive. There are three methods of accessing a policy's cash value while the insured is living. The first choice is to surrender the policy. If the policy is surrendered and the cash value is greater than the total premiums paid, the difference is subject to ordinary income tax. A policy owner must ask his agent and give careful consideration before surrendering because if done improperly a portion of the surrender vales may be taxable, plus, once surrendered, the policy no longer exists.

What if you want to access a portion of the cash value but not lose the coverage? There are two methods, withdrawals and loans, to accomplish this. A withdrawal, also called a partial surrender, does not cause the policy to terminate, but it does lower the death benefit of the policy by the amount of the withdrawal. If a withdrawal is requested, then under the current first in first out (FIFO) accounting rules, the total amount of premiums paid into the policy are removed first, and more importantly, without any income tax liability. Any withdrawals removed in excess of the gross premium paid would be income taxable.

Because withdrawals beyond a policy's basis are taxable, loans are often used at this point, because in most cases policy loans are not taxable. If the insured dies while a loan is outstanding, the insurance company repays the loan from the death proceeds, and the remaining death benefit goes to the named beneficiary. In other words, the death proceeds will decrease by an amount equal to each loan. Also, unless the interest charged on the loan balance is paid annually, the size of the loan will increase as the interest accrues to the loan. So when withdrawals and loans are combined, a significant portion of a policy's cash value can be accessed while the policy is still in-force.

VIOLATING THE 2 OUT OF 3 RULE

Another common mistake involves an issue of gift taxation. Violating the 2 out of 3 rule can result in a policy owner unwittingly making a sizable gift of the entire death benefit and wasting a major portion of his/her unified credit as a consequence. The *three* refers to the parties to the policy: the insured, the policy owner, and the beneficiary. *Two* of these *three* parties should almost always be the same.

POLICY REPLACEMENT: SECTION 1035 EXCHANGES

If a policy owner intends to replace an existing policy with a new policy, he/she has two choices regarding the existing policy. Once the new policy is issued, the policy owner can simply surrender the first policy and receive the cash value, if any. Income taxes will be due if there is a gain in the policy.

However, most policy owners would rather transfer the cash value from the old policy into the new policy, rather than actually receive it. If this is the case, the policy owner can take advantage of an Internal Revenue Code Section 1035 exchange. This section of the tax code allows a policy owner to transfer cash value from one life insurance policy *directly* to a new policy. The main advantage of a Section 1035 exchange, unlike a regular surrender, is that the transfer is tax free, even if the first policy had a large gain.

Section 1035 exchanges have a definite procedure that requires the insurance companies to conduct the exchange of money, much as in the trustee-to-trustee transfer of qualified funds. Additionally, this procedure only permits the transfer of a life insurance policy to (A) another life insurance policy or (B) an annuity policy. Annuities can *only* be transferred to annuities.

Unfortunately, policy replacement is probably recommended more often than it is really necessary. If replacement and a Section 1035 exchange are recommended, the medical professional or healthcare practitioner should carefully review the proposal. Ensure that the assumptions made for projecting the old policy into the future are consistent with those assumptions for the new policy. Also, if replacement is warranted, a policy owner should never cancel an existing policy until the new policy is in force. Replacement will be covered again later in this section.

MODIFIED ENDOWMENT CONTRACTS

MEC is the last tax issue to be addressed with regard to life insurance policies. Because the cash values inside of a life insurance policy grow tax-deferred, many policy owners recognized this advantage and deposited large, single premiums into their policies. Unfortunately, it was perceived as abusive by Congress. It was clear these people were buying life insurance primarily as a means of escaping income taxation and not actually for the life insurance death benefit.

As a result, the laws were changed in 1984 to discourage putting very large amounts of money into life insurance contracts in the early years. Based on the age, sex, and size of the death benefit, a MEC premium (also referred to as the TAMRA 7-pay guideline) is established for each policy. For the first 7 years of the policy, the policy owner cannot have paid cumulative premiums greater than the cumulative MEC premium.

If a policy is classified as a MEC, then it is treated as an annuity contract, and not a life insurance policy, for any and all lifetime withdrawals or loans. Taxable interest earnings are removed before basis is recovered, that is, all funds removed from the policy in excess of basis will be immediately taxable. If the insured is under 59½, there will also be a 10% tax penalty. Thus, one of the basic tax benefits of life insurance is destroyed. Remember from our previous example that withdrawals of non-MEC policies are not taxable until the withdrawals exceed the cumulative premiums. Finally, once an MEC... always an MEC!

TAX WARNING!

According to fee-only life insurance expert Peter C. Katt of Kalamazoo, Michigan, doctors should be on guard against believing in the existence of perfect retirement vehicles funded through springing cash value life insurance plans. These plans reportedly feature payments of very large premiums while the policy is subject to favorable tax treatment, and then transferring the policy to the insured doctor when it appears to have no taxable value, after which the cash value *springs* to life.

Unfortunately, in the real world, tax deductible contributions and tax-free benefits do not exist without resorting to fraud or deception. Particularly notorious are the so-called continuous group insurance and Voluntary Employee Benefit Association (VEBA) prepaid retiree plans, despite the fact that the latter has been mistakenly endorsed by state medical societies in certain cases.

So, always remember that no matter how professional and sincere insurance agents and marketers appear, there are no life insurance policies that can legitimately provide tax-deductible insurance with tax-free retirement benefits. Therefore, you should always consult a qualified professional for further information regarding your specific needs.

OVERHEARD IN THE ADVISOR'S LOUNGE: ON
CHILDHOOD LIFE INSURANCE POLICIES

When Susan came into the world in 1974, of course her physician parents wanted the best for her. At that time, one of the loving things many parents did for their children was to purchase life insurance policies on them. Her parents had two reasons for these policies. The first was to pay for the funeral if a child were to die prematurely. The second was to build a little nest egg that the child might use later in life for college or a down payment on a home.

When Susan was 6 months old, her parents bought a $2500 whole life policy on her. That amount would actually have purchased two funerals in 1974. The premium was $38 a year. If we adjust these numbers for inflation, they are comparable to a current policy with a death benefit of $12,000 and an annual premium of about $180.

The insurance agent explained they could purchase term insurance on Susan for $12 a year, but this would not accumulate anything to help Susan with a down payment on a home or college tuition. For an additional investment of $26 a year, Susan's policy would grow and accumulate dividends, giving her the cash she would need for that down payment. But, Susan never did tap her policy for college or her first home. Instead she let it grow and accumulate, doing nothing but toss her annual statements into a file folder. Even so, Susan's parents dutifully paid the premiums every year.

This year, Susan became curious about her policy and dug out her most recent annual statement. She learned that if she died today her death benefit would be $2945.90. This was the original $2500 face value of the policy, plus dividends of $445.90 that had accumulated over 39 years. If she wanted to cancel the policy, the company would send her a check for the "surrender value" of $1120.45.

Susan grabbed a calculator and figured that the total premiums paid were $1482. At first glance it would appear the policy may not have been a great investment, since the cash value in the policy was less than the sum of the payments. But, to make a fair comparison, she needed to subtract the cost of providing the insurance ($12 a year, or a total of $468) from the total premiums. Only $26 a year, or a total of $1014, had gone toward accumulating the cash value. It was actually the $1014 that grew to $1120.45, which represented an annual return of about 0.25%.

Susan was curious what the $26 a year might have grown to if her parents had purchased only the term insurance and invested the difference in a stock mutual fund. She did some research and found there was a reasonable chance stocks might have returned 8% annually, meaning she would have $6212 today. That would make a down payment on a small house and might pay for one semester of tuition at a state school. The death benefit of almost $3000 from the term life policy would pay about half the cost of a proper funeral.

She realized canceling the policy and adding the money to her savings or investment portfolio would be the best financial decision. She was surprised at how difficult it was to carry out that decision. The policy had "always been there." Canceling it felt like rejecting a loving gift from her parents, especially since her father had died a few years earlier. The policy was part of her security. Giving it up was an emotional as well as a financial decision.

Susan said, "It was like saying goodbye to an old friend."

Rick Kahler, MS, CFP®, ChFC
www.KahlerFinancial.com

ANNUITY OVERVIEW

Annuity contracts transfer the financial risk of living too long, that is, outliving one's savings. Annuities are deferred or immediate, fixed or variable, and tax-qualified or non tax-qualified.

DEFERRED ANNUITIES

The deferred annuity contract, like a permanent life insurance policy, has been found by some to be a convenient method of accumulating wealth. Funds can be placed in deferred annuities in a lump sum, called Single Premium Deferred Annuities, or periodically over time, called Flexible Premium Deferred Annuities. Either way, the funds placed in a deferred annuity grow without current taxation (tax-deferred).

Fixed Deferred Annuity

Fixed deferred annuities provide a guaranteed minimum return of return (usually around 3% per year) and typically credit a higher, competitive rate based on the current economic conditions. Fixed annuities are usually considered conservative investments.

Variable Deferred Annuity

Recently, variable deferred annuities have become very popular. Like fixed annuities, variable deferred annuities offer tax-deferred growth, but this is where the similarities end. Variable deferred annuities offer separate accounts (similar to mutual funds) that provide different investment opportunities. Most of the separate accounts have stock market exposure, and therefore, variable annuities do not offer a guaranteed rate of return. But the upside potential is typically much greater than that of a fixed annuity.

The value of a variable deferred annuity will fluctuate with the values of the investments within the chosen separate accounts. Although similar to mutual funds, there are some key differences. These include

- A variable annuity provides tax deferral whereas a regular mutual fund does not.
- If a variable annuity loses money because of poor separate account performance, and the owner dies, many annuities guarantee at least a return of principal to the heirs. It is important to note that this guarantee of principal only applies if the annuity owner dies. If the annuity value decreases below the amount paid in, and the annuity is surrendered while the owner is alive, the actual cash value is all that is available.
- When money is eventually withdrawn from a deferred annuity, the amount withdrawn that is investment gain is taxable at ordinary income tax rates. Taxable mutual funds can be liquidated and the gains, if held longer than 12 months, are taxed at lower capital gains rates.
- There is also a 10% penalty if the annuity owner is under 59 ½ when money is withdrawn. There is no such charge for withdrawals from a mutual fund.
- The fees charged inside of a variable annuity (called mortality and expense charges) are typically more than the fees charged by a regular mutual fund.

Variable deferred annuities are sensible for people who want stock market exposure while minimizing taxes during the accumulation phase of their lives. Most financial planners recommend regular mutual funds when the investment time horizon is under 10 years. But if the time horizon is more than 10 years, variable annuities may become more attractive because of the additional earnings from tax-deferral.

Both types of deferred annuities may be subject to surrender charges. Surrender charges are applied if the annuity owner surrenders the policy during the surrender period, which typically run for 5–10 years from the purchase date. The charge usually decreases each year until it reaches zero. The purpose of the charge is to discourage early surrender of the annuity. Surrender charges may be eliminated if the annuity purchased is a "no-load" annuity.

IMMEDIATE ANNUITIES

Immediate annuities provide a guaranteed income stream that starts at the date of purchase. An immediate annuity can be purchased with a single deposit of funds, possibly from savings or a pension distribution, or it can be the end result of the deferred annuity, commonly referred to as annuitization. Just like deferred annuities, immediate annuities can also be fixed or variable.

Immediate annuities can be set up to provide periodic payments to the policy owner annually, semiannually, quarterly or monthly. The annuity payments can be paid over life or for a finite number of years. They can also be paid over the life of a single individual or over two lives.

Immediate Fixed Annuity

Immediate fixed annuities typically pay a specified amount of money for as long as the annuitant lives. They may also be arranged to only pay for a specified period of time, that is, 20 years. Either way, they often contain a guaranteed payout period such that, if the annuitant lives less than the guaranteed number of years, the heirs will receive the remainder of the guaranteed payments.

Immediate Variable Annuity

Immediate variable annuities provide income payments to the annuitant that fluctuates with the returns of the separate accounts chosen. The theory is that since the stock market has historically risen over time, the annuity payments will rise over time and keep pace with inflation. If this is indeed what happens, it is a good purchase, but it cannot be guaranteed. Some companies will, at a minimum, provide a guarantee of a low minimum monthly payment no matter how poorly the separate accounts perform.

QUALIFIED ANNUITIES

The term "qualified" refers to those annuities which permit tax-deductible contributions under one of the Internal Revenue Code (IRC) sections, that is, § 408 Individual Retirement Accounts (IRA), § 403(b) Tax Sheltered Annuities, § 401(k) Voluntary Profit Savings Plans. Qualified annuities can also result from a rollover from such a plan.

Nonqualified annuities, then, do not permit deductible contributions.

There is much debate as to whether an annuity, which is tax-deferred by nature, should also be used as a funding vehicle within a tax-qualified plan, that is, a tax-shelter within a tax-shelter. Since the investment options within the annuity are also generally available to the plan participant without the additional management expenses of the annuity policy, it is felt this could be a breach of fiduciary responsibility, and both the National Association of Securities Dealers (NASD), FINRA and the Securities and Exchange Commission (SEC) have gone on record as criticizing these sales.

ANNUITY TAXATION

The tax treatment of annuities is extremely dependent on whether it is a qualified or nonqualified annuity. Although both permit the tax-deferred growth of the investment and both have penalties for early distributions, they are governed under different sections of the IRC. Since qualified annuities were just discussed, we will start with them.

QUALIFIED ANNUITY TAXATION

Qualified annuities are treated no different than any other tax-qualified retirement investment. Growth of the investment, whether fixed interest or variable; escapes current taxation under one of the 400-series IRC sections. Additionally, if the funds are withdrawn prior to age 59½, there is a 10% penalty. As the money is withdrawn, every dollar is taxed as ordinary income. Finally, fund distributions must begin no later than April 1 of the calendar year following the year in which the owner turns age 70½. In addition, withdrawals from the annuity may be subject to the surrender fee charged by the annuity company.

NONQUALIFIED ANNUITY TAXATION

The taxation of nonqualified annuities is generally contained within IRC § 72. Again, the annuity is provided tax-deferred growth and the 10% penalty for early withdrawal. The manner in which distributions are taken, however, will determine the nature of their taxation.

Since the tax act TEFRA of 1982; if nonannuitized funds are withdrawn, they are taxed under Last In First Out (LIFO) accounting rules. Under these rules, the first funds withdrawn are considered the investment earnings, that is, the last funds credited to the annuity. Ordinary income tax will be paid until all earnings are removed, at which time only the original principle remains. This principle, having already been taxed, can then be withdrawn without any further income taxation.

On the other hand, if annuitization, the choice for a guaranteed monthly payment option is chosen, an exclusion-ratio is developed by the insurance company using governmental tables. This technique causes a portion of each payment to be considered a return of principle and thus only a portion of each payment is taxable. Generally, the option to annuitize is permanent. This exclusion ratio remains in effect until the insurance company has returned all of the original principle to the owner. After that, each payment received will be considered 100% earnings and totally subject to ordinary income taxation.

Wealth Transfer Issues

Regardless of whether the physician has a qualified or nonqualified annuity, extreme care must be given when specifying beneficiaries. Although these investments have great potential for appreciating sizable amounts of wealth during a lifetime, they are, unfortunately, very poor vehicles for the transfer of this wealth to successor generations after death.

Upon the death of an annuity owner, an annuity can be subject to both federal estate and federal income taxes. This double taxation may result in a 40–70% loss of annuity value before the heirs can receive it. The retired doctor should seek wealth transfer advice if he/she holds a large portion of their wealth in annuities or other qualified plans such as IRAs. One good strategy to consider is the Stretch IRA, which spreads the income and the tax liability over a period as long as the life expectancy of the beneficiary.

HEALTH INSURANCE OVERVIEW

Health insurance transfers the potential financial hardship caused by severe or chronic health conditions resulting from accidents or illnesses (morbidity), whereas life insurance is concerned with death (mortality). Health insurance, like life insurance, also has families of policies. There are medical expense/hospital policies, disability income policies, and long-term care policies. Although the medical professional or Financial Advisor should be familiar with the medical expense/hospital family of insurance policies, as well as changes brought about by the Patient Protection and Affordable Care Act (PP-ACA) recently passed into law, they are rapidly changing and will be briefly reviewed here.

What Types of Traditional Health Coverage Are Still Available?

Rising healthcare costs have driven the demand for, and the price of, medical insurance sky-high. The availability of group coverage through employment has helped many Americans face such costs. However, people who are not currently covered by their employers have few affordable sources for group coverage currently. Generally, those seeking personal medical coverage can explore purchasing an individual private health insurance policy. And, those aged 65 and older may qualify for Medicare coverage.

There are three general classifications of medical insurance plans: fee-for-service (indemnity), managed care (e.g., HMOs and PPOs), and high-deductible healthcare plans (HD-HCP).

Fee-for-Service

With a basic fee-for-service (indemnity) insurance plan, healthcare providers (such as physicians, nurse practitioners, surgery centers, and hospitals) are paid a fee for each service, on a per-unit basis (Current Procedural Terminology (CPT®) and/or Diagnostic Related Group®) provided to insured patients. However, this leads to the quantity-of-care *versus* quality-of-care conundrum that exists today. In other words; more DRG® and CPT® coded procedures lead to additional physician/facility reimbursement. This is, rightly or wrongly, recapitulated by the "malpractice phobia" crisis of increased medical testing leading to physician/facility reduced liability, but forcing the cost-curve upward!

Indemnity plans normally cover hospitalization, outpatient care, and physician services in or out of the hospital. You select the healthcare provider for consultation or treatment. You are then billed for the service and reimbursed by the insurance company, or you can "assign" direct payment to the provider from the insurance company. Indemnity plans typically require the payment of premiums, deductibles, and coinsurance. Limits on certain coverage or exclusions may apply. Lifetime limits on benefits are prohibited and limits on annual benefits were prohibited beginning in 2014.

MANAGED CARE

Managed-care plans became popular in the 1990s as a way to help rein in rising medical costs. In managed-care plans, insurance companies contract with a network of healthcare providers to provide cost-effective health care. Managed-care plans include health maintenance organizations (HMOs), preferred provider organizations (PPOs), and point-of-service (POS) plans.

Health Maintenance Organizations

A HMO operates as a prepaid healthcare plan. You normally pay a monthly premium in addition to a small copayment for a visit to a physician, who may be on staff or contracted by the HMO. Copayments for visits to specialists may be higher. The insurance company typically covers the amount over the patient copayment amount.

Each covered member chooses or is assigned a primary-care physician from doctors in the plan. This person acts as a gatekeeper for his or her patients and, if deemed necessary, can refer patients to specialists who are on the HMO's list of providers. Because HMOs contract with healthcare providers, costs are typically lower than in indemnity plans.

Preferred Provider Organizations

A PPO is a managed-care organization of physicians, hospitals, clinics, and other healthcare providers who contract with an insurance company to provide health care at reduced rates to individuals insured in the plan. The insurance company uses actuarial tables to determine "reasonable and customary" fees for each type of service, and healthcare providers accept the PPO's fee schedule and guidelines.

The insured can see any healthcare provider within a preferred network of providers and pays a copayment for each visit. Insured individuals have to meet an annual deductible before the insurance company will start covering healthcare services. Typically, the insurance company will pay a high percentage (often 80%) of the costs to the plan's healthcare providers after the deductible has been met, and patients pay the balance.

Although insured individuals can choose providers outside the plan without permission, patient out-of-pocket costs will be higher; for example, the initial deductible for each visit is higher and the percentage of covered costs by the insurance company will be lower. Because PPOs provide more patient flexibility than HMOs, they may cost a little more.

Point-of-Service Plan

A POS healthcare plan mixes aspects of a PPO and HMO to allow greater patient autonomy. POS plans also use a network of preferred providers whom patients must turn to first and from whom patients receive referrals to other providers if deemed necessary. POS plans recommend that patients choose a personal physician from inside the network. The personal physician can refer patients to other physicians and specialists who are inside or outside the network. Insurance companies have a national network of approved providers, so insured individuals can receive services throughout the United States. Copayments tend to be lower for a POS plan than for a PPO plan.

High-Deductible Healthcare Plans

HD-HCPs provide comprehensive coverage for high-cost medical bills and are usually combined with a health-reimbursement arrangement that enables participants to build savings to pay for future medical expenses. HD-HCPs generally cover preventive care in full with a small (or no) deductible or copayment. However, these plans have higher annual deductibles and out-of-pocket limits than other insurance plans.

Participants enrolled in a HD-HCP can open a health savings account (HSA) to save money that can be used for current and future medical expenses. There are annual limits on how much can be invested in a HSA. The funds can be invested as you choose, and any interest and earnings accumulate tax deferred. HSA funds can be withdrawn free of income tax and penalties provided the money is spent on qualified healthcare expenses for the participant and his or her spouse and dependent children.

Remember that the cost and availability of an individual health insurance policy can depend on factors such as age, health (pre-existing conditions), and the type of insurance purchased. In addition, a physical examination may be required.

U.S. Medicare

Medicare is the U.S. government's healthcare insurance program for the elderly. It is available to eligible people aged 65 and older as well as certain disabled persons.

Part A provides basic coverage for hospital care as well as limited skilled nursing care, home health care, and hospice care. Part B covers physicians' services, inpatient and outpatient medical services, and diagnostic tests. Part D prescription drug coverage is also available.

Medicare Advantage is a type of privately run insurance that includes Medicare-approved HMOs, PPOs, fee-for-service plans, and special needs plans. Some plans offer prescription drug coverage. To join a Medicare Advantage plan, you must have Medicare Part A and Part B and you have to pay the monthly Medicare Part B premium to Medicare, as well as the Medicare Advantage premium.

Medicare Supplement Insurance (MSI), or Medi-Gap, is sold by private insurance companies and is designed to cover the deductibles and copayments that Medicare doesn't cover. At one point, there were more than 200 different policies available. Then the National Association of Insurance Commissioners (NAIC) stepped in and created 10 standard packages of coverage, designated by the letters A through J. Since June 2010, plans E, H, I, and J have not been sold, although you are able to keep your plan if you already had one of these plans before June 2010. There are also two new policies (plans M and N) that offer different benefits and premiums. Plans D and G bought on or after June 1, 2010, have different benefits than D and G plans bought before June 1, 2010 (although the benefits won't change for those who participated in these plans prior to June 1). Only Medigap insurers are able to offer these plans. Although each standardized plan is identical from insurer to insurer, prices may differ and all these plans may not be available in every state.

Medicare Premiums and Deductibles for 2014–2015

A premium is the monthly amount paid for Medicare coverage. It changes each year. The Centers for Medicare and Medicaid Services (CMS) publishes Medicare Part A and Part B rate changes for the following calendar year in the middle of October or November. New premium rates for Medicare Part D and Medicare Advantage Plans become available October 1st, when sponsors are allowed to start marketing their plans.

Medicare Part A Premiums

Most beneficiaries do not pay a monthly premium for Medicare Part A coverage if they or their spouse paid Medicare taxes while working. In fact, according CMS, approximately 99% of Medicare beneficiaries do not have to pay Medicare premiums on Part A because they have more 10 years (or 40 quarters) of Medicare-covered employment. The small percentage of people who do have to pay Medicare premiums will pay up to $426 each month. The monthly amount depends on the number of quarters of Medicare-covered employment the person (or his/her spouse) has

- Those with 30–39 QTRS of covered employment paid a monthly rate of $234 in 2014.
- Those with less than 30 quarters employment and who are not eligible for free or reduced Medicare premiums paid a monthly premium of $426 in 2014.
- Premium amounts may change for 2015.

Medicare Part B Premiums

The Medicare Part B premium is set each year at a level calculated to pay for 25% of the average cost of coverage. The standard premium—the premium for most enrollees—applies to those with annual household incomes that do not exceed a set threshold amount. For 2014, the standard Part B premium was $104.90, and the threshold was $85,000 for single filers or married couples who file separately and $170,000 for couples who file jointly, based on 2012 tax returns.

Although most beneficiaries pay the standard rate, there are three provisions that alter the premium rate for certain Part B enrollees:

1. There is a premium surcharge for those who enroll after the initial enrollment period.
2. A "hold-harmless" provision can lower the premium rate for those who have their premiums deducted from their Social Security check. This provision limits the dollar increase in the Part B premium to the dollar increase in Social Security benefits.
3. There are higher "income-related" premiums for those whose annual income exceeds the threshold amount.

2014–2015 Part B Income-Related Premium Amounts

(Individual Tax Return)	(Joint Tax Return)			
$85,000 or less	$170,000 or less	25%	$104.90	$123.10
$85,001–$107,000	$170,001–$214,000	35%	$146.90	$156.90
$107,001–$160,000	$214,001–$320,000	50%	$209.80	$224.20
$160,001–$213,000	$320,001–$426,000	65%	$272.70	$291.50
More than $213,000	More than $426,000	80%	$335.70	$358.70

Note: If your annual income is percent of cost covered actual premium estimated 2015 premium.

Medicare Part D Premiums

The monthly Medicare Part D base premium is set to pay 25.5% of the cost of standard coverage, established by bids submitted annually by Part D plans. CMS releases the Medicare Part D base premium in early August each year. Actual premiums are based on this set premium, but can vary greatly. The premium for 2014 was $32.42.

As of 2011, beneficiaries with higher incomes must pay a premium adjustment based on their income. This premium adjustment is called the Income-Related Monthly Adjustment Amount

(IRMAA), and is paid directly to the Federal government (deducted from Social Security, Railroad Retirement Board, or Office of Personnel Management benefits).

MEDICARE PART A DEDUCTIBLES

Medicare Part A pays all covered hospital, skilled nursing facility, and home healthcare services for each benefit period except for the deductible. For 2014, this deductible was $1216, and the overall cost for coinsurance ranges based on the length of hospital stay:

- 1–60 days: $0
- 61–90: $304 per day
- 91 and beyond: $608 per day

For those on Medicare who receive care in a skilled nursing facility, Medicare will cover days 1 through 20 in full. In 2013, there was a copayment of $148 per day for days 21 through 100, and no coverage after day 100 in a benefit period.

MEDICARE PART B DEDUCTIBLE

Medicare Part B included a yearly deductible of $147 in 2014. This deductible was applied to healthcare costs that involve physician services, outpatient hospital services, certain home health services, and durable medical equipment. Once the deductible is met, you are required to pay 20% of the Medicare-approved amount charged by providers for healthcare services. Because of the new healthcare law, many preventive services are provided at no cost. These free benefits are not subject to a deductible.

MEDICARE PART D DEDUCTIBLE

The annual deductible for the standard Medicare Part D benefit was $310 in 2014, which is a decrease of $10 from the 2013 deductible. No Medicare drug plan may have a deductible more than $310 in 2014, although some plans may have a lower deductible or no deductible at all.

THE PATIENT PROTECTION AND AFFORDABLE CARE ACT

The opening date was October 1, 2013. And now, the competition is lined-up and ready to go after bronze, silver, gold, and even platinum plans. These competitors aren't athletes, but insurance providers. The field they are entering is the new Health Insurance Exchanges (HIEs) as mandated by Obamacare (PP-ACA). Beginning January 1, 2014, nearly everyone in the United States was required to have health insurance or pay a tax penalty. Those not insured through their employers can apply for coverage through these health insurance exchanges, also called "marketplaces." Enrollment began October 1, 2013 for coverage that started in January, 2014. The exchanges were intended to make it easier to find insurance providers and compare coverage and costs. Each state's exchange website lists all the policies available in that state, with prices and policy provisions. So far, over half of the states have opted to use exchanges managed by the federal government instead of setting up their own. But, state and national changes, modifications and exceptions abound by political fiat with this ever changing law.

THE FOUR BASIC (COLORS) HEALTH PLAN CATEGORIES

Bronze, silver, gold, and platinum describe the four basic categories of policies that will be available through the exchanges at different costs. Here is a very brief summary of each category.

Bronze

The least expensive option is a bronze plan, which might be the best choice for younger people with lower incomes and good health. The plan will pay 60% of healthcare costs and the insured will be responsible for 40%.

Silver

The second level, silver, will pay 70% of healthcare costs.

Gold and Platinum

Gold covers 80%, and a platinum plan covers 90%. Obviously, the categories with higher benefits also will have higher premiums.

Copper Plans?

To add to the above, a recent copper plan legislative proposal would cover 50% of medical costs, compared to the 60% actuarial value for bronze plans, 70% for silver plans, 80% for gold plans, and 90% for platinum. The proposal holds the potential for low-deductible, but inexpensive plans, with very high cost sharing.

THE ESSENTIAL BENEFITS

All these plans are required to cover 10 "essential health benefits." These include preventive and wellness care such as cancer screening, chronic disease management, pediatric care, many prescription drugs, injury rehabilitation, mental health and addiction treatment, maternity and newborn care, hospitalization, and emergency services. Companies are not allowed to deny coverage or charge more for those with pre-existing conditions. There are no lifetime benefit limits.

THE CARROT AND STICK APPROACH

The PP-ACA requirement to have health insurance coverage, the "stick" of Obamacare, is accompanied by a "carrot" in the form of federal subsidies to help pay insurance premiums. It's estimated that two-thirds of Americans are eligible for subsidies, which are figured on a sliding scale. The upper limit for qualifying is four times (400%) the federal poverty level, which amounts to about $88,000 a year for a family of four.

To find out more about the PP-ACA, it's a good idea to spend some time online, especially at two sites that offer more helpful information.

1. The first site is the federal government website at www.HealthCare.gov. It provides links to the state exchanges, plus detailed information that for the most part is explained in straightforward, plain English (beware-the site is not totally secure, and the integrity of website "navigators" may be suspect).
2. The second site is the Henry J. Kaiser Family Foundation at kff.org; an especially useful tool available here (http://kff.org/interactive/subsidy-calculator/). It has a calculator to determine the federal subsidy for specific income levels.

WHO GETS GOVERNMENT AID THROUGH THE HEALTH INSURANCE EXCHANGES?

According to LonJefferies, MBA, CFP® of the financial advisory firm Net-Worth-Advice in Salt Lake City Utah, the Premium Assistance Tax Credit (PATC) was designed to help "lower" income individuals and families pay for health insurance plans purchased through the new healthcare exchange program. However, more people may qualify for government assistance when purchasing health care through the Health Information Exchange (HIEs) than may realize (personal communication).

UNDERSTANDING THE PREMIUM ASSISTANCE TAX CREDIT

The program defines "lower" income as households that earn less than 400% of the Federal Poverty Level (FPL), which is based on the number of individuals in the home. In 2013, the FPL for a single individual was $11,490. Similarly, the FPL for a household of two people was $15,510 and the FPL for a home of four individuals was $23,550.

Consequently, at least some premium assistance credit is available for individuals earning less than $45,960, couples earning less than $62,040, and a household of four earning less than $94,200. It's important to note that for the purposes of the assistance program, income is defined as modified adjusted gross income (MAGI). This means that a taxpayer's adjusted gross income will include all Social Security benefits received (whether it was taxable or not), and all bond interest (tax-exempt or not). This factor will reduce a person's eligibility for aid if he begins receiving Social Security before age 65 (at which point he qualifies for Medicare and can no longer participate in the healthcare exchange).

The amount of aid the government will provide is essentially calculated in reverse—the maximum amount that an individual or family can owe is calculated, and the government will pay the remaining premium. Single persons who don't purchase health insurance will have to pay a tax equal to 1% of their income, or $95—whichever amount is greater.

The table below shows the *Premium Assistance Tax Credit* thresholds based on income relative to the Federal Poverty Level:

Income Relative to FPL:	Premiums Limited to:
Up to 133% of FPL	2% of household income
133–150% of FPL	3–4% of income
150–200% of FPL	4–6.3% of income
200–250% of FPL	6.3–8.05% of income
250–300% of FPL	8.05–9.5% of income
300–400% of FPL	9.5% of income

EXAMPLE 7.1

Assume John LPN is a single 62-year-old man living in Utah and making $30,000 per year. (Again, remember that when calculating the PATC, it really doesn't matter whether John's $30,000 of income is from employment, a Social Security benefit, or a combination of the two.) John's income is 261% of the FPL amount for singles ([$30,000/$11,490]*100), so this puts his threshold between 8.05% and 9.5% of his income. His exact threshold is 11/50ths of the way between 250% and 300% of the FPL, so his maximum premium is 11/50th of the way between 8.05% and 9.5%, which means his maximum premium is 8.37% of his $30,000 income, or $2511 per year ($210 per month). This is the most John will need to pay for an adequate health insurance plan.

What is deemed an adequate health insurance plan? The next relevant figure in the calculation involves determining the cost of the *second least expensive Silver plan in the state*. This can be determined by obtaining a quote at www.healthcare.gov. Assuming John lives in Salt Lake County, the second least expensive Silver plan available to him cost $5100 per year ($425 per month). Whether or not John decides to purchase this exact policy, the $5100 annual cost of the plan is significant.

Since the second least expensive Silver plan available to John cost $5100, but the most John will be required to pay is $2511 per year (8.37% of his income), the PATC program will cover the cost difference of $2589. This amount will be the tax credit available to John for purchasing any health insurance policy through the exchange.

However, this does not mean that John is required to actually purchase and utilize the second least expensive Silver plan available to him. If John is so inclined, he can purchase a less expensive policy and he will still receive the $2589 tax credit determined to be available to him. Nevertheless, since the policy is less expensive, John would need to cover less of the cost of the inferior policy out of his own pocket. Similarly, John could also purchase a more expensive policy, but his tax credit would still be $2589 and he would need to cover the additional cost of the superior policy with his own money.

The bottom line is that the PP-ACA may well mark the beginning of the end of tying health insurance decisions to employment status, which ultimately will reshape important career, retirement, and other financial planning decisions that clients make. Some may find a new freedom in the job decisions that they make—whether changing jobs, starting a new business, or retiring altogether—but they will also need help to content with affordability of health insurance and how to pay for it, including maximizing the PATC. In addition, many clients—and small business owners—will need help in the coming years handling the transition from employer-based to individual-based health insurance, as the system slowly shifts. In the long run, arguably a system where people can make employment and job decisions without being constrained to access to health care may be a huge plus, but there will be much planning to be done, including helping clients to change their mindset, during the coming transition years!

HEALTH SAVINGS ACCOUNT

The High Deductible-Health Care Plans (HD-HCPs) mentioned earlier are becoming more common. With a qualifying high-deductible plan comes the chance to contribute pretax dollars to a HSA. Compared with health Flexible Spending Accounts, HSAs have higher contribution limits—$6550 for a family compared with $2500 for a health FSA—and there's no limit to how much can be rolled over year to year. So, sheltering $6550 with a tax rate of 25% could result in annual savings of $1500 on a tax bill.

Disability Income Insurance

Disability income insurance is designed to transfer the financial risk of lost wages due to an accident or illness to an insurance company. The actual benefits may be received for as short a period as 6 months in some short-term group policies, to age 65 in both group long-term and many individual policies, and possibly even to lifetime for some individual "professional" policies. The length of the benefit period is one of the main factors in determining the premium to be charged by the insurance company.

Disability Defined

Arguably, the most important issue when purchasing disability insurance is the definition of disability found within the policy. Disability insurance pays a monthly benefit to the insured if he/she satisfies this definition of disability. Unlike a life insurance policy death claim, a disability income claim can be a far more difficult issue. Different policies from the same insurance company can define disability differently, and a medical professional or healthcare practitioner must be sure they are comfortable with the definition found in the policies that they are considering for purchase.

The more liberal the definition of disability in any given policy, the easier it will be to meet that definition, and the more likely the insurance company will pay benefits. Consequently, these are also the most expensive policies. Many agents and financial planners recommend paying the extra premium so that you have a higher chance of receiving benefits. The last thing an insured wants to do after becoming seriously injured is having to fight an insurance carrier over benefits.

There are two common definitions of disability:

- The ability to perform the substantial and material duties of your occupation
- The ability to perform any gainful occupation for which you are reasonably trained

Some aggressive insurance companies have even gone so far as to define the disability in terms of occupational and/or medical specialties. Regardless, the definition will almost always end with the words "and under a physician's care."

Some polices will pay benefits under the first definition for a couple of years, and then use a second definition thereafter. This design permits the insured full monthly benefits immediately after a disability and then time to rehabilitate and establish a new career.

Partial Disability

Some policies also allow fractional benefits for a partial or residual disability. Partial benefits can be available under two circumstances:

1. During a disability where the insured cannot perform some of the duties of his/her occupation, or
2. When the insured can still perform all the duties of his/her occupation, but for a limited period of time during recuperation.

The doctor should pay particular attention to the partial disability benefit language in their policy. Some companies require total disability prior to any partial claims payment. Other companies may have no such provision and, in fact, even pay a full benefit for the first 3 months of partial disability. This gives the insurance company the opportunity to give an incentive for the claimant-doctor to recover and go back to full time work.

Elimination Period

Another aspect used in the development of a disability income insurance premium is the waiting period, that is, that period of time which elapses, at the beginning of a disability, prior to the payment of any benefits during which the insured must generally be continuously disabled. This is also referred to as the elimination period and in individual contracts is usually specified as 30, 60, 90, 180, or 365 days.

The shorter the elimination period is, the higher the potential premium. In short-term group policies, the standard elimination period is the first day for accidents and the seventh day for sickness. Long-term group policies traditionally begin after 6 months. Medical professionals and healthcare practitioners with ample savings should consider a longer elimination period in order to save premium dollars, but those with less-savings should obviously choose a shorter elimination period. A personal emergency fund can provide the cash flow needed during the elimination period. This emergency fund makes it feasible for a doctor to select a longer elimination period, thus reducing the premiums.

Coordination of Benefits

Coordination between short-term group and both long-term group and individual contracts is often possible to complete an overall portfolio of coverage. Since most long-term group policies have a provision for coordination of benefits (insurance-speak for "reduction of benefit payments") with individual coverage purchased subsequent to the group policy effective date, many financial service professionals will look for the opportunity to place substantial amounts of individual coverage prior to writing the group coverage.

Monthly Benefit Amount

Yet, another aspect to be taken into consideration for developing the premium to be charged is the monthly benefit amount. The amount of coverage that can be initially purchased is dependent on the current level of predisability earnings. Insurance companies have usually been willing to insure up to 50% of current income (for the highest wage earners), to up to 70% of current income (for moderate to lower-income workers).

Occupation

The hazard category of the insured's occupation is also important to develop an adequate premium. Obviously bus drivers, fire fighters, cardiovascular surgeons, and financial service professionals face different risks during their typical day. These occupation classifications also take into account the claims experience related to that occupation. For example, dentists at one time were in the same top classification as physicians. However, because of poor claims experience, many companies have since lowered their classification, that is, raised their premiums.

Inflation Protection

When purchasing a disability income policy, it is strongly recommended that it include an inflation rider. In the event of disability, this rider will increase the benefit each year in an attempt to keep pace with inflation. Without this rider, if a young insured becomes totally disabled, their monthly benefit will certainly lose its purchasing power over the years. If the insured is young enough, a level benefit may become almost meaningless 20–30 years in the future. An inflation rider will cost extra, but it is money well spent.

Renewability

The last major issue to be considered when purchasing a disability policy is the renewal feature of the policy. The typical renewal features are

- Conditionally Renewable
- Guaranteed Renewable
- Noncancelable

Conditionally renewable policies allow the insurance company a limited ability to refuse to renew the policy at the end of a premium payment period. The insurance company may also increase the premium. Most policies sold to doctors will not contain this limitation.

Guaranteed renewable means the insurance company cannot cancel the policy, except for non-payment of premium, but it can change the premium rates for an entire class of policies.

Noncancelable means the insurer cannot cancel the policy nor can it change the rates. This added level of security means noncancelable policies are more expensive than guaranteed renewable policies.

Although redundant, many disability income policies specify that they are both "Non-cancelable and Guaranteed Renewable."

Disability Income Taxation

The general rule for taxation of disability benefits is that if the policy owner pays the premiums from his/her own funds, and then any benefits received as a result of the disability are income tax free. If the policy owner's employer pays the premiums as an employee benefit then any benefits are taxable. Therefore, when choosing a monthly benefit amount, the physician should always factor his/her individual tax status of the benefits into the calculations.

Disability Income Statistics

Risk of Disability:

- At age 30, long-term disability is 4.1 times more likely than death
- At age 40, long-term disability is 2.9 times more likely than death
- At age 50, long-term disability is 2.2 times more likely than death

Risk of Disability within Groups of People:

- At age 30, there is a 46.7% chance of any one person having a 90-day disability before age 65
- At age 40, there is a 43% chance of any one person having a 90-day disability before age 65

- At age 50, there is a 36% chance of any one person having a 90-day disability before age 65
- At age 30, there is a 71.6% chance of any one person out of any two people having a 90-day disability before age 65
- At age 40, there is a 67.5% chance of any one person out of any two people having a 90-day disability before age 65
- At age 50, there is a 59% chance of any one person out of any two people having a 90-day disability before age 65

Source: 2012–13 National Underwriter Field Guide.

LONG-TERM CARE INSURANCE

Long-Term Care Insurance (LTCI) was considered one of the newer forms of personal coverage insurance. LTCI insurance is designed to transfer the financial risk associated with the inability to care for oneself because of a prolonged illness, disability, or the effects of old age. In particular, it is designed to insure against the financial cost of an extended stay in a nursing home, assisted living facility, adult day care center, hospice, or home health care. It has been estimated that two out of every five Americans now over the age of 65 will spend time in a nursing home. As life expectancy increases, so does the apparent need for LTCI.

MEDICARE

Currently, the only nursing home care that Medicare covers is skilled nursing care and it must be provided in a Medicare-certified skilled nursing facility. Custodial care is not covered. Most LTCI policies have been designed with these types of coverage, or the lack thereof, in mind. To qualify for Medicare Skilled Nursing Care, an individual must meet the following conditions:

1. Be hospitalized for at least three days within the 30 days preceding the nursing home admission
2. Be admitted for the same medical condition which required the hospitalization
3. The skilled nursing home care must be deemed rehabilitative

Once these requirements are met, Medicare will pay 100% of the costs for the first 20 days. Days 21–100 are covered by Medicare along with a daily co-payment, which is indexed annually. After the initial 100 days, there is no additional Medicare coverage.

Medicare Home Health Services cover part-time or intermittent skilled nursing care, physical therapy, medical supplies and some rehabilitative equipment. These are generally paid for in full and do not require a hospital stay prior to home health service coverage.

CRITICAL LTCI POLICY FEATURES AND MARKETS

According to the U.S. Department of Health and Human Services and the Health Insurance Association of America, there are seven features that should always be included in a good long LTCI policy.

1. Guaranteed renewable
2. Covers all levels of nursing care (skilled, intermediate, and custodial care)
3. Premiums remain level (individual premiums cannot be raised due to health or age, but can be raised only if all other LTCI policies as a group are increased)
4. Benefits never reduced
5. Offers inflation protection

6. Full coverage for Alzheimer's disease
7. Waiver of premium (during a claim period, further premium payments will not be required)

In addition, there are another seven features considered to be worthwhile and are included in the better LTCI policies:

1. Home healthcare benefits
2. Adult day care and hospice care
3. Assisted living facility care
4. No prior hospital stay required
5. Optional elimination periods
6. Premium discounts when both spouses are covered
7. Medicare approval not a prerequisite for coverage

Top 25 Most Expensive Markets for Long-Term Care Insurance Coverage

Market	Nursing Home Private Room Annual Rate
Bridgeport–Stamford–Norwalk, CT	$159,359
Anchorage, AK	$156,950
New York–Northern New Jersey–Long Island, NY–NJ	$155,180
Poughkeepsie–Newburgh–Middletown, NY	$155,180
Hartford, CT	$154,118
Boston–Worcester–Lawrence, MA	$146,372
Rochester, NY	$141,244
San Diego, CA	$135,554
Seattle–Tacoma–Bremerton, WA	$131,750
San Francisco–Oakland–San Jose, CA	$130,283
Philadelphia–Wilmington–Atlantic City, PA-NJ-DE	$129,239
San Jose–Sunnyvale–Santa Clara, CA	$127,130
Albany–Schenectady–Troy, NY	$126,932
Portland, ME	$121,910
Honolulu, HI	$121,154
Washington–Baltimore, DC–MD	$120,709
Sacramento–Yolo, CA	$120,322
Boise, ID	$118,475
Milwaukee–Racine, WI	$118,005
Manchester–Nashua, NH	$117,264
Miami–Fort Lauderdale, FL	$116,931
Buffalo–Niagara Falls, NY	$116,577
Los Angeles–Riverside–Orange County, CA	$115,165
Detroit–Ann Arbor–Flint, MI	$114,716
Portland–Salem, OR	$111,909

Source: NYLIC (New York Life Insurance Company 2014).

ADLs

Most LTC policies provide benefits for covered insured's with a cognitive impairment or the inability to perform a specified number of Activities of Daily Living (ADLs). These ADLs generally include the inability to perform two of six, in order to file a claim: bathing, dressing, toileting, transferring, eating, and continence.

Another issue is whether the covered insured requires "hands-on" assistance or merely needs someone to "stand-by" in the event of difficulty. Obviously, policies that read the latter are more liberal, and costly.

Long-Term Care Insurance Taxation

Some LTCI policies have been designed to meet the required provisions of the Kassenbaum–Kennedy health reform bill, passed in 1996, and subsequently are "Tax Qualified Policies." Insured's who own policies meeting the requirements are permitted to tax deduct some of the policy's premium, based on age, income, and the amount of total itemized medical expenses. The major benefit of the tax-qualified LTC policy is that the benefit, when received, is not considered taxable income.

Selecting Nursing Homes

The following will allow the FA to assist appropriate clients in choosing a nursing home.

The Checklist

1. Review the client's requirements. An assisted-living facility may suffice instead of a true nursing home, which is required by the frail and elderly needing daily medical care.
2. Pick a location close to home and relatives. Frequent visits are crucial, not only to combat loneliness but also to ensure resident receives proper attention.
3. Read inspection report (state survey). If the financial advisor encounters difficulties in obtaining a current report, he or she should assume that the home has something to hide. Don't expect perfection. Nursing homes provide a difficult service for difficult residents. If a home is unresponsive to inquiry regarding items in a report, assume a similar response to concerns about the quality of care being provided in the future.
4. Tour the facility on an unannounced basis at different times on different days. Stroll through corridors and look and listen. Trust senses and instincts. Items to consider should include
   - *Appearance of residents' rooms.* Outward decor of facility can be misleading, so the FA should inspect the residents' rooms. To what extent can the rooms be personalized? If rooms are shared, how are good roommate matches made?
   - *Smells.* High-quality homes have no lingering stench of urine or air freshener to cover up bad care and unusually high incidences of incontinence due to lack of attention by staff.
   - *Safety hazards.* Be especially aware of items in corridors that can be obstacles to those with unsteady gait and poor eyesight.
   - *Sufficient staff members who are pleasant and respectful to residents.* Are staff members responsive to residents' needs? Are staff members warm in their interactions with all residents, even those requiring the heaviest supervision? Are aides helping residents with walking or exercise of their arms and legs?
   - *Residents' attitudes toward facility's service.* Talk with residents and staff to determine attitudes toward the facility's service. Does the facility have a family counsel to provide it with input?
   - *Grooming.* A clear sign of neglect is failure to keep residents clean, well dressed, and well groomed.
   - *Physical restraints.* Nursing homes that have eliminated restraints also have improved quality of life and more social contact among residents. Ties, belts, vests, and high bed rails are an easy but unsatisfactory solution to managing residents. Count number of residents that are restrained; ask what percentage are restrained and why.

- *Food.* Visit at meal time and sample the food to make sure it is palatable. The setting for meals should be attractive and pleasant, and food should be served at the proper temperature. Staff should be available to help residents who are not able to feed themselves. Review menus and determine the amount of concern for nutrition.
- *Activities.* A wide variety of activities should be provided, and the participation level should be high. Bored residents in front of a television may be a sign of a home's failure to stimulate its residents.
- *Dignity.* Residents should be handled in ways that respect their dignity. For example, are residents properly clothed in public?
- *Bed sores.* Bed sores are a sign of poor care. Review inspection reports and see if they are mentioned, or talk to residents or their families about this topic.
- *Special care units.* Such units are often used as an expensive marketing device. The special care units may not be designed well and may indicate a lack of outdoor facilities.

5. Review the facility's policy on medical care. Will residents be seen by their personal doctors or by staff physicians? Does the home have good infection control and immunization plans? What sort of access to dentists and eye doctors is there?
6. Perform financial analysis. The planner should gain a complete understanding of what the client's and/or his or her family's financial commitments are and how they will be met:
    - Determine the financial strength of the nursing home, particularly if client funds are to be advanced.
    - Consider a single lifetime payment in lieu of monthly rental payments.
    - Consider exclusions in contract. For example, nursing home insurance coverage should include loss of personal property and personal injury.
    - Determine what services the client will require, what is covered under the facility's general fee, and what services are provided for an extra fee. Determine what the extra fee will be for each additional service that will be required. Family members should not agree to pay these charges because this could delay Medicaid funding.
    - Analyze pricing structure in general and what the pattern of increases in fees has been.
    - Determine residents' rights in eviction proceedings for nonpayment of rent, in returning to nursing home after hospital stay, and in having Medicaid make payments on behalf of resident.
    - Determine residents' rights to appeal decisions and what the appeal procedures are.
7. Obtain and check references, including families of current residents, local hospitals, doctors, and government agencies, particularly the ombudsman at state departments for aging.

New Thoughts on LTCI

To be sure, physicians and FAs are aware that there is a sometime need to recommend a LTCI policy to clients. Of course, in such cases, it is a good idea to work with a low load provider (or the physician or client's agent). Yet, most LTCI policies are sold, not bought, and that most statistics used to sell LTCI policies are fear-based and half-truths. Even the Department of Health and Human Services (DHHS) gets into the fear mongering on their website quoting that "about 70% of people over age 65 require some type of long-term care services during their lifetime" (http://www.longtermcare.gov/LTC/Main_Site/Planning/Index.aspx).

This may be a deceptive statistic as it omits the length of long-term care needed in these 70% of cases. And, it is not 3+ years in all these cases (our estimate is closer to 2.5). With the recent stamp of approval by the Supreme Court of the United States SCOTUS on the PP-ACA, we may be looking at social LTCI in the United States like other social medicine countries and give up on private LTCI insurance altogether. Germany introduced mandatory long-term care insurance in 1995. Japan and France also have a LTCI tax funded insurance plan. And, the poor utilization and growing risks associated with long-term care insurance, are leading a growing number of financial advisors and CMPs™ to recommend alternatives to their clients.

To be a thought-leader ahead of the curve, the newest aging trend is away from LTCI and toward *sheltering at home*—living at home and dying at home. Perhaps, this is the way it should be. Dying should not be a for-profit industry.

GENERAL TYPES OF INSURANCE POLICIES COVERING POSSESSIONS

Unlike those insurance policies covering people, where it is mostly a matter of personal choice, most coverage's discussed are virtually required by law.

HOMEOWNERS (AND RENTERS) INSURANCE OVERVIEW

The basic model of the homeowners contract began in 1958 and contains three areas of coverage: property, theft, and liability. There are seven standard forms of homeowner contracts and their coverage's are contained in two sections.

Section I is for property and theft coverage and typically includes coverage for the

- Structure itself (commonly called the dwelling)
- Appurtenant structures (unattached buildings, fences, swimming pools, etc.)
- Unscheduled personal property (commonly just called contents within the structures and only those not itemized by endorsement)
- Additional living expenses (the increased cost of living during the period after damage occurs while the structure is uninhabitable)

"Contents coverage" is typically 50% of the dwelling coverage for on premises losses. Off premises coverage is typically worldwide but limited to 10% of the limit for contents coverage. Typically, there are other restrictions, with some types of personal property being totally excluded and others having a dollar limitation applied against them.

A common mistake is to not have a basic inventory of your property in an off-site location, possibly a safe deposit box. This is often conveniently accomplished by periodically taking photographs of each of the rooms in the house. Should there be a fire that damages that section, the picture may assist in bringing to mind property which was destroyed and for which a claim needs to be filed.

Section II is the liability protection section and covers personal liability for bodily injury to others, or for damage to their property, and includes reasonable medical payments for their injuries. Section II is identical in all seven forms. Liability protection often begins at $100,000 with medical payments at $1000 per person.

Briefly, the seven forms are as follows:

1. *HO-1: The Basic form* insures against fire, lightening, removal, vandalism or malicious mischief, glass breakage, and theft. It also provides what is called Extended Coverage for damage from wind, civil commotion, smoke, hail, aircraft, vehicles, explosion, and riot. The dwelling protection is specified as a dollar amount, while the contents are covered at 50% of this amount and the additional living expenses are covered at 10%.
2. *HO-2: The Broad form* gets its name from broadening the Extended Coverage perils of the HO-1. Coverage is now extended to include damage from falling objects; weight of ice, snow or sleet; accidental damage to steam or hot water heating systems; accidental discharge of water or steam from those systems or domestic appliances; freezing of those systems or appliances; and electrical surge damage. Again, the dwelling protection is specified and the contents are covered at 50%. Additional living expenses are increased to 20% of the dwelling coverage amount.

3. *HO-3: The Special form,* also called the "all-risk" form, expands on the HO-2 by provid-ing coverage for the dwelling, appurtenant structures and additional living expenses on an all-risk basis. Rather than naming each peril to be covered, this form covers all perils not specifically named as an exception, such as flood, earthquake, war, and nuclear accidents. Coverage for the dwelling, contents, and additional living expenses are identical to the HO-2.

4. *HO-4: The Tenants form* is basically the same as the HO-2 and provides a named perils basis for the contents of renters. Additional living expenses are provided at 20% of the amount of coverage purchased for the contents.

5. *HO-5: The Comprehensive form* is seldom seen anymore. It is identical to the HO-3 except contents are covered at 50% of the dwelling amount and provides this level for both on and off premises.

6. *HO-6: The Unit Owners form* is also referred to as the Condominium form. It is very simi-lar to the tenants form except additional living expenses are provided at 40% of the amount of coverage purchased for the contents. There are other unique differences with regard to insuring additions and alterations by the unit owner and the availability of optional cover-age to protect against the exposure to losses from assessment by the condominium associa-tion for uninsured property damage or liability claims.

7. *HO-8: The Modified Coverage form* is designed specifically to provide coverage for older dwellings. Many older homes contain elaborate carvings and specialty features that would cause the replacement value to substantially exceed current market value. This form of coverage has no replacement cost provision, but substitutes a "functional replacement" concept for any losses.

REPLACEMENT COST VERSUS ACTUAL CASH VALUE

Actual cash value settlements provide payments for claims that generally start with the cost today to replace a lost, stolen, damaged, or destroyed item. However, it then takes into account the length of time the item was owned or in service, to develop a deduction for depreciation. Often, this deprecia-tion amount is substantial and severe.

Under replacement cost coverage, insured's are able to collect for their losses without the deduc-tion for appreciation, up to the limits of the policy. This is an automatic but optional provision of all homeowner forms. To take advantage of this provision, the amount of insurance on the dwelling must be at least 80% of its replacement cost at time of claim.

INFLATION PROTECTION

The easiest way for a homeowner to assure replacement cost coverage is with the addition of a rider which automatically adjusts the value of the dwelling coverage by the inflation rate for their com-munity as calculated by the insurance company. This coverage adjusts policy limits periodically to maintain appropriate levels of coverage.

OTHER HOMEOWNER POLICY ENDORSEMENTS

The homeowner is well advised to also consider a multitude of endorsements and/or potential increases in policy limits. Examples include

- Scheduling personal property, such as jewelry, furs, art, golf equipment and computers, which have been exempted from coverage, or coverage has a severe dollar limitation.
- Increasing liability coverage to take advantage of the minimums needed for "Umbrella Liability" to be covered shortly.

- Theft extension endorsement to remove the exclusion for loss of unattended property from a motor vehicle, trailer, or watercraft.
- Earthquake and/or sinkhole collapse coverage.
- Increasing the deductible from the standard $250 to a convenient self-insurance amount.

TITLE INSURANCE

As a routine part of any home purchase, a history of the title to the property, as well as any liens or conveyances, is completed. This is referred to as title insurance, and typically protects the mortgage lender from any title defects. If a title defect causes loss, the title insurance company will indemnify the lender, not the homebuyer, to the extent of the loan. These are single premium policies of indefinite duration, but can terminate when the loan is retired.

The physician should also inquire about the cost of personally owned title insurance policy. This second policy would protect them rather than the mortgage lender. Although it would undoubtedly add to the expense of closing, there is no harm in requesting that the seller be responsible for providing this protection to the purchaser as well.

RENTER'S INSURANCE

Renters insurance can protect you from damage caused by weather events like wind, rain, snow, or lightning, as well as fire, vandalism, or theft. Some policies also include liability protection. This would be valuable if someone got injured in your home and sued you. Renters insurance tends to be cheap. For a low payment, usually annually, you can often get replacement coverage for your belongings and living expenses if you are displaced. This means that you can get money to replace a damaged or stolen item as well as paying for a hotel or alternative rent if you are forced to leave your home because of damage.

BOAT INSURANCE OVERVIEW

Watercraft and small pleasure boats are usually covered within a homeowner policy, but generally only for $1000. More expensive boats are often insured either under a separate Inland Marine policy or as a Personal Articles Floater (attachment) to the homeowner's policy. The decision between these two alternatives usually involves the liability risk element. There is no provision in the Personal Article Floater for liability, and although it could be increased on the homeowners, it is usually preferable to use a separate policy. Other items to consider are the size of the craft, maximum speed, engine horsepower, waters navigated, and special uses, such as water skiing or racing.

AUTOMOBILE PURCHASE AND INSURANCE OVERVIEW

With the possible exception of the handgun, the automobile represents the greatest single item of ownership that is capable of inflicting death, injury, and damage. America's fascination with the automobile has resulted in a marked increase in the power and potential speed of our vehicles. The latest trend in sports utility vehicles (SUVs) has also witnessed a substantial increase in damage due to their higher ground clearance and heavier frames. The owners and operators of any vehicle must be financially able to respond to any resulting claims, or they need to transfer the risk through insurance. All states require some minimal coverage for personal vehicles.

PURCHASING THE VEHICLE

Typically, car buyers who wait until the end of the year can score a deal. Buying at the end of the month can also increase negotiating power as dealerships look to move volume, and shoppers in the late summer and early fall may be able to get a deal when the new-model-year vehicles enter inventories. Also, cold or rainy weather can work to a doctor's advantage, since bad weather can discourage people from walking around a lot to look at vehicles, potentially giving those who do show up a bit more negotiating power. Even a serious buyer who goes to a dealership near the end of the day may receive a better price as the dealer makes concessions to speed things up so everyone can go home. So, if you time your car purchase right, and you aren't buying one of the more popular models or colors, you might save $500–$2000 just by waiting until the end of the month or day to make your purchase.

INSURING THE VEHICLE

The most frequently used policy to insure individual private passenger vehicle risks is the Family Automobile Policy (FAP). It provides two major types of coverage: liability and physical damage. Liability coverage includes both bodily injury and property damage. Physical damage, on the other hand, includes comprehensive and collision coverage.

Liability Coverage

The liability section of the FAP is contained within most policies as Part A—Liability and Part B—Personal Injury Protection.

Bodily Injury

Bodily injury liability coverage generally includes sickness, disease, and death, and is expressed in dual limits—per person and per occurrence. Nearly half of the states require minimums of $25,000 per person and $50,000 per occurrence. Higher limits of $100,000 per person and $300,000 per occurrence are often a prerequisite for consideration of umbrella coverage.

Property Damage

Property damage liability is coverage for damage or destruction to the property of others and includes loss of use. Liability coverage limits usually include property damage limits as the third number, that is, $100/300/25. The coverage here would be for $25,000 of property damage. As automobiles become more expensive, however, coverage to $50,000 is not considered excessive.

Personal Injury

Personal injury coverage is provided for medical expenses, funeral expenses, and loss of earnings for anyone sustaining an injury while occupying your vehicle, or from being struck by your vehicle while a pedestrian.

Liability insurance follows the vehicle, not the driver. Coverage is extended to the vehicle owner and any resident in the same household. It also covers anyone using the insured vehicle with the permission of the owner *and* within the scope of that permission.

Newly acquired vehicles are usually covered automatically for liability for 30 days after acquisition, but physical damage must have been on all currently covered vehicles to be included. Coverage is also typically extended to a temporary substitute automobile, but only if this vehicle is used in place of the covered automobile, because of its breakdown, repair, servicing, loss, or destruction.

Physical Damage Coverage

Comprehensive

Comprehensive physical damage includes coverage for theft, vandalism, broken windshields, falling objects, riot, or civil commotion, and even damage from foreign substances, such as paint. Comprehensive is often described as coverage for all those hazards other than collision.

Collision

Collision involves the upset of the covered vehicle and collision with an object, usually another vehicle, and not enumerated in the discussion of comprehensive. Colliding with a bird or animal is considered under the comprehensive coverage.

The distinction between comprehensive coverage and collision coverage is more than technical. The deductible provisions of the FAP often show a considerable difference in these areas, with the collision deductible typically being much greater.

Damage to tires can be covered by provisions in either comprehensive or collision. Exclusions typically include normal wear and tear, rough roads, hard driving, or hitting or scraping curbs.

Repairs after the Accident

Following a collision, the insurance company will assign a claims adjuster to determine the extent of damage and the cost of repairs. If these repairs exceed the estimated value of the vehicle, it may be "totaled." Experience tells us that the value of the vehicle to the owner nearly always exceeds that estimated by the insurance company.

The physician is therefore strongly urged to consider purchasing replacement cost coverage rather than accepting actual cash value, which is the depreciated value of the vehicle. The cost may be higher for this coverage, but accepting a larger deductible will often make up the difference. Paying a little more towards the deductible could easily be worth it, if the damage is extensive.

Uninsured/Underinsured Motorists Coverage

Uninsured motorist coverage provides protection from the other driver who is operating his/her vehicle without any insurance coverage. It covers expenses resulting from injury or death as well as property damage. There are currently a dozen states where it is estimated that over 20% of the vehicles on the highway are being operated without any insurance. This is not coverage that should be rejected when buying automobile insurance.

Underinsured motorist coverage provides protection from the other driver who purchased only the state-mandated minimum liability insurance coverage. Again, this is not coverage that the medical professional or healthcare practitioner should thoughtlessly reject when buying automobile insurance.

Tip: By failing to check once a year, you might be overpaying for some insurance needs. For example, get quotes online and approach your current insurer about lowering their rate when coverage and quality of insurers are comparable. Also mention life changes, such as an adult child no longer needing auto insurance or a new home-security system. Other discounts can typically be had for school-age drivers with good grades or for those who take a defensive-driving class. And, those with older vehicles worth under $1000–$3000 should consider dropping comprehensive and collision coverage. For example, school-age drivers with good grades can save up to 25% on average, depending on the company and the state. Defensive-driving classes can yield about 10% savings depending on the state. Using the national average annual auto-insurance payment of $797, these discounts could yield annual savings of about $199.25 and $79.70, respectively. And, dropping some coverage on an old car could bring savings of 15–40%, although do not drop liability insurance on your car. Of course, there's always the option of switching to a higher deductible—increasing a homeowners deductible to $1000 from $500, for instance, can save 25% on annual premiums. This strategy amounts to annual savings of $244.50 based on the national average premium of $978 in 2011, the latest year the statistic is available from the insurance institute.

The Most Expensive Cars to Insure in 2014

1. Nissan GT-R Track Edition	$3169
2. BMW M6	$3065
3. Mercedes-Benz CL550 4Matic AWD	$3019
4. Mercedes-Benz SLS AMG GT	$2986

5. Porsche Panamera Turbo S	$2970
6. Audi R8 5.2 Spyder Quattro	$2917
7. Mercedes-Benz G63 AMG	$2887
8. Audi A8 L 6.3 Quattro	$2869
9. Jaguar XKR Supercharged	$2854
10. Jaguar XK	$2610

Source: Edmunds.com

UMBRELLA LIABILITY INSURANCE OVERVIEW

Umbrella policies should be considered anytime the doctor has substantial current income or has accumulated a sizable estate, and is concerned about asset protection from potential litigation. Umbrella policies vary greatly in structure so care should be taken to examine all of the various aspects of the policy carefully. Not only do umbrella policies vary in structure, but they can also be arranged with many different endorsements to meet the specific needs of the doctor. A few examples would be

- The addition of personal injury coverage (to include libel, slander, and defamation of character)
- Incidental business pursuits (to include coverage to personal automobiles where the business activity was incidental and not the primary purpose of the use of the car)
- The broadening of personal automobile coverage (to the insured regardless of whose vehicle they were driving and the coverage afforded that vehicle)

NEEDS ANALYSIS APPROACH TOWARD LIFE INSURANCE

Needs analysis is a generic term used to help quantify the financial need for life insurance. And, whereas a broker or agent may use a simple needs analysis designed to pinpoint a certain life insurance amount, a CMP's™ model should include a more thorough review of insurance needs and a long and short term financial analysis The CMP™ or insurance agent assisting the physician should request

- An in-depth discussion of your goals, both financial and personal
- A review of your current insurance (life, health, disability, property and casualty, etc.), and financial holdings, investment assets and their projected growth potential
- A review of your current estate plan, including any current wills and trusts
- Any personally owned business information

Keep in mind there is a difference between using an agent or broker for this service and using a CMP™. An agent or broker will not normally charge a fee for this service. A CMP™ will generally charge a set amount, depending on the size of the estate being analyzed. Finally, as each of your life and practice evolves, an in-depth re-analysis should periodically be performed. This will assure an accurate, up-to-date plan for the future.

BUSINESS USES OF LIFE INSURANCE

KEY PERSON INSURANCE

Hospitals, a local family practice office, a pharmaceutical company, all likely have one thing in common. Somewhere within these companies or partnerships, there are key employees or profit makers. Due to their expertise, management skills, knowledge, or "history of why," they have become indispensable to their employers.

If this key employee were to die prematurely, what would potentially happen to the company? In many cases, especially in smaller companies, it would have a devastating effect on the bottom line, or even precipitate a bankruptcy. In these circumstances, a form of business insurance, called key person coverage, is recommended in order to alleviate the potential financial problems resulting from the death of that employee.

The business would purchase and own a life insurance policy on the key person. Upon the death of the employee, the life insurance proceeds could be used to

- Pay off bank loans
- Replace the lost profits of the company
- Establish a reserve for the search, hiring and training of a replacement

BUSINESS CONTINUATION FUNDING

See the section on buy–sell agreements in the chapter on estate planning.

EXECUTIVE BONUS PLAN

An executive bonus plan (or § 162 plan) is an effective way for a company to provide valued, select employees an additional employment benefit. One of the main advantages to an executive bonus plan, when compared to other benefits, is its simplicity. In a typical executive bonus plan, an agreement is made between the employer and employee, whereby the employer agrees to pay for the cost of a life insurance policy, in the form of a bonus, on the life of the employee.

The major benefits of such a plan to the employee are that he or she is the immediate owner of the cash values and the death benefit provided. The only cost to the employee is the payment of income tax on any bonus received. The employer receives a tax deduction for providing the benefit, improves the morale of its selected employees, and can use the plan as a tool to attract additional talent.

NONQUALIFIED SALARY CONTINUATION

Commonly referred to as deferred compensation, this is a legally binding promise by an employer to pay a salary continuation benefit at a specific point in the future, in exchange for the current and continued performance of its employee. These plans are normally used to supplement existing retirement plans.

Although there are different variations of deferred compensation, in a typical deferred compensation agreement, the employer will purchase and own a life insurance policy on the life of the employee. The cash value of the policy grows tax deferred during the employee's working years. After retirement, these cash values can be withdrawn from the policy to reimburse the company for its after-tax retirement payments to the employee.

Upon the death of the employee, any remaining death benefit would likely be received income tax free by the employer. (Alternative Minimum Taxes could apply to any benefit received by certain larger C corporations). The death benefit could then be used to pay any required survivor benefits to the employee's spouse, or provide partial or total cost recovery to the employer.

In a typical plan, the terms of the agreement are negotiated as to the amount of benefit received by the employee, when retirement benefits can begin, how long retirement benefits will be paid, and if benefits will be provided for death or disability. The business has established what is commonly referred to as "golden handcuffs" for the employee. As a result, the benefit will only be received if the employee continues to work for the company until retirement. If the employee is terminated or quits prior to retirement, the plan would end and no benefits would be paid.

SPLIT DOLLAR PLANS

Split dollar arrangements can be a complicated and confusing concept for even the most experienced insurance professional or financial advisor. This concept is, in its simplest terms, a way for a business to share the cost and benefit of a life insurance policy with a valued employee. In a normal split dollar arrangement, the employee will receive valuable life insurance coverage at little cost to them. The business pays the majority of the premium, but is usually able to recover the entire cost of providing this benefit at termination of employment, death, or surrender of the policy.

Following the publication of IRS Notices 2002–8 and 2002–59, there are currently two general approaches to the ownership of business split-dollar life insurance: Employer-owned or Employee-owned.

Employer-Owned Method

In the employer-owned method the employer is the sole owner of the policy. A written split-dollar agreement usually permits the employee to name the beneficiary for most of the death proceeds. The employer owns all the cash value and has the unfettered right to borrow or withdraw it as necessary. At the end of the formal agreement, the business can generally (1) continue the policy as key person insurance, (2) transfer ownership to the insured and report the cash values as additional income to the insured, (3) sell the policy to the insured, or (4) use a combination of these methods. This is commonly referred to as "rollout."

Practitioners should be careful not to include rollout language in the split-dollar agreement. The reason the rollout should not be included is that if the parties formally agree that after a specified number of years—or following a specific event—related only to the circumstances surrounding the policy, that the policy will be turned over to the insured, the IRS could declare that the entire transaction was a sham and that its sole purpose was to avoid taxation of the premiums to the employee, generating substantial interest and penalties in addition to the additional taxes due.

The death proceeds available to the insured employee's beneficiary are considered a current and reportable economic benefit (REB), and it is an annually taxable event to the employee. If an individual policy is involved, the REB is calculated by multiplying the face amount times the government's Table 2004 rates or the insurance company's alternative term rates, using the insured's age. If a Second-to-Die policy is involved, the government's PS38 rates or the company's alternative PS38 rates will be used. Any part of the premium actually paid by the employee is used to offset any REB dollar-for-dollar.

Employee-Owned Method

With the employee-owned method, the insured-employee is generally the applicant and owner of the policy. Any premiums paid by the business are deemed to be loans to the employee and the employee reports as income an imputed interest rate on the cumulative amount of loan based on Code § 7872. A collateral assignment is made for the benefit of the business to cover the cumulative loan amount. In some cases, the assignment may allow the assignee to have access to the cash values of the policy by way of a policy loan. This method is unavailable for officers and executives of publicly held corporations because of the current restrictions on corporate loans (the Sarbanes-Oxley Act of 2002).

The employee-owned method is somewhat similar to the older collateral assignment form of split-dollar. The benefits for the employee are both the ability to control large amounts of death proceeds as well as developing equity in the policy. Whether or not this new method catches on will depend greatly on the imputed interest rate published by the IRS every July. If set low enough, this may be an excellent opportunity for the employee to use inexpensive business dollars to pay for life insurance.

OTHER MEDICAL PRACTICE BUSINESS-RELATED INSURANCE

There are other important medical practice, and business related, insurance products that physicians should be aware including the following.

GENERAL COMMERCIAL PROPERTY INSURANCE

Commercial or business insurance protects against those perils and losses that a healthcare practitioner routinely faces in their practice of medicine. These exposures are both wide and varied and include aspects that may never affect most practitioners, such as the explosion of boilers, or aviation mishaps, or ship's hulls failing. However, many risk exposures should be considered.

COVERED PROPERTY

- Buildings
- Business personal property which may be the practice/business
- Property and equipment used in the business
- Personal property of others in the care and custody of the policy owner

COVERED PERILS

This topic defies clear summarization because it usually defines the exposures unique to the healthcare practice. The risks of loss for a radiology practice are different from those of an obstetrician/gynecology office. Within numerous policy forms, "named perils" are identified in addition to the "all-risks" form that generally cover common perils such as crime or fire. In addition, just like with the individual Homeowner's policies, endorsements can be obtained to cover unique and specific risks, such as earthquakes in California and hurricanes in Florida.

LOSS SETTLEMENT

This special provision of commercial policies provides for the settle of losses on a cash value basis. Most policies are subject to a deductible amount, although "Full loss replacement value" coverage is usually available. Typically, the deductible is 20% of the covered value, with the insurance company only covering the balance. As with personal lines of coverage, the amount of the deductible effects the premium charged.

COMMERCIAL GENERAL LIABILITY INSURANCE

Commercial general liability (CGL) provides coverage for a wide variety of risks that a medical/healthcare facility may face. In brief, these exposures will include (there are others in a general liability policy that may be "endorsed out" for the particular practice)

- Premises liability—injuries on the property owned or occupied by policy owner
- Business operations liability—losses caused by business activities of employees
- Contractual liability—litigation arising from oral or written contracts

Unfortunately, for the medical practitioner, as with many property and liability contracts, liabilities that occur "from the rendering or failure to render professional services" are standard exclusions from this section of liability coverage.

Often, insurance companies offer "packaged" programs or, Business Owners Policy (BOP) especially for small to medium practices. These policies include "all-risks" coverages for the property and limited liability. Most BOP programs include such coverages as

- Debris removal
- Fire Department service charges
- Pollutant cleanup and removal
- Water damage

Most importantly, BOP contracts will cover

- *Loss of Business Income* (it is difficult to run the practice if half of it was destroyed by water damage from the fire in the office upstairs)
- *Extra Expense Coverage* (the cost of renting substitute property while the covered property is being repaired)
- *Payroll Expense* (the need to retain specialists or key employees while the property is being rehabilitated)

Although the latter is limited in amounts and period of coverage, it is valuable coverage, especially for professional practices. Finally, the BOP will cover losses due to crime (such as, forgery and alteration). As with Commercial Liability coverage, professional liability is excluded from BOPs.

PROFESSIONAL LIABILITY (MEDICAL MALPRACTICE) COVERAGE

For liability protection not covered under the General Liability Provisions, the healthcare professional can obtain *Professional Liability Coverage*. This coverage is generally defined as insurance to protect against failures to use the degree or skill expected of a person in a particular profession. This coverage is also known as *malpractice insurance.*

A discussion of the current issues regarding this particular coverage is unnecessary. The debate continues, even among healthcare professionals, as to the causes of the dramatic increases in premiums and claims in recent years. Insurance company underwriting losses (generally speaking—claims) increased to 160–170% of the premiums collected in 2012. Combine this with poor investment returns in 2007 and 2008, and the result is substantially increased insurance premiums, which will probably continue to do into the future. Fortunately, professional liability coverage is universally offered through professional organizations and associations. It would be prudent to investigate coverage through these groups because the policies are often structured and created for the specific requirements of the specialty and are frequently more financially attractive.

Professional Liability coverage is specified in an Endorsement to the General Liability policy. The doctor policy owner should take care in specifically reviewing this provision of the contract with their insurance professional, especially one with thorough knowledge and experience in this significant area. The terminology used in the policy language may have long-reaching effects on the practitioner and their practice.

Since most insurance companies develop unique policies with specialized language for the medical profession, policies are, therefore, quite varied. The general provisions typically include

Covered Acts: Although the language will vary widely among insurers, this agreement generally covers acts, errors, or omissions that occur while performing professional services.

Coverage—Occurrence versus "claims made": This area needs particular scrutiny and discussion with your insurance professional. The confusion here concerns what coverage (particularly, what insurance company) was in-force when the event causing the liability *occurred* versus what coverage was in-force when the *claim is made*. Review this language to ensure that the contract contains the proper endorsements. If the coverage is on a "claims made" form, an extended reporting period—also known as "tail coverage"—option should be included. Some states restrict the premium that can be charged for this feature and it is often not included. Secondly, new limits on the coverage are often offered, and the period of any "tail coverage" varies. The new limits and period of coverage are important issues since extended coverage is considered "long tail" and should be reviewed carefully to ensure that the healthcare professionals policy meets your risk management tolerance.

The policyholder should attempt to get unlimited tail coverage and consider 36 months to be the minimum acceptable period.

Definition of "medical services" or "professional liability:" This definition is the foundation of the policy and must fit the practitioner's level of comfort.

Definition of Incident: Each policy provides a broad definition of "incident" thereby providing coverage for claims that arise while the healthcare professional is doing their job.

Defense Coverage: This provision identifies that the cost of defending against a civil action suit, proceeding or demand by any person arising out of any actual or alleged act, error or omissions will be covered by the policy. Defense coverage may be provided even if the allegations of the claim are groundless, false, or fraudulent. The contract may also include the costs of depositions, and peripheral legal expenses. This would include the loss of income, extraordinary expenses incurred for the practice. The medical practitioner should review these provisions carefully, since some policies include these costs under the "total limits" of the policy (rather than an additional benefit) while other companies may cover this provision only by an additional endorsement.

Personal Injury Protection: This provision may also be included in any individual malpractice policy. This coverage protects the healthcare professional for any lawsuit resulting from allegations of personal injuries like breach of a patient's privacy or confidentiality, slander and libel during the performance of your professional services. This coverage part is usually consistent with the professional liability coverage limits.

Broad Range of Limits of Liability: All insurance programs offer a wide range of limits the healthcare professional can select to fit their professional liability exposure. Limits typically range anywhere from a minimum of $250,000/$500,000 (Limit per Claim/Annual Aggregate Limit) to a more typical $2,500,000/$5,000,000. Some locations, where Malpractice coverage has been difficult to maintain, have limits nearing $10,000,000.

The following are buying tips for healthcare professionals who are shopping for medical professional liability (malpractice) insurance coverage:

- Shop well in advance of your renewal or expiration date. Your agent should have all of the necessary information to the insurer at least 6–8 weeks before your coverage expires. See the attached checklist for the types of information your agent will need.
- If you do not know an agent who can place your coverage, the Bureau of Insurance has a list of agencies that are licensed and appointed with at least one of the insurers on the Bureau's list of "Insurers Writing New Business for Physicians and Surgeons."
- Contact one or two agents and be sure to ask each agent which insurer will be contacted for a quote. Ask the agent if an application will also be submitted to a surplus lines broker. If so, ask for the name of the surplus lines broker and ask which surplus line insurers will be contacted. Provide this information to the other agent to avoid multiple applications being submitted to one insurer from different agents. If the application is being submitted to a surplus lines broker, be sure to ask the agent for information on the coverage provided and specifically request information on exclusions.
- If the agent recommends coverage through an unlicensed company (such as a surplus lines insurer or a risk retention group), be aware that, in the case of insolvency, the insured will not have coverage through the (State) Property and Casualty Insurance Guaranty Association. However, if the healthcare professional has had several claims or an open claim, they may only be able to obtain coverage through a company not licensed in their state.
- Ask the agent for information on the financial rating of the company and if the surplus lines insurer has its own guaranty fund. Also, if shopping, the medical professional should feel free to check with the Insurance Bureau of their respective state to see if the company and agent are licensed or authorized to do business.
- The agent should fully understand the healthcare professional's business. If incorporated, ask the agent what coverage is needed to protect the corporation as well as any individual doctors.

- Ask the agent about the availability of "tail coverage" or if the new insurer will provide coverage for "prior acts." If coverage is offered with two insurers, ask the agent what each insurer charges for "tail coverage." This information may help in deciding which insurer has the most competitive price.
- Complete the application for coverage in its entirety. Don't omit any information and be sure to provide as much detail as possible, especially about prior claims. Many insurance companies want 10 years of information. They may also request information about any risk management practices and procedures.
- Discuss deductible options with your agent. These may help lower your premium.
- Find out if the insurance company offers any risk management or loss prevention programs. Such programs may lower the premium and help reduce exposure to losses.

WORKER'S COMPENSATION

While medical practitioners and facilities can operate without Professional Liability coverage, one business related insurance that cannot be avoided is Worker's Compensation. Employers in all but seven states—so-called "monopolistic" states because they have their own state funds, are under statutory obligation to provide coverage for their employees. Historically, Worker's Compensation pre-dates Social Security entitlements and well before the emergence of employer sponsored group benefits.

The coverage under worker's compensation provides for lost income due to on-the-job accidents or work-related disability or death and the amount of benefits vary by state. In some instances, the coverage will reimburse the employee for medical expenses incurred with the accident. The four general benefits covered under Worker's Compensation are

Medical Care—for expenses incurred usually without limitations on amount or period of care.

Disability Income—payable for both total and partial disability and is usually based on 66 2/3% of their wage base.

Death Benefits—generally fall into two categories; one, a flat amount for "burial" insurance; and two, survivor benefits. Though varying by state, these benefits are similar to the disability payment (a percentage of weekly base wages) but may be capped as to total benefit, such as $50,000 or a period, such as 10 years.

Rehabilitation Benefits—which includes not only medical rehabilitation, but vocational rehabilitation, vocational counseling, retraining or educational benefits, and job placement.

Traditionally, the secondary purpose of Worker's Compensation was to reduce potential litigation because employees accepting the benefits from a Worker's Compensation claim generally waived their right to sue their employer. However, in our litigious society, this "protective shelter" has been severely tested and is crumbling.

Employers may provide their Worker's Compensation three ways:

- Private commercial insurance
- State government funds
- Self-insurance

Very few factors drive the premium structure—the occupation of the workers is the single most important determinant of premiums. An office worker may have premiums as low as $.10 per hundred of wages and a coal miner may exceed $50.00 per hundred of wages. Generally speaking, however, Worker's Compensation premiums for the medical profession or healthcare worker are among the lowest available.

Therefore, for the medical practice some physicians may consider self-insurance because the weekly benefits are typically below $500, thus making this decision attractive. Alternatively, because officers and owners can elect not to be covered by Worker's Compensation, the decision to purchase coverage from a private insurance company may afford inexpensive assurance that the benefits will be conveniently provided and administered by a private insurance company for their employees.

OTHER FORMS OF PROPERTY AND LIABILITY COVERAGE

Obviously, not all forms of coverage can be described in detail, however the medical practitioner should consider other forms of commercial property and liability coverage.

DIRECTORS AND OFFICERS LIABILITY INSURANCE

The officers and directors of large practices, or healthcare facilities can be held personally accountable, and thus liable, for breaches of their duties by a number of parties.

COMMERCIAL AUTOMOBILE/VEHICLE INSURANCE

As the name suggests, this coverage provides protection for any commercial (not personal) vehicles owned and operated by the healthcare corporation. If the practice or facility owns automobiles or other vehicles that are used in the "usual and customary" business activities, this coverage is required. The policy owner should be aware of the nine classifications of automobiles insured to ensure that coverage is appropriate.

COMMERCIAL UMBRELLA LIABILITY INSURANCE

This coverage is very similar to the personal umbrella coverage discussed under the personal coverage area. Again, risks above the limits established by the underlying commercial liability coverage trigger the umbrella policy. The word of caution for this coverage is "Read the Provisions Carefully" as there is little standardization among insurance companies. Make sure the umbrella policy covers what you want it to cover, with the right limits of benefits and "trigger" points, with proper exclusions, and proper endorsements (if being used specifically for a medical practice.)

ASSUMPTIONS

- A claimant won a $1,500,000 judgment against the insured
- The insured's CGL policy and excess liability (umbrella) policy both covered the claim
- Each policy had an "each occurrence" limit of $1,000,000

$2,000,000 total limit

$500,000 from
umbrella policy

$1,000,000 malpractice

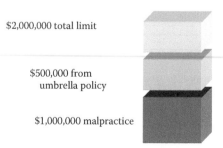

MISCELLANEOUS INSURANCE POLICIES

The following insurance policies should be carefully considered before purchase, since they may be unnecessary, too expensive, provide only minimal benefits, or be duplicated in your other policies.

These include credit life or home mortgage insurance (decreasing term), life insurance for children, accident policies for students, hospital indemnity policies, dread disease insurance, credit card insurance, pet health insurance, life insurance for the elderly, funeral insurance, flight insurance, prepaid legal insurance, and most extended warranties on automobiles, televisions, stereos, home computers, and the like.

On the other hand, the following types of coverage may be important, in selected cases: trip cancellation insurance, termite insurance, and flood and earthquake insurance.

ASSESSMENT

Traditionally, the physician protected his family with whole-life, disability, and long-term care insurance, and his practice with malpractice liability and business interruption insurance. For modern physicians however, a comprehensive financial plan must acknowledge more risks than ever before and in an economically sound manner not counterproductive to individual components of the plan.

For example, with the acceleration of private, state, and federal managed care initiatives, and the PP-ACA, physicians may be facing the ultimate personal contingent liability by selecting the *wrong profession,* as suggested by Yale University economist Robert J Shiller, PhD. In his book, *The New Financial Order: Risk in the 21st Century,* Shiller states that a new risk-sharing paradigm to protect us from "gratuitous random and painful inequality" is required.

The solution! *Livelihood insurance,* framed as a risk management insurance contract?

CONCLUSION

Doctors, like most people, tend to experience losses more intensely than gains, and evaluate risks in isolation. So it's no surprise that goaded physicians might prefer vehicles like the guaranteed minimum death benefit of variable annuities, or the assurance that comes with disability or long-term care insurance, or traditional cash value life insurance policies, despite their decidedly higher costs and commissions. Now, after reading this chapter, you may know better.

For insurance professionals on the other hand, this is an exciting time to work with the medical sector because there is much research and creative enlightenment occurring in academic and practitioner communities. But one must be willing to abandon ancient thoughts and remain open to new ideas that identify and provide solutions to the contemporaneous problems of physicians.

As an example of this epiphany, the economist Christian Gollier (2005) revisits the *raison d'être* of insurance, by asking: "Should one even buy insurance since the industry itself is so skilled at exploiting human foibles?" Although this emerging work is descriptive, it is not yet time tested since some of it aspires to be normative, as developing modern models of savings and consumption hint that insurance may deserve a smaller role in personal risk management than previously believed.

So, physicians should always consult a trusted fee-only CFP®, CMP™, insurance agent, owner, producer, broker, or Certified Insurance Counselor (CIC) to get a second opinion before the purchase of any policy product.

COLLABORATE

Discuss this chapter online with others at www.MedicalExecutivePost.com.

ACKNOWLEDGMENTS

To Matthew Lawrence DeSantos, JD; Matthew D. Rogers, CFP®, CLU, ChFC; Hope Rachel Hetico, RN, MHA, CMP™; and Lon Jefferies, MBA, CFP® of NetWorthAdvice.com.

REFERENCE

Gollier, C, Schlesinger, H, and Eeckhoudt, L: *Economic and Financial Decisions under Risk*. Princeton University Press, Princeton, NJ, 2005.

FURTHER READING

Abraham, KS: *Insurance Law and Regulation*. Foundation Press, New York, 2010.

Dogra, A: Four things everyone should know about end of life planning. In www.KevinMD, March 9, 2014.

Kinder, J and Kinder, G: *Secrets of Successful Insurance Sales*. Napolean Hill Foundation, Hammond, IN, 2012.

Kunreuther, HC and Pauly, MV: *Insurance and Behavioral Economics*. Cambridge University Press, New York, 2013.

Marcinko, DE and Hetico, HR: *Dictionary of Health Insurance and Managed Care*. Springer Publishing, New York, 2008.

Muldowney, TA, Marcinko, DE and Hetico, HR: Financial Planning for the Elderly. In: Margolis, HS, Esq. (editor): *Elder Law Portfolio Series*. Wolters-Kluwer and Aspen Publishers, New York, 2007.

Muldowney, TA, Marcinko, DE and Hetico, HR: Postmortem Estate Planning. In: Margolis, HS, Esq. (editor): *Elder Law Portfolio Series*. Wolters-Kluwer and Aspen Publishers, New York, 2007.

Reavis, MW: *Insurance: Concepts and Coverage*. Friesen Press, Victoria, BC, Canada 2012.

Rejda, G and McNamara, M: *Principles of Risk Management and Insurance (Pearson Series)*. Prentice Hall, New York, 2013.

8 Modern Risk-Management Issues for Physicians

It's Not Just about Medical Malpractice Liability Insurance Anymore!

Charles F. Fenton III and David Edward Marcinko

CONTENTS

Most traditional books on financial planning for medical professions limit their discussion of risk management to life insurance planning, occasionally some property casualty issues, usually asset protection management and perhaps those methods to avoid medical malpractice claims. Defensive medicine and risk management were often synonymous terms. However, limiting medical risk management to these issues is completely misplaced in modernity; for both medical practitioner and his/her financial advisor.

INTRODUCTION

In today's medico-legal environment, the physician faces risks from many directions. Risks come from the federal government (including the *Centers for Medicare and Medicaid Services,* the

Occupational Safety & Health Administration, the *Drug Enforcement Agency,* the *HHS Office of Civil Rights [HIPAA],* the *Environmental Protection Agency*), state government (including state medical boards), insurance companies (including *Health Maintenance Organizations, Preferred Provider Organizations,* indemnity plans, and the *Patient Protection and Affordable Care Act*), patients, and even one's own employees and prospective employees. The practicing physician almost needs to have a law degree to keep track of the rules and regulations attendant with practicing.

MEDICARE RECOUPMENT RISKS

Historically, the main risk any physician faced that would place personal assets at risk was the threat of a Medicare recoupment. Although many are surprised upon receipt of a notice of recoupment, the majority of requests were preceded with a request for copies of medical records to determine the necessity of care. Many doctors, upon receiving a request to forward copies of such records simply assign the task to a clerk and forget about the incident; or attempt to change the records. Both actions are misguided; but it does not mean that you cannot "complete" your medical records. Medical records should be completed according to your office's previously established written medical record policy.

But, DO NOT ALTER THE MEDICAL RECORDS!

If unsuccessful at demonstrating medical necessity and the recoupment letter still is received, then the practitioner should retain an attorney to preserve all the legal rights. Generally, there is a right to request a *Fair Hearing* before a *Hearing Officer.* At the Fair Hearing, the practitioner is given the opportunity to present justification of the treatments to the impartial Hearing Officer. If the Fair Hearing results are adverse to the practitioner, there is a right to request a hearing before an *Administrative Law Judge.* Even if the practitioner is unsuccessful at that level, there may be additional appeal rights. So be aware that some malpractice insurance policies may contain an Administrative Defense rider that might assist you in such an instance.

HEALTH CARE FRAUD RISKS

The greatest risk to the practicing physician's fiscal fitness in the current medico-legal environment is the fraud risk. Yet, it is relatively easy for an administrative billing error to be labeled as fraud. In this manner, an innocent act becomes a criminal act, which the practitioner must now defend.

MEDICARE FRAUD

The federal government has many weapons in its arsenal to investigate and prosecute Medicare and Medicaid fraud. Some of these include: the *Medicare and Medicaid Anti-Fraud and Abuse Statute,* the *RICO* statute, the *Federal False Claims Act,* money laundering laws, and civil asset forfeiture laws.

INSURANCE FRAUD

The federal government now has the power to investigate and prosecute fraud involving private insurance companies. The new federal crime of *Health Care Fraud* authorized in 1996 gives the federal government wide scope of authority. A practitioner being investigated for Medicare fraud may also end up defending against a charge of private health care fraud.

MISREPRESENTATION

Let's say a physician decided to sell his practice and move to another state. The value of the sale was based, in part, on the yearly gross of the practice. The physician accepted installment payment terms from the buyer and moved to the new state. The buyer began to practice medicine at his new office. Although he was busy, his gross never approached the gross of the prior physician. Eventually, the buyer defaulted on the loan. The selling physician sued for the deficit. The defaulting physician performed in-depth evaluation of the seller's practice. The buyer noticed some discrepancies in the billing patterns and practices of the seller. Considering these discrepancies to constitute Medicare and insurance billing fraud, the seller counter-sued the buyer on the grounds of misrepresentation, alleging the gross receipts of the practice purchase price, was grossly inflated. Therefore, the buyer determined that the seller had fraudulently misrepresented the potential of the practice. He also notified state and federal authorities and filed complaints of insurance fraud against the seller. The seller thought that he would move to the good life in the new state, but his old practice kept him in constant legal trouble.

PROVIDER HEALTH CARE FRAUD CONSIDERATIONS

Fraud in the health care arena has become a high priority for the *United States Department of Justice;* for 2014–15 and beyond. Health care fraud ranks close behind terrorism and drug crimes, as one of the Department's top priorities. Because physicians are engaged in delivering health care services, and because a high percentage of those services are delivered to patients covered by federal plans (e.g., Medicare, Medicaid, TRICARE-CHAMPUS, etc.), many physicians may soon find themselves subject to a federal investigation. As the investigators seek to uncover health care fraud, many innocent or unsuspecting physicians may find themselves the subject of investigation.

In the past practitioners feared an audit because it meant the possibility of paying back prior reimbursements. Often this repayment placed a financial burden on the practitioner. Now, with the PP-ACA and an increased emphasis on fraud, the repayment of such amounts will seem insignificant compared with the burden of paying back those amounts, paying civil penalty fines, paying lawyer fees, being subject to forfeiture, and being placed in jeopardy of going to jail. The government has always had an arsenal of laws to deal with health care fraud. These included the *Medicare and Medicaid Anti-Fraud and Abuse Statute*, the *Stark Amendments,* the *Federal False Claims Act*, mail and wire fraud laws. Recently, the federal government's arsenal has been significantly augmented.

THE KENNEDY–KASSEBAUM (HIPAA) ACT

The Health Insurance Portability and Accountability Act (HIPAA) of 1996, also known as the Kennedy–Kassebaum health care bill, provides a whole section to fight health care fraud. In particular, it increases the civil money penalties from $2,000.00 *per line item* to $10,000.00 per line item! Even ONE erroneous item can be devastating for the provider. Add 20 or 30 such items and many physicians will see their net worth drop to near zero! The Bill also made it easier for money laundering charges and civil asset forfeiture to be brought against health care professionals. Furthermore, unlike the past when the federal government concerned itself with fraud in federal programs, the law now extends the federal government's power to include ALL health plans, public and private! The practitioner could potentially face civil asset forfeiture for alleged claims of fraud involving an HMO, PPO, or MCO.

The Bill also authorized the usage of bounty hunters in the pursuit of health care fraud. If an individual provides information to the government that results in a recovery of only $100.00, then the whistle-blower will share in the recovery. The frightening fact is that now your own patient (or their relatives) or employee may become a bounty hunter against you. Additionally, the Bill authorizes CMS to contract with private entities to pursue health care fraud on a wide scale. Private entities will now have financial incentives to investigate health care providers in an attempt to uncover health care fraud. The practitioner will find their activities under scrutiny from different sides.

The above provisions are commonly termed HIPAA, part one to distinguish them from HIPAA, part two—those provisions dealing with the recently required Privacy Rule and Transaction Standards.

BALANCED BUDGET ACT

The Balanced Budget Act of 1997 provided some additional tools that the federal government can use in their fight against health care fraud. In particular, physicians convicted of three-heath care crimes can be permanently prohibited from Medicare.

FEDERAL FALSE CLAIMS ACT

A civil war era law, titled the False Claims Act (*qui tam* [in the name of the king]), is increasingly popular with prosecutors who pursue inappropriate billing mishaps by physicians. This Act allows a private citizen, such as your patient, your employee, or a competing doctor, to bring a health care fraud claim against you, on behalf of and in the name of the United States of America. The "relator" who initiates the claim is rewarded by sharing in a percentage of the recovery from the health care provider. Essentially, this Act allows informers to receive up to 30% of any judgment recovered against government contractors (Medicare, Medicaid, TRICARE-CHAMPUS, prison systems, American Indian reservations, or the VA systems). With a low burden of proof, triple damages, and penalties up to $10,000 for each wrongful claims submission, these suits are the enforcement tools of choice for zealous prosecutors pursuing health care fraud. All that must be proven is that improper claims were submitted with a reckless disregard of the truth. Intentional fraud is irrelevant to these cases, even if submitted by a third party, such as a billing company.

MONEY LAUNDERING

Charges of money laundering may seem foreign to the practice of medicine. The term "money laundering" evokes visions of a suitcase of drug cash being brought into a legitimate business and being transformed into that business's receipts and later tunneled through legal channels. In medicine the route beings with receipt of a claim payment check (i.e., a check as opposed to the drug dealer's cash). The check is then deposited into the professional corporation's checking account. The funds are then paid to the physician in the form of wages. Those wages are then deposited into the physician's personal checking account. Those funds and other similarly situated funds are then accumulated until a check is written to pay for a sports utility vehicle. The money received from the alleged fraudulent insurance claim has successfully been "laundered" into a hard asset (e.g., a new SUV).

CIVIL ASSET FORFEITURE RISKS

Civil asset forfeiture is a "seize now, ask questions later" activity. This appears on the surface to constitute punishment without due process. However, in civil asset forfeiture there is due process, it just comes AFTER the seizure. Civil asset forfeiture is to property like an arrest is to the person. A warrant is issued stating in essence that the property did something wrong. The property is "arrested" (i.e., seized) and then a hearing or trail will follow at some later date to determine the facts.

SELF-REFERRAL RISKS

The Federal and state governments have enacted several overlapping laws to deal with the issue of financial inducement in the referral of patients. These laws create a virtual maze of laws and regulations, which can easily snare the unwary.

FEDERAL BACKGROUND

The extent of the federal regulation in the area of self-referral includes the *Medicare Anti-Fraud and Abuse Statute,* the *Medicare Safe Harbor Regulations*, and the *Stark Amendment.*

MEDICARE ANTIFRAUD AND ABUSE STATUTE

This antifraud statute applies to persons receiving kickbacks for referring Medicare or Medicaid patients. There are many examples of physicians who run afoul of the law. These included chiropractors that were paid "handling fees" for collection and transmission of lab specimens to a certain laboratory. In another case, cardiologists who received "interpretation fees" for referring patients to a certain cardiac lab were found guilty of violating the statute. Additionally, a hospital administrator was found guilty when he received perks from an ambulance company to whom he had referred patients. Succinctly, any benefit given or received in exchange for referral of a Medicare or Medicaid patient will violate the statute.

MEDICARE SAFE HARBOR REGULATIONS

The *Medicare Safe Harbor* rules were passed in an effort to identify areas of practice that would not lead to a conviction under the antifraud statute. The Safe Harbor regulations provide for 11 areas where providers may practice without violating the antifraud statute. Areas of safe practice under these regulations are briefly highlighted below:

- *Large Entity Investments*—Investment in entities with assets over $50 million. The entity must be registered and traded on national exchanges.
- *Small Entity Investments*—Small entity investment entities must abide by the 40–40 rule. No more than 40% of the investment interests may be held by investors in a position to make referrals. Additionally, no more than 40% of revenues can come through referrals by these investors.
- *Space and Equipment Rentals*—Such lease agreements must be in writing and must be for at least a one-year term. Furthermore, the terms must be at fair market value.
- *Personal Services and Management Contracts*—These contracts are allowable as long as certain rules are followed. Like lease agreements, these personal service and management contracts must be in writing for at least a one-year term, and the services must be valued at fair market value.
- *Sale of a medical practice*—There are restrictions if the selling practitioner is in a position to refer patients to the purchasing practitioner.
- *Referral services*—Referral services (such as hospital referral services) are allowed. However, such referral services may not discriminate between practitioners who do or do not refer patients.
- *Warranties*—There are certain requirements if any item of value is received under a warranty.
- *Discounts*—Certain requirements must be met if a buyer receives a discount on the purchase of goods or services that are to be paid for by Medicare or Medicaid.
- *Payments to Bona Fide Employees*—Payments made to bona fide employees do not constitute fraud under the Safe Harbor Regulations.
- *Group Purchasing Organizations*—Organizations that purchase goods and services for a group of entities or individuals are allowed: provided certain requirements are met.
- *Waiver of Beneficiary Co-Insurance and Deductible*—Routine waiver would not come under the safe harbor.

A physician's actions that come under the Safe Harbor Regulations will not violate the Medicare Fraud and Abuse Statutes. However, the provider must still abide by the Stark amendments and must also abide by applicable state law.

THE STARK AMENDMENT

The *Stark Amendment* to the *Omnibus Budget Reconciliation Act of 1989* was a step by the federal government to prohibit physicians from referring patients to entities in which they have a financial interest. Originally, the Stark Amendment applied only to referral of Medicare patients to clinical laboratories in which the physician had a financial interest. The Amendment provides that if a physician (including a family member) has a financial interest in a clinical laboratory, then he may not make a referral for clinical laboratory services if payment may be made under Medicare. A financial interest is an ownership interest, an investment interest, or a compensation arrangement.

There are certain *exceptions* to the *Stark* Amendment. They include if a physician personally provides the service or if a physician or employee of a group provides the services. Like the Safe Harbor Regulations, the Stark Amendment permits physician investment in large entities and provides an exception for rural providers. Under the Stark Amendment, large entities are defined as publicly traded entities with assets greater than $100 million. There are certain other exceptions that are similar to the Safe Harbor Regulations. They include items such as provision for rental of office space, employment and service arrangements with hospitals, and certain service arrangements. These arrangements must be at arms-length and at fair market value.

Stark II was passed in 1993 to modify and expand the *Stark I* Amendment. In particular, it acts to bring numerous other entities, besides clinical laboratories, within the prohibitions of the Stark Amendment. Self-referral and overutilization may become less of a problem as managed care makes further inroads in medical practice control and quasisubrogation. Future legislation is likely to address the concerns of the financial incentives toward underutilization of ancillary medical services.

And, *Stark III* suggests that "under arrangement" transactions occur when a hospital contracts with a third party (typically a joint venture owned, at least in part, by physicians who may refer) to provide a hospital service, and the hospital then bills and is reimbursed by Medicare for those services and pays the supplier, or joint venture. As the "entity" to which the physicians refer patients is the hospital, not the joint venture (i.e., the "entity" is deemed to be the entity that submits the reimbursement claim to Medicare), this type of "arrangement" is permitted under Stark. However, buried in the 2008 Medicare Physician Fee Schedule rules, CMS broadened the definition of "entity" to include the person or entity that performs the designated health services and prohibits space and equipment lease arrangements where per-click payments are made to a physician lessor who refers patients to the lessee. These self-referral prohibitions (as well as arrangements where the physician is the lessee and rents space from a hospital) appeared in the Final Rules of 2008. CMS also passed restrictions related to independent diagnostic testing facility (IDTF) arrangements. For example, IDTFs are no longer allowed to share practice locations, operations, and diagnostic testing equipment with other Medicare-enrolled providers, including leasing and subleasing agreements.

OCCUPATIONAL SAFETY AND HEALTH AGENCY RISKS

The Occupational Safety and Health Administration (OSHA) has several standards with which the physician must comply. Physicians are covered generally under OSHA simply by the fact that they have employees, but they also have two specific standards that they must follow. These include the Bloodborne Standard and the Hazardous Communication Standard and General provisions.

DRUG ENFORCEMENT AGENCY RISKS

The Drug Enforcement Agency (DEA) controls the issuance of DEA numbers that permit the physician to prescribe controlled substances to their patients. The use of controlled substances is important to almost all medical specialties. Family practitioners use codeine to treat coughs and surgeons use narcotics to manage pain. There will always be a rogue physician willing to sell narcotic prescriptions. These physicians cause the DEA to cast a jaundiced eye toward all physicians. However, there are simply too many stories of physicians who "overuse" controlled substances in a practice designed to ease the suffering of their patients. The physician never knows when a patient comes into the office complaining of pain and asking for pain medication whether that patient is truly in pain or is an undercover agent for the DEA. This risk and paranoia (combined with the risk of a malpractice claim of "hooking" the patient) causes mainly physicians to actually underprescribe pain medication.

ENVIRONMENTAL PROTECTION AGENCY RISKS

The practitioner may not think about the *Environmental Protection Agency (EPA)* when thinking about the possible risks of practicing. But that agency could be a nightmare for the unsuspecting physician. For example, a doctor who improperly disposes of developing fluid, silver wastes, bodily fluids or bio-hazardous materials, and/or other wastes, may become a target of the EPA.

HEALTH AND HUMAN SERVICES (OFFICE OF CIVIL RIGHTS) RISKS

According to Part II of HIPAA, patients must be informed of their privacy rights and physicians must adhere to certain regulations in order to safeguard the privacy of their patients. A failure to do so can result in civil money penalties of $100.00 per incident, up to a maximum of $25,000.00 per year. There are also substantial criminal penalties (jail and fines) for certain transgressions of the HIPAA Privacy Rule.

ANTITRUST RISKS

- *Monopolistic* risks are reduced when more than a few networks or contracts are available in the local area for excluded providers to join.
- Fee schedule MCO contracts, *per se,* are not generally considered price fixing, provided the providers have not conspired with one another to set those prices. Moreover, the network pricing schedule should not spill over into the nonnetwork patients.
- Individual providers may be excluded from a network if there is a rational reason to do so. It is much more difficult to exclude a *class* of providers, than it is to exclude an *individual* provider.
- A *safety zone* can be created if networks or other contractual plans require a substantial amount of financial risk-sharing among plan participants, since Stark II laws have been relaxed. Such zones have been created by the *Department of Justice (DOJ)* and *Federal Trade Commission (FTC),* in recent policy statements.
- The FTC and DOJ are not likely to challenge an exclusive provider IPA that includes no more than 20–25% of the doctors within the panel, who share financial risk. Such panels are likely to fall within a *Safe Harbor.*
- *Tying arrangements* (e.g., the requirement to buy one item/service in order to buy another item/service) are suspect if not reasonably justified. For example, a patient should not be required to obtain a brace prescription from a specific provider, in order to purchase the device from a laboratory that the doctor owns.

- *Nonexclusive* provider panels will not usually be challenged if no more than 30% of the providers are included (another Safe Harbor provision).
- Physician networks are often analyzed according to *four criteria:* (1) anticompetitive effects, (2) relevant local markets, (3) pro-competitive effects, and (4) collateral agreements.

Further antitrust considerations consist of analyzing *Market Power*. This consists of two factors: (1) Geographic Power, and (2) Product Power.

Geographic Power is difficult to define in today's environment. In the past, the geography that was analyzed when medical practices merged was the immediate neighborhood. Currently, the geographical area could consist of an entire metropolitan area. In the past, individual patients would often seek a physician whose office was close to work or home. Now they seek a physician based on inclusion in a health plan. Now, health plans choose physicians based on needs within an entire metropolitan area.

Product Power relates to the specific service being performed. There are two products in today's environment: (1) Primary Care and (2) Specialty Care. Since there are so many primary care physicians in practice, it would be difficult for all but the largest group to acquire product power.

It is easier for specialists to develop product power. However, certain specialists may never be able to obtain product power. For example, foot care is provided by many types of physicians. Primary care physicians, emergency physicians, chiropractors, physical therapists, orthopedic surgeons, nurse practitioners, and podiatrists all provide foot care. Therefore, it would be difficult, even for a large group of podiatrists to obtain significant product power.

BUSINESS PRACTICE LITIGATION RISKS

A recent report stated that 25% of all suits filed in *Federal District Court* relate to a growing field of law loosely called "Business Practices Litigation." That percentage is only likely to grow in the coming years. Business Practices Litigation encompasses a wide variety of issues, but they mostly resolve around the relationship between a business and its employees and customers. The issues include, for example, racial and sexual discrimination, sexual harassment, wrongful termination, and violations of the *Americans with Disabilities Act*. These claims are not confined to big corporations, but can affect the sole proprietor physician.

For example, a Georgia physician recently paid $5000 in settlement of an employment claim. Apparently, the physician would have won the claim, but only after paying over $20,000.00 in legal fees. That $5000.00 settlement was not paid by the malpractice insurance carrier, but was paid by the individual physician himself.

PATTERNS OF PRACTICE RISKS

One of the next big areas of risk that will surface in the near future is the *Pattern of Practice Risk*. Pattern of Practice refers to the way that a particular physician practices medicine. With computers, eHRs, standardized diagnosis and treatment codes, and the budgetary restraints inherent in medical practice, it is becoming easy to analyze a physician's method of practice. The treatment and diagnosis codes that a physician uses and submits to third-party payers can be quantified and compared to colleagues in the same or similar specialties. Statistical *outliers* can be identified. These outliers will then be further audited and required to justify their treatments. If no rational basis exists for the statistical differences, the outlier may find himself the subject of a fraud investigation.

MANAGED CARE CONTRACT RISKS

Attorneys are becoming more aggressive in suing HMOs and other managed care companies. Historical bars to such suits are declining simultaneously with recent Federal ERISA protection erosion. The upshot is that more litigation against managed care companies, their affiliates, and their health care providers are likely. The health care provider needs to be aware of these trends, needs to evaluate his/her own situation, and may need to take certain steps to limit these new evolving risks and potential liabilities.

For example, the usual method of protection for the practicing physician, the use of the corporate form of business, is usually no benefit when signing managed care contracts. Most managed care companies credential the individual physician and, hence, require that the individual physician and not the professional corporation sign the contract. *This puts all of the physician's personal assets at risk.*

HISTORIC BARS TO MANAGED CARE LAWSUITS

Historically, managed-care companies have been afforded immunity from negligence and malpractice lawsuits. Several state and federal bars, including *Employee Retirement Income Security Act of 1974 (ERISA)*, have insulated managed-care companies from liability relating to the treatment of patients. Likewise, managed-care companies have historically been immune from malpractice committed by a health care member of its panel of providers. On a state laws basis, the *Corporate Practice of Law* often insulated managed-care companies from such liability. The theory underlying this protection was essentially uncomplicated; since corporations are prohibited under the Corporate Practice of Law Doctrine from practicing medicine, they should not be held liable for medical negligence and malpractice.

However, in recent years, it has become apparent that managed-care companies do in fact "practice medicine." These companies tell their panel of providers how to practice, whether it is in a generalized or specific field of medicine. They establish a formulary of approved drugs, limiting those medications available to their subscribers. They review and then approve or deny needed medical care. They create economic incentives for patients to be under treated or treated in a predetermined manner. They effectively minimize referrals to specialists, often at the peril of the patient subscriber and the health care provider seeking that consultation.

In the Federal arena, ERISA has been the primary deterrent to suits against managed-care companies. Under the theory of Federal preemption, even the lowest Federal regulation takes precedence over any and all state laws. ERISA has however been described as possessing "*Super-preemption.*" That term was coined to evince the special deference that courts have displayed to potential defendants who allege defensive protection based upon ERISA. In the past, most providers ran into the ERISA preemption when a health plan governed by ERISA was contrary to a state law, such as state anti-discrimination law (i.e., a state law prohibiting insurance payment discrimination based on degree). In the context of this chapter, the reader should understand that liability claims, such as medical malpractice claims, are state law causes of action. Since the Federal ERISA law trumps state laws, bringing a medical malpractice action against an ERISA entity is almost impossible.

THE CONTRACT CAPITULATION DILEMMA

The dilemma that a provider will have to consider when facing the adverse effects of a Hold Harmless Clause is the prospective detriment to his/her practice if he/she does not capitulate to the managed care company's demand to provide indemnification for a settled case. The provider has the option to fight the issue in court. In some cases, the provider may prevail, but it is likely to be a futile and expensive effort in most scenarios. In any event, if the provider does not indemnify the managed-care company, most likely, he/she will find himself/herself deselected from the panel. Such a deselection is likely to create a domino effect of deselection from other panels. Such events could destroy the provider's practice.

EMPLOYEE RISKS

Practice employees have *inside information* concerning the practice and the physician's patterns of practice. In most cases the staff is trained by the doctor. The staff's frame of reference is thereby limited to what they have been taught. However, more credit should be given to the office staff. Staff members deal everyday with insurance companies (including Medicare) and they field a wide array of patient questions and complaints. An astute staff member will soon realize if the physician is miscoding insurance submission.

An informed, irate employee can be your biggest risk. Many medical malpractice lawsuits have been brought by patients because terminated employees have informed the patient that "something was wrong" with their treatment. Likewise, OSHA investigations have been instituted by disgruntled employees. In these cases the employee had nothing to gain but revenge against real or perceived injustices from their former employer. Now, an employee also has a financial incentive to bring health care fraud charges against their former physician–employer.

VICARIOUS RISKS

In certain situations, the doctor may at risk for vicarious fraud charges, even if he never submitted a questionable claim. The two classes of practitioners that may have such risk involve physicians who are members of a group practice and employed (or contracted) physicians.

Employed Physician

You may think that as an employed physician that you are not at risk. However, in some cases your risk could be greater. For example, if you work for a physician who employs you to see patients at a contracted nursing home and you either get paid per patient or per day, realize that Medicare is being billed under your name as the provider of services. Although you may never get receipt of the money, since the billing was done under your name, if there is a question of fraud, you would be the one liable! The point is that whether you are a self-employed, a member of a group, or an employed physician, you should personally ensure that the billing being conducted under your name and signature is proper.

GROUP PRACTICE

If you are a member of a group and your income is at all dependent upon the income of another member of a group (e.g., expense sharing or production-based income), then you may be liable for the fraud of another member of your group. The rationale is because every member of the group benefits financially from the money received secondary to the fraudulent activity. This can put a practitioner in a very difficult position. One must choose whether to continue in practice with a practitioner employing questionable billing techniques or whether to dissolve the group.

Certificates of Medical Necessity

Physicians are asked daily to sign Certificates of Medical Necessity (CMN). Under the new law, you may be liable if you sign a CMN and the product or service is later found to be not medically necessary. In most cases, a physician should have no problem with this rule. The practitioner should be careful in signing CMNs that come into your office unsolicited. For example, you may be asked to sign a CMN for transportation of a Medicaid patient to your office. But was that transportation or the particular level of transportation medically necessary? Extreme caution should be employed when signing a CMN for transportation. In most cases, transportation to your office will be nonemergency transportation of an ambulatory patient. Unscrupulous transportation companies have been known to bill for stretcher transportation of ambulatory patients. Do not allow yourself to be swept into another's fraudulent scheme. Be careful what you certify as medically necessary!

CONTRACT DESELECTION RISKS

In the current medical environment, a physician's practice does not consist of a collection of individual patients or of the "charts." A physician's practice consists of a number of managed care contracts that allows the physician to be a member of a panel and listed in the individual subscriber's insurance book. The patients merely flow from those managed-care contracts. Without the contracts, there will be no patient flow. Therefore, the physician faces the risk of being deselected from an individual, or several, managed care panels. Each deselection will have an adverse effect on the physician's practice. In actuality, the revenue lost from deselection will come disproportionally from the net revenue of the practice. Often one deselection will snowball into several deselections, until the physician barely has a practice remaining.

COLLATERAL CONSEQUENCES RISKS

Many risks inherent in medical practice also have collateral consequences. For example, making a payment in response to a medical malpractice claim requires reporting to the *National Practitioner Data Bank*. Often such a report instigates an investigation by state boards and hospital staffs. The result is that the medical license of staff privileges can be placed in jeopardy.

MEDICARE 5-YEAR EXCLUSION RISKS

Medicare rules provide for a mandatory exclusion of a provider who has been convicted of certain crimes. For example, a physician who is convicted of insurance fraud (unrelated to the Medicare program) could also be excluded from Medicare participation during a 5-year period.

STATE BOARD ACTION RISKS

Many of the State Medical Board actions are "piggy-back" actions. That means a disciplined physician may find himself subject to action by an out-of-state State Board where he holds an additional license. The grounds will be that the practitioner had been disciplined by the practitioner's home state and therefore, the foreign state has grounds for action against the medical license in that state. Some states investigate all closed malpractice cases, even cases that have settled. The investigation in these cases is to determine whether the practitioner is engaging in practice patterns that would be adverse to the public benefit. It is easy to see how one incident can snowball. The risk is great.

Take the example of a physician who settles a malpractice claim. The physician's state board investigates the matter and determines that there is enough evidence for a reprimand. Next, an out-of-state board takes action simply because of the action taken by the home state. All of these actions are subsequently reported to the National Practitioner Data Bank. When the physician's local hospital appointment is up for re-appointment, the hospital (as required by law) checks the National Practitioner Data Bank. Seeing the adverse actions taken against the physician, the hospital restricts the physician's privileges. Finally, the managed-care companies, of which the physician is a panel member, learn of all these actions and deselect the physician. The physician's ability to earn a living is therefore significantly impaired. The legal risks today are just too great!

OVERHEARD IN THE DOCTOR'S LOUNGE: ON INSURANCE POLICIES

I currently have no fewer than ten separate insurance policies associated with my plastic surgery practice. I understand very little about the policies and risk management other than somebody at some point told me I needed each and every one of them, and each made sense when I bought it.

But, am I over-insured and thus wasting money? Am I under-insured and thus at risk for a liability or other disaster? I never really had the means of answering these questions.

Lloyd M. Krieger, MD, MBA
(Rodeo Drive Plastic Surgery)

MEDICAL FRAUD AND ABUSE BILLING RISKS

The following actions can be taken by the practitioner in an attempt to limit charges of fraud.

STATISTICAL ANALYSIS AND FRAUD INVESTIGATIONS

The CMS compiles data concerning fee charges and payments by all physicians. This data is broken down into various categories, such as by CPT® code, physician specialty, and state. Each and every physician should obtain a copy of this report and review it thoroughly. This data is available through CMS or can be downloaded from its Internet web site. The report contains valuable yearly statistical information concerning the rendering of services to Medicare beneficiaries. By comparing the statistics of this report with the statistics of your office, you can determine your risk of an audit.

Since the likelihood of an audit is dependent upon "where the money is," then the nationwide average and the placement of your state in the table can indicate the likelihood of your being audited. Therefore, the risks are that many physicians in high reimbursement states will be audited and few physicians in low reimbursement states will be audited. This is not as arbitrary as it may seem. There must be a reason why the average physician's Medicare charge in one state is higher than that of the national average. Unfortunately only an audit will determine the reason why, whether the reason is due to valid treatments or health care fraud. These statistics are available to Medicare. Since "knowledge is power," you should familiarize yourself with the data that Medicare will use in targeting audit candidates. By knowing where a likely audit will take place, the practitioner can alter procedures and documentation to ensure that such has the ability to withstand an audit.

THE BELL-SHAPED NORMALIZATION CURVE

Although a bell-shaped normalization curve will not ensure that you will not be audited, it can go a long way to disprove any intent to defraud a third-party payer. Understanding your options is the first step in visualizing the bell curve.

For example, take these five patient E/M codes (99201, 99202, 99203, 99204, and 99205) and five established patient E/M codes (99211, 99212, 99213, 99214, and 99215). A normal bell curve for most physicians would probably see most of the visits spread fairly evenly over the different levels of codes of each group, with a smaller amount in the level one and five codes. You can use your computer to evaluate whether your CPT® codes especially the E/M codes and the other codes all fall within a bell curve. If these codes do not fall within a bell curve, then you should consider whether to adjust your coding patterns to bring them into a bell curve. Staying within the Bell Curve is a prudent defensive step.

APPROPRIATE CONTRACTS

The provider should read every managed care contract. Most providers simply sign and return every contract that comes across their desk. In recent years, with so much of the population participating in some form of managed care, many providers feel that they have no choice but to sign the contract. Remember that even if the terms are not negotiable, you still have a choice of not signing the contract. If you do sign the contract, you should fully understand the risks that you are undertaking. It is okay to assume a risk, BUT only if you understand the risk you are assuming and are willing to assume that risk. It is often not reasonable to expect that the provider will fully understand the import of many of the clauses in current managed care contracts. For that reason, it is prudent to have an attorney review every contract that you intend to sign. Although it costs more initially to pay legal fees to review the contract, it could potentially save a lot of problems and money at a later date. Once you become aware of a risk or a clause in the managed care contract that is contrary to your interests, your first defensive step is to attempt to negotiate the clause out of the contract. Unfortunately, the individual provider has very little leverage in negotiating such contracts and the clause is likely to remain.

The next defensive step to take is to "Just Say NO!" Many readers will balk at that statement and will declare: "I don't have a choice. If I don't sign the contract, I will not have any patients!" The point is that you do have a choice. If you choose to sign the contract, then what becomes important is what you do after you sign the contract.

If you choose to sign the contract, then you should sign the contract in the name of your Professional Corporation and as agent of your Professional Corporation (*i.e., do not sign the contract in your personal capacity*). By signing the contract on behalf of your corporation, your liability (in most cases) becomes limited to your equity in the corporation.

Unfortunately, the usual method of protection for the practicing physician, the use of the corporate form of business, is usually no benefit when signing managed-care contracts. That is because most managed-care companies credential the individual physician and hence require that the individual physician and not the professional corporation sign the contract. This puts all of the physician's personal assets at risk. Nonetheless, the provider should attempt to sign all such contracts in the name of the corporation. Some contracts are likely to be accepted by the managed-care company. When the company requires the provider to sign in his individual capacity, then the provider can make the decision at that time.

It is important to realize that the risks delineated above apply not only to affluent physicians, but to any physician who signs a managed-care contract. A typical example resonates when the provider requests legal analysis of the contract and is quoted a fee for this professional service. More often than not, the health care provider will reject this as costing too much, yet in reality the fee, when juxtaposed to the fees charged for medical services, is generally fair and equitable. A young physician with an unpaid student debt loan that finds herself on the wrong end of a Hold Harmless Agreement with a managed-care company may find herself forced into bankruptcy.

PRACTICING BARE

Many providers in practice would not think of "practicing bare." In the past, the term practicing bare meant that the provider did not have malpractice insurance. Current managed-care contracts often require that the provider not only have certain limits of malpractice, but also that the provider shows evidence of such insurance. Therefore, many providers are under the impression that they are not practicing bare. As can be seen from the example clauses above, most providers are in effect practicing bare. Most providers have no protection from adverse results arising out of a Hold Harmless Clause in an agreement. Most malpractice insurance companies do not provide such coverage. If your malpractice insurance company does not provide coverage for such events, it is incumbent upon you and your associations to lobby the malpractice insurance carriers to provide such coverage. An additional rider, at an additional premium, for Hold Harmless coverage would help the practitioner sleep better at night.

The first question that the provider should ask is: *Would I consider practicing without malpractice insurance?* If the answer to that question is *"no",* then the next question that the provider should ask is: *"Why am I assuming the risk under the Hold Harmless Clause?"* If the provider cannot provide a lucent answer to that question (stating: "I have no choice," is not a lucent answer!), then the provider should not sign the managed care contract. Nonetheless, if the provider has signed managed-care contracts, then the provider should understand that he is practicing bare and should take steps to reduce his exposure. In effect, the provider should attempt to become "judgment-proof." Such a step does present its own risks. Ultimately, the first step for every physician who signs a managed-care contract with a hold harmless agreement is to read the contract and then consult an attorney or other professional. Plaintiff attorneys are beginning to make inroads in suing managed care companies. The managed care attorneys foresaw such events and provided protection for the company in the contracts most providers have signed.

As plaintiffs become successful in suing and recovering from managed-care companies, those companies are going to seek indemnity from the provider. Unless the provider protects himself, the provider is likely to become a collateral casualty of events. The current practice of medicine presents risks to the provider. The provider may not be able to insure against these risks and therefore should take defensive steps to avoid future problems.

Staff Education and Training

The medical staff is an extension of the physician. Furthermore, several federal regulations, including HIPAA and OSHA, have specific staff training requirements. Failure to provide the required training not only subjects the physician to the risk of employee transgression, but also to the risk of administrative discipline for failure to conduct proper training of staff.

Elimination of Risky Treatments

One of the methods most often overlooked in malpractice risk management is an evaluation of the risk-reward ratio of treating certain patients or performing certain surgical procedures. Managed care has effectively reduced the reimbursement of treatments and surgeries across the board. In the past, the physician could demand a reasonable fee for the risk involved. Now, that fee is determined by someone other than the physician. Although the resource-based view (RBV) values include a malpractice component, sometimes that component does not adequately reflect the risk of certain procedures or the increased risk of certain patients. Therefore, the physician should evaluate their own practice and identify those procedures and those patient types that carry a high risk of malpractice and for which the physician is not adequately reimbursed for that risk. The physician then should tailor his or her practice so that he no longer provides those services. The revenue lost will be worth the risk of the malpractice suit and the collateral consequences. This is simply the unintended consequence of insurance company and other managers reducing the physicians' reimbursement. If the reward is high enough, people will take the risk. If the reward is reduced and the risk remains the same, fewer people will be willing to engage in that behavior, simple free market economics. A physician need not feel bad for turning away patients or dropping certain procedures from one's practice. That is simply part of risk management.

MEDICAL WORKPLACE VIOLENCE RISKS

We can define the meaning of workplace violence as "violent acts including assaults and threats which occur in, or are related to the workplace and entail a substantial risk of physical or emotional harm to individuals, or damage to an organizations resources or capabilities." More specifically it includes

- Actual violence that causes or is intended to cause injury or harm to a person or property
- Threatening remarks and/or behavior in which intent to harm is stated or implied or indicates a lack of respect for the dignity and worth of an individual
- Verbal abuse
- Mobbing, bullying, emotional abuse
- Possession of a weapon while working or on company property

THE STATISTICS

Let's begin with some historical data on the cost of workplace violence.

- In 1995 the National Council of Compensation Insurance found $126 million in workers compensation claims for workplace violence.
- A study released by the Workplace Violence Research Institute in April 1995 showed that workplace violence actually resulted in a $36 billion annual loss.
- According to the Bureau of Justice Statistics, about 500,000 victims of violent crime in the workplace lose an estimated 1.8 million workdays each year. This presents an astounding $55 million in lost wages for employees, not including days covered by sick and annual leave and a loss of productivity that has direct consequences for an employer's bottom line.
- Lawsuits in the area have been impacting cost substantially. The average out-of-court settlement for this type of litigation approaches $500,000 and the average jury award of $3 million. A few awards have reached as high as $5.49 million.
- The Bureau of Labor Statistics reported a rate of 8.3 assaults per 10,000 hospitals workers occurred in 1999. This rate is much higher than the rate of nonfatal assaults for all private sector industries, which is 2 per 10,000 workers.
- According to the 1997 NIOSH Fact sheet—Violence in the Workplace—64% of all nonfatal assaults occurred in service industries and of these over 38% occurred in heath care related operations.
- The Fact Sheet further reported that 48% of nonfatal assaults in the workplace are committed by a health care patient.
- Staff working in psychiatric and long-term care settings is at high risk. A stunning 50% of all long-term care staff and 46–100% of nurses, psychiatrist, and other therapists in psychiatric facilities experience at least one assault during their careers.

MEDICAL WORKPLACE PREVALENCE

Less than five years after Army psychiatrist Nidal Hasan MD went on a shooting rampage at Fort Hood, the military base was shaken by another shooting. Dr. Hasan, convicted in the November 5, 2009 tragedy, left 13 dead and 31 wounded, and sentenced to death by a military jury in August 2013. He was convicted on 13 counts of premeditated murder and 32 charges of attempted premeditated murder.

Yet, on April 3, 2014, and at the same base in Kinilleen, Texas, Specialist Ivan Lopez, age 34, was accused of killing three people before committing suicide. Sixteen more were injured when he allegedly opened fire on the sprawling military base. He was engaged by military police before he fatally shot himself in the head.

The Statistics

An October 2003 survey of doctors conducted by Health Policy and Economic Research Unit of BMA also reported that half of all doctors believe violence is a problem in the workplace. Of the almost 1000 doctors who responded to the survey, the key findings were

- Violence is a problem in the workplace for almost half of doctors.
- 1 in 3 respondents had experienced some form of violence in the workplace last year—this was the case for both hospital doctors and general practitioners.
- The majority of violent incidents took place in the doctors' office or hospital ward. Among GPs the majority of incidents took place in their office or waiting room, while for hospital doctors, the most frequently cited location was the hospital ward.
- Among hospital doctors those working in accident & emergency and psychiatry were more likely to experience patient violence.
- Among doctors who reported some experience of violence, almost all (95%) had been the victim of verbal abuse in the past year.
- The main cause of violence was perceived to be health-related/personal problems, dissatisfaction with service provided and/or drugs/alcohol.

Focusing on Prevention

Zero Incidents is a comprehensive approach, process, and system characterized by an emphasis on prevention of violence and/or injury to employees. The focus is on early identification of individual and organizational warning signs by assessing facility risk, level of individual threat, and organizational violence prone factors. The goal is to identify and eliminate or mitigate risk factors that are known to contribute to increasing the likelihood of a violent incident occurring. In addition, to focusing on Zero Incidents this approach typically incorporates a Zero Tolerance for threats and acts of violence and subjects employees that violate the policy to disciplinary action up to and including termination.

Implementation of a "Zero Incident" approach often involves the following:

- Focus on eliminating "at-risk" behaviors
- Establish a workplace violence prevention policy
- No weapons in the workplace policy
- Define the nature of the risk to the company
- Facility risk assessments
- Organizational violence assessments
- Individual threat assessment
- Enhance physical security
- Synchronize your personnel, security, and safety policies
- Develop crisis response procedures
- Emergency protocol with police
- Enhance hiring procedures
- Promote your employee assistance program
- Train managers, supervisors, doctors, nurses, and employees
- Involve health care employees in the prevention effort

Disastrous Planning Mistakes

According to W. Barry Nixon SPHR MS, one of the cruelest myths in physical crisis management and medical workplace violence prevention planning is the belief that plans adopted, but not tested, will actually work as planned (personal communication).

Another costly fallacy for health care organizations is to forget their people and focus solely on protecting their hard assets, for example, facilities, technology, information, and networks. It is one thing to test your alarm systems, system recovery processes, backing up information protections, and another to have your people improperly or not trained in what they need to do or worse; what they have been told to do causes confusion because it has never been tested to have the kinks worked out. You need to prepare your people for crisis because they will make the difference in how quickly and effectively you are able to return to normal business operations.

The third myth regarding crisis planning is the belief that you can effectively insure losses in a disaster. Ken Smith, former vice president of consulting operations for SunGard Planning Solutions, Wayne, Pennsylvania, an expert in handling crisis claims says "settling claims after a disaster is not a pretty process." Insurers trying to mitigate casualty losses often lock horns with executives trying to recover quickly (personal communication).

ACKNOWLEDGMENT

To W Barry Nixon, SPHR, founder of the National Institute for the Prevention of Workplace Violence, Inc., Lake Forest, California.

SEXUAL HARASSMENT RISKS

There are positive reasons to consider medical practice climate. Preventing discrimination and sexual harassment boosts worker morale and productivity. But, there are also costly negatives to avoid. Discrimination and harassment lawsuits cost companies more and more each year. For example, a study released in January 2002 by Jury Verdict Research, Inc., found that

- The national median jury award for employment-practice liability cases, which include discrimination and retaliation claims, rose 44%—from $151,000 to $218,000—between 1999 and 2000. The median award had stayed level at about $150,000 between 1997 and 1999.
- Of all discrimination types, age discrimination plaintiffs won the most money from 1994–2000.
- The overall median jury award in discrimination cases was $150,000 for the 7-year span.

The study also showed an increase in public awareness and jury sympathy for the plaintiffs in discrimination cases:

- In 2000, 62% of plaintiffs in sex discrimination cases (including sexual harassment) won their cases, compared with only 43% in 1994.
- 67% of race discrimination plaintiffs won their cases in 2000, compared with 50% in 1994.

In 1999 survey of 496 companies published by the Society for Human Resource Management, was found that

- Sexual harassment complaints increased at those companies by almost 140% between 1995 and 1998.
- Small businesses averaged nearly one claim per 100 employees in 1998—five times higher than the rate of one claim per 500 among large businesses.
- Only 51% of small businesses said that they offered sexual harassment prevention training, while 76% of large companies did.

DEFINITIONS

The courts have defined sexual harassment as unwelcome sexual advances, requests for sexual favors, and other verbal or physical conduct of a sexual nature, when

- Submission to such conduct is an explicit or implicit term or condition of employment;
- Submission to such conduct is used as the basis for a favorable employment decision or the employee's rejection of such conduct is used as the basis for an adverse employment decision; or
- Such conduct unreasonably interferes with an employee's work or creates an intimidating, hostile, or offensive working environment.

According to Vicki L. Buba, JD, although accurate from a legal perspective, this definition offers little or no guidance to a physician trying to articulate to his/her office staff what behavior is prohibited and what is acceptable (personal communication, Louisville, KY). Unfortunately, there is no clear-cut line to provide an answer to the relevant question: What specific acts are classified as sexual harassment? Therefore, the two-pronged test may be useful in this definitional determination.

TWO-PRONGED TEST FOR OFFENSIVE BEHAVIOR

This test asks first whether the conduct was severe and pervasive enough to create a hostile and abusive work environment; and then whether this victim subjectively perceived the environment to be hostile or abusive. In other words, would a "reasonable" person be offended and was this particular person offended? Both questions must be answered yes before the behavior will be classified as sexual harassment.

GENDER-BASED ANIMOSITY

A sexually hostile work environment often results from comments or actions that contain some sort of sexual connotation. However, this cause of action stems from actions that are based on gender. Consequently, sexual content is not required. Acts that fall into this category are easily recognized because they are generally based on negative stereotyping.

SAME SEX HARASSMENT

Before 1998, courts around the country were split on the issue of whether sexual harassment claims could be asserted only if the behavior occurred between a male and a female. In 1998, the U.S. Supreme Court settled the issue in its ruling in *Oncale v. Sundowner Offshore Services, Inc.* when it ruled that sexual harassment is behavior based on gender and it applies whether the parties are different sexes or the same sex. The Court also said that the relevant question was whether there was a hostile work environment because of gender and, therefore, the sexual orientation of the parties was not to be considered.

With this ruling, the Court expanded the body of law previously delineated as sexual harassment. The Court emphasized that male-on-male horseplay is not prohibited. However, when it rises to the level of more serious acts, such as genital grabbing, threatened sexual acts or severe language which offends or frightens the victim to the extent it interferes with the victim's work performance, it is prohibited under the law governing sexual harassment (*Oncale v. Sundowner Offshore Services, Inc.*, 523 U.S. 75 [1998] and *Faragher v. City of Boca Raton*, 524 U.S. 775 [1998]).

Doctor Employer Liability

A key question is under what circumstances will the physician employer be liable for sexual harassment in the workplace? The rules vary, according to whether the harassing party is a supervisor or a nonsupervisor. For many years, the courts held that where the harasser is also a supervisor, the employer would be absolutely liable. This liability is based on the premise that a doctor employer must have notice of the harassment in order to be liable and that since supervisors are agents of the employer, there is notice. The Court outlined an affirmative defense that would permit the employer to avoid or limit liability. An affirmative defense exists where the employer exercised reasonable care to prevent and promptly correct harassing behavior and where the victim unreasonably failed to take advantage of any preventive or corrective opportunities to avoid harm. And, it is not sufficient to merely have a policy in place and to disseminate it to employees. The physician employer must be prepared to uniformly enforce the policy once it has been established.

Disciplinary Actions

Many events may contribute to a sexual harassment claim, but even though each of them standing alone may be insufficient to prevail in a court of law. However, because the threshold for a sexual harassment claim falls in a gray area, employers have the right to protect themselves by establishing rules which may be more stringent than those imposed by a court. Disciplinary action may be something as simple as a verbal conversation explaining to the alleged harasser that these things do offend some people and the harasser should avoid such behavior in the future. Obviously, more serious violations may warrant more serious disciplinary action, up to and including termination of employment. The bottom line is that doctor employers must be able to show they have done everything within their power to prevent sexual harassment and when complaints are made, they have immediately investigated and, when necessary, taken corrective action. Such is the only way in which a doctor employer may avoid liability for sexual harassment complaints.

Using a Common Sense Approach

Any hospital or medical workplace, even a small- to mid-sized doctor's office or clinic, should always be viewed as a professional environment. Employees should be viewed as just that. When an individual walks through the office door in the morning, that individual is not a female, not a Jew, not a black, but is simply an employee there to do a job. A physician employer who makes attempts to enforce such an attitude will go far in eliminating sexual harassment in the medical work place.

NEW-WAVE CLINICAL RISKS

It seems that the potential liability associated with medical practice is limitless, as the following three additional risks have recently been identified.

Expert Witness Risks

In the past, a physician expert witness for the plaintiff was merely an opposing opinion by a learned and/or like colleague. Today, it is becoming a risk management minefield as the AMA and other groups are urging state medical licensing boards to police expert witnesses, which might require expert testimony be considered the practice of medicine. This seems especially true with the Rolling Meadows, Illinois-based American Association of Neurological Surgeons (AANS). Currently, a member of the AANS can file a complaint against any fellow member for testimony as either an expert witness for the plaintiff, or defense witness for the doctor. A committee then reviews the court records and requires the accuser to face the accused in a formal review. Sanctions range from three months to a year, to complete expulsion from the association. Since 2001, the courts have been beginning to take the AANS process seriously. So always remember, if you testify falsely, or too far from the norm, you may be at risk.

Peer Review Risks

The Center for Peer Review Justice is a group of physicians, podiatrists, dentists, and osteopaths who have witnessed the perversion of medical peer review by malice and bad faith. Similar to the AANS, they have seen the statutory immunity, which is provided to "peers" for the purposes of quality assurance and credentialing, used as cover to allow those "peers" to ruin careers and reputations to further their own, usually monetary agenda of destroying the competition. Therefore, the group is dedicated to the exposure, conviction, and sanction of doctors, and affiliated hospitals, HMOs, medical boards, and other such institutions that would use peer review as a weapon to unfairly destroy other professionals. PeerReview.org is a rallying point and resource center for any medical professional that finds himself in the midst of an unfair and bad faith attack by unethical, malicious "peers."

On-Call Risks

On call is getting more expensive these days to take hospital calls as physicians are electing not to take this responsibility because of decreased reimbursement rates. Others opt out because of a desire to spend more time with family, and/or scheduling conflicts. Regardless, there is a growing revolt of specialists against hospital on-call duties that threatens to violate Federal law and lose status as trauma centers. Specialties most likely to refuse include plastic surgery, ENT, psychiatry, neurosurgery, ophthalmology, and orthopedics. Refusing to respond to an assigned call is a violation of Federal law and carries fines as much as $50,000 per case. In contrast, refusing to sign up for call does not violate the law, and more physicians are taking this option.

PERSONAL MEDICAL REPUTATION RISKS

Medical professionals, financial advisors, and management consultants can now get instant online reputation management services. Patients, people, and clients are posting new content on the Internet every day. Keeping tabs on a personal or professional reputation may be vital to your advisory reputation and medical practice success. Why would you need Internet monitoring?

- Finds existing posts about YOU online
- Sends alerts whenever new posts appear
- Finds exposed personal info in databases
- Identifies and alerts you to damaging posts

No one asks for job references, patient or client referrals, or background information anymore; they ask Google or some other search engine. If your name turns up negatively in news, malpractice verdicts or CRD reports, patient complaints, messy divorces, bankruptcies, legal filings, embarrassing photos, or other questionable material, you're likely to get passed over. So, check out www.Reputation.com.

MEDICAL MALPRACTICE AND THE PP-ACA

The health care reform law will reduce liability payouts by insurers for auto and workers' compensation claims by nearly $1.7 billion annually while increasing medical malpractice claims by $120 million a year, according to a study released by the RAND Institute for Civil Justice. The RAND researchers looked at the anticipated impact on insurance claims under the ACA in 2016, when the law is expected to be fully implemented.

While the law's most obvious impact will be on health insurance policies, researchers found that it will also have minor but financially significant effects on claims paid by other common types of insurance policies. *Source*: http://www.rand.org/health.html.

CONCLUSION

Medical Risk Management is no longer just about medical malpractice anymore—it has not been for some time now, despite the recent resurgence of liability fears. In fact, since most practicing physicians have malpractice insurance, then a malpractice suit should be viewed as a mere inconvenience and the practitioner and his financial advisors should realize that the lawsuit is mainly about someone else's money.

A shift in thought paradigm is needed. The medico-legal landscape has changed. The physician in practice today is faced with many legal challenges that have the potential to destroy the medical practice and the individual's personal assets. These have been briefly reviewed in this chapter. Therefore, every practice should have a qualified health care specific attorney on retainer.

Be aware, the legal risks are only going to increase, going forward!

COLLABORATE

Discuss this chapter online with others at www.MedicalExecutivePost.com.

ACKNOWLEDGMENTS

To Edward J. Rappaport, JD, LL.M, Atlanta, Georgia; Vicki L. Buba, JD, Philadelphia, Pennsylvania; and Dr. Steven D. Chinn, MS, MBA, CPHQ, Millbrae, California.

REFERENCES AND READINGS

1. Workplace Violence in Health Services, Joint ILO/ICN/WHO/PSI research, 2002.
2. Fatal Choices online at: www.Washington.edu, University of Washington, Seattle, WA.
3. Smith MH., Legal considerations of workplace violence in healthcare environments, *Nursing Forum*, 36(1), 5–14, Jan-Mar 2001.
4. Duane F., Detective, Minneapolis Police Department.
5. Distasio CA., Protecting yourself from violence in the workplace, *Nursing* 32(6), 58–64, June 2002.
6. Fatal occupational injuries by event or exposure, US Department of Labor, Bureau of Labor Statistics, Census of Fatal Occupational Injuries, 1991–2002.
7. Bureau of Justice Statistics, http://www.ojp.usdoj.gov/bjs/.
8. Helge H., Sparks K., and Cooper CL., The Cost of Violence/Stress at work and the Benefits of a Violence/Stress-Free Working Environment, Report Commissioned by the International Labor Organization (ILO), University of Manchester Institute of Science and Technology, Geneva.
9. Jones S., Work Stress Taking Larger Financial Toll, August 9, 2000.
10. Richard HG., Apocalypse Maybe, *Controller Magazine*, June 1998.
11. Dan D., Ph.D., Dana Mediation Institute, Inc., The Dana Measure of the Financial Cost of Organizational Conflict: An Interpretive Guide, 2001, www.mediationworks.com.

FURTHER READING

Bode, GL: Internal medical practice controls. In Marcinko, DE (Ed), *Business of Medical Practice*. Springer Publishing, New York, 2010.
Buba, V: Sexual harassment in healthcare. In Marcinko, DE (Ed), *Insurance Planning and Risk Management for Physicians*. Jones and Bartlett Publishing, Sudbury, MA, 2006

Fenton, CF: Medical practice sales contract. In Marcinko, DE (Ed), *Business of Medical Practice*. Springer Publishing, New York, 2010.

Fenton, CF: Medical risk management issues. In Marcinko, DE (Ed), *Insurance Planning and Risk Management for Physicians*. Jones and Bartlett Publishing, Sudbury, MA, 2006.

Trites, P: Medical records, insurance billing and coding guidelines. In Marcinko, DE (Ed), *Business of Medical Practice*. Springer Publishing, New York, 2010.

9 Personal Financial Accounting and Income Taxation

The Ethical Pursuit of Tax Reduction and Avoidance

Perry D'Alessio

CONTENTS

The objective of tax planning is to arrive at the lowest overall tax cost on the activities performed. Inasmuch as physicians constitute 14% of the so-called and often maligned "one-percenters" ($388,905 earned, not passive income/per year), this chapter will address some methods and strategies to reduce federal and state income taxes. It is applicable to all physicians and medical professionals, as independent practitioners or employees.

So, how much in income taxes do the wealthy pay? According to the Tax Foundation, a think tank that advocates for lower taxes, the top 10% of taxpayers paid over 70% of the total amount collected in federal income taxes in 2010, which is the latest year figures available. That's up from 55% in 1986. The remaining 90% bore just under 30% of the tax burden and 47% of all Americans pay hardly anything at all.

You should realize that is just federal income tax and does not include payroll tax for Social Security and Medicare (which the vast majority of people pay), plus state taxes, and all of the other taxes we face, and when you add them all together, using figures from the Tax Policy Center and the Institute on Taxation and Economic Policy. Earners in the top 1% pay about 43% of their incomes in tax. People in the middle quintile pay 25% while the poorest fifth pays 13%.

Finally, before you assume these 1- and 10-percenters are living on luxury yachts and in million-dollar mansions, consider how little money it takes to be a top wage earner. According to 2011 IRS data, the top 1% have adjusted gross incomes (AGI) of $388,905 per year or more. To be in the top 10%, you need an AGI of just $120,136 or more. These are good incomes to be sure, but definitely not enough to be out of work or the medical office for more than a few weeks each year.

Now, consider the following more specifically:

- 42% of all federal tax revenue came from individual income taxes in 2010 and it has been the largest single source of revenue since 1950.
- Individuals paid more than $2.2 trillion in 2010.
- Bush-era tax cuts have finally expired, giving us the twentieth century tax rates with the top income tax rate of 39.6%; we have not seen rates this high in almost 15 years.
- 39.6% tax rate kicks in at $400,000 for individual taxpayers and $450,000 for married couples filing jointly.
- Taxpayers who make over $200,000 ($250,000 for married taxpayers) will be subject to the Medicare surtax. If that's you, Medicare surtax will be tacked on to your wages, compensation, or self-employment income over that amount. The amount of the surcharge is 0.9%.
- Net investment income tax (NIIT), new as of 2013; if you have both net investment income and modified adjusted gross income (MAGI) of at least $200,000 for an individual taxpayer and $250,000 for taxpayers filing as married, an additional 3.8% of the net investment income is an added tax.

INTRODUCTION

There are many books written on tax planning and financial strategy for individuals. These texts all derive their information from the Internal Revenue Code and related regulations, along with the body of case law that has served to provide additional guidance for taxpayers. Unfortunately, most of these books become dated rather quickly with the passing of new tax bills and the settlement of court cases. Moreover, most healthcare professionals are not as wealthy as they think, because of their silent partner, Uncle Sam.

For example, according to A. Westhem and S. Weissman, authors of *Tax Smart Investing*, suppose longtime employee Betty Jones, RN, built up a one million dollar balance in her tax-deferred retirement plan at Memorial Hospital, and is gratified to know that she is now a millionaire. However, is she really? To get her hands on the money, she will likely have to pay over $400,000 to the IRS; depending on her city, state, and local government.

Susan Smith, RPT, has also been aggressively investing regularly in mutual funds, but outside of her retirement account. In the aggregate, she has contributed $100,000 into her account, which is valued at more than $250,000 because of a bull market in equities. Although the account is worth a quarter of a million dollars, it is not worth that much to her. When she cashes in her shares to pay for her son's medical school education, she will owe tax on her $150,000 capital gain of at least $30,000 (20% of $150,000). Thus, her hot portfolio is cooled down to $220,000. In addition, we now have a NIIT if you have both net investment income and MAGI of at least $200,000 for an individual taxpayer and $250,000 for taxpayers filing as married, an additional 3.8% of the net investment income is added, resulting in an additional $5700 in this case.

The above personal examples are not unusual in the healthcare industry, as virtually all investments have taxation consequences that can reduce the amount of money left over to enjoy; so too, in the U.S. income tax system. The vital notion is that it is important to learn as much as possible to reduce your individual burden in a legal manner. The number of tax planning ideas is limited only by the imagination and unique circumstances of the healthcare professional.

ADJUSTED GROSS INCOME

The U.S. individual tax return is based around the concepts of AGI and taxable income (TI). AGI is the amount that shows up at the bottom of page one of Form 1040, the individual income tax return. It is the sum of all of the taxpayer's income less certain allowed adjustments (like alimony, one-half of self-employment taxes, a percentage of self-employed health insurance, retirement plan contributions and IRAs, moving expenses, early withdrawal penalties, and interest on student loans). This amount is important because it is used to calculate various limitations within the area of itemized deductions (e.g., medical deductions: 10% of AGI; miscellaneous itemized deductions: 2% of AGI).

When a healthcare professional taxpayer hears the phrase "an above-the-line deduction," the line being referenced is the AGI line on the tax return. Generally, it is better for a deduction to be an above-the-line deduction, because that number helps a taxpayer in two ways. First, it reduces AGI, and second, since it reduces AGI, it is also reducing the amounts of limitations placed on other deductions as noted above.

Obviously, if there is an above-the-line deduction, there is also a "below-the-line" deduction. These below-the-line deductions are itemized deductions (or the standard deduction if itemizing is not used) plus any personal exemptions allowed. AGI less these deductions provides the TI on which income tax is actually calculated. All of that being said, it is better for a deduction to be above-the-line. Although this is a bit dry, it helps to understand the concepts in order to know where items provide the most benefit to the medical professional taxpayer.

PERSONAL TAXATION CALCULATIONS

Gross income (all income, from whatever source derived, including illegal activities, cash, indirect for the benefit of, debt forgiveness, barter, dividends, interest, rents, royalties, annuities, trusts, and alimony payments)

Less nontaxable exclusions (municipal bonds, scholarships, inheritance, insurance proceeds, social security, unemployment income [full or partial exclusion], etc.)
Total income
Less deductions for AGI (alimony, IRA contributions, capital gains, 1/2 SE tax, moving, personal, business and investment expenses, penalties, etc.)
Adjusted gross income (bottom form 1040)
Less itemized deductions from AGI (medical, charitable giving, casualty, involuntary conversions, theft, job, miscellaneous expenses, etc.) or
Less standard deduction (based on filing status)
Less personal exemptions (per dependents, subject to phase outs)

Taxable income
Calculate regular tax
Plus additional taxes (AMT, etc.)
Minus credits (child care, foreign tax credit, earned income housing, etc.)
Plus other taxes

Total tax due

Tax Planning Tip
Many healthcare professionals provide services both as a wage earner, in which case they receive a W-2, and as an independent contractor receiving a 1099-misc.

For example: A healthcare professional's main employment is for a hospital yielding a W-2, and on a few occasions a month will make speeches for a pharmaceutical company or provide medical opinions in court matters yielding a 1099-misc.

Expenses for wage positions are presented in the section of itemized deductions called unreimbursed work-related deductions subject to an offset of 2% of AGI, alternative minimum tax (AMT) phase out, and limitation reductions (should your AGI be over $250,000 single, $275,000 head of household, $300,000 married filing jointly, or $150,000 married filing separately), which in most cases these deductions yield no tax benefit.

The deductions for the independent position(s) are allowed directly against the income associated with it, no hurdles or phase outs of any kind; this is an *above-the-line deduction*.

Consideration and effort need be taken to properly pair your deductions with the nature of the services you provided, whether as a wage earner or independent. Simply listing all your expenses and providing this listing to your preparer can cost you thousands.

Are the deductions particular to the above-the-line deduction or to your wage position?

FILING STATUS AND TAX RATE BRACKETS

One of the questions most frequently asked by doctors and healthcare professionals revolves around the filing of a joint tax return versus the filing of a separate return. This question comes up because of the so-called marriage penalty that is built into the standard deduction and into the tax rates for married couples filing a joint return. The penalty exists because the standard deduction for couples is not twice the amount allowed to a single taxpayer. Albeit there is a penalty built into the above areas, joint filers do get the highest standard deduction, the lowest tax rates at any level of income, and the highest phase outs for credits, deductions, and personal exemptions.

On the other hand, married persons filing separate returns pay tax at the most unfavorable mix of rates of any taxpayer. Therefore, although there is a real marriage penalty built into the tax process, eliminating the penalty by filing separate only works under certain circumstances. The main area where this strategy works is when one spouse has significantly less income but a high level of itemized deductions (e.g., medical expenses for a chronic condition requiring significant outlays of cash). Remember, a lower AGI produces a lower deductible threshold for medical and miscellaneous expenses. This particular scenario can generate tax savings that make it worthwhile to consider filing separately; however, the numbers should be run both ways, jointly and separately, to see what that actual impact would be before making a final decision.

Tax Planning Tip
Often emphasis on planning is only on the federal tax position when considering married filing separate versus filing jointly. Many states permit you to file separately even though you may have filed jointly on your federal return. In many cases, considerable tax savings exist here. Make certain you tax professional reviews your options on a state level as well and calculates these potential savings.

Caution!
For those healthcare professionals living in either community property or common law states, special care needs to be taken in making the above filing decision. Extra care in the documentation of income and deductions (and their "ownership") is a must to assure a realistic result. In community property states, most items of both income and deduction will be split 50/50. However, each community property state has its own rules as to how income from separate property (property owned by one spouse or the other, not jointly, e.g., inherited property) is treated. For common law states, income is traced to ownership and deductions claimed by one spouse must be paid from that spouse's separate funds.

TAX BRACKETS

Currently, the income tax has seven marginal income tax rates: 10%, 15%, 25%, 28%, 33%, 35%, and 39.6%.

2013 Individual Income Tax Rates, Standard Deductions, Personal Exemptions, and Filing Thresholds

If Your Filing Status Is Single

Taxable Income

Over—	But not Over—	Marginal Rate
$0	$8925	10%
$8925	$36,250	15%
$36,250	$87,850	25%
$87,850	$183,250	28%
$183,250	$398,350	33%
$398,350	$400,000	35%
$400,000	and over	39.6%

If Your Filing Status Is Married Filing Jointly

Taxable Income

Over—	But Not Over—	Marginal Rate
$0	$17,850	10%
$17,850	$72,500	15%
$72,500	$146,400	25%
$146,400	$223,050	28%
$223,050	$398,350	33%
$398,350	$450,000	35%
$450,000	and over	39.6%

If Your Filing Status Is Head of Household

Taxable Income

Over—	But Not Over—	Marginal Rate
$0	$12,750	10%
$12,750	$48,600	15%
$48,600	$125,450	25%
$125,450	$203,150	28%
$203,150	$398,350	33%
$398,350	$425,000	35%
$425,000	and over	39.6%

If Your Filing Status Is Married Filing Separately

Taxable Income

Over—	But Not Over—	Marginal Rate
$0	$8925	10%
$8925	$36,250	15%
$36,250	$73,200	25%
$73,200	$111,525	28%
$111,525	$199,175	33%
$199,175	$225,000	35%
$225,000	and over	39.6%

Standard Deduction

	Standard	Blind/Elderly
Single	$6100	$1500
Married filing jointly	$12,200	$1200
Head of household	$8950	$1500
Married filing separately	$6100	$1200

Standard Deduction for Dependents

Greater of $1000 or sum of $350 and individual's earned income

Personal Exemption	$3900
Threshold for Refundable Child Tax Credit	$3000

Filing Threshold

	Number of Blind/Elderly Exemptions				
	0	1	2	3	4
Single	10,000	11,500	13,000		
Head of household	12,850	14,350	15,850		
Married filing jointly	20,000	21,200	22,400	23,600	24,800

Source: Internal Revenue Service, Revenue Procedure 2013–15, downloaded January 30, 2013 from IRS.

Note: Long-term capital gains—that is, gain on the sale of assets held more than 12 months—and qualified dividend income are taxed at lower rates.

MARGINAL TAX RATES

Keep in mind that the tax rates listed in these tables are marginal rates. That means that you do not owe your rate on all of your income.

For example, if you are single, you earn $100,000 per year, *you would not owe 28% on all of your income*—you would not owe $28,000 to the federal government. You would owe 10% of $8925, 15% of $27,325 (the difference between the top and the threshold of the second tax bracket), 25% of $51,600, and 28% of $12,150 (the difference between your income and the threshold of the third tax bracket).

That calculation results in $21,293, or an effective (not marginal) tax rate of 21.2%.

That will be further reduced by any credits, assuming your TI is the same as your gross income. Your effective tax rate could be much lower if deductions have already reduced your TI to $100,000 from a larger gross income. For example, if a 401(k) contribution reduced your TI from $115,000 to $100,000, you would still use the same tax calculation I've described here, but your effective tax rate would be 18.5%.

The limits for tax brackets have been increased for inflation by less than 2.5%. So, on joint returns, for example, the 28% rate will not apply until TI exceeds $43,850, and the 31% rate will not apply until TI exceeds $105,950.

Let's suppose that Dr. David Suppan's effective marginal federal tax rate is 41%, he lives in a city where state and local income tax must be paid, and his marginal rates for those two taxes are 8% and 4%, respectively, for a total of 12%. But he does receive a federal tax deduction for every dollar paid in state and local income tax. Now, perform the following mathematical calculations:

1. Multiple 41% times 12%, to obtain 4.92% or his effective tax savings.
2. Subtract 4.92% from 12% to obtain 7.08%, which is his effective additional cost for state and local taxes.
3. Add the 7.08% (state and local) to 41% (federal) to obtain his true effective tax bracket of about 48%.

The point of running the numbers is not precision but simply the realization that in a nearly effective tax bracket of almost 50%, the true economic benefit of every $1000 of annual investment interest or dividends, is only about $500, after tax.

PERSONAL AND DEPENDENCY EXEMPTIONS

Each personal or dependency exemption you claim reduces TI by $3900.

For estates, simple trusts, and complex trusts, this is $600, $300, and $100, respectively.

You can claim an exemption for yourself, your spouse, and each of your dependents.

Higher-earning medical professionals lose some or all exemptions according to a phase-out schedule where personal exemptions are reduced by 2% (4% for married filing separately) for each $2500 of AGI over $267,200 for joint returns, $222,700 for heads of households, $178,150 for single taxpayers, and over $133,600 for married filing separately.

For example, Dr. Joe Miller, a DO surgeon and joint filer, with an AGI of more than $389,700 ($122,500 above the joint threshold) will lose 100% of the personal exemption.

STANDARD DEDUCTION

Married filing jointly and surviving spouses	$12,200
Single taxpayers	$6100
Heads of households	$8950
Married filing separately	$6100
Dependents who file	$1000

Medical professionals who are blind or aged 65 and older may obtain an additional standard deduction of $1200 if married (whether filing jointly or separately), or $1500 if single or head of household! If a healthcare worker is both over 65 and blind, double these amounts.

WHO HAS TO FILE

Married, filing jointly, both under 65	$20,000
Married, filing jointly, one spouse 65 or older	$21,200
Married, filing jointly, both 65 or older	$22,400
Married, filing separately	$3900
Qualifying widow(er) with dependent child	$16,100
Qualifying widow(er) with dependent child 65 or older	$17,300
Head of household, under 65	$12,850
Head of household, 65 or older	$14,350
Single taxpayers, under 65	$10,000
Single taxpayers, 65 or older	$11,500

Remember, the above, as well as certain other thresholds and limits, are indexed for inflation each year. The above amounts relate to tax year 2013 filings.

TAXPAYER RELIEF ACT OF 1997

The current tax code includes more than 2.8 million words. The Taxpayer Relief Act of 1997 (The "Act") was 2 inches thick and added another 3000 pages of material to the subject. The following significant changes are highlighted below.

CAPITAL GAINS AND LOSSES

First, you must understand tax basis. When a medical professional reports capital gains, the taxable gain is the amount received minus the basis, or cost for tax purposes. When cash has been received (constructive receipt), the gain is said to be *recognized*. Gain is said to be *realized* when a transaction has taken place but cash has not yet been received. Gain is said to be *unrealized* when a transaction has not yet taken place, for example, when the gain exists in an investment portfolio only on paper.

The Act created a large amount of confusion regarding the holding period to be considered a long-term capital gain and the applicable capital gains tax rate. Much of this confusion is now gone since the transition period has passed. The rules are now more clear-cut. When a taxpayer sells an asset held less than 12 months, the gain is short term and is taxed as ordinary income (the same rate the taxpayer would pay on wages or interest and dividends). Assets sold after being held more than 12 months will generate long-term capital gains (or losses). Long-term capital gains are taxed at 10% if the taxpayer is in the 15% bracket, and at 20% if the taxpayer is in any higher tax bracket. For real estate that has been depreciated, the tax rate on the gain up to the amount of depreciation taken is 25%, with the remainder taxed at 20%. Collectibles (art, coins, jewels, etc.) are yet a different story being taxed at 15% or 28%, depending upon whether the taxpayer's tax bracket is 15% or higher.

Now, there are several strategies that can be adopted to utilize capital gains and losses. The obvious strategy is to periodically review any investment portfolio and cull the securities that are down without hope of a quick turnaround. These losses can be used to offset gains taken during the period. The main disadvantage to this strategy is that the taxpayer does not get the maximum bang for the deduction buck by eliminating a gain at 20% tax rate. The alternative is to plan to use capital losses to offset short-term capital gains and in years when there are no long-term capital gains. Recall that the maximum *net* capital loss, after offsets and deductions each year, is limited to $3000, so this strategy has its limitations.

New as of 2013 we have added NIIT. If you have both net investment income and MAGI of at least $200,000 for an individual taxpayer and $250,000 for taxpayers filing as married, an additional 3.8% of the net investment income is an added tax.

SALE OF A PERSONAL RESIDENCE

For many medical professionals, a home is their largest asset. In addition, it is their largest tax shelter as well. Certain costs of the purchase and ownership of the home are deductible expenses if the taxpayer itemizes (i.e., interest with total loan balance not to exceed one million dollars, interest on home equity loan interest up to $100,000, and property taxes). The law regarding the sale of a personal residence changed in mid-1997. This change in the tax law has been one of the most overlooked by all taxpayers. The new law states that the first $250,000 ($500,000 for married taxpayers filing jointly) of gain from the sale of a residence will be free of federal income tax. To qualify for this exclusion, the medical professional taxpayer must have owned the residence and occupied it for at least two of the last five years prior to the sale. In addition, if the taxpayer does not meet the above requirement due to change in employment, health or various other reasons, s/he may receive an "exclusion" for a portion of the above amount. An added bonus is that the taxpayer may take advantage of this same exclusion again after a two-year waiting period.

Compared to the old law where a taxpayer had to "buy up" into a higher priced home in order to defer the gain on the sale of the old residence, this is a huge benefit. For healthcare professionals, this is an especially fortuitous change in the law. Depending on the state you reside in, a residence is for the most part creditor proof; this tends to be one of the investments that is maximized. The potential to reap rather large tax-free treatment is something to keep in mind.

SMALL BUSINESS STOCK

If you own a qualified small business stock (stock in a corporation capitalized with $1 million or less), you may exclude from income 50% of any capital gain realized from the sale or exchange of the stock, provided you have held the shares for more than 5 years. The remaining gain is taxed at a top rate of 28%. You may also elect to roll over a gain from the sale or exchange of a small business held for more than 6 months by investing in other qualified small business stock, within 60 days of the sale of the original stock.

ESTIMATED TAX RULES

The IRS wants income taxes throughout the year; the system is often described as a "pay as you earn." Most employees pay the required estimated income taxes throughout the year via withholding as wages are paid. Estimated tax is the method used to pay tax on income that is not subject to withholding. Self-employed individuals or independent contractors are required to make estimated tax payments to the IRS each quarter. Otherwise, the IRS may assess a penalty for failure to timely pay taxes throughout the year. The IRS looks at each quarter independently to determine whether a penalty applies. Hence, you can't "catch-up" in later quarters to avoid the penalty.

Penalties can be avoided by basing estimated tax payments on

- 90% of the current's year's tax
- 100% of the prior year's tax (unless AGI is over $150,000)

However, when a taxpayer's AGI for a prior year exceeds $150,000 ($75,000 for married filing separately), the safe harbor percentage will either be 90% of current's year's tax or 110% of the tax shown on the prior taxable year.

Penalties

The following penalties apply to all the U.S. taxpayers:

1. Failure to file return: 5% per month (maximum 25%)
2. Accuracy-related penalties: 20% of underpayment attributable to the following:
   Negligence
   Substantial understatement: greater of 10% of tax or $5000
3. Civil tax fraud: 75% of underpayment with burden of proof on the IRS

Deductions

Paying a deductible expense is less costly than paying a nondeductible expense since, in a 31% tax bracket, for example, a $1000 deductible expense will only cost the medical professional $690.

Taxpayers with an AGI over $300,000 ($150,000 for married filing separately) must also reduce their itemized deductions by 3% of the excess over the threshold amount, up to a maximum of an 80% reduction. Deductions for medical expenses, investment interest, casualty, and the like are exempt from the reduction.[*]

For example, Dr. Goodyear, a surgeon with married filing joint AGI of $400,000 ($100,000 over the threshold) would have to reduce her itemized deductions by $3000, unless that amounts to more than an 80% reduction. These reductions have the practical effect of increasing the top tax rate for high-income taxpayers by several percentage points. The amounts are adjusted each year for inflation.

Home Equity Loans

This vehicle allows the healthcare professional to take advantage of the equity in his or her home (personal or second residence) to obtain an interest deduction on items that may otherwise not be deductible. There are certain restrictions in general, such as the total amount cannot exceed $100,000 ($50,000 for married taxpayers filing separately) and not exceeding the fair market value of the residences. However, especially for healthcare professionals, there are hidden traps to be considered. Depending on the state you reside in, a residence is for the most part creditor proof; it is one place that the healthcare professional can invest in without the fear of losing the asset in a malpractice action. Utilizing the residence as collateral on another loan can place an unnecessary risk on one of the only safe harbors the healthcare professional has available. Use home equity loans with great care.

Business Automobiles

A medical professional can claim deductions on business-related use of an automobile, using either the standard mileage rate methods or the actual expense method. The standard mileage rate for operating your passenger car is 56.5 cents per mile in the year 2013. If the former method is used, you may separately deduct business parking fees and tolls, the business portion of state and local personal property taxes, and the business portion of auto loan interest.

If you own and operate only one business vehicle, you should choose the method that yields the greatest deduction. However, once you've claimed accelerated depreciation for a business car in prior years under the expense method, you cannot switch to the standard mileage rate method for

---

[*] See the site www.forbes.com/sites/greatspeculations/2013/01/09/pease-limitation-puts-a-lid-on-itemized-deductions-for-wealthy-folks/.

that car in a subsequent year. The IRS now allows use of the standard mileage rate for a lease business automobile.

MEALS AND ENTERTAINMENT

The IRS allows only 50% of meals and entertainment expenses to be deducted for federal income tax purposes. The other 50% is considered a permanent difference that increases TI.

However, like most expenses, if done right, medical professionals can deduct part of their dining and entertainment costs. This can occur if bona fide business discussions occur directly preceding or following the dinner or entertainment. Be ready to justify the motivation for entertainment was business in nature, and not purely social.

For example, Dr. Simon Smith meets with business associates during the day. In the evening, he entertains the group and their spouses at a restaurant and then a theater production. Even though the purpose of the entertainment is goodwill, the expenses are still partially deductible (50%). Further, the IRS concedes that it may be appropriate for a medical professional's spouse to assist in entertaining a business associate also accompanied by a spouse. Meals of the medical professional while entertaining away from home on a business trip would be deductible at 50%.

Whether you structure business trips around vacations, or vacations around business trips, the IRS allows for some rest and relaxation. The entire airfare to a business location outside of the United States is deductible if the entire trip took less than a week. A deduction is also allowed even if the trip lasts longer than a week provided less than 25% of the time was spent on personal activities. If you cannot comply with these regulations, then only a pro rata portion of the airfare is deductible. A few modifications to a planned business and vacation trip can qualify much of the expenses for a business deduction. Generally, any temporary overnight business trip made away from home, which is primarily for business purposes, entitles the medical professional for a full deduction of the transportation costs incurred, even if a portion of the trip involves leisure time activities. You must keep good records of the date, destination, purpose, and amounts spent on each trip.

Tax Planning Tip
Since medical professionals can benefit from the flexibility of deducting entertainment expenses, take care to ensure that proper documentation is completed. Valid documentation should include the name(s) of person(s) entertained, amount, time, place, and business purpose involved. Expenses must be "directly related" or "associated with" the active conduct of the taxpayer's trade or business. In general, "directly related" usually refers to the context of active business discussions, or a clear business setting for such discussions. On the other hand, "associated with" refers to expenses incurred for the purposes of building goodwill, following or preceding business meetings or discussions. In each case, only the portion of the expenses "directly related" or "associated with" the medical professional's trade or business is deductible. Strict scrutiny is exercised by the IRS where the medical professional exhibits a pattern of abusive or undocumented entertainment. Although you do not have to prove income or other benefit from the entertainment, it would help to substantiate the business purpose.

Caution!
The Internal Revenue Code states that where no distinction can be made between the commingling of expenses that are fully deductible with those that are only partially deductible, all expenses within that category will be considered only partially deductible. The bottom line here is that each entity should segregate its meals and entertainment expenses from other expenses.

Tax Planning Tip
You do not have to save receipts or paid bills to substantiate travel expenses less than $75 unless the expenditure is for lodging! You must retain proper documentation of all your lodging expenditures, regardless of the amount.

Simple Charitable Giving

For the healthcare professional wanting to include charitable giving in a tax strategy, the contribution of securities with large gains can generate a double benefit. By giving the security (i.e., stock, bond, etc.) directly to the charity, the healthcare taxpayer can obtain a tax deduction for the fair market value of the stock without having to pick up the capital gain into income.

Although people say they give from the heart and not for tax reasons, a recent Gallup survey[*] showed that people who itemize their deductions gave an average of $1277, or 2.1% of household income last year. Those who didn't claim the tax benefit averaged $367, or 1.1% of income.

Tax Planning Tip

If giving to a charity this year is desired, but no cash is available at year end, put the contribution on a credit card. A pledge is not enough to get a deduction but the credit card contribution will qualify for a current year gift, even though the credit card bill is paid in the next year.

Complex Charitable Giving

Charitable remainder trusts and charitable lead trusts are two areas used in long-term planning strategies. With a charitable remainder trust, the donor gets the income from the economic value of the property given and upon the donor's death, the remainder goes to charity.

For example, Dr. Duke gives $100,000 in zero coupon bonds (the bonds pay no interest and are sold at a discount) to his favorite charity through a charitable remainder trust. He bought the bonds for $32,000 (a steep discount) and they are now worth $150,000. The bonds are then sold inside the trust and reinvested in a stock portfolio paying a handsome dividend. Dr. Duke gets the income from this portfolio during his life, along with a deduction for the present value of the remainder (the value of the trust at the end of the trust agreement with the charity), and the charity gets the assets upon the death of Dr. Duke.

A charitable lead trust works on the opposite concept of the charitable remainder trust. Using the example from above, the charity would get the trust's income, Dr. Duke would get a deduction for the present value of the trust's income and Dr. Duke's heirs get the remainder at the end of the term of the trust's agreement with the charity.

Charitable trusts are supported by many organized charities that have programs available where they can provide all of the details necessary for setting up the trust.[†]

Education Student Loan Interest

Up to $2500 of interest paid on qualified higher education is potentially deductible. However, the student loan deductions begin to phase out for AGI incomes above $155,000 on a joint return, and $75,000 for singles.

For example, Joe, a radiology technician, had already made 5 months of timely payments on his college loan when he started graduate school to begin work on his MHA. No payments are required on the loan while he is in school, but when he graduates and resumes making payments, the interest he is required to pay for up to 55 months is potentially deductible.

Employer-Paid Educational Assistance

Now is a good time for healthcare workers to take advantage of any educational assistance offered by a hospital, MCO, HMO, ACO, or other employer. If certain requirements are met, up to $5250 of employer-paid assistance is excluded from taxable wages.

---

[*] Gallup, A: *The Gallup Poll Cumulative Index*. Gallup Press, Princeton, NJ, 2000, or see www.gallup.com.

[†] Vanguard Charitable Endowment Program (888-383-4483) and Fidelity Investments' Charitable Gift Fund (800-682-4438).

State and Local Taxes

When looking at your individual tax picture for the year, special care should be given to state and local taxes. A traditional strategy (if a taxpayer is itemizing deductions) would be to make sure all of these taxes are paid by year end. This allows them to be deducted in the current year's federal income tax return. The alternative is to pay them early in the succeeding year and then wait another whole year before being able to take the deduction. If income is expected to go up significantly in the next year and put the taxpayer in a higher tax bracket, then he or she may want to hold off because that deduction will be worth more on the next year's tax return. Also, if the taxpayer is barely able to exceed the standard deduction in the current year, including the taxes, he or she should pay these taxes in the beginning of the year and pay next year's taxes before the end of next year. This "bunching" of deductions will allow for a higher amount of itemized deductions to be taken next year. Note that if you are subject to the AMT, these prepayments do not help.

One of the impacts from the fiscal cliff legislation to be felt by high-income earners is the reintroduction of the Pease limitation (Donald J. Pease, Ohio congressman), that reduces the amount of itemized deductions that certain taxpayers are allowed.

For the higher-income medical professional, you must reduce your itemized deductions by 3% of the excess amount over a threshold. The limitation for 2013 will kick in on AGI levels that exceed $300,000 for joint filers and $250,000 for individuals, indexed for inflation. Income over the applicable amount will trigger an itemized deduction limitation that is the lesser of

a. 3% of the AGI above the applicable amount
b. 80% of the amount of the itemized deductions otherwise allowable for the taxable year

EXAMPLE 9.1

Assume a married couple has an AGI of $670,000 and the 2013 applicable amount is $300,000. The couple's itemized deductions come to a total of $45,000 and they are broken down as follows:

- Mortgage interest deduction—$5000
- Property tax deduction—$5000
- State income tax deduction—$20,000
- Charitable deduction—$15,000

Based on the fact pattern and the calculation methods listed above for limiting the itemized deductions, option (a) would result in a $11,100 reduction of the couple's itemized deductions, while option (b) would reduce the couple's itemized deductions by $36,000:

a. 3% × $370,000 ($670,000–$300,000) would reduce the couple's itemized deductions by *$11,100*.
b. 80% × $45,000 would reduce the couple's itemized deductions by *$36,000*.

Since option (a)'s 11,100 reduction is the lesser of the two limitations, the couple's itemized deductions would *only* be reduced by 25%, taking their total itemized deductions of $45,000 down to $33,900 ($45,000–$11,100).

Tax Planning Tip
While there aren't many practical roads that high-income earners can take to avoid the Pease limitation in 2013 and beyond, the following can help reduce the impact:

a. Lower "above-the-line" income through contributions to retirement plans or health savings accounts.

b. Refinance or pay down your mortgage to lower the "deductible" amount of interest.
c. Have your tax advisor do multiyear tax projections, so you can do a better job of spreading deductions over multiple years to minimize the impact.

FRINGE BENEFITS

Most healthcare employers offer some sort of benefit package to their employees (and themselves). These benefits are among the best tax planning areas for an employed individual taxpayer. Many of these benefits (i.e., health insurance, group term life insurance up to $50,000, disability insurance, retirement plan contributions, etc.) create a tax deduction for the employer and are not included in the TI of the taxpayer. This is a win–win for both employer and employee, and one of the few areas within the Internal Revenue Code where the taxpayer benefits without having to pick up income. Even where an employee contribution or salary reduction is required, as is the case within a "cafeteria plan" (CP) (so called because there is a "menu" of employee benefits available for participation on an individual choice basis via salary reduction) or "flexible spending account" (FSA), it is typically made on a pretax basis (e.g., 401(k) contribution, dependent care, unreimbursed medical expenses, and educational expenses). Therefore, these benefits should be maximized by the individual taxpayer wherever possible.

For example, Jane, an LPN, has a child in daycare at a cost of $75 per week and estimates that she and her daughter will have a total of $600 of either uncovered or unreimbursed medical expenses during the year. Under her employer's CP, Jane elects to have a salary reduction of $4350. This amount will cover 50 weeks of daycare at $75/week and the $600 estimate of unreimbursed medical expenses. It is deducted evenly from her gross wages. When she incurs an expense for either daycare or out-of-pocket medical expenses, she turns the receipt in to her employer and is given reimbursement for that expense. The effect is to pay for these benefits with pretax dollars. The benefit to the employee is that the amount of salary reduction is not included in TI; therefore, Jane saves the income tax on the $4350.

Tip: Opt for Flexible Spending Accounts

One way to put aside pretax dollars for certain expenses is an FSA. The two most common FSAs are health FSAs, which can be used for qualified medical expenses, and dependent-care FSAs, used for qualified child-care and elder-care costs. As an example for dependent-care FSAs, a speech pathologist making $60,000 with a 30% tax rate could see $1500 in tax savings in just 1 year by contributing the annual maximum of $5000. One thing to keep in mind is that dependent-care FSAs can't be rolled over at the end of the year. But a recent change in the rules on health FSAs allows contributors to carry over up to $500 at the end of any given plan year.[*]

Caution!

Care should be used when estimating these costs since any amounts not used will be forfeited. Also, it is difficult to discontinue participation in the CP during the year once the election to participate in the plan has been made.

Tax Planning Tip

Estimate the amount to reduce salary by only those costs certain to be incurred. For instance, if Jane's child will be in daycare, these costs should be included. In addition, if the child has braces that will be on all year, including the monthly orthodontic fees would be reasonable. However, do not include laser vision correction costs that might happen at the end of the year. Include this procedure's cost when it becomes a certainty, rather than risking several thousand dollars on the possibility that it might get done this year.

---

[*] Source: WageWorks.com.

For the small employer, the rule of thumb on providing a CP or FSA is that the plan pays for itself at employee participation of about 10 employees. Before that amount of participation, the amount of employment tax savings will not cover the cost of annual administration and tax preparation costs.

Tax Planning Tip
In years of a large AGI, consider postponing itemized deductions that have a deductible floor, such as medical and miscellaneous expenses, until the next tax year. Likewise, a taxpayer can accelerate deductions and/or defer revenue-generating transactions (should a taxpayer have such control) until early the following year if it will reduce the overall income tax impact.

HOME OFFICE

A taxpayer's business use of his or her home may give rise to a deduction for the business portion of expenses related to operating the home. The basic requirements are

1. There must be a specific room or area that is set aside for and used exclusively on a regular basis as
   a. The principal place of any business, or
   b. A place where the taxpayer meets with patients, clients, or customers in the normal course of their trade or business, or
   c. A separate structure that is used in the taxpayer's trade or business and is not attached to their house or residence
2. An employee can take a home office deduction if he or she meets the regular and exclusive use test and the use is for the convenience of the employer.

Deductable expenses include business portions of mortgage interest, property taxes, depreciation, repairs, and maintenance to the overall home that help the business use area, janitorial services or maid, utilities, insurance, as well as other expenses directly related to the operating the remainder of the home.

Safe Harbor

The self-employed get something of a break in 2014: There is an option to claim a new, simplified deduction for a home office. The deduction is equal to $5/square foot of home office space—up to a maximum of 300 square feet ($1500). It's an easy calculation ($5 × the number of square feet) and beats figuring out your own expenses and pro-rating them though that's still an option if that works out better for you. The per-square-foot calculation is intended to save hours more than dollars. The deduction made its first appearance in 2013, but you can also take the deduction in 2014.

Tax Planning Tip
When a home office deduction is claimed on a pro-rated basis, it is important to make careful calculations and be prepared to back them up in the event of an IRS tax audit. Drawing up a floor plan that clearly documents the square footage used for personal and business purposes is a good idea. Alternatively, rooms used for business divided by total rooms in the house can be used to calculate the business use percentage. The taxpayer can choose the method that generates the largest business percentage. Then, apply office deductions based on the chosen percentage. Overstating the claim about which portions of the home you're using for business can easily backfire. So, do not try to claim shared spaces like bathrooms or kitchens. Taking several photographs of your file cabinets or the room strictly reserved for your business purposes will further support your case for the home office deductions.

Caution!

One reason the IRS has eased the business use of home standard is to turn an otherwise tax-free gain, generated by the sale of a personal residence, into at least a partially taxable transaction. The portion of a residence claimed as business property by the homeowner is viewed as business property by the IRS and not as a residence. As a result when the home is sold, the business use portion does not qualify for the $250,000 ($500,000 for married taxpayers filing jointly) exclusion of gain and will be subject to federal income tax. The question becomes, "Is the annual office in home deduction worth more than the eventual TI generated from the sale of the 'business' portion of the home?"

COMPUTERS

To qualify for a deduction when you purchase a computer to use for business purposes while at home, healthcare employees must pass a two-pronged test. First, the computer must be a "condition of employment," which means it must be essential to properly perform your job. Second, the computer must be for the convenience of the employer. These are very tough rules to overcome, according to Robert Trinz, an editor at the *RIA Group*, a publisher of tax guidelines for accountants and lawyers in New York (personal communication).

HOBBY DEDUCTIONS

If you have a sideline business, like selling vitamins, telecommunication cards, magnets, and the like, you may need to take some year-end steps to ensure the IRS treats your sideline like a real business and not just a hobby. If deemed a hobby, you'll be able to deduct expenses only to the extent of income from your sideline job. In order to write off more of your business expenses, you will need to demonstrate that your sideline is a profit-motivated enterprise and not just a pleasurable coincident to your healthcare profession.

Tax Planning Tip

The best way to achieve this goal is to be profitable. The IRS will presume your sideline is a business and not a hobby if you show a profit in three of five consecutive years (two of seven for horse racing). If you cannot make a profit, you can still convince the IRS by offering evidence that you are operating the entity like a real business and attempting to make a profit.

INVESTMENT TAXATION

CAPITAL LOSSES

Short- and long-term capital gains and losses must be offset against one another to produce a net short- or long-term figure. Net capital losses in excess of gains are fully deductible, dollar for dollar, against ordinary income, up to a $3000 annual limitation. Any excess capital losses may be carried forward indefinitely.

Tax Planning Tip

Capital losses on securities can offset capital gains on other passive investments, such as art or real estate. Capital gains and losses from all passive investments can be combined in figuring net capital gains and losses. Publicly traded securities are reported in the year the trade occurs, even if settled in the following year.

Zero Coupon Bonds

Although no cash is received on zero coupon bonds, a portion of the original issue discount (OID) must be reported each year as taxable (phantom) interest. This accretion increases the medical professional's cost basis. Of course no tax is due if held in a tax-deferred account.

Tax-Exempt Bonds

A tax-exempt bond bought at a premium must be amortized over the life of the bond or to the earliest call date. The premium cannot be deducted because it is an expense of earning tax-exempt income. The basis of the tax-exempt bond is reduced by the amount of the premium attributable to the period for which the bond is held. If the bond is held to maturity, no capital loss results from the purchase of a tax-exempt bond at a premium.

Stock Splits

When a medical professional receives additional shares as the result of a stock split, cash paid in lieu of the fractional shares is treated as if received from the sale of the fractional shares and reportable as a capital gain.

Wash Sale Rule

The wash sale rule applies when a medical professional sells a security at a loss and repurchases securities substantially identical to those sold within 61 days, beginning 30 days before the sale and ending 30 days after the sale. A deduction is denied for losses realized under these circumstances. Instead, the disallowed loss is added to the basis of the substantially identical securities acquired. The holding period of the securities sold at a loss is added to the holding period of the newly acquired security.

A wash sale may be avoided by purchasing the replacement security outside of 30 days. Alternatively, the medical professional investor could reinvest in securities that are not substantially identical, such as those in another company in the same industry.

Short Sales

The taxable event of a short sale (a sale of securities not currently owned by a taxpayer) occurs when the securities are delivered to the lender (brokerage firm) by the seller to close the short sale. Whether a capital gain or loss on a short sale is long term or short term depends on how long the seller held the stock that was used to close the short sale. These rules prevent the conversion of a short-term gain into a long-term gain or the conversion of a long-term loss into a short-term loss.

This "constructive sale rule" eliminates the deferral on the gain from "short sales against the box." Medical professionals must now recognize the gain when they enter into a short sale. The immediate recognition of gain can be avoided if the following occurs:

- The medical professional remains at risk for the loss on the identical security (long position) for at least 60 days after closing the short position.
- Identical securities are purchased in the open market to close (cover) the short sale on or before the 30th day of the following year.

WORTHLESS SECURITIES

To turn worthless securities into a tax write-off, you usually must sell or exchange the securities to establish a tax loss. However, you may be able to deduct the loss on worthless stocks or bonds, without a sale, if you can prove the securities became worthless during the taxable year. You can deduct the loss only in the year the security becomes completely worthless. Unfortunately, it is up to the medical professional to prove the securities have no value and became worthless in the year claimed.

VACATION HOMES

A vacation or second home can be a tax benefit if you are willing to rent it out. The tax benefit depends on how much you use the home. If rented for less than 15 days during the entire calendar year, then all rental income is tax free. However, you are only allowed to deduct the real estate taxes, mortgage interest, and any casualty losses. If you rent the home for 15 or more days throughout the year, then the rent must be included in your income. The offsetting benefit is that you can deduct maintenance and repairs. This analysis assumes that you use the home for vacation for no more than 14 days a year, or 10% of the rental days. This assumption is not harsh when you consider that a fix-up day does not count toward the 14 days, even if the family comes along.

NANNY TAX

Although not deductible for income tax purposes, the reporting of a nanny is required as part of the medical professional's individual tax return. The IRS has foreclosed all opportunity to call the nanny an independent contractor. If a nanny could be considered an independent contractor, then no payroll withholding taxes, in the form of social security, Medicare, and state and federal unemployment insurance premiums, would be required. Thus, as an employee, the nanny's wages are subject to payroll withholding taxes and reported on Schedule H of an individual tax return.

However, one opportunity exists for the medical professional that employs a nanny. Allocate some part of the nanny's day to helping your office practice. For example, relaying business faxes or phone messages received at home is a justifiable expense. The business-related responsibilities of the nanny can then be deducted as a business expense.

Note however that in most states converting even a portion of your nanny services from domestic employee to regular employee requires additional payroll insurances, namely, worker's compensation and disability insurance.

INVESTMENT INTEREST EXPENSE

Investment interest expense deductions are limited to net investment income, which is investment income (interest, dividends, and short-term capital gains) minus investment expenses. An exception is that such net capital gains may be included in net investment income, to the extent the medical professional elects to reduce the amount of net capital gains eligible for the 20% and 28% maximum capital gains tax rates. In the case of either a taxable or nontable bond, bought at a premium, the medical professional can either amortize or deduct the premium each year, with a corresponding reduction in cost basis, over the remaining life of the bond. Other complicated tax rules may also apply, depending on the specific year the bond was purchased.

Tax Planning Tip
Segregate consumer, business, and investment activities since, with the exception of home equity interest expense, the deductibility of interest depends on the use of the loan proceeds. For example, if securities are margined and the loan proceeds are used to purchase a new car, the margin interest is considered consumer interest and not investment interest. The IRS requires that the loan

proceeds be traceable to the actual use of funds. Therefore, be sure to trace credit transaction so that each can be allocated to the proper activity.

MUNICIPAL BOND MARGIN

Margin interest expense used to purchase municipal bonds or similar investments is not tax deductible. In addition, the IRS may infer a relationship between interest expense and the carrying of tax-exempt securities. A medical investor who borrows to finance a stock or bond portfolio, while owning tax-exempt bonds, may have an apportioned amount of the interest deduction disallowed. Similarly, interest expense is not deductible if loan proceeds are used to purchase or carry single premium insurance, or annuity contracts. Interest expense incurred to purchase other life insurance contracts are considered consumer interest expense, and not deductible.

MUTUAL FUNDS

The IRS allows four methods to determine cost, also known as the adjusted tax basis, for mutual funds:

1. FIFO (first-in, first-out): The holding period and cost for the first share sold is based on that of the first share purchased, and so on. The IRS assumes this method, if one of the other three is not specified, because more tax is collected in this manner.
2. LIFO (last-in, first-out): This is the opposite of FIFO and results in a lesser tax burden.
3. Specific identification: The cost basis of each specific share is tracked, and reported.
4. Average cost method: This is probably the most common method, as seen in the example below:

Average Cost Method Calculations for Mutual Fund Shares

(A medical investor makes three share purchases)

Transaction	Price	Shares	Total	Cumulative Cost
1/1/92 Purchase $2000	$20	100	100	$2000
6/1/93 Purchase $5000	$25	200	300	$7000
2/1/00 Purchase $10,000	$50	200	500	$17,000

LISTED STOCK OPTIONS

Writing stock options offers timing advantages for medical professionals because the premium becomes taxable only upon the close of the position by exercise, or a closing transaction. The premium income is considered a short-term capital gain if the option expires unexercised.

BROAD-BASED INDEX OPTIONS

Broad-based index options open at year end must be marked to the market, and unrealized capital gains and losses are taxed as if the position had been closed at year end. Under special rules, 60% of the capital gain or loss is treated long term, and 40% is treated as short term, regardless of the actual holding period.

LIKE-KIND EXCHANGES

An often ignored technique is a like-kind exchange. Whenever you sell business or investment property and you have a gain, you generally have to pay tax on the gain at the time of sale. IRC

Section 1031 provides an exception and allows you to postpone paying tax on the gain if you reinvest the proceeds in similar property as part of a qualifying like-kind exchange. Gain deferred in a like-kind exchange is tax-deferred, but it is not tax free. It is not available for securities or other types of assets.

INSTALLMENT SALE

Generally, an installment sale is the disposition of property where at least one loan payment is to be received after the close of the taxable year in which the disposition occurs. The installment method of accounting provides an exception to the general principles of income recognition by allowing a taxpayer to defer the inclusion of income of amounts that are to be received from the disposition of certain types of property until payment in cash or cash equivalents is received.

This tends to lower the overall tax paid on the gain by spreading the gain over the term of the note(s) to be collected as a result of the sale. The notes due you resulting from the sale usually carry attractive interest rates when comparing to bank interest rates and risk tends to be low since default simply yields you the property sold back to you.

If the liquidity from a sale of property is not required for you to make a pending investment, installment sales are great tools for tax savings and yielding higher than normal interest rates on your money.

REAL ESTATE

Generally, most healthcare professional's participation in real estate will be considered passive; losses from passive activities that exceed the income from passive activities are disallowed for the current year. Disallowed passive losses are carried forward to the next taxable year. A similar rule applies to credits from passive activities.

Passive activities include trade or business activities in which you do not "materially participate." You materially participate in an activity if you are involved in the operation of the activity on a regular, continuous, and substantial basis. In general, rental activities, including rental real estate activities, are always passive activities, even if you do materially participate.

However, rental real estate activities in which you materially participate are not passive activities if you qualify as a "real estate professional." Additionally, there is a limited exception for rental real estate activities in which you "actively participate." The rules for active participation are different from those for material participation.

Guidelines for determining material participation, the rules for a real estate professional, active participation, and the special rules that apply to the income and losses from a passive activity held through a publicly traded partnership (PTP) can be found in Internal Revenue Service Publication 925, *Passive Activity and At-Risk Rules*.

Generally, you may deduct in full any previously disallowed passive activity loss in the year you dispose of your entire interest in the activity. In contrast, you may not claim unused passive activity credits upon disposition of your entire interest in the activity. However, you may elect to increase the basis of the credit property in an amount equal to the portion of the unused credit that previously reduced the basis of the credit property.

Tax Planning Tip

Have a complete plan for your real estate holding that includes a sell date of the property. This enables you to view your investments from two perspectives:

1. A holding period rate of return (one in which usually no operating losses are permitted but deferred)

2. A disposition point of view (when you dispose of the interest and take advantage of your accumulated losses that release upon sale)

What makes this difficult in most cases? The exit date for sale of your investment is not always known. The taxing system is designed to provide benefits in the short term for material participation and for passive participation benefits in the disposal of the interest.

TAX CREDITS

CHILD TAX CREDIT

Healthcare workers can claim a $1000 tax credit for each qualifying child, who is a son or daughter, a stepson or stepdaughter, or an eligible foster child who is a dependent, is a U.S. citizen, and is under the age of 17.

For joint filers with AGI from $110,000–159,001, $75,000–$124,001 for singles or heads of households, and over $55,000–104,001 for married filing separately, the credit is reduced by $50 for every $1000, or fraction thereof, in excess of these limits.

LIFETIME LEARNING CREDIT

As its name implies, this tax credit is not restricted to the first 2 years of postsecondary education for the healthcare professional. Undergraduate, graduate, and professional degree courses can qualify. The maximum credit is $2000 per taxpayer return (20% of expenses up to $10,000), regardless of the number of students. The Lifetime Learning credit amount that a taxpayer may otherwise claim is phased out beginning at $53,000 ($107,000 for joint returns) MAGI and is eliminated at $63,000 ($127,000 for joint returns) MAGI in 2013.

If there is a choice between this credit and a Hope Scholarship it is better to choose the more generous Hope credit. It will not prevent you from also electing a lifetime earning credit for another eligible family member's expenses.

As an example, a married couple who are both LPNs, have a daughter who is a college freshman and a son who is a senior they can elect a Hope credit for their daughter and a lifetime learning credit for their son (assuming all other requirements are met).

NONBUSINESS ENERGY PROPERTY CREDIT

You may claim a credit of 10% of the cost of certain energy-saving property that you added to your main home. This includes the cost of qualified insulation, windows, doors, and roofs. In some cases, you may be able to claim the actual cost of certain qualified energy-efficient property. Each type of property has a different dollar limit. Examples include the cost of qualified water heaters and qualified heating and air-conditioning systems. This credit has a maximum lifetime limit of $500. You may only use $200 of this limit for windows and your main home must be located in the United States to qualify for the credit.

Not all energy-efficient improvements qualify, so be sure you have the manufacturer's credit certification statement. It is usually available on the manufacturer's website or with the product's packaging. The credit was to expire at the end of 2011. A recent law extended it for 2 years through the end of 2013.

RESIDENTIAL ENERGY-EFFICIENT PROPERTY CREDIT

This tax credit is 30% of the cost of alternative energy equipment that you installed on or in your home. Qualified equipment includes solar hot water heaters, solar electric equipment, and wind turbines.

There is no limit on the amount of credit available for most types of property. If your credit is more than the tax you owe, you can carry forward the unused portion of this credit to next year's tax return. You must install qualifying equipment in connection with your home located in the United States and it does not have to be your main home. The credit is available through 2016.

DO IT YOURSELF, ELECTRONIC, OR PROFESSIONAL PREPARATION

Online filing of your own income taxes is quicker, easier, and cheaper than ever before; however, owing to the complex nature of most physicians' returns, it is not a perfect system. While working to create a draft of your income tax return and being involved with the preparation process is educational, self-preparing without professional review can create compliance problems due to lack of familiarity with the timing and content of forms that are required.

The Internal Revenue Service audits returns based on your return presentation as it relates to others in your given industry sector, relationship of particular expenses to your income, and for incompleteness. An experienced professional review will help insure accuracy, reasonableness, and completeness as well as highlight tax financial planning opportunities.

ALTERNATIVE MINIMUM TAX

The aim of a tax planning strategy for the healthcare professional is to generate the lowest possible tax within each taxpayer's unique set of circumstances. However, as noted earlier, Uncle Sam has a "safety net" to make sure that every taxpayer pays some tax and does not take advantage of the government by overutilizing the tax loopholes available. This safety net is called the AMT. This is a separate tax calculation based upon regular TI and adding back certain itemized deductions plus certain other tax deductions claimed in a year to see if the taxpayer has received too much benefit from these items, which include tax exempt interest from private activity bonds, issued after 8/7/86, bargain element in incentive stock options, and certain other accelerated depreciation items. No AMT deductions are available for personal exemptions, state and local income, personal property and real estate tax payments, medical expenses not exceeding 10% of AGI, and miscellaneous expenses subject to the 2% of AGI floor.

This calculation generates AMT income. This AMT income number has its own tax rate and, if the tax derived from this calculation is higher than the regular tax rate, the taxpayer pays according to the AMT calculation. Unlike the ordinary tax rates, the AMT has only two tax brackets of 26% and 28%. AMT income consists of AGI, plus the preference income, minus certain itemized deductions, and an exemption based on the filing status for 2013 are as follows:

- Married, filing jointly, surviving spouses: $80,800
- Single taxpayers, heads of household: $51,900
- Married filing separately, trusts, estates: $40,400

The individual medical professional must pay the higher of the minimum tax or the income tax computed in the regular fashion.

For 2013, the exemption amount is completely phased out if AMT TI exceeds $477,100 for joint return filers, $323,000 for single tax payers and heads of households, and $229,550 for married professionals filing separately.

Tax Planning Tip
Medical professionals are increasingly becoming targets of the AMT and should try to incur as much ordinary income as possible until they reach a crossover point where their regular tax liability equals their AMT liability. Recall that each dollar subject to the AMT is taxed at either at 26% or 28%, both of which are lower than the current top three regular tax rates (31%, 36%, and 39.6%).

Therefore, try to accelerate ordinary income by

- Converting municipal bond (tax exempt) investments into taxable investments
- Redeeming CDs, Treasury paper, and Series E or Series EE bonds to generate interest income
- Considering the withdrawal of money from IRAs, if not subject to the 10% or other penalties
- Exercising nonqualified stock options, since their bargain element is taxed as ordinary income at the time of exercise
- Exercising incentive stock options and selling option stock in the same calendar year to recognize additional ordinary income and eliminate a like amount of tax preference

Additionally, the medical professional should try to defer certain deductions that reduce regular taxes, but do not reduce the AMT. These tactics and tips include

- Postponing miscellaneous deductions, when possible, to the following tax year
- Limiting estimated payment of state and/or local income taxes in the current year to an amount sufficient to avoid penalties

Obviously, the idea is to avoid the AMT if possible. The additional tax from this calculation mitigates the work involved in planning for the lowest liability possible. This tax is calculated on Form 6251 and is becoming much more common as the difference between regular tax rates and the AMT rates get closer together.

Medical professionals may take a credit against their regular tax for any AMT paid in prior years, but they may not be used to reduce the AMT tax liability. The credit is limited to the portion of the AMT attributable to items that defer, rather than cause a permanent exclusion of income, such as items of accelerated depreciation.

TAX "GAP"

The tax gap is the difference between true tax liability in any year and the amount of tax that is paid voluntarily and on time; this gap amounted to an estimated $450 billion in tax year 2006. Underreporting accounted for an estimated $376 billion, while underpayment and nonfiling amounted to $46 billion and $28 billion, respectively. Considering the total tax liability was $2.66 trillion, the compliance rate was only 83.1% (or a net rate of 85.5%). Whether noncompliance is due to ignorance or fraudulent intent, you can bet that Uncle Sam wants his piece of your hard-earned pie.

TAX PLANNING TIP: ON ELECTRONIC HEALTH RECORDS

The following is taken from the CMS website:

Q: Are payments from the Medicare and Medicaid Electronic Health Record (EHR) Incentive Programs subject to federal income tax?

A: Nothing in the Act excludes "meaningful use" payments from taxation or as tax-free income. Therefore, incentive payments are treated like any other income *in other words* (*IOW*): EHR incentives are considered "gross income" to an "eligible medical provider."

IRS AUDIT STATISTICS

The chance of receiving a tax audit generally changes based upon income level and filing type. Below are IRS statistics that are broken down by individual, income level, and business type. These are the overall numbers provided by the IRS, but realize that there are many factors that go into determining if the IRS is going to audit. IRS audits are rarely random and can be avoided by understanding how the IRS audit process works and what the common red flags are for an audit.

Total Amount of IRS Audits on Individual Tax Returns

	FY 2009	FY 2010	FY 2011
Total returns filed prior CY	138,949,670	142,823,105	140,837,499
Total audits conducted	1,425,888	1,581,394	1,564,690
Percentage audited	1.03%	1.11%	1.11%

IRS Audit Rates by Income Level for Individuals (2009)

	Percentage of Total Returns Filed (%)	Percentage of Returns Audited (%)
No adjusted gross income	2.13	2.15
$1–$24,999	40.51	0.90
$25,000–$49,999	24.31	0.72
$50,000–$74,999	13.44	0.69
$75,000–$99,999	7.99	0.69
$100,000–$199,999	8.69	0.98
$200,000–$499,999	2.25	1.92
$500,000–$999,999	0.43	2.98
$1,000,000–$4,999,999	0.23	4.02
$5,000,000–$9,999,999	0.02	6.47
$10,000,000+	0.01	9.77

IRS Audit Rates/Statistics by Tax Filing Type FY 2011

	Returns Filed (Prior Calendar Year)	Returns Audited	Percentage Audited
Small corporation	1,931,008	19,697	1.02%
Large corporation	59,291	10,459	17.64%
Subchapter S	4,444,154	18,519	0.42%
Partnership	3,434,905	13,770	0.40%
Individual	140,837,499	1,564,690	1.11%

Overall, the odds that you are going to get picked for an audit is low each year. Generally speaking, the IRS does audit individuals with higher income because they only have limited resources to go after people and they get more "bang" for their buck going after the higher-income individuals. Higher-income individuals are also more likely to have things on their tax returns that create IRS red flags than individuals with lower income. Considering the fact that you file a tax return each year and have about a 1% chance each year, it is more likely than not that you will get audited at some point in your life.

PAPER OR ELECTRONIC TAX FILING?

Some CPAs suggest filing the old-school way if you're worried about an audit. Why? Paper filing means more work for the IRS to access all the information in your return. Other experts disagree as follows.

Philosophy in Favor of Paper Returns

Some suggest that a paper tax return might reduce your chance of an audit because the IRS must transcribe your information into a computer by hand. The IRS does not transfer all of the information in your return as a result of the prohibitive cost of transcribing returns. When you file a return electronically, a computer instantly analyzes your return for errors and discrepancies. *Source*: http://www.ehow.com/info_8488086_filing-increase-chances-irs-audit.html#ixzz2yh9m8pEy.

Philosophy in Favor of Electronic Returns

Filing an electronic tax return reduces the number of math mistakes on your return and the chance that the IRS makes a mistake when it transfers data by hand. Overall, electronic returns contain fewer errors than paper returns, which increase the chance of audits. Also, the IRS performs an automatic audit when its electronic scanning system cannot read your handwriting. *Source*: http://www.taxdebthelp.com/tax-problems/tax-audit/irs-audit-statistics#ixzz2yLVTp0l1.

Filing Extensions

No one knows for sure what triggers an audit. Yet, according to filelater.com, many financial professionals and accountants suspect the Internal Revenue Service has an "audit quota," which begins to fill around mid-April. Thus, if you file an extension, a large percent of the "audit quota" may be filled, making your chance of an audit less likely later than had you filed on time. Regardless of the quota, there's little evidence that filing an extension will increase the chance of being audited.

Nevertheless, tax pundits like Stephen Ohlemacher believe the chance of getting audited by the IRS is the lowest it has been in years because it has fewer agents auditing returns than at any time since the 1980s. Remember, your duty as a taxpayer is to be truthful and accurate, but you don't have to make it easy for the IRS. *Source:* http://news.msn.com/us/chances-of-getting-audited-by-irs-lowest-in-years.

ASSESSMENT

Most very busy medical professionals realize the importance of making their money grow through investment in business, the financial markets, and in real estate. Most are also aware that without a good understanding of how the tax systems affects these investments, their efforts to grow their money will not be fruitful, riddled with complexity and surprise tax bills.

Understanding some of the principles in this chapter are an important foundation, but the need is there to take time out to meet with tax professionals to understand your particular taxes and how they will affect your potential investments. Organizing your efforts in a material way will improve your effective tax rate and help your money work for you.

Be certain however that your efforts in business, the financial markets, and real estate will not be well received by the taxing authorizes if presented in an incomplete or unprofessional way. If you are starting a business, it should have the attributes of a business, a mission statement, business card, website, and separate phone number, and bank account, for example.

Therefore, your only defense is proper documentation. IRS agents are like most medical practices; a good image improves confidence. For example, an audit of your tax return is really an audit of your records. The benefit of the doubt will be given where information is well organized and easy to understand. All audits start with random verification of deductions. If the random testing raises suspicion, then full verification is inevitable. On the other hand, if the random test proves accurate, then a full verification is typically waived.

Another benefit to focusing on documentation is the risk of losing deductions. Many deductions are lost because of failure to remember the expenditures. For example, medical professionals can document and deduct all charitable contributions, even if receipts aren't available, as illustrated in the scenarios below:

- Donations to a church during a visit
- Mileage used during the year to transport Boy Scouts
- The portion of a fund-raising dinner expenses that benefit the charity
- Donations of personal property to charities   .

Note that substantial documentation is typically required for contributions of $250 or more. Substantiation does not include a canceled check, but does include a receipt from the organization.

Also, do not forget such deductible items as state taxes, property taxes, business-related phone bills, medical expenses not reimbursed by insurance to the extent they exceed 10% of AGI, and other miscellaneous deductions such as professional association dues, subscription renewals to investment and trade publications, uniforms and laundry, and tax preparation-related computer software. Unfortunately, healthcare employee business expenses may become harder to write off each year because these miscellaneous expenses are deductible only to the extent that they exceed 2% of AGI.

Finally, tax planning is a very personal task for the healthcare professional, and it is unique based upon the characteristics each one possesses. Do not be lulled into the follower syndrome. Just because a colleague in the lounge has used a tax planning strategy, do not assume that the same strategy will provide a similar benefit. A custom-fit suit always provides a better fit than an off-the-shelf item, and the same goes with tax planning. Review the unique facts and circumstances surrounding the subject of the tax planning and find those deductions, credits, and strategy that fit the best for your individual circumstances.

CONCLUSION

The objective of tax planning is to arrive at the lowest overall tax cost on the activities performed. And this chapter addressed methods and strategies to reduce federal and state income taxes.

COLLABORATE

Discuss this chapter online with others at www.MedicalExecutivePost.com.

ACKNOWLEDGMENTS

To Thomas P. McGuiness, CPA, CVA of Reimer, McGuinness & Associates, PC in Houston, Texas and Thomas Bucek, CPA, CVA in Houston, Texas; Dr. David Edward Marcinko, MBA, CMP™; and Richard S. Bryson, JD, Suwanee, Georgia.

FURTHER READING

Ernst & Young Tax Guide. Wiley, New York, 2014.
J.K. Lasser's *Your Income Tax 2014: For Preparing Your 2013 Tax Return*. Wiley, New York, 2014.
McGuinness, TP and Bucek, T: Income taxation. In Marcinko, DE (editor): *Financial Planning for Physicians*;
     JB Publishing, Sudbury, MA, 2004.
Piper, M: *Taxes Made Simple: Income Taxes Explained in 100 Pages or Less, Simple Subjects*. John Wiley & Sons,
     New York, 2014.
Westhem, A and Weissman, S: *Tax Smart Investing*. John Wiley & Sons, New York, 2012.

10 Basic Medical Office Tax Reduction Strategies

Executing Innovative Techniques

Perry D'Alessio

CONTENTS

The formulation and implementation of tax reduction strategies for the medical office shouldn't be an all-consuming activity. Medical professionals should concentrate on what they know and do the best, providing services to their patients. This is how they earn their living and should always be their primary focus. However, all physician executives can better their financial position by keeping more of the money they earn. This is one reason office tax planning should be an important part of each physician's short-term and long-term strategy.

INTRODUCTION

The objective of tax planning is to arrive at the lowest overall tax cost on the activities performed. This means pushing as much income as possible beyond Uncle Sam and into personal or business accounts to stay. Some have stated that income tax planning is like playing a game and those who best know the rules of the game "win." This section will address items to be aware of and methods and strategies to use to reduce federal and state income taxes. Winning is a relative term when dealing with income taxes. A healthcare professional doesn't have to force fit every tax planning tool available in order to win. Winning is achieved each time a tip or strategy is utilized to help reduce taxable income or increase a credit that can be taken to reduce taxes to be paid.

A former Commissioner of the Internal Revenue Service (IRS) once stated on national television that the IRS wanted each taxpayer to pay no more to the government than what he or she actually owed. The meaning was that each person or entity should take advantage of every deduction legally available in order to arrive at the lowest possible taxable income. For those in the healthcare professions, this is a most important concept since, for many, managed care has had an extremely negative effect on income. This being the general case, it is imperative to be frugal when dealing with Uncle Sam at tax time.

BUSINESS TAX PLANNING PROCESS

Organization

To ensure your entities success, breaking down the process that creates your year-end compliance and planning is necessary. Sourcing the components separately can help save fees, and lends itself to more timely information.

> *Bookkeeping*—This area is often underserved and at times improperly combined with year-end tax services. Bookkeeping should be performed on a perpetual basis; it provides clarity and timely management information to adjust your business. Current bookkeeping

software packages like QuickBooks® and Peachtree® provide an affordable and easy to use platform. The software allows users to participate in the bookkeeping process having only select access making the break down process easy so long as you take the time to design your bookkeeping effort to examine safeguarding and segregation of duties to help prohibit misappropriations.

If you outsource this function off premises, maintain control of this effort by utilizing cost effective online solutions to remotely access your computer where the accounting software resides. Having outside bookkeepers log in to perform regular bookkeeping services on your terminal ensures data is always with you as you need it and provides a time clock for your bookkeeping effort as they log in and out to perform work.

Payroll Processing and Human Resources—We are in an era of very active Department of Labor disputes and audits. Know that your employees are aware of the law and capitalize on it when inadequacies in payroll reporting or overtime rules are violated. These claims lien the business owners personally and are not dischargeable in bankruptcy. The claims awarded are devastating to a business, but easily avoided with basic know how and proper compliance.

Outsourcing to the larger payroll providers is a great way to get low-cost high value-added services. Be certain to take advantage of your ability to screen potential employees. This low cost effort can save you considerable in employee litigation and provide a more harmonious work environment.

Tax Planning and Tax Compliance Services—A reputable Certified Public Accountant (CPA) should be engaged to review the bookkeeping effort for appropriateness and perform year-end compliance. Having your efforts segregated as we discussed provides fast and timely information for tax planning and greatly reduces time to prepare year-end compliance.

Orderly, timely, and competent information lends itself to planning tax events, avoiding tax problems, and maximizing your legal tax deductions.

Tax Planning Tip

Set up one file at the beginning of the tax year to store all potential tax information. During the year, as tax-sensitive information is received from whatever source (i.e., receipts, paycheck stubs, charitable donation letters, stock purchase or sale information, etc.), put it in the "Tax File." At year-end, the tax-gathering process is already done. More importantly, as potential opportunities arise during the year, all of the pertinent tax information is already in one place for easy access and review of current tax status. This process can get much more detailed by segregating different types of tax information into separate files or setting up spreadsheets to track this information, but those additional processes are a matter of personal preference.

Information is the lifeblood of good decision-making. This is just as true in the tax planning process as it is in any healthcare practice. Consider the above tax file being analogous to the history and physical portion of the examination process. Every healthcare professional always wants it to be up-to-date in order to allow for good decision-making when the opportunity or need arises.

Tax Planning Tip

If you are concerned that you may not have saved all tax documents mailed to you, a comprehensive accumulation of your entities income tax reporting information can be obtained six to eight months after the tax year-end by calling the Internal Revenue Service and requesting a "wage and income summary" for your entity. This summary report provides a reference point to compare your information gathered to the Internal Revenue Service records to help ensure completeness of tax filings and will greatly reduce Internal Revenue Service correction letters.

A Quick Accounting Lesson

Although this may be boring, it is the one accounting lesson that will assist in making cash flow and tax planning decisions that can save untold dollars. There are two basic methods of accounting in healthcare practice entities: the cash basis and the accrual basis of accounting.

The Cash Basis of Accounting

First of all, most healthcare practices utilize the cash basis (or cash method) of accounting. The cash basis of accounting recognizes revenue when cash is received and recognizes expenses when they are paid. This is the easiest concept to grasp because, with few exceptions, the income or loss for a particular period can be roughly estimated by looking at the change in the practice's bank account from the beginning to the end of that period. The exceptions, to name a few, would include asset purchases and payments that are not deductible for tax purposes (i.e., penalties and fines, one half of entertainment expense, or principal payments on loans) and those items that are noncash in nature (i.e., depreciation and amortization expenses).

The terms "tax basis" or "income tax basis" of accounting may also be heard. These are the same thing and are basically the same as the cash basis with modifications that are allowed by tax law. For example, various retirement plan contributions are allowed to be deducted in the current year (typically at the entity's year-end) and paid in the following tax year, up to the due date of the entity's tax return plus any valid tax return extensions filed. The exception is that IRAs must be deposited by April 15 in order to be counted as a contribution for the prior year.

Cash Basis Revenue Example

A physician sees a patient in the office on December 1st and the charge for the visit is $75. The patient pays a $10 copay and two months later the patient's insurance carrier pays $40 of the accounts receivable balance and disallows the rest due to a contractual adjustment. The practice will recognize revenue of $50 (the $10 copay plus the $40 insurance payment), $10 in the current year and $40 in the subsequent year.

Cash Basis Expense Example

The telephone bill of $675 comes in on December 15 for this calendar year entity. If the bill is paid by December 31 it is an expense for the current year. If it is paid on January 1 or any time thereafter, it will be an expense of the next year and the entity will have to wait over a year to take advantage of that deduction.

The Accrual Basis of Accounting

The accrual basis of accounting states that income goes on the books when it is earned and expenses are booked when they are incurred.

Accrual Basis Revenue Example

Using the same facts as in the above example, under the accrual method of accounting, the entire $75 is recognized as income at the point the physician has performed "substantially all functions necessary to earn the revenue." In this example, that means once the physician has completed the examination of the patient.

This is very unappealing for several reasons. First, most patients do not pay the entire bill at the time of the visit. Therefore, the majority of the charge ($65) goes into the accounts receivable sub ledger. Second, if this is an insurance charge, most insurance carriers pay the charge based upon their usual, customary and "reasonable" fee schedule rather than the physician's fee schedule. For income tax purposes, the entire $75 is considered revenue for the physician when the patient has been seen. This creates a scenario where the physician is paying income tax on income that will never be realized.

Eventually, when the insurance carrier provides a correct explanation of benefits (EOB), the practice will be able to write off the remaining $25 ($75 charge less the $10 copay and $40 insurance payment) as an adjustment against revenue. However, cash flow will have been used to pay income tax on "phantom" revenue. In the real world there will always be timing differences between the time a service is provided and when payment is received. When a year-end falls in between the two events, the practice pays tax on the "paper income" represented in that timing difference.

Accrual Basis Expense Example

The physician or office manager orders influenza vaccine from the office's typical supplier. When the vaccine is delivered to the office, the practice has incurred the expense of that vaccine.

This part of the accrual basis of accounting is more appealing, as it acts as somewhat of an offset to the recognition of income per above. However, since most practices are "for profit" entities, it is hoped that there will be more revenue than expenses in the practice.

Bottom line, under accrual basis accounting, most healthcare practices will typically pay more money in both federal and state income taxes sooner than on the cash basis of accounting. In addition, the practice will probably pay somewhat more in accounting related costs for keeping up with an accrual basis set of books. The accounts payable sub ledger, the year-end search for accrued expenses and the potential of having to pay more for a staff person with a heavier accounting background are the factors that will generate the additional cost.

This is the extent of accounting knowledge needed in order to understand the effects of various tax planning strategies.

PRACTICE ENTITIES UTILIZED BY HEALTHCARE PROFESSIONALS

Healthcare professionals practice within many different legal structures and there are various differences in tax planning techniques depending upon how the entity or entities you practice within are structured. The various entities and types of returns that are filed for those entities are as follows:

Entity	Type of Return
Sole proprietor	Schedule C, Form 1040
C Corporation (Inc. or Corp.)	Form 1120
S Corporation (Inc, Corp., P.A. or P.C.)	Form 1120S
Professional Corporation (P.C.)	Form 1120, or 1120S
Professional Association (P.A.)	Form 1120, or 1120S
General Partnership	Form 1065
Limited Partnership	Form 1065
Limited Liability Partnership (L.L.P.)	Form 1065
Limited Liability Company (L.L.C.)	
More than one owner	Form 1065, Form 1120 or 1120S
One owner	Form 1040
Professional Limited Liability Company (P.L.L.C.)	Form 1065, Form 1120 or 1120S
Foundation Model	Form 990
Tax Exempt, Not for Profit Corp.	Form 990

Each state is responsible for enacting its own legal statutes on the organization of physician corporations. Therefore, if a practice entity is a corporation, it could be an Inc., Corp., P.A., or P.C., depending on the state in which the practice entity is organized. In addition, many states have enacted legislation to create limited liability entities that provide the liability protection afforded a corporation, while having the attributes of a partnership. These entities have become very popular with professional practices (physicians, lawyers, accountants, engineers, architects, etc.) because they allow more flexibility with regard to buy-ins and buyouts, and in the allocation of income and deductions. Since limited liability entities differ from state to state, the healthcare professional should seek out either an attorney or accountant familiar with the nuances of limited liability entities in the particular state. For federal income tax purposes these entities having more than one owner are viewed as partnerships unless an election is made to be treated as a corporation. The election is made on federal Form 8832 and is also known as a "check the box" election.

Corporations

Within the C Corporation status, there is a distinction between entities providing personal services and those that provide goods and services that are not personal in nature. A physician corporation (C Corporation) is considered to be what is called a "Personal Service Corporation" for federal income tax purposes. A personal service corporation pays federal income tax on every dollar of taxable income at a rate of 35%. All other C Corporations follow the progressive tax rate structure that taxes corporate income below $100,000 at lower tax rates (15% on the first $50,000 and 25% on the next $25,000 and 34% on the following $25,000). The IRS believed that professionals had too much ability to manipulate their year-end income and, therefore, the tax they paid. The IRS asked Congress to close this loophole. Congress created the Personal Service Corporation designation to remove this tax planning opportunity. This is now one of the disadvantages of being organized as a C Corporation for those providing personal services.

The difference between a C Corporation and an S Corporation is strictly a federal tax consideration. The S Corporation was created by Congress to allow small business corporations the flexibility of a partnership while retaining the limited liability advantages of the corporate structure. Therefore, for federal income tax purposes the S Corporation reports its income, deductions, expenses and credits to its shareholders more along the lines of a partnership. This is important to note since C Corporations are taxpaying entities, while, all of the other entities are generally considered to be tax reporting, or passthrough entities. S Corporation status is achieved by filing Form 2553 with the IRS either within 75 days of when the practice is incorporated or when business is actually started or within 75 days of the beginning of a corporation's fiscal year. This election can be made even if an entity has been a C Corporation for many years; however, there are potential tax traps (known as the "built-in gains" tax) in a C Corporation conversion to an S Corporation for those unaware of the law. This is an area where the assistance of a qualified tax professional would be well worthwhile since the tax cost of falling into the traps can be very significant.

Passthrough Entities and Favored Tax Status

Partnerships, S Corporations, and Limited Liability entities (LLPs or LLCs) are all generally considered to be passthrough entities. The term "passthrough" entity is based upon the way in which the tax attributes of the entity (e.g., income, expenses, deductions and credits) flow through to the owners and are taken into account in the owners' individual tax returns. This treatment allows the owner to avoid the potential of double taxation that exists in a C Corporation.

Sole Proprietors

A sole proprietor is an individual business owner whose business is accounted for on a separate schedule of the owner's individual income tax return. Typically, owners filing their business returns via the use of Schedule C of Form 1040 have the lowest level of reporting requirements and also (in general) do the poorest job of keeping good records of business activity. There is only one level of tax for the sole proprietor. The net profit (or loss) from the Schedule C business is reported on page one of Form 1040 and is combined with all of the other income items reported to arrive at gross income. Different from interest and dividend income, or investment income that is typically considered passive in nature, self-employment income is income considered to be generated by ones own actions. There is "Self Employment" tax to be paid on virtually all self-employment income reported in the tax return. Many sole proprietors get into trouble because they neglect to take this tax into account when estimating their tax liability for the year and this tax is significant as noted below.

Self-employment tax is paid on 92.35% of all self-employment net profits. This tax is the equivalent of the combination of the employer's and employee's Social Security tax and Medicare tax. Social Security tax is 12.4% of the first $117,000 (in 2014) in net income and Medicare tax is paid 2.90% of net income without any upper income limit. There is also no maximum for the 9% additional Medicare tax under the PP-ACA [Obamacare] that applies when adjusted gross income exceeds $250,000 for joint filers, $200,000 for single filers, or $125,000 on married-filing-separate returns. The Social Security income limit is indexed and adjusted (upward) annually. The sole proprietor is allowed to deduct one half of the self-employment tax against income; however, this deduction is worth far less than the actual tax.

EXAMPLE 10.1

Dr. Soloman is a sole proprietor with a self-employment tax liability of $11,500. She gets to deduct $5750 (50% of $11,500) against her income. Now, she is in the 31 percent tax bracket, therefore, her deduction is worth $1782.50 in actual income tax dollars ($5750 × 31). The discrepancy between one half of the self-employment tax, $5750 and the tax deduction is $3967.50 in tax. Therefore, although Dr. Soloman received a 50 percent deduction for her self-employment tax, she actually pays $9717.50, or 84.5 percent of the self-employment tax. This is not the bargain that the Congressional spin doctors made it out to be when it was being sold to the general public. However, it is still better than paying the entire $11,500 in self-employment tax.

Tax Planning Tip
If the healthcare professional's core service entity operates on cash basis, by setting up a separate corporation for management and choosing the accrual method of accounting for the new entity litigation protection and tax timing on short-term profitability can be better managed.

Owing to the healthcare professional's core service entities considerable accounts receivable assets, the risk of litigation is high as plaintiff attorneys have little concern over judgment collectability. By placing the nonpatient care risk outside of the core entity, litigation is discouraged.

Furthermore, by defining the relationship between the managing entity and the core entity, contractually cost containment is obtained. The managing entity employs all nonmedical staff, assumes lease and rental commitments, and pays utilities as well as all other operating expenses other than the doctors. Contracts can contain clauses that indicate the costs of operations cannot exceed a percentage of the core entities gross receipts.

Systematically, checks are drafted to the management company for its efforts and ,when matched to revenue, quickly alert the core service entity of any cost creep that requires consideration and adjustment.

The core service entity should operate as a calendar year S Corporation and the managing entity as a C Corporation on a fiscal year (noncalendar year), as such profits in the S Corporation can be at least partially recognized in the C Corporation. This allows for the timing of tax on short-term profitability to be stretched out to the due date of the C Corporation.

Review of Internal Revenue Section 267 "Losses, expenses, and interest with respect to transactions between related taxpayers" is required to structure the core service entities transactions with the management entity so that they are considered "nonrelated."

GENERAL TAX PLANNING ISSUES

The following issues apply to all business entities. There may be minor differences in the section of the Internal Revenue Code (IRC) or nuances in the way that the Code section applies to the entity, but, in general, these areas are worthy issues not to be missed.

Purchased Accounts Receivable

Recently, some practices were selling out to Public Practice Management Companies (PPMC) or other buyers. However, many of those transactions have soured since the PPMCs or other network models were not able to generate the earnings Wall Street or some other market force wanted to see. Many of those same practices are now being bought back by the same physicians that sold out several years earlier. If an entity is being bought back and accounts receivable is being purchased, be careful not to pick this item up as income twice. The costs can be immense to the practice or other business unit.

EXAMPLE 10.2

A family practice recently purchased itself back from a PPMC. Part of the mandatory purchase price, approximately $200,000 (the approximate net realizable value of the accounts receivable), was paid to the PPMC to buy back accounts receivable generated by the physicians buying back their practice. The office administrator unknowingly began recording the cash receipts specifically attributable to the purchased accounts receivable as patient fee income. If left uncorrected, this error could have incorrectly added $200,000 in income to this practice and cost it (a C Corporation) approximately $70,000 in additional income tax ($200,000 in fees × 35% tax rate).

The error in the above example is that the PPMC must record the portion of the purchase price it received for the accounts receivable as patient fee income. The buyer practice has merely traded one asset, cash, for another asset, the accounts receivable. When the practice collects these particular receivables, the credit is applied against the purchased account receivable rather than to patient fees.

Tax Planning Tip

The above types of hidden costs lurk in many, if not all, business purchase and sale transactions of healthcare entities. The costs of incorrect accounting and tax treatment in such transactions can be very high, as in the above actual example. Uncovering and removing this type of unnecessary transaction cost can make it easy to justify the hiring of competent tax counsel. In fact, the cost differential is usually the difference between a viable transaction and a bad deal.

Organization Costs

When any entity is organized as other than a sole proprietorship, it will incur some costs associated with the start-up of the business called organization costs, and typically include legal and or accounting fees to establish the entity.

An entity may deduct in the taxable year in which a taxpayer begins an active trade or business, an electing taxpayer may deduct an amount equal to the lesser of the amount of the start-up expenditures that relate to the active trade or business, or $5000 (reduced [but not below zero] by the amount by which the start-up expenditures exceed $50,000). The remainder of the start-up expenditures is deductible ratably over the 180-month period beginning with the month in which the active trade or business begins. All start-up expenditures that relate to the active trade or business are considered in determining whether the start-up expenditures exceed $50,000, including expenditures incurred on or before October 22, 2004.

EXAMPLE 10.3

Expenditures of $5000 or less. Corporation X, a calendar year taxpayer, incurs $3000 in start-up expenditures after October 22, 2004, that relate to an active trade or business that begins on July 1, 2011. Under paragraph (b) of this section, Corporation X is deemed to have elected to amortize start-up expenditures under section 195(b) in 2011. Therefore, Corporation X may deduct the entire amount of the start-up expenditures in 2011, the taxable year in which the active trade or business begins.

EXAMPLE 10.4

Expenditures of more than $5000 but less than or equal to $50,000. The facts are the same as in *Example 10.3* except that Corporation X incurs start-up expenditures of $41,000. Under paragraph (b) of this section, Corporation X is deemed to have elected to amortize start-up expenditures under section 195(b) in 2011. Therefore, Corporation X may deduct $5000 and the portion of the remaining $36,000 that is allocable to July through December of 2011 ($36,000/180 × 6 = $1200) in 2011, the taxable year in which the active trade or business begins. Corporation X may amortize the remaining $34,800 ($36,000 − $1200 = $34,800) ratably over the remaining 174 months.

Asset Expensing Election

Purchases of furniture, fixtures, machinery, equipment, and other personal property are typically not allowed to be expensed when purchased. Rather, the entity is required to capitalize and depreciate these assets over their useful lives. The Internal Revenue Service publication 946 provides asset lives to be used for tax purposes.

Type of Asset	Depreciable Life in Years (In General)
Computers and peripherals	5
Office machinery and equipment	5
Transportation equipment	5
Furniture and fixtures	7
Leasehold improvements	27.50
Real property, nonresidential	31.50

These tax lives typically do not agree to the actual useful lives of the assets and that should not be of any concern. There are also various methods of depreciating equipment and these methods do generate different amounts of expense. However, most healthcare entities wish to maximize the current deduction for depreciation. This strategy brings the entity closer to a pure cash in/cash out business.

IRC § 179 allows an entity to expense a certain amount of asset purchases each year that would otherwise have to be depreciated over their tax lives. This deduction is available for tangible personal property only, not real estate or leasehold improvements, and is a big benefit to most businesses.

The § 179 election is subject to three important limitations:

First, there is a dollar limitation. Under §179(b)(1), the maximum deduction a taxpayer may elect to take in a year is $500,000 in 2010, 2011, 2012, and 2013, and $25,000 for years beginning after 2013 [2014–15].

Second, if a taxpayer places more than $2,000,000 worth of section 179 property into service during a single taxable year, the § 179 deduction is reduced, dollar for dollar, by the amount exceeding the $2,000,000 threshold. This threshold is reduced to $200,000 for years beginning in 2014.

Finally, § 179(b)(3) provides that a taxpayer's § 179 deduction for any taxable year may not exceed the taxpayer's aggregate income from the active conduct of trade or business by the taxpayer for that year.

Also, the depreciation expense created by this election cannot create or increase a tax loss for the practice. Any amount unable to be used in the current period can be carried forward to future periods to offset income in those periods.

Year	Amount of Deduction
2008	$250,000
2009	$250,000
2010	$500,000
2011	$500,000
2012	$500,000
2013	$500,000
2014	$25,000

There are various tricks to use in choosing the equipment to elect for § 179 depreciation. For instance, if the entity is adding assets in excess of the yearly limit, it would be wise to make the expensing election on those assets the entity fully intends to hold for that asset's entire tax life. Otherwise, the entity will have to recapture (pick up as income) the unused portion of the depreciation deduction that was taken early via the use of the election. Recapture can mitigate the tax benefit of this planning opportunity and should be avoided whenever possible.

EXAMPLE 10.5

An obstetrics practice purchases four exam room set ups for $20,000 along with an ultrasound machine for another $20,000. The practice makes the expense election on the ultrasound machine because it is easier to take the deduction on one asset. After being in practice one year, the physicians agree that they don't like their current ultrasound machine. They opt to sell it and buy another one they all prefer. In the year of sale the practice must recapture 80 percent ($16,000) of the expense election they made when they purchased the first ultrasound machine. This adds $16,000 to their current year's taxable income. Had they used the expense election on the four exam room set ups, they would be much better off for tax purposes.

Tax Planning Tip
If the entity does not already have a policy, it should set a capitalization policy for purchases of assets. This policy should state that any purchase below a certain dollar value will be expensed and items over that threshold amount will be capitalized and depreciated. Even the IRS signs off on this one because it views this policy on a cost–benefit basis. No purpose is served by creating additional accounting work capitalizing the cost of a trash can, calculator, or coffee maker when there is no significant accounting or tax difference between expensing and depreciating the item. The method used to set this policy should be to review the types of purchases that are made within the entity. There is typically a break off point between office supply items and larger items. In most healthcare-related entities this break off is between $100 and $250, but a higher number could be used if there is adequate reasoning to support a larger number. By setting this policy and following it consistently, the entity will reduce its chance of having the policy challenged in the case of an audit. The entity also reduces the number of "assets" it must track. The only caution here is not to get carried away with the threshold number.

Purchase of an Entity

When a corporate entity is purchased, whether it is a physician's practice, an ancillary service provider, a durable medical equipment entity or a hospital, it may be thought that the deal is done when agreement has been reached on the purchase price. However, for tax planning purposes, this is just the beginning of the exercise.

For starters, most buyers want to purchase assets because their investment in those assets can be recovered via depreciation or amortization over some period of time. The purchase of stock is considered a capital transaction and does not allow for the depreciation of the investment. Buyers of healthcare entities typically don't want to buy stock for another reason; namely, there is the potential acquisition of unknown and unwanted liabilities (e.g., legal problems including, product liability, malpractice lawsuits, other torts alleged under prior ownership, etc.).

Sellers on the other hand, want to sell the stock of a corporation to obtain favorable capital gains tax treatment on the sale. Sellers do not like to sell assets of the corporate entity because the sales proceeds end up flowing into the corporation where they are either subject to double taxation or flow out to the shareholders in the form of salaries. This is very unappealing for tax purposes. This creates a real problem that in many cases can be a deal breaker.

Caution
This is not a simple transaction to be crafted at home with a piece of do-it-yourself software. This is a complex area of the law and competent legal and tax counsel should be engaged. The tax benefit in

most cases will far outweigh the cost of hiring the experts. In addition, this type of transaction can wreak havoc at the state tax level if care is not taken to review all of the ramifications.

EXAMPLE 10.6

A recent third party billing company sale in Texas of approximately $9 million, handled in the above manner, saved the sellers significant dollars and avoided the ordinary tax treatment deal breaker. This transaction had a Texas State Franchise Tax consequence to the sellers of approximately $450,000. Even after the impact of the franchise tax, there was enough benefit for the buyers to consider the transaction a good deal. The bottom line is that this type of transaction has a place and can save many thousands of dollars, but just as with a patient, the healthcare professional wants to review all of the information to "diagnose" whether this strategy could work in the entity's specific tax circumstances.

Caution

When an entity is being purchased (or sold), there is one important detail that is overlooked in many transactions. The purchaser needs to formally allocate the purchase price among the various classes of assets bought. This is a required function by both the purchaser and seller of a business for federal tax purposes. According to Internal Revenue Regulations, this allocation must be documented in the tax returns of both purchasing and selling entities in the year of the transaction on Form 8594.[*] In addition, the allocation reported must be the same on both returns. Therefore, both parties must agree to the allocation.

Red Flag!

It can be very detrimental to miss this detail. The IRS has ways of identifying purchase and sale transactions that have taken place with an entity (like the filing of a final or initial return, seeing large increases in assets on the tax return balance sheet of an ongoing entity, etc.). Should the entity not spend the time to go through this exercise and allocate the price on its own behalf, or file the tax return without the proper disclosure, the IRS has the right to step in after the fact and reallocate the purchase price. Their allocation will be based upon what the IRS thinks the allocation should have been in the first place. This allocation will most assuredly be a favorable allocation to the IRS rather than the purchaser and seller.

Amortization of Goodwill

In many cases, the hard assets (furniture, fixtures, and equipment) you obtain in a purchase transaction make up only a small portion of the purchase price. At least part of the price will be allocated to "goodwill." Goodwill, or "blue sky" as it has also been called, is a premium paid for the reputation of the owner or the business, the company name, or other intangible assets identified within the entity. This goodwill, along with most other intangible assets, is amortizable over 15 years using the "straight-line" method. The straight-line method is a ratable method calculated by dividing the asset's value by 180 months (15 years × 12 months). The importance of the asset allocation between asset classes (noted in the Caution above) becomes evident at this point since most other assets can be depreciated over much shorter periods of time, thus providing larger annual deductions to the business. It is preferred to allocate as much of the purchase price as reasonably possible to assets that can be depreciated over shorter periods of time.

Caution

An unreasonably high allocation of a purchase price to assets is likely to be challenged by the IRS. When making the allocation, be sure to document the reasoning behind the allocation. Keep any documentation or research that supports the allocation methodology. This documentation will be

---

[*] See www.irs.gov or Form 8594.

vital to upholding the entity's allocation should it have to be defended somewhere down the road. The IRS has three years from the date the return (including the allocation) is filed to challenge the allocation. Furthermore, most states have a sales tax on the resale of fixed assets making proper valuation necessary to diminish the changes of review for sales tax payment adequacy.

Lease versus Purchase of Assets

Looking back to the initial premise of tax planning, the idea is to put more net dollars into the entity's pocket. Leasing is a financing strategy that can have some advantages in healthcare practices. However, don't believe everything being stated about the tax advantages of leasing. If leasing entities weren't making a lot of money leasing assets, there would be no such thing as a leasing industry. Typically, an entity will pay more to lease an asset over its useful life than it would have had it purchased the asset outright. With that being said, if the entity can tailor a lease to conform to its own needs, pay only for the portion of the asset the entity uses and be able to return the property without large penalties, there may be a place for leases within the entity's tax planning strategy.

For each buy-versus-lease decision the healthcare professional should look at the total cost (including all potential fees and charges) of each option. Obtain answers to the following questions (in writing) and evaluate the additional cost each item adds to the property being considered before making a final decision.

1. What are the upfront costs of each transaction (i.e., down payment, loan origination fees, first and last months rent, sales tax, documentation fees, or other deposit structures)?
2. What is the monthly lease payment versus monthly principal and interest payment on a loan?
3. Who is responsible for personal property tax payments on the asset while it is being leased?
4. What adjustments are made on the back end of a lease should the entity decide to return the leased property?
   a. Make up payment to leasing company if actual residual value is less than estimate.
   b. Cost for excess mileage above annual limits specified in the contract (for vehicles).
   c. Cost of excess copies for a copy machine.
   d. "Damage" estimates that can be assessed by the lessor on leased property that must be paid by lessee.
   e. Shipping or delivery costs to put the leased assets in the location specified at the end of the lease.
5. What costs are incurred on the back end of a lease should you decide to keep the leased property (i.e., "purchase price," which can be anywhere from $1.00 to approximately 20% of the original cost of the leased property, potential sales tax on sale)?

Once all of these questions have been answered, the healthcare professional can quantify the total cost of each alternative and can make an informed decision on which route is best for the entity.

There may also be overriding factors involved in the decision-making process. These factors may include the entity's inability to find a lender that will loan funds to a healthcare entity. This has been a very real problem for healthcare professionals in some parts of the country. In such cases, leasing may be the only viable alternative. In these situations the prudent healthcare professional would still go through the exercise to understand all of the costs involved. In addition, there can be competition created by obtaining bids from various lessors for the property being leased. The end result, even in less than optimal circumstances, will be the best deal the entity can obtain on lease of property.

Working Capital Loans

For those entities that have lenders willing to accommodate line of credit arrangements, care should be taken to understand the underlying costs of borrowing. It is always a good idea to have a working capital credit line available in the event of collection slow downs or necessary asset acquisitions. Some lending institutions charge what is called a loan commitment fee on the total working capital amount committed to the entity. This fee is obviously in addition to the interest cost that will be charged on any amounts borrowed against the credit line.

EXAMPLE 10.7

A practice thinks that it may need a $100,000 credit line to provide safe coverage for the operation of the business in the event of collection slow downs. However, the bank offers the practice $250,000 because of its "good credit standing." The bank also charges a commitment fee in the amount of ½ percent of the committed funds, not the amount actually borrowed. Therefore, if the practice sticks to its plan of $100,000, the cost for the privilege will be $500 ($100,000 × 005). However, if the practice goes with the flattering bank proposal, the commitment cost will be $1,250 ($250,000 × 005). In this instance, the bank may be padding its own bottom line at the expense of the healthcare entity's bottom line.

Be sure to shop around before even thinking of paying a commitment fee on a credit line. Not every lending institution charges such fees, and, although deductible in nature, these fees reduce the entity's bottom line.

Capital Contribution versus Loans to Your Entity

When starting or operating an entity, the need to capitalize the operation is always a concern to the owners. How should the owners put money into the entity? Most states require some minimum amount of cash or property contribution to be considered viable by statute. This amount is typically between $100 and $1000. However, beyond the minimum amount there are planning opportunities available to business owners. When loaning additional cash flow requirements to the entity, Internal Revenue Service requires interest be charged at applicable federal rates ("AFRs").

These are interest rates published monthly by the Internal Revenue Service. These rates are used for various purposes under the Internal Revenue Code including determining the minimum interest rates that can be charged for certain loans to avoid the IRS "inputing" interest on low or no interest loans. These rates are published for short-term loans (3 years or less), mid-term loans (3–9 years), and long-term loans (more than 9 years). In practice, these rates are often referenced to determine appropriate interest rates for private business loans, shareholder/partner or intercompany loans, and loans between family members.

The interest paid is a deduction to the entity when it is paid and is income to the owners when received. These payments avoid being considered compensation to the corporate shareholder or self-employment earnings for owners of unincorporated entities. The savings from this strategy can be between 2.9% and 15.3% depending upon whether the individual owner has met the Social Security minimum for the year.

GENERAL TAX PLANNING ISSUES: INCOME STATEMENT ACCOUNTS

The above dealt with general tax planning issues that could appear on the balance sheets of most healthcare entities. This chapter will continue the review of general tax planning issues available for virtually any entity; however, the items below will appear on the income statement. The following information provides insight to income and expenses that require better classification to take advantage of "special" tax rules. Segregating these items will give your entity the best chance to utilize the tax planning and saving opportunities that already exist within the entity.

INTEREST INCOME

Most interest income earned within a business entity will be taxable. However, if the entity has excess cash in one or more accounts, it would be wise to consider investment of the excess funds in tax-exempt issues. Tax-exempt issues, in general, pay a lower rate of interest than do taxable issues because of the built-in tax advantage. In addition, the entity's tolerance for risk in the investment of these funds should be very low (the entity doesn't want to lose any part of this money), therefore it won't be looking for the highest return on these excess funds anyway. Interest from tax-exempt sources should be segregated into a separate account from otherwise taxable interest on the practice's books to highlight the tax advantage.

Tax Planning Tip
If not segregated, this tax advantage is easily forgotten and lost at year-end. Tax-free income is often subjected to taxation along with the rest of the taxable interest income due to laziness associated with the failure to set up a separate general ledger account to identify the tax advantaged income. This happens all too often. Don't allow the entity to be a victim of this laziness.

Tax Planning Tip
If the entity is investing in tax-exempt securities, be sure to invest, whenever possible, in issues that are also exempt from state income tax. Ask the practice's investment advisor before the purchase, or even better, set this double exemption as a prerequisite for any investment in tax exempt issues within the entity. This will save the entity from the unpleasant surprise of finding out that only half of the tax-planning job was accomplished. Some care will also want to be taken to limit the tax-exempt income from "private activity" bonds. The interest on these bonds is subject to the AMT. The AMT tax is a safety net for the IRS to make sure that every person or entity pays some tax on the income it earns. The AMT tax catches those who make too much use of certain deductions, credits, and tax exemptions to avoid paying tax.

MEALS, ENTERTAINMENT, AND TRAVEL EXPENSES

The IRS only allows 50% of meals and entertainment expenses to be deducted.

Tax Planning Tip
Certain meals can be deducted at 100% rather than the 50% as noted above. Providing a meal for company employees while they remain on the premises exempts the expenditure from the 50% reduction. This might be the case where a staff meeting is held through the lunch hour or when dinner is brought in when the staff is working late. Although 50% of the expense in these instances may not be significant individually, they can add up to a significant amount throughout the course of a year. Therefore, these expenditures should be classified to a separate general ledger account "Meals—100 percent deductible." This will help to identify the qualifying expenditures and take advantage of the entire deduction where it is available.

Prior to this change in the lax law, travel and entertainment expenses were typically combined into one account in the general ledgers of many healthcare entities. When the law changed to reduce the deductible portion of meals and entertainment expenses, many entities changed the classification within their general ledger accounts to coincide with the tax law change. However, many did not make the change and still classify travel and entertainment expenses in the same account.

Caution
The IRC states that where no distinction can be made between the commingling of expenses that are fully deductible with those that are only partially deductible, all expenses within that category will be considered only partially deductible. The bottom line here is that each entity should segregate its meals and entertainment expenses from other expenses.

PAYING EMPLOYEE BONUSES WITHOUT WITHHOLDING

It is easy to come up with an amount to give a person as a Christmas or merit bonus. However, many healthcare professionals feel that taking taxes out of this amount cheapens the thought. Although this may seem like a small issue to most, it is one of the areas that the IRS looks for in business returns. Healthcare professionals are very susceptible to this trap.

Caution

In most states, the State Unemployment Agency is required to audit each business periodically. This may be every three or four years. The auditor will request information on employee salaries. He will also look at several other accounts on the general ledger, if not the entire general ledger. This investigation usually uncovers these compensation items and the auditor will assess the tax and penalties on any items considered to be compensation. In addition, all of these state agencies share information with the IRS, so the additional wages will be reported to the IRS and the employer ends up paying all taxes due on the bonus amounts, including the employee's portion. The IRS will also charge interest and penalties on these delinquent wages. The point of this issue is to always withhold taxes. It will save time, money, and a lot of hassle in the long run.

PENALTIES AND FINES

Penalties and fines are usually assessed by a government agency (like the IRS) or municipality. These expenses are not deductible for income tax purposes. However, there is a common misnomer that late payment "penalties" on invoices are penalties as well and are not deductible. These charges are more accurately considered to be interest or finance charges. These are deductible items and should not be overlooked. Therefore, before accepting a "penalty" at face value and chalking it up to a nondeductible expense, see who issued the penalty or fine and reclassify where appropriate, to finance charges or an interest expense account.

DISABILITY INSURANCE

Some entities offer disability insurance to their employees on a group basis as part of an employee benefit program. The expense for this coverage is typically deducted as an ordinary and necessary expense by the employer entity. However, many entities also purchase additional disability insurance for the owners. This additional disability insurance expense should not be deducted on the entity's tax return for two reasons. First, it would probably be considered a discriminatory benefit to the owners and, therefore, not be allowed as a deduction anyway. Second, and more importantly, when a person becomes disabled and qualifies for disability benefits whose premiums have been deducted as a business expense by the entity, the disability insurance proceeds are considered taxable income to the person receiving them. This can be personally catastrophic since disability insurance covers only a portion (~60%) of regular earnings. This coverage was designed to be paid on an after tax basis. The benefits would be tax free to the beneficiary and would be close to the disabled person's net take home pay before being disabled. This is one of those instances where the traditional tax planning thought process is overridden by a long-term (potential) tax cost/benefit decision.

OFFICERS OR OWNERS LIFE INSURANCE

Premium payments for life insurance on the owners of an entity are typically not deductible unless they are part of a group term life insurance policy covering all eligible employees of the entity and then only up to a maximum of $50,000.* Any amount above $50,000 will generate fringe benefit income to the owner or other employee. Therefore, if the entity is paying large premiums for life insurance on the medical professional, be prepared for the taxable income that will show up at tax time, according to the table below:

---

* IRC § 79.

Age[a]	Monthly Cost per $1000
Under 30	$0.08
30–34	0.09
35–39	0.11
40–44	0.17
45–49	0.29
50–54	0.48
55–59	0.75
60–64	1.17
65–69	2.10
70–	3.76

[a] Age determined on the last day of the taxable year.

PROFESSIONAL AND TRADE ASSOCIATION DUES

Several years ago the IRS required professional organizations and trade associations to disclose to their constituents the percentage of their dues that were being expended for political lobbying purposes. That portion of the dues payment associated with lobbying activities is not considered deductible for federal income tax purposes. This portion of dues should be segregated into a separate account along with dues to country clubs, hunting leases, athletic facilities, and so on, since these dues are not allowed as deductible expenses to the taxpayer. Only the charges associated with direct entertainment are considered to be deductible, and then only at the 50% amount mentioned earlier.

POLITICAL CONTRIBUTIONS

Political contributions are not deductible for income tax purposes, even though there might be the need from a business perspective to contribute to a specific candidate or Political Action Committee (PAC). These items should be segregated from other contributions being made by the entity to accurately identify the deductible versus nondeductible variety of contribution.

RETIREMENT PLANS

Several tax planning strategies utilizing retirement plan vehicles can generate large tax deductions while providing continuing benefits to the entity and its employees. Retirement plan contributions can be accrued (even in a cash basis entity) and paid in the next year. This accrual can provide a large, one time deferral that can have significant impact on the income of the entity. In addition, many of the plans currently available allow for flexible contributions, thus providing entities the ability to contribute based upon the availability of cash flow.

401(k) Plans

Primary and matching contributions to a 401(k) plan, as well as its earnings, are tax deferred. The 2013 maximum employee contribution for a medical professional is $ 17,500 per year.

403(b) Plans

Healthcare professionals employed by hospitals or other tax-exempt organizations may participate in their employer's 403(b) plan, also known as a tax-sheltered annuity. Both contribution limits and tax deferral status are similar to that of a 401(k) plan.

SIMPLE Plans

The Savings Inventive Match Plan is a retirement savings plan available to most small businesses including most healthcare practices. For 2013 employees who are eligible to participate can contribute up to $12,000 of pay per year, on a pre-tax basis. For 2013, employers are required to contribute 3% of employee wages up to a maximum of $12,000 per year. The employer matching percentage must be communicated to employees by November 1 of each year. The advantage of this type of plan is that there is no requirement to test for discrimination against the non-highly compensated employees. The disadvantage is that the maximum contributions available on an annual basis are lower than for other qualified retirement plans.

Traditional IRAs

For 2014, an individual may contribute up to $5500 to an IRA if you're under age 50 or $6500 if you're age 50 or older. However, you can't contribute more than you earned during the year, and for Roth IRAs, there may be additional limits based on income.

The table below helps further compare Roth and Traditional IRA rules.

Eligibility	Roth IRA	Traditional IRA
Is there a minimum income limit?	Yes. In addition to being subject to IRS limits, the amount of your contribution can't exceed the amount of income you earned that year. This also applies to minors who want to start contributing to an IRA, with limits based on their own income, not their parents'. Also, if you're married and filing a joint tax return, a spouse who isn't working may still be able to contribute to an IRA. But the total contribution for both spouses can't exceed the amount of income earned by the working spouse.	Yes. In addition to being subject to IRS limits, the amount of your contribution can't exceed the amount of income you earned that year. This also applies to minors who want to start contributing to an IRA, with limits based on their own income, not their parents'. Also, if you're married and filing a joint tax return, a spouse who isn't working may still be able to contribute to an IRA. But the total contribution for both spouses can't exceed the amount of income earned by the working spouse.
Is there a maximum income limit?	Yes. Your modified adjusted gross income (MAGI) for the year may affect the amount you can contribute or—if high enough—make you ineligible.	No.
Does it matter how old I am?	No. You can contribute at any age.	Yes. You must be under age 70½ to contribute.

Caution

The choice of the right retirement plan for an entity is a very important decision. Do not choose a particular plan just because of the current year tax benefit that can be obtained. Review each of the retirement plan alternatives for their respective benefits, responsibilities, and obligations. Once instituted, modification of these documents can be difficult without triggering unwanted results. This is a very complex area of law and can generate very bad results when improperly utilized. Seek the counsel of a competent tax or retirement plan specialist prior to committing. In addition, many brokerage houses have prototype retirement plan documents available for the set up of a retirement plan. Although this may be the most economical means of setting up a "boiler plate" retirement plan, it does not mean that the stockbroker has the knowledge to guide the healthcare professional to the right plan, much less through the elections to be made in a plan document.

Tax Planning Tip

If contributing to a standard IRA is in an individual's plans, making that contribution at the beginning of the tax year (early January) can put that money to work as much as 15½ months earlier than making the deposit in mid-April of the following year, when the individual's tax return is due. This hypothetical IRA contribution, at a 8% return (which would be a conservative return in the stock market over the past 10 years) would earn an additional $227 if contributed at the beginning of the tax year as in the above example. That is just for that one contribution over a 15½-month period. When this one change in thought process (or strategy) is evaluated over 20 years, the numbers become staggering.

Investing $2000 on January 1, 2013 and each year thereafter for 20 years, at the above 8% rate of return, generates $132,037 at December 31, 2033. Investing this same $2000 starting on April 15, 2014 and each year thereafter for 20 years at a 8% rate of return generates $113,175 or a difference of $18,862.

The above tip is what tax planning is all about and what it can do for any person willing to take advantage of the strategy. The opportunities are available and waiting to be utilized. It is up to each healthcare professional to identify the opportunities that apply to their situation and to act upon them. This section is organized to help identify such opportunities.

OVERHEARD IN THE DOCTOR'S LOUNGE: PHYSICIANS AND TAXES

I read a poll on SERMO (a doctor-only web forum) asking what percentage of income was paid in taxes. The lowest option was <20%. I thought it ridiculous since I make about an average salary and paid about 8% in Federal tax, 3.5% in payroll tax, and 4% in state income taxes. So, I spoke up about it.

After a few days of correspondence, it became evident that most doctors have no idea what they pay in taxes, or that they pay far too much in taxes. For example, of 58 responses on the poll, I was the only one who was paid less than 20% in taxes. Keep in mind that more than half of doctors make less money than I do.

I found it hilarious that 4 doctors thought they paid more than 50% in taxes. I can't quite figure out how to pull that off; even if you are single, make a ton of money, take a standard deduction, are self-employed, and pay ridiculous state and local income taxes. Really … more than 50%! You're either mistaken or stupid … hopefully; just mistaken.

Or is the problem simply that doctor's have no idea what their effective tax rate is?

D.J. Morgane, DO
(Internal Medicine)

PERMANENT VERSUS TIMING DIFFERENCES IN TAX RETURNS

When reviewing income and expense items, it is important to understand whether the benefit being obtained is a temporary (a difference in the timing of the taxation of an item) or permanent tax benefit, or cost. Obviously, tax benefits are much better than tax costs. Permanent differences are better than temporary differences, when they are in your favor.

An example of a timing difference would be accelerated depreciation rather than straight-line depreciation. Eventually, the asset will be fully expensed under either method, the only difference revolves around when and how much of a deduction is available. Examples of permanent differences would be penalties and fines. Fines and penalties are paid out of business cash flow but are never deductible for income tax purposes.

Tax Planning for C Corporations

For those healthcare C Corporations that are not considered personal service corporations, tax planning can be fairly easy. The progressive tax rate structure allows certain tax breaks for C Corporations with less than $100,000 in taxable income. The following table provides the tax brackets for corporate taxpaying entities.

2013 Taxable Income Is			
Over	But Not Over	The Tax Is	Of Excess Over
$ 0	$ 50,000	$ 0 + 15%	$ 0
50,000	75,000	7500 + 25%	50,000
75,000	100,000	13,750 + 34%	75,000
100,000	335,000	22,250 + 39%	100,000
335,000	10,000,000	113,900 + 34%	335,000
10,000,000	15,000,000	3,400,000 + 35%	10,000,000
15,000,000	18,333,333	5,150,000 + 38%	15,000,000
18,333,333	—	6,416,667 + 35%	18,333,333

The above tax brackets do not take into account the potential effects of the alternative minimum tax, if applicable.

The use of bonuses, retirement plan contributions, and relevant combinations of the other items noted above can be used to reduce corporate tax liability into the preferred tax bracket. As mentioned earlier, the tax planning process requires action and some forethought on the part of the entity to position itself to optimize its tax situation.

Of course, with no tax planning at all, the corporation will still end up in one of the above tax brackets. The unpleasant part of this surprise is that the bracket will typically be higher and the tax will definitely be more than it could have been.

In general, shareholders in a personal service corporation (C corporation) want to keep taxable income of the corporation as close to a break-even as possible. Any income retained in the corporation will be taxed at 35% for federal income tax purposes as noted above plus any applicable state income taxes. Shareholders typically pay out the excess cash flow in the form of salaries or bonuses at year-end to reduce taxable income and, therefore, the potential income tax. This is what is called "gutting" the income of the corporation. Although there is a tax advantage to gutting the entity on an annual basis, there are some very distinct disadvantages to this tax planning strategy.

Pulling out all of the profit from the entity on an annual basis leaves no cash flow within the entity to carry on day-to-day operations of the business. Likewise, this strategy leaves no funds available for needed capital expenditures (updating or adding to facilities or systems). This deficit usually requires the shareholders to loan funds back into the entity to fund operations. In many cases these funds are the same funds that were paid out as bonuses to remove profits. Does this sound familiar? It should be easy to see how the continued use of this strategy year after year will require larger annual loans to fund the deficits.

Many shareholders find the above strategy to be very frustrating and don't understand how they end up in the deficit position each year with only two alternatives seemingly available:

1. The continued funding of higher loan amounts
2. Payment of a large tax bill

When unwanted tax surprises occur in a C corporation, it is usually due to nondeductible expenses (permanent differences) or limitations in otherwise deductible expenses reducing the offsets to current period income. In addition to the items listed above, there is one income exclusion item and several deduction limitations that need to be considered in arriving at estimated taxable income.

Dividend Income

If a C Corporation owns stock in a taxable domestic corporation, it is entitled to a reduction in the amount of income it has to pick up on its tax return. The dividends received deduction (DRD) is an allowed exclusion from income and is a percentage of the dividends received. A base exclusion rate of 70% is allowed in most circumstances and, depending upon the type of corporation issuing the dividend, the exclusion can increase to 80% or even 100% of the dividends received. This exclusion is calculated on page two of Form 1120 and cannot exceed 70% of the receiving corporation's income (after certain adjustments including the DRD itself). Any DRD amount not used due to this limitation is lost, period. Dividends from mutual funds do not qualify for the DRD.

Capital Gains and Losses

Capital gains and losses are generated by the sale of capital assets. These assets include stocks, bonds, and other assets held for investment purposes, real estate and personal property used in the business. The gain from the sale of such assets is treated the same way for all entities: it is included in income in the year of the sale. However, capital losses are a different story. A capital loss in a C Corporation is allowed only to the extent that it can offset a capital gain. Put differently, a capital loss cannot be used to offset ordinary income. Unused capital losses can be carried back three years and carried forward five years to offset capital gains in those periods. Any unused capital losses remaining after the five-year carry-forward period expire and are lost.

Tax Planning Tip
Where available, a corporation considering the sale of a capital asset that will generate a capital loss should coordinate the sale of other assets generating capital gains to create an offset.

Charitable Contributions

Many physicians tend to give to charities through their corporations thinking that the contributions will reduce the income of the corporation. However, there is a limitation placed on the amount of deductible contributions a corporation may take in any year. The limitation is 10% of the corporation's taxable income before the charitable contribution deductions are taken into consideration.

EXAMPLE 10.8

C Corporation has book income of $26,000 at year-end. This income includes contributions of $4500 that C Corporation made during the year to various recognized charities. For federal and (most) state income tax purposes, taxable income would be as follows:

Book income	$26,000
Contributions	4500
	30,500
Contribution limitation	10%
Allowable contributions	$3050
Excess contributions disallowed	1450
Book income	26,000
Taxable income	$27,450

The excess amount of contributions can be carried over to future periods to offset income. Any amount(s) carried over must be used to offset income within the next five years or they will expire and be lost forever. This becomes a trap for those who annually give through their corporation, but also try to minimize income.

Tax Planning Tip

If reducing the corporation's tax liability to zero is your strategy, do not make any charitable contributions through the corporation. Likewise, if the entity's income is close to zero on an annual basis, use up contribution carryovers before making additional contributions out of the C Corporation. This will minimize the potential of turning a timing difference into a permanent difference and losing a deduction forever.

There are several points to be taken from the above example. First, much of the standard tax planning that takes place to gut the corporation actually works against the deduction of charitable contributions. For that reason, the disallowance of charitable contributions in C Corporations is very common. Second, in order to be deductible, the contribution needs to be made to a "recognized" charity. A recognized charity is one that has filed the necessary documents with the IRS to be exempt from federal income taxes. Merely giving to a needy individual or organization is not enough to make the contribution deductible.

When all is said and done, the C Corporation is not the optimal entity to use for charitable giving, especially for small or personal service corporations.

Tax Planning Tip

The limitation for deductibility for (cash) charitable contributions at the individual taxpayer level is 50%. Therefore, it makes sense to generate charitable gifts at the individual rather than the corporate level. In most individual tax instances the income limitation will not be an issue. In the event contributions have already been made during the current year, the corporation can reclassify those contributions to the owner employee as compensation and the individual can take the entire deduction at the individual level.

C Corporation Summary

Several of the income statement items mentioned above generate tax benefits for the entity while most generate tax costs and provide unwanted income tax surprises at year-end. It is important to keep all of the above items and their respective amounts in mind as the year progresses because decision-making opportunities do present themselves all during the year. The ability to identify an opportunity and act upon it in a timely manner will allow the healthcare professional to position the corporation for the best outcome available in its unique set of circumstances.

There is no "ones size fits all" tax planning strategy. The entity can remove the uses of corporate cash flow that do not generate a deductible expense for tax purposes. It can require the shareholders to annually fund the deficits caused by zeroing out income. Or, it can adopt a strategy that requires the payment of some tax each year but will reduce the constant escalation of year-end borrowings needed to fund deficits that one day have to culminate in the corporation paying a lot of tax. The following Tax Planning Worksheet can be used to estimate the C Corporation's taxable income.

C Corporation Tax Planning Worksheet

	Gross Amt.	Pct.	Net Amount	
Book income <loss> before taxes				
Less:				
Dividends Received Deduction			<	>
Tax exempt interest			<	>
Contribution carryover from prior period			<	>
Section 179 Depreciation			<	>
Accrued retirement plan contribution			<	>
Other				

continued

C Corporation Tax Planning Worksheet (continued)

	Gross Amt.	Pct.	Net Amount
Add Back:			
Capital losses			
Penalties and fines			
Excess charitable contributions			
Meals and entertainment		50%	
Nondeductible dues			
Political contributions			
Officers' life insurance			
Disability insurance			
Other			
Taxable income <loss>			

Tax Planning/Awareness for Passthrough Entities and Their Owners

Passthrough entities report their income, deductions, expenses, and credits to their owner/shareholders via a form called a K-1. The K-1 is each owner/shareholder's pro rata share of items coming from Schedule K of the respective return (either Form 1065 or 1120S).

Various items of income and expense are reported as separate line items on Schedule K-1. The reason for this presentation is that these items flow into the owner/shareholder's individual tax return and are either subject to a limitation at that level or are used to calculate a limitation on the individual return. Examples of these amounts are § 179 depreciation, charitable contributions, interest, dividend and royalty income, and capital gains and losses.

There are not many tax planning opportunities specifically available to taxpayers organized within these entities. Rather, there are a number of special rules that affect the owner/shareholders of passthrough entities. Several of these rules will be discussed below.

The § 179 depreciation (expense election deduction) is limited for each individual to the same amount per year as noted above for corporations. Therefore, those individuals involved in many passthrough entities that are also able to exercise some level of control over the expensing election may have planning opportunities available.

EXAMPLE 10.9

Dr. James owns a medical practice as a sole proprietor and has $50,000 in asset purchases during the year 2013 (per the table above, $25,000 in § 179 expense election is available). He is also a 50 percent owner (and an active participant) in an ambulatory surgical center (ASC) partnership with $200,000 in asset purchases and a 10 percent owner in five additional unrelated oil and gas partnerships that each utilized their $20,000 section 179 deduction in the year 2013. Dr. James cannot do anything to influence the expense election in each of the five oil & gas partnerships. Therefore, he already has $10,000 in § 179 deduction before taking into account the acquisitions in his practice and the ASC. Dr. James can maximize the expensing election in the ASC of $10,000 ($20,000 × 50% ownership) and have his practice depreciate the new assets over their useful lives. Or, if all entities maximize the expensing election, Dr. James ends up with a § 179 carryover of $25,000 ($25,000 × 100% ownership in his practice).

EXAMPLE 10.10

Assume the same facts as above except that the practice purchases $520,000 in assets in the year 2013. Because the asset purchase limitation has been exceeded, Dr. James will not be able to deduct any § 179 expense in his practice. In addition, if any other entity has reported § 179 depreciation to him, he will lose that deduction because his practice's purchases have made him ineligible to take any § 179 deduction in the year 2013. Therefore, he loses the $10,000 deduction from the oil & gas partnerships and whatever the ASC elects in the year 2013.

Several problems exist where partners or shareholders are concerned. Namely, they also have opinions about whether to take such deductions or not and their tax situations may all be different from one another. This can create problems when planning for maximizing such deductions without generating unreasonable carryovers or losses. Although the § 179 expense election carryover does not expire after some finite period of time, it is still not wise to generate large annual carryovers unless there is some assurance they will be used within the foreseeable future.

Charitable contributions flow through to the individual tax returns of the respective partner or shareholder. The limitation for the contribution deduction is applied to each individual at his individual level. Each individual's tax scenario is unique; therefore, the ability to deduct a contribution may differ from taxpayer to taxpayer.

Interest, dividends, annuities, and royalties are among the income items stated separately on the K-1. The reason these items flow through to the individual taxpayer is that investment income is the reference point for the limitation to the deduction of investment interest expense. If the passthrough entity has excess cash in an operating account, the movement of the excess above operational necessity could be invested to generate additional income to flow through to the owners and increase their individual ability to deduct investment interest.

Capital gains and losses flow through to the individual's return to allow for the calculation of the net capital loss limitation at the individual taxpayer level. This is an area where periodic updates by the passthrough entity can be beneficial to the individual owners in year-end planning for capital gain and loss offsets.

Owners of a C Corporation can receive health coverage on a tax-free basis.

The corporation can fully deduct its premiums. In contrast, S Corporation shareholders must report the benefit as income and then deduct the premiums from gross income on their personal returns—this is merely a wash. Self-employed individuals also deduct their premiums from gross income on their personal returns; they cannot reduce their business income by the premiums allocable to their personal coverage and wind up effectively paying self-employment tax on the premiums.

A C Corporation can also set up medical reimbursement plans to pay fixed dollar amounts for out-of-pocket medical costs of employees. As long as the plan is nondiscriminatory (i.e., does not favor owners), the reimbursements are not taxable to employees, while they are deductible by the corporation. One client of mine who had a severe disability was able to handle many of his medical costs through the reimbursement plan that covered his corporate employees—himself and his wife.

Caution

Cafeteria plans are another area that owners of passthrough entities need to be aware of when planning for deductions. The owners of these entities usually look to see the individual benefit available to them before agreeing to provide such a plan for the benefit of all employees. However, the rules associated with cafeteria plans apply "discrimination rules" to see whether the owners are receiving a disproportionately high amount of the cafeteria plan benefits. If this is the case, the ability for owners to participate will be limited.

Caution

Owners need to take care in the type of retirement plan being utilized since the participation of the owners is limited to a percentage of the participation of the nonowners. This is a simplified explanation, but provides the notice that close review is required before choosing a retirement plan within a passthrough entity. In addition, owners are not allowed to make loans against retirement plan balances while nonowner employees are allowed to borrow from the plan, if provided for in the plan document.

OTHER POTENTIAL DEDUCTIONS

The goal of paying less income tax requires some up front analysis to identify all business expenses and capture them within the entity's accounting system. In addition to the typical business expenses deducted by the entity, list all personally paid expenses that benefit the practice. The following is a partial list that may appropriately be allocated to the practice:

- Cellular phone: many medical professionals completely deduct the cost where the number is given to the answering service.
- Internet access: where time is spent communicating with the office, other medical professionals or performing research.
- Home computer, telephone lines, periodicals, and books: to the extent used for the practice.
- Automobile expenses: it is almost always more beneficial for an entity to own a vehicle and charge personal use back to an individual owner. These rules are complex and should be discussed with a tax advisor for specifics in each state. One disadvantage has to do with the purchase of commercial auto insurance, which can be significantly more expensive than personal auto insurance. There are also liability issues to review. Therefore, care needs to be exercised before acting in this area.

The core deductions for passthrough entities are similar to the basic business deductions allowable for every entity. The rules noted above are different for passthroughs and, although not all inclusive, the noted items cover the most common differences faced by healthcare professionals. Most of the tax planning issues with passthroughs flow to the tax returns of the taxpayers they affect.

CONCLUSION

The objective of tax planning is to arrive at the lowest overall tax cost on the activities performed. This chapter addressed methods and strategies to reduce federal and state income taxes.

COLLABORATE

Discuss this chapter online with others at www.MedicalExecutivePost.com.

ACKNOWLEDGMENTS

To Thomas P. McGuinness, CPA, CVA of Reimer, McGuinness & Associates, PC in Houston, Texas; Thomas Bucek, CPA, CVA in Houston, Texas; and Dr. David Edward Marcinko, MBA, CMP™.

FURTHER READING

Ernst & Young: *Tax Guide 2014*. Wiley, New York, 2014.
Lasser, JK: *Your Income Tax 2014: For Preparing Your 2013 Tax Return*. Wiley, New York, 2013.
McGuinness, TP and Bucek, T: *Income Taxation. In Financial Planning for Physicians*. JB Publishing, Sudbury, MA, 2004.
2014 Master Tax Guide CCH Incorporated, Chicago, Illinois, 2014.

ADDITIONAL REFERENCES

From the Internal Revenue Service website (www.IRS.gov)

- How Obamacare Affects HSAs and Cafeteria Plan Accounts
- Health Insurance Tax Breaks for the Self-Employed
- Self-Employed/S Corporation Compensation and Medical Insurance Issues
- Internal Revenue Section 267

From the Small Business Administration's website (www.SBA.gov)
- Five reasons to be a C Corporation

11 Introduction to Major Investment Vehicles and Concepts
A Primer on Securities with Risk and Return Analysis

Timothy J. McIntosh, Jeffrey S. Coons,
and David Edward Marcinko

CONTENTS

Any medical professional who wants to save money for retirement or plan for a child's education needs to understand the basic tenets of investing. It allows them to improve the prospects of meeting future financial goals.

INTRODUCTION

This chapter offers an introduction to a wide range of investment categories and alternative ideas. The diverse types of investments, including fixed income, equities, exchange traded funds (ETFs), mutual funds, and so on will be defined at the beginning of each section. Various security selection strategies will also be reviewed.

FIXED INCOME SECURITIES

An investment can take the form of a "real" asset, such as art, real estate, baseball cards, and so on, or "liquid" asset such as a bond. The first and one of the most basic liquid assets are fixed income securities.

As a vital part of a well-balanced portfolio, fixed income securities afford opportunities for safety and predictable cash flow. Fixed income instruments also provide for capital preservation of assets and limit the volatility of an investor's diversified portfolio. A fixed income investment is a debt security, similar to an IOU. When you purchase a fixed income investment, you are simply lending money to an entity. This entity could be a government, municipality, or corporation. In return for the funds lended to the entity, the issuer provides you with a promise to pay a specified rate of interest during the life of the fixed income security and to ultimately repay the face value (also known as the principal) when it matures, or comes due. Among the most popular types of fixed income investments are U.S. government securities (bills, notes, and Treasuries), mortgage- and asset-backed securities, municipal bonds, corporate bonds, and foreign government bonds.

Here is a list of the major fixed income securities:

1. *Treasury Securities.* The U.S. Treasury owns the printing press for the dollars it borrows. Treasury securities are considered the most creditworthy or, in other words, the most likely to be paid back. In fact, the yield on a Treasury security is often referred to as the "risk-free" rate of return, since the probability of default is practically nonexistent. Treasury bills have a maturity of less than 1 year and, like zero coupon bonds, are sold at a discount to par value in lieu of paying interest payments. Treasury notes have a maturity of 1–10 years and Treasury bonds have a stated maturity in excess of 10 years.

2. *Agency Bonds.* In contrast to Treasury bonds, agency bonds tend to be backed by loans or other revenue generating activities of that specific governmental agency. While agency bonds are typically backed by the "full faith and credit of the U.S. government," there is slightly less certainty regarding the coupon and principal payments. Examples of agencies issuing fixed income securities include Government National Mortgage Association (GNMA), Federal National Mortgage Association (FNMA), and Federal Home Loan Mortgage Corporation (FHLMC).

3. *Municipal Bonds.* A municipal bond is a fixed income security issued by a state or local governmental institution, and may represent a general obligation backed by the taxation powers of the municipality or a revenue bond backed by the revenue generated from a specific project. Examples of projects used to back revenue bonds include water and sewer, hospitals, housing, and airports. Since revenue bonds are typically backed only by one source of the municipality's total revenue sources, general obligation bonds tend to have stronger creditworthiness than revenue bonds. One characteristic of most municipal bonds is that their coupon payments are often exempt from federal income taxes, as well as state taxation for taxpayers in the state of issue, which is why these securities are also generally referred to as tax-exempt securities.

4. *Corporate Bonds.* Corporate bonds are a debt security issued by a corporation and sold to investors. The backing for the bond is usually the payment ability of the company, which is typically money to be earned from future operations. Corporate bonds are considered a higher risk than government bonds. As a result, interest rates are almost always higher, even for top-flight credit quality companies. Corporate bonds are issued in blocks of $1000 (also known as par value). Corporate bonds may also have call provisions to allow for early

prepayment if prevailing rates change. Most corporate bonds provide taxable interest to investors. Fixed income corporate securities with a maturity of less than 1 year are generally referred to as short-term debt securities that include commercial paper and corporate certificates of deposit (CD).

5. *Foreign Bonds.* A foreign bond is a debt security issued by a borrower from outside the country, whose currency the bond is denominated, and in which the bond is sold. For example, a bond denominated in U.S. dollars that is issued in the United States by the government of Canada is a foreign bond. A foreign bond allows an investor a measure of international diversification without subjection to the risk of changes in relative currency values.

FIXED INCOME RETURNS AND HISTORY

The average U.S. government bond return since 1926 is 5.40% (Table 11.1). However the returns are highly unstable. Bond returns are most dependent on the starting interest rate and the changes in general interest rates over time; that is, when interest rates increase, the value of bonds decrease, or vice versa. This fact may have a dramatic impact on future expected returns. Throughout the Great Depression of 1929–1933, bond yields declined as economic growth and inflation turned negative. Under the New Deal in the 1930s, the U.S. Treasury issued new bonds at low interest rates to fund public works and America's preparation for and entry into World War II. This kept yields in check for the decade.

The 10-year U.S. Treasury bond yielded 3.29% at the start of 1930, but declined to 2.21% by the end of the decade. Interest plus gains in price appreciation resulted in a total return of 4.48%. Over the decade of the 1940s, inflation picked up averaging 6.1% while 10-year Treasury yields averaged only 2.33%. The total return during the 1940s was a mere 1.82%, a quote below the average rate of inflation. During the 1950s, economic growth was strong and interest rates began the slowly climb higher. By the end of the decade, 10-year U.S. Treasuries were yielding 4.72%. In fact, the 40-year period from 1940 to 1979 provides an example of an extended stage of rising bond yields. Again, changes in yields have a hefty impact on bond prices.

As bond yields first rise in a low-interest rate environment, capital losses are more pronounced as lower interest payments only partially offset the capital losses. As yields increase to greater amounts, higher annual interest payments are more successful in offsetting the price declines. This latter concept was demonstrated in the 1970s when bond yields and inflation both increased dramatically. Yields on 10-year Treasury Bonds increased from 7.79% in 1970 to 10.8% by 1980. The annualized return for the decade was an above average 6.97%. However, much of the return

TABLE 11.1
Compound Annualized Total Returns (%) Ending March 2012

	IA SBBI Interterm Government Bond	IIA SBBI Long-Term Government Bond
1 year	2.24	4.32
5 year	5.17	7.79
10 year	6.31	8.20
20 year	7.39	9.61
30 year	8.57	9.93
January 1926–March 2012	5.40	5.60

Source: Adapted from Loughran, T: *Journal of Financial and Quantitative Analysis* 32, 249–268, 1997.

earned from interest was offset by price loss due to increasing inflation. Inflation averaged 7.8% during the 10-year period. Again the return is comprised of a capital loss of 4.5% offset by interest earned of 10.5%.

The 1970s marked the end of rising interest rates and led to one of the great bull markets in history. Federal Reserve Chairman Paul Volcker raised interest rates to as high as 20% to tame inflation during 1981. In the years that followed, inflation and interest rates declined rapidly, pushing up bond prices. The 10-year Treasury yield, which reached a high of 15.8% in September 1981, fell to as low as 2.05% on December 30, 2008. Investors reaped the rewards, getting both interest alongside capital appreciation from declining bond yields. The average annual gain for 10-year Treasury bonds was 10.36% through the 1980s. For the 1990s, the annualized return was 7.53%. The return over the previous decade matched the long-term average, at 5.7%. In 2014, the 10-year Treasury bond yields slightly under 2%. Thus, after five decades, we have returned to a similar interest rate period as in the late 1940s. This does not augur well for the future.

Most of the longer-term returns from bonds over the preceding 80 years have come from the four-decade period from 1960 to 2000. It is during this time phase that bonds provided a higher than average yield component. Combined with the capital appreciation factor from declining yields during the 1980s, bonds produced outsized returns for investors for nearly half a century.

GAZING INTO THE FUTURE

Given that government bond yields today are at historical lows, the opportunity for price appreciation is minimal. More likely, the collection of interest payments will provide most, if not all, of market returns. Additionally, interest rates could also trend up over the ensuing decade. This would result in capital losses as bond prices decline, reducing total return further. Much like the decade of the 1940s, total returns from bonds will most likely be subdued as either market interest rates remain constant or interest rates trend upwards. Most certainly investors cannot expect an average long-term return of 5.40%. A 3% total return over the ensuing decade is most probable. The problem with this examination is that most individual investors have a substantial portion of their assets in bonds, especially of the government sort. As the average total portfolio-return target for most investors is 6–8% on an annualized basis, investors must expect either a substantial decline in interest rates from the current historic lows, or that stocks will make up the difference.

Although bonds do present moderate investments returns for today's investor, without bonds as part of a portfolio, investment losses could be a much higher percentage if invested in stocks alone. Although stocks do generate a higher rate of return over a long period, in short or immediate term, they may well be outperformed by bonds, especially at critical periods in the economic cycle. Bonds in general are known for the stability and predictability of returns. Bonds, especially those of the government kind, have a low standard deviation (volatility). In fact, bonds are one of the least risky asset classes an investor can own. When combining bonds in a diversified portfolio, you will lower your overall risk. The tradeoff, of course, is the return will be lower than an all stock portfolio. Most investors have money parked in bonds of the government type, that is, notes, bills, or bonds. The reason for this has to do with risk and diversification. Government bonds have one of the lowest risk profiles of any asset class, and have generally produced consistent returns. Government bonds are also thought to maintain a very low correlation (a statistical measure of how two securities move in relation to each other) with equities. The long-term average correlation is about 0.09.

However, this verity has to be examined on a long-term framework. In fact, correlations between the U.S. stocks and treasury bonds have swung widely over the past 80 years. The correlation was positive for most of the late 1930s and throughout the 1940s. In the 1950s, the correlation was actually negative as stocks advanced strongly and bonds suffered from declining prices (due to increasing interest rates). From the mid-1960s until 2000 there was a positive correlation, averaging about 0.50. The correlation turned negative once gain during the past decade. This was primarily due to the fact that stocks struggled mightily with two large bear market declines (2002, 2008), while bonds rallied strongly as interest rates declined. So much of the supposed low or negative correlation depends upon what time period you examine. The principal problem with owning government bonds is the negative correlation an investor is looking for only appears sporadically throughout history.

There are a number of risk variables to consider when investing in bonds as they may affect the value of the bond investment over time. These variables include changes in interest rates, income payments, bond maturity, redemption features, credit quality, and priority in capital structure, price, yield, tax status, and other provisions.

Here are some of the most common risks associated with fixed income securities.

Interest Rate Risk

The market value of the securities will be inversely affected by movements in interest rates. When rates rise, market prices of existing debt securities fall as these securities become less attractive to investors when compared to higher coupon new issues. As prices decline, bonds become cheaper so the overall return, when taking into account the discount, can compete with newly issued bonds at higher yields. When interest rates fall, market prices on existing fixed income securities tend to rise because these bonds become more attractive when compared to the newly issued bonds priced at lower rates.

Price Risk

Investors who need access to their principal prior to maturity have to rely on the secondary market to sell their securities. The price received may be more or less than the original purchase price and may depend, in general, on the level of interest rates, time to term, credit quality of the issuer, and liquidity. Among other reasons, prices may also be affected by current market conditions, or by the size of the trade (prices may be different for 10 bonds vs. 1000 bonds), and so on. It is important to note that selling a security prior to maturity may affect actual yield received, which may be different than the yield at which the bond was originally purchased. This is because the initially quoted yield assumed holding the bond to term. As mentioned above, there is an inverse relationship between interest rates and bond prices. Therefore, when interest rates decline, bond prices increase, and when interest rates increase, bond prices decline. Generally, longer maturity bonds will be more sensitive to interest rate changes. Dollar for dollar, a long-term bond should go up or down in value more than a short-term bond for the same change in yield. Price risk can be determined through a statistic called duration, which is featured at the end of the fixed income section.

Liquidity Risk

Liquidity risk is the risk that an investor will be unable to sell securities due to a lack of demand from potential buyers, sell them at a substantial loss, and/or incur substantial transaction costs in the sale process. Broker/dealers, although not obligated to do so, may provide secondary markets.

Reinvestment Risk

Downward trends in interest rates also create reinvestment risk, or the risk that the income and/or principal repayments will have to be invested at lower rates. Reinvestment risk is an important consideration for investors in callable securities. Some bonds may be issued with a call feature that allows the issuer to call, or repay, bonds prior to maturity. This generally happens if the market rates fall low enough for the issuer to save money by repaying existing higher coupon bonds and issuing new ones at lower rates. Investors will stop receiving the coupon payments if the bonds are called. Generally, callable fixed income securities will not appreciate in value as much as comparable noncallable securities.

Prepayment Risk

Similar to call risk, prepayment risk is the risk that the issuer may repay bonds prior to maturity. This type of risk is generally associated with mortgage-backed securities. Homeowners tend to prepay their mortgages at times that are advantageous to their needs, which may be in conflict with the holders of the mortgage-backed securities. If the bonds are repaid early, investors face the risk of reinvesting at lower rates.

Purchasing Power Risk

Fixed income investors often focus on the real rate of return, or the actual return minus the rate of inflation. Rising inflation has a negative impact on real rates of return because inflation reduces the purchasing power of the investment income and principal.

CORPORATE BOND ADVANTAGES

One higher yielding security to consider is corporate bonds. Corporate bonds are debts issued by a wide type of the U.S. and foreign corporations. Surprisingly, in terms of total face value of bonds outstanding, the corporate bond market is bigger than each of the markets for municipal bonds, the U.S. treasury securities, and government agencies securities. Unlike government bonds, corporate bonds are subject to credit risk, which refers to the probability of, and potential loss arising from, a credit event such as defaulting on scheduled payments, filing for bankruptcy, or restructuring. Physician-investors in corporate bonds have an extensive range of selections when it comes to bond maturity, interest rates, credit quality, and provisions. The corporate bond market is generally divided into two markets, those that are investment grade and those marked as junk. An investment grade rating that indicates that a corporate bond issuer has a relatively low risk of default. Bond rating firms, such as Standard & Poor's or Moody's, use different designations consisting of upper- and lower-case letters "A" and "B" to identify a bond's credit quality rating. For example, S&P utilizes AAA and AA as its high credit quality rating and, A and BBB for its medium credit quality rating. These ratings are all considered investment grade. Credit ratings for bonds below these designations (BB, B, CCC, etc.) are considered low credit quality, and are commonly referred to as speculative (junk) bonds (Table 11.2).

Here are some features of corporate bonds:

1. Corporate bonds are hybrids, that is, maintaining a dual nature: equity and bond. As debt, its value is closely linked to the quality of the issuer, its earnings and revenue, and the reasonability of default. This risk is indicated through the interest rate paid by the issuer.

TABLE 11.2
Standard & Poor's, Moody's, and Fitch's Have the Following Credit Ratings Scale

	Standard & Poor's	Moody's	Fitch's
Investment Grade	AAA	Aaa	AAA
	AA	Aa	AA
	A	A	A
	BBB	Baa	BBB
Speculative (junk) Grade	BB	Ba	BB
	B	B	B
	CCC	Caa	CCC
	CC	Ca	CC
	C	C	C

2. Corporate bonds are generally less sensitive to a rise in interest rates.
3. Corporate bonds have less liquidity in the capital markets. The lack of liquidity gives rise to market distortions between the value of the bond and its market price. The more uncertain in the markets or economy, the greater is the potential distortion in corporate bond pricing.

Historically, the promised yield on the U.S. corporate bonds rated by S&P as AAA (the highest quality bonds issued only by blue chip companies) has been 0.7% higher (also known as yield spread) than on similar maturity U.S. Treasuries. BBB bonds, the lowest grade bonds deemed by S&P still to be considered investment grade, have a historical yield spread of 1.9% above Treasuries. Credit Suisse Company publishes a yearbook that examines the long-term returns of various asset classes, including corporate bonds. As the U.S. has consistent corporate bond data going back to 1900, the return subset is quite large. Credit Suisse has found that the long-term return of corporate bonds over 111 years, from 1900 to 2010, was 2.52% per year. This was 0.68% per year more than on the U.S. Treasuries. The firm finds these returns very close to the generalized promised yields of AAA bonds, which has averaged 0.70% above Treasury Bonds. Published academic research in the past 5 years also reports the advantage of favoring corporate bonds over Treasury Bonds.

Alexander Kozhemiakin (2007) demonstrated in his study published in *The Journal of Portfolio Management* that the excess return of corporate bonds over treasuries is consistent over time. Furthermore, he found that as investors move to lower quality bonds, the return differentials become more pronounced. This is especially true in the BB category, where the excess return is the highest of any grade. The lower tier of the investment-grade spectrum (A/BBB) accounts for two thirds of the investment-grade market capitalization and trading activity in market is active. The excess returns over the U.S. Treasuries are listed in Tables 11.3 and 11.4.

TABLE 11.3

Corporate Bonds Historical Returns and Risk%, January 1985–December 2005

Annualized Excess Return over the U.S. Treasuries	Return	
AAA/AA Rating	8.9%	1.4%
A Rating	9.2%	1.7%
BBB Rating	9.3%	1.8%
BB Rating	11.0%	3.3%
B Rating	9.7%	2.0%
CCC Rating	2.8%	−2.7%

Source: Kozhemiakin, A. 2007. The risk premium of corporate bonds. *The Journal of Portfolio Management*, 33, 101–109.

TABLE 11.4

Performance of BB High-Yield Bonds versus Index

Historical Returns and Risk (%)	5 Year (%)	10 Years (%)	20 Years (%)
BB Rated Bonds	9.29	8.78	9.63
Barclays Aggregate Bond Index	6.52	5.74	6.80
Barclays Govt. Bond Index	5.62	4.87	5.76

An investor should expect corporate bonds to trade at higher yields than Treasury bonds over extended periods of time. The primary difference between the two yields is known as the credit spread. However, credit risk is not the only factor in determining the excess returns of corporate bonds over government bonds. Other key factors include tax treatment, illiquidity, and the unique provisions that are included in the contracts of corporate bonds. These are characteristics that government bonds do not share. Although most investors will look at the excess returns as coming from pure credit risk, academic research has concluded otherwise.

Credit risk is in fact not the primary factor in explaining excess returns. Jing-zhi Huang of Penn State University and Ming Huang of Stanford University found that within the investment grade bond arena, less than one-third of the excess return was associated with default risk. Additional studies confirm these findings. Professors Gordon Delianedis and Robert Geske of The Anderson School at UCLA found that for AAA rated firms, only a small fraction (5%) could be attributed to actual default risk. For BBB-rated firms, which are those rated just above junk, only 22% of the credit spread can be attributed to default risk. The team further concluded that credit risk and credit spreads above government bonds are not primarily explained by default, leverage, or a firm's specific risk—but are primarily attributable to taxes, jumps, liquidity, and market risk factors.

It is interesting to view whether these studies are consistent with actual default rates. According to the aforementioned Credit Suisse yearbook, default rates for all rated corporate bond issuers since 1900 has averaged 1.14% per year, while for riskier high-yield bonds the average was 2.8%. Of course over certain chaotic economic periods the default rate has reached much higher extremes. Default rates were at the highest levels following the Great Depression, at 8.4% in 1933 for high-grade bonds, while high-yield bonds had a default rate that year of 15.4%. The default rate for all corporate bonds reached 3.7% in the recession of 2001. The second worst episode for default rates followed the recent credit crisis and, in 2009, the default rate on all rated bonds was 5.4%, while that on high-yield bonds was just over 13%. Given the low default rates over history, a long-run return premium of 0.68% per year for the highest grade, AAA, seems puzzlingly high. For the riskier element of the corporate bond market, a 3% plus premium for BB bonds seems downright generous, given the fact that the annual default rate for these bonds is less than 3%.

Furthermore, many researchers have found the 3% default rate on the edge of junk status, BB, are overstated. Stephen Kealhofer, Sherry Kwok, Wenlong Weng found that true default rates for AAA bonds were only 0.13% while even the riskier BB rating category only showed a default rate of 1.42%. Part of this credit premium is undoubtedly a risk of default premium, but given that the actual risk of nonpayment has been quite low, it seems likely that other factors are at work.

One primary theory for why the wide yield spread for corporate bonds persists is the typical illiquidity of these bonds. The foundation for excess returns is that the illiquidity of corporate bonds has a larger than customary effect. While corporate bonds are traded widely on markets such as the New York Stock Exchange, the volume of transactions is far less than for government bonds. Since increased liquidity is an attractive quality of any investment, investors will thus demand extra remuneration for holding securities that are less liquid and thus more expensive to sell. For corporate bonds, this illiquidity premium shows up in higher interest rate spreads over otherwise comparable government securities. That is the theory of several prominent researchers.

Patrick Houweling, Albert Mentink, and Ton Vorst (2005) analyzed the effect of liquidity risk on corporate bond credit spreads based on a sample of 999 investment-grade corporate bonds. In their paper, they controlled two common factors (1) the excess return from the stock market and (2) the excess return of long-term corporate bonds over long-term Treasury bonds in addition to the rating and maturity of each bond. They found that liquidity risk is priced into credit spreads and does explain a significant portion of observed credit risk spreads.

In addition to liquidity risk, corporate bonds also have a substantial amount of volatility risk. This is due to the fact that although actual default risk is below expectations, default is most likely to take place in recessions. While relatively protected for most economic periods, corporate bonds thus become a far riskier asset in severe recessions. This has been demonstrated emphatically in the deep recession of 2008/2009. Corporate bonds returned a negative 21% in 2008, while the Barclays U.S. 5–10 Year Treasury Index returned 16.77%.

Many financial advisors argue the corporate bond asset class is less appropriate for long-term investors who hold a substantial portion of equity in their portfolio because other fixed income asset classes (namely government bonds) do a better job reducing the risk of the overall portfolio. In 2008, holding treasury bonds over corporate bonds would have resulted in a substantial reduction in portfolio volatility. However, in 2009, corporate bonds excelled and rebounded strongly alongside stocks. If an investor can withstand the extra volatility, especially during recessions, then corporate bonds will ultimately be the best asset class to own. It is especially rewarding if investors concentrate their corporate bond holdings within the BBB and BB ratings universe. These bonds typically will reward a bond investor with a 3% annualized premium over the same duration government bond.

INTERNATIONAL BOND ADVANTAGES

International bonds now account for more than 35% of the world's investable assets, and yet many investors have little or no exposure to these types of securities. International fixed income securities make up a noteworthy portion of the global investable market.

While investors in international bonds are exposed to the hazard of interest rate movements and political risks, the principal factors driving international bond prices are actually uncorrelated to the most common U.S. risk factors. This indicates a true diversification benefit for any investor. International bonds have become more prominent and attractive due to the increase in globalization and the pervasive expansion of debt issuance overseas, primarily by governments. There has been a near doubling of the relative weight of the non-U.S. bond market from approximately 19% in 2000 to approximately 37% in 2011. Thus, there is more selection of international bonds than ever for the U.S. investors.

Investing in international bonds involves contact to the movements of global currencies. This is the primary component of determining international bond returns. Alternations in currencies create an extra layer of volatility in these types of securities. However, that volatility actually enhances diversification benefits. One of the key considerations of any purchase of international bonds is whether or not to hedge the currency impact. These deviations create return volatility above the level inherent to the underlying investment. An allocation to an unhedged international bond does reflect an investor's bearish view of the U.S. dollar. This is because as the dollar depreciates against a foreign currency, an international bond will gain in value. The past 25-plus years have witnessed a long-term decline in the U.S. dollar, actually providing a tail wind for international bond investors. In fact, according to data from Vanguard, unhedged international bonds outperformed hedged bonds by 2.2 percentage points a year since 1987. The diversification benefit from international bonds is also attractive. From January 1, 1992 to March 31, 2012, the correlation between the Citigroup World Government Bond Index ex-U.S. 1–3 Years index and 5-year U.S. Treasury notes was a mere 0.35. An allocation to international bonds can amplify portfolio diversification across economies, currencies, and yield curves.

Purchasing Bonds

Trading individual bonds is not like trading stocks. Stocks can be bought at uniform prices and are traded through exchanges. Most bonds trade over the counter, and individual brokers price them. Price transparency has gotten better in the last decade. In 1999, the bond markets gained clearness from the House of Representatives' Bond Price Competition Improvement Act of 1999. Responding to this pioneering law, the site www.investinginbonds.com was established. This site provides current prices on bonds that have traded more than four times the previous day. With the advent of Investinginbonds.com and real-time reporting of many trades, investors are much better off today. Many well-regarded brokers including Schwab, Ameritrade, and Fidelity Investments now have dedicated websites devoted to bond trading and pricing. Fidelity Investments chose to disclose its fee structure for all bonds, making it clear what it will cost you per trade. Fidelity charges $1 per bond trade. Some online brokers charge a flat fee as well, ranging from $10.95 at Zions Direct to $45 at TD Ameritrade. Depending on the number of bonds trading, one may be more complimentary than another. The trading fee disclosures, however, do not divulge the spreads between the buy and sell price embedded in the transaction that some dealer is making in the channel. Keep in mind that only by comparison shopping can assist you in finding the best transaction price, after all fees are taken into account. Other sites may not charge any fee, but rather embed the profit in the spread.

Despite the difficulty in pricing and transparency, investing in individual bonds offers several rewards over purchasing bond mutual funds. First, you know exactly what you will be receiving in interest each year. You will also know the exact maturity date. Furthermore, your individual investment is protected against interest rate risk, at least over the full term to maturity. Both individual bonds and bond funds share interest-rate risk—mentioned above (the risk of locking up an investment at a given rate, only to see rates rise). This pushes bond prices down. At least with an individual bond, you can re-invest it at the higher market rate once the bond matures. But the lack of a fixed maturity date on a bond mutual fund causes an open-ended problem; there is no promise of the original investment back. Short of default, an individual bond will return all principal and pay all interest assuming you hold it to maturity. Bond funds are not likely to default as most funds maintain positions in hundreds of individual bonds. The force of interest rate risk to individual bond or bond mutual fund prices depends on the maturity of a bond investment: the longer the maturity of a bond or bond fund (average), the more the price will drop due to rising rates. This is known as duration.

Duration is a statistical term that measures the price sensitivity to yield; it is the primary measurement of a bond or bond fund's sensitivity to interest rate changes. Duration indicates approximately how much the price of a bond or bond fund will adjust in the reverse direction given a rise in interest rates. For instance, an individual bond with an average duration of 5 years will fall in value approximately 5% if rates rise by 1% and the opposite is accurate as well.

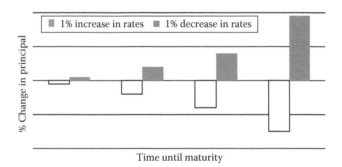

Source: Ibbotson Associates/Morningstar (2012), Chicago, Illinois.

Although stated in years, duration is not simply a gauge of time. Instead, duration signals how much the price of your bond investment is likely to oscillate when there is an up or down movement in interest rates. The higher the duration number, the more susceptible your bond investment will be to changes in interest rates. If you have money in a bond or bond fund that holds primarily long-term bonds, expect the value of that fund to decline, perhaps significantly, when interest rates rise. The higher a bond's duration, the greater its sensitivity to interest rates alterations. This means fluctuations in price, whether positive or negative, will be more prominent. For example, a bond fund with 10-year duration will diminish in value by 10% if interest rates increase by one percent. On the other hand, the bond fund will rise in value by 10% if interest rates descend by one percent. The important concept to remember is once you recognize a bond's or bond fund's duration, you can forecast how it will react to a change in interest rates.

Duration Primer

1. To locate your bond fund's duration, look for it in the mutual fund's fact sheet or the statistics section.
2. There are also online calculators (located at Appendix 1) available that compute an individual bond's duration.
3. Duration measured the general movement of interest rates and the impact on the prices of bonds. Corporate, municipal, and agency bonds are also impacted by various other factors such as credit risk, economic growth, state and city financing.

Fixed Income Summary

In summary, fixed income securities are promises from an issuer to pay a combination of periodic coupon payments and/or par value at maturity. In the simplest sense, the issuer of a fixed income security is borrowing money from the holder of the fixed income security. Assuming that an issuer does not default on the coupon or principal payments and that the security is held to maturity, then a bondholder will receive a total return over the life of the investment equal to the market yield when the security was purchased. In the interim, however, the total return will fluctuate depending upon such factors as changes in the perceived credit quality of the issuer and changes in market interest rates.

EQUITY SECURITIES

If a security represents legal title to a future stream of cash flows, then equity of a company designates ownership of earnings or profits after accounting for normal operating expenses, interest payments (e.g., coupon payments to bond holders), and taxes. In contrast to bondholders, holders of equity securities (i.e., shareholders) are considered owners of the company as opposed to creditors of the company. Typically, the primary benefit of being a shareholder in a company is that the investor benefits from the company's ability to generate profits. Thus, one way of analyzing the decision to acquire equity in company is to ask: "How much can the company earn above its fixed obligations?" If instead an equity investment is considered on a termination value basis, then equity represents title to corporate assets after payment of all debts. The latter viewpoint offers almost a "worst case" evaluative question: If the company was to shut its doors and discontinue operations, what is the value of the assets less liabilities?

When physician-investors talk about equities, most of the time they are referring to common stocks, which represent title to income after all other obligations of the corporation have been satisfied (including interest payments to bondholders). Common stock is the least senior of all securities issued by a corporation in that the obligations represented by all other securities and debts are expected to be paid before the common stock owner has a right to the assets or earnings. From a different perspective, a common stock holder has the ownership of all earnings after payment of expenses and taxes. Thus, if the company is extremely profitable, the common stockholder's upside is not limited by a fixed rate of return.

LOCATION OF THE ISSUER

Key differentiating features of equity securities include the issuer's location, size, and industrial classification. Domestic stocks are simply equity securities issued by corporations based in the United States, while foreign stocks are equities issued by companies headquartered outside of the United States. Foreign stocks are typically further divided into developed and emerging markets, with developing markets generally representing countries with relatively well-developed economies, financial markets, and property rights. In contrast, emerging market countries are typically characterized by smaller economies and relatively underdeveloped financial markets.

The U.S.-based investors can acquire foreign stocks in several ways. First, certain foreign stocks are traded directly on the U.S. stock exchanges or traded as American Depository Receipts (ADRs). An ADR is a security issued by a domestic financial institution, is traded on a U.S. exchange, and represents a specified number of shares of a foreign stock held in trust at an affiliated financial institution abroad. Second, with accelerating globalization of financial markets and improved transactional efficiency of foreign stock exchanges, investors can often make direct foreign investment by actually investing in shares of companies that are traded on exchanges outside of the United States. While the separation between domestic and foreign stocks is generally thought of as a way to identify greater or lesser sensitivity to the U.S. economy, this mindset fails to recognize that most corporations operate in an increasingly global economy. Many foreign and domestic multinational companies have as much exposure to foreign economies as the companies have to their home economy. On the other hand, the earnings of foreign corporations must be translated to the U.S. dollars for a U.S. investor, so sensitivity to the currency of the foreign stock's home country remains. Thus, investors must consider the risk of unfavorable currency fluctuations (i.e., currency risk) when investing in foreign stocks.

Size of the Issuer

Another differentiating feature among common stocks is the size of the company issuing the equity. Size is often measured by a stock's market capitalization, which is defined as the aggregate market value of the corporation's outstanding stock and calculated by multiplying outstanding shares by the current price per share. In general, companies are considered to be large capitalization stocks if their market capitalization exceeds $5.0 billion, while companies with a market capitalization of less than $1.5 billion are referred to as small cap stocks. Companies whose market capitalization falls between $1.5 billion and $5.0 billion are commonly referred to as midcap stocks, although these thresholds should only be used as rough guides since there are no universally accepted breakpoints used in the investment industry today.

Another classification that is related to size of a company is its seasoning, which is a concept related to the length of time over which a company has an operating history. The spectrum of seasoning runs from blue chip stocks to IPOs. Blue chip stocks are the equities of high quality, large, established companies. Many of the stocks included in the Dow Jones Industrial Average are considered to be blue chip stocks. In contrast to large, well-established companies, Initial Public Offerings or IPOs are stocks of relatively new companies that generally lack a long-term corporate earnings track record. While blue chip stocks have historically been considered safe stocks due to their large size and strong positions in their respective industries, it is important to remember that all investment decisions should be based on future expected returns. Just because a company is large and well established does not guarantee that the company's stock will make a good investment. For example, not too long ago Bethlehem Steel was considered a high-quality blue chip stock that investors could not go wrong; owning. However, as the 1980s showed, even a once dominant stock like Bethlehem Steel can fall on extremely hard times. Likewise, while the medical professional will often hear anecdotes of IPOs that turned out to be exceptional investments, many of these stocks may be considered speculative at best with significant risk of losing all of its value. Thus, it is important for investors to remember that there may be changes in a stock's fundamentals, as well as the market and economic environment. This means that any equity investment, even in blue chip stocks, need to be consistently evaluated and monitored. As an example, the strong stock market rally of the late 1990s was driven by a handful of large, well-established, blue chip and technology companies. Like the Nifty Fifty period of the mid-1970s; these stocks were hardest hit in the ensuing correction.

Industrial Classification

The final classification of common stocks discussed here is the separation of companies by the industry or economic sector in which their primary business operates. In fact, there are 11 economic sector classifications and 115 industry subclassifications according to Standard & Poor's. Stocks in the same industry tend to move together, because the companies' revenue and earnings tend to be influenced by common industry-wide factors. Just as the overall economy experiences periods of expansion and contraction (i.e., recession), specific industries experience periods of growth and decline that generally affect all companies in that industry. Likewise, some industries are more affected by economy-wide business cycles.

The distinction between cyclical stocks and defensive stocks lies in how closely related the stock's performance is to industry and economic cycles. Thus, stocks that operate in industries that are highly correlated to the strength of the domestic economy are considered to be cyclical stocks. For example, the construction and automobile industries are generally considered cyclical industries given that demand for their products is highly related to the current economic environment. In periods of weak or declining economic growth, demand for automobiles and new construction products decline, thus resulting in a decline in earnings for companies operating within those industries. Defensive stocks are viewed as being less susceptible to fluctuations in the overall economy. For example, since demand for food products is generally considered to be less dependent on the strength or weakness of the overall economy, food stocks are generally considered defensive stocks.

Dividends

If the definition of a security is title to a stream of cash flows, then the dividends a company is expected to pay to equity shareholders on a periodic basis (e.g., quarterly) are a clear source of return for an investor. A dividend is simply a distribution of (some portion of) the company's earnings to equity shareholders. Like a bond yield, a stock's dividend yield can be used to measure the income return on the stock. To determine a stock's dividend yield, the trailing year's dividends per share paid are divided by the current stock price. However, a key difference between a dividend yield and a bond yield is the level of certainty that can be assumed regarding future payments, since a bond's coupon is generally predetermined and its payment is expected to be senior to the payment of dividends.

After a company has determined that it has earned a profit, management has to decide what to do with those profits. One choice is to distribute the earnings to shareholders in the form of dividends, while another option is to reinvest the profits in the company. A company's management may determine that the shareholders interest is best served by using the earnings to pursue growth opportunities (capital expansion, research & development, etc.) at the corporate level. Thus, when management believes that its investment opportunities are likely to produce a higher return than what investors' could generate with their dividends or that reinvestment is needed to maintain its financial strength, the company will retain the earnings.

One of the biggest myths in investing is that capital appreciation accounts for the largest part of investors' gains. Dividends, or cash payments to shareholders actually account for a substantial part of an equity investor's total return. In fact since 1926, dividends have accounted for more than 40% of the total return of the S&P 500 stock index. In the past decade (2000–2009), the S&P 500's total return of −9% would have been a heftier loss of −24% had it not been for the 15% contribution from dividends.

History has shown that dividends have been a powerful source of total return in a diversified investment portfolio, especially during periods of market turbulence. In examining the prior eight decades of stock market performance (Table 11.5), dividends often account for more than 2/3 of the total return (1930s, 1940s, 1970s, and 2000s). If an investor avoided dividend paying stocks during these elongated time periods, most of the total gains would be lost.

During those decades such as the 2000s where the stock market struggled to advance, dividends were a significant element for investor survival. This is not only due to the dividends alone, but also

TABLE 11.5

Dividend Contribution of S&P 500 Return by Decade

Years	S&P 500 Price % Change	Dividend Contribution[a] (%)	Cumulative Total Return (%)	Dividends % of Total Return	Average Payout Ratio[b] (%)
1930s	−41.9	56.0	14.1	>100	90.1
1940s	34.8	100.3	135.0	74.3	59.4
1950s	256.7	180.0	436.7	41.2	54.6
1960s	53.7	54.2	107.9	50.2	56.0
1970s	17.2	59.1	76.4	77.4	45.5
1980s	227.4	143.1	370.5	38.6	48.6
1990s	315.7	117.1	432.8	27.0	47.6
2000s	−24.1	15.0	−9.1	>100	35.3
2010s	27.9	8.4	36.3	23.1	28.4

Source: Strategies as of December 31, 2012, Ibbetson Associates/Morningstar.

[a] DC.

[b] APR.

TABLE 11.6

Downside and Upside Capture Ratios of High Dividend Stocks, 1927–2011

The lower the number, the better	Downside Capture Ratio
Since 1927	81.53
50-year	67.45
30-year	65.86
20-year	65.83
10-year	81.61

Source: Kenneth French, December 31, 2011.

the risk element of stocks that pay dividends. Dividend stocks have historically provided lower overall volatility and stronger downside protection when markets decline. Since 1927, dividend stocks have consistently held up better than the broader market during downturns. You can measure downside risk through a statistic known as downside capture ratio. Downside capture ratio is a statistical measure of overall performance in a down stock market. An investment category, or investment manager, who has a down-market ratio less than 100 has outperformed the index during a falling stock market. For example, a down-market capture ratio of 80 indicates that the portfolio measure declined only 80% as much as the index during the period. The downside capture ratio of high-dividend-yielding stocks, since 1927, has been 81% or lower over various long-term periods (Table 11.6). Put a better way, during months that the S&P 500 stock index fell, dividend stocks declined by nearly 19% less than the broader market.

STOCK VALUATION

If investments are the reallocation of today's dollars for expected dollars in the future, why would an investor buy a common stock that does not pay a dividend? The simple answer is that the investor expects to be able to sell the stock later at a higher price as a result of some combination of higher valuations on the company's existing earnings power and/or growth in future earnings. While the

TABLE 11.7

Sample Stock Statistics

Stock	Price-to-Earnings Ratio	Price-to-Book Ratio	Price-to-Sales Ratio	Dividend Yield (%)	Consensus Earnings Growth Rate (%)	Market Cap ($MM)	Price-to-Earnings Growth Ratio
Dominion	56.2	3.3	2.8	3.5	6.0	$36.9	2.5
Boeing	23.7	11.2	1.2	1.5	11.4	$100.5	2.3
Ford	11.8	3.1	0.5	2.4	12.3	$64.3	0.6
Cisco	11.1	1.8	2.2	3.2	9.9	$108.2	2.8
McDonalds	17.1	6.2	3.4	3.3	9.1	$93.9	1.9
Microsoft	13.7	3.8	3.9	2.6	8.5	$306.3	1.2

Source: Morningstar, September 30, 2013.

safety of knowing that a company has been paying a dividend is comforting, the lack of dividend does not necessarily mean that investors will not be rewarded for owning stocks with either low dividend yields, or no dividend at all. An investor purchasing stocks is usually attempting to buy stocks that not only may pay dividends, but that will also increase in value over time.

Table 11.7 contains various statistics for a handful of stocks to illustrate that there can be dramatic differences in these statistics across different stocks. The primary statistic used by investment professionals to measure a corporation's earnings power is known as EPS or earnings per share, which are simply the company's per-share profits distributable to the common stockholders (i.e., what is left over after accounting for expenses, including interest payments on debt obligations, taxes, and preferred stock dividends).

The three most common measures used to quantify a stock's valuation are the price-to-book ratio, price-to-earnings ratio, and price-to-sales ratio. A stock's book value is generally defined as the accounting value of the firm's assets less its liabilities. Thus the price-to-book ratio identifies how much investors are willing to pay per dollar of net assets. Similarly, the price-to-earnings ratio indicates how much investors are willing to pay for a dollar of earnings. Unfortunately, a corporation's earnings are very easily manipulated by adjusting certain accounting "assumptions." Therefore, some investors prefer to use price-to-sales as a measure of a firm's value since revenues or sales are generally subject to fewer accounting assumptions. However, it is important for medical professionals or those who advise them to remember that, just because one stock may have a higher growth rate (or any other statistic) than another stock, it does not necessarily mean that the stock will produce a higher return.

Another key element for evaluating a firm is known as the PEG ratio. The PEG ratio (also known as the price/earnings to growth ratio) is a valuation metric for determining the trade-off between the earnings per share (EPS) and the company's expected future growth rate. In general, the P/E ratio is higher for a company with a higher growth rate. Thus using just the P/E ratio would make high-growth companies appear overrated in relation to competitive firms. It is assumed that by dividing the P/E ratio by the earnings growth rate, the resulting ratio is better for contrasting firms with different growth rates. PEG is an extensively employed indicator of a stock's feasible stock value. The PEG ratio of 1 is sometimes said to represent a good trade-off between the growth value and earnings. In general, the lower the PEG value, the more the firm is considered a good potential investment.

VALUATION APPROACHES

There are basically two different approaches for common stock valuation; top–down and bottom–up. Under either of the two fundamental approaches, an investor will have to work with individual company data. In reality, each of these approaches is used by investors and security analysts when doing fundamental analysis. With the bottom–up approach, investors focus directly on a company's prospects. Analysis of such information as the company's products, its competitive position, and its financial status leads to an estimate of the company's earnings potential and, ultimately, its value in the market. Considerable time and effort are required to produce the type of detailed financial analysis needed to understand a firm's standing. The emphasis in this approach is on finding companies with good long-term growth prospects, and making accurate earnings estimates. The top–down approach is the opposite of the bottom–up approach. Investors begin with the economy and the overall market, considering such important factors as interest rates and inflation. They next consider likely industry prospects, or sectors of the economy that are likely to do particularly well (or particularly poorly). Finally, having decided that factors are favorable for investing, and having determined which parts of the overall economy are likely to perform well, individual companies are analyzed.

Growth Stocks: Catching the Momentum

The growth style of investing focuses on companies with strong earnings and accelerating capital growth. A growth investor will make investment decisions based on forecasts of continuing growth in earnings. Growth investing emphasizes qualitative criteria, including value judgments about the company, its markets, its management, and its ability to extract future earnings growth from the particular industry. Quantitative indicators of interest to the growth investor include high Price/Earnings ratios, Price/Sales ratios, and low dividend yields. A high P/E ratio suggests that the market is prepared to pay more per share in anticipation of future earnings. A low dividend yield suggests that the company is reinvesting rather than distributing profits. These indicators are considered in relation to the company's immediate competitors. The companies with the highest P/E ratios relative to their industry will often be dominant within their market segment and have strong growth prospects. Growth investors will generally focus on premium and leading-edge companies.

Some industry sectors by their nature have stronger growth characteristics, particularly more innovative and speculative industries. For example, during the bull market run on the U.S. stock markets during the late 1990s, the technology sector was a major area of growth investment. On observing strong earnings growth, a growth investor will decide whether to buy shares based on whether the company's growth is going to continue at its present rate, to increase, or to decrease. If it is expected to increase, the growth investor will consider it a candidate for purchase. The key research question is: at what point will the company's growth flatten out, or fall? If a company's growth rate slows or reverses, it is no longer attractive to a growth investor. Growth investors are normally prepared to pay a premium for what they believe to be high-quality shares. The potential downside in growth investing is that if a company goes into sudden decline and the share price falls, you can lose capital value rapidly.

Growth stocks carry high expectations of above-average future growth in earnings and above-average valuations. Investors expect these stocks to perform well in the future and are willing to pay high P/E multiples for this expected growth. The danger is that the price may become too high. Generally, once a company sports a P/E ratio above 50, the risk significantly escalates. Many technology growth stocks traded at a P/E ratio of above 100 during 1999. This is unsustainable. No company in the history of the stock market has been able to maintain such a high P/E level for a sustained period of time.

Value Stocks: Looking for Bargains

The bargain-hunting value style is looking for shares that are underpriced in relation to the company's future potential. A value investor will invest in a company in the expectation that its shares will increase in value over time. Value investing is based essentially on quantitative criteria; asset values, cash flow, and discounted future earnings. The key properties of value shares are low Price/Earnings, Price/Sales ratios, and normally higher dividend yields.

On observing a company's earnings growth, a value manager will decide whether to buy shares based on the company's consistency or recovery prospects. The key research questions are: (1)

Does the current P/E ratio warrant an investment in a slow growth company or, (2) Is the company a higher growth candidate that has dropped in price due to a temporary problem. If this is the case, will the company's earnings growth recover, and if so, when? The key to value investing is to find bargain shares (priced low historically or for temporary and/or irrational reasons), avoiding shares that are merely cheap (priced low because the company is failing).

The buying opportunity is identified when a company undergoing some immediate problems is perceived to have good chances of recovery in the medium to long term. If there is a loss in market confidence in the company, the share price may fall, and the value investor can step in. Once the share price has achieved a suitable value, reflecting the predicted turnaround in company performance, the shareholding is sold, realizing a capital gain. A potential risk in value investing is that the company may not turn around, in which case the share price may stay static or fall.

Performance of Growth and Value Stocks

Although many academics argue that value stocks outperform growth stocks, the returns for individuals investing through mutual funds demonstrate a near match. A 2005 study *Do Investors Capture the Value Premium?*, written by Todd Houge at The University of Iowa and Tim Loughran at The University of Notre Dame, found that large company mutual funds in both the value and growth styles returned just over 11% for the period of 1975–2002. This paper contradicted many studies that demonstrated owning value stocks offers better long-term performance than growth stocks. These studies, led by Eugene Fama, PhD, and Kenneth French, PhD, established the current consensus that the value style of investing does indeed offer a return premium. There are several theories as to why this has been the case, among the most persuasive being a series of behavioral arguments put forth by leading researchers. These studies suggest that the outperformance of value stocks may result from investors' tendency toward common behavioral traits, including the belief that the future will be similar to the past, overreaction to unexpected events, "herding" behavior which leads at times to overemphasis of a particular style or sector, overconfidence, and aversion to regret. All of these behaviors can cause price anomalies that create buying opportunities for value investors. Another key ingredient argued for value outperformance is lower business appraisals. Value stocks are plainly confined to a P/E range, whereas growth stocks have an upper limit that is infinite. When growth stocks reach a high plateau in regard to P/E ratios, the ensuing returns are generally much lower than the category average over time. In addition, growth stocks tend to lose more in bear markets. In the last two major bear markets, growth stocks fared far worse than value. From January 1973 until late 1974, large growth stocks lost 45% of their value, while large value stocks lost 26% . Similarly, from April 2000 to September 2002, large growth stocks lost 46% versus only 27% for large value stocks. These losses, academics insist, dramatically reduce the long-term investment returns of growth stocks.

However, the study by Houge and Loughran reasoned that although a premium may exist, investors have not been able to capture the excess return through mutual funds. The study also maintained that any potential value premium is generated outside the securities held by most mutual funds. Simply put, being growth or value had no material impact on a mutual fund's performance. Listed below in the table are the annualized returns and standard deviations for return data from January 1975 through December 2002.

Index	Return (%)	SD (%)
S&P 500	11.53	14.88
Large Growth Funds	11.30	16.65
Large Value Funds	11.41	15.39

Source: Houge/Loughran Study.

The Hough/Loughran study also found that the returns by style also varied over time. From 1965 to 1983, a period widely known to favor the value style, large value funds averaged a 9.92% annual return, compared to 8.73% for large growth funds. This performance differential reverses over 1984–2001, as large growth funds generated a 14.1% average return compared to 12.9% for large value funds. Thus, one style can outperform in any time period. However, although the long-term returns are nearly identical, large differences between value and growth returns happen over time. This is especially the case over the last 10 years as growth and value have had extraordinary return differences—sometimes over *30 percentage points* of underperformance. Table 11.8 indicates the return differential between the value and growth styles since 1992.

Between the third quarter of 1994 and the second quarter of 2000, the S&P Growth Index produced annualized total returns of 30%, versus only about 18% for the S&P Value Index. Since 2000, value has turned the tables and dramatically outperformed growth. Growth has only outperformed value in 2 of the past 8 years. Since the two styles are successful at different times, *combining them in one portfolio* can create a buffer against dramatic swings, reducing volatility and the subsequent drag on returns. In our analysis, the surest way to maximize the benefits of style investing is to combine growth and value in a single portfolio, and maintain the proportions evenly in a 50/50 split through regular rebalancing. Research from Standard & Poor's showed that since 1980, a 50/50 portfolio of value and growth stocks beats the market 75% of the time. Due to the fact that both styles have near equal performance and either style can outperform for a significant time period, a medical professional might consider a blending of styles. Rather than attempt to second-guess the market by switching in and out of styles as they roll with the cycle, it might be prudent to maintain an equal balance your investment between the two.

TABLE 11.8
Yearly Returns of Growth/Value Stocks

Year	Growth (%)	Value (%)
1992	5.1	10.5
1993	1.7	18.6
1994	3.1	−0.6
1995	38.1	37.1
1996	24.0	22.0
1997	36.5	30.6
1998	42.2	14.7
1999	28.2	3.2
2000	−22.1	6.1
2001	−26.7	7.1
2002	−25.2	−20.5
2003	28.2	27.7
2004	6.3	16.5
2005	3.6	6.1
2006	10.8	20.6
2007	8.8	1.5
2008	−38.43	−36.84
2009	37.2	19.69
2010	16.71	15.5
2011	2.64	0.39
2012	15.25	17.50

Source: Ibbotson.

STOCK SPLITS

One final equity concept that medical professionals should be aware of is the idea of stock splits. In a stock split, a corporation issues a set number of shares in exchange for each share held by shareholders. Typically, a stock split increases the number of shares owned by a shareholder. For example, XYZ Corp. may declare a 2-for-1 split, which means that shareholders will receive two shares for each share that they own. However, corporations can also declare a reverse stock split, such as a 1-for-2 split where shareholders would receive 1 share for every 2 shares that they own.

While stock splits can either increase or decrease the number of shares that a shareholder owns, the most important thing to understand about stock splits is that they have no impact on the aggregate value of the shareholder's position in the company. Using the XYZ Corp. example above, if the stock is trading at $10 per share, an investor owning 100 shares has a total position of $1000. After the 2-for-1 split occurs the investor will now own 200 shares, but the value of the stock will adjust downward from $10 per share to $5 per share. Thus, the investor still owns $1000 of XYZ stock. While stock splits are often interpreted as signals from management that conditions in the company are strong, there is no intrinsic reason that a stock split will result in subsequent stock appreciation.

COMMON VERSUS PREFERRED STOCK

A common stock is the least senior of securities issued by a company. A preferred stock, in contrast, is slightly more senior to common stock, since dividends owed to the preferred stockholders should be paid before distributions are made to common stockholders. However, distributions to preferred stockholders are limited to the level outlined in the preferred stock agreement (i.e., the stated dividend payments). Like a fixed income security, preferred stocks have a specific periodic payment that is either a fixed dollar amount or an amount adjusted based upon short-term market interest rates. However, unlike fixed income securities, preferred stocks typically do not have a specific maturity date and preferred stock dividend payments are made from the corporation's after tax income rather than its pre-tax income. Likewise, dividends paid to preferred stockholders are considered income distributions to the company's equity owners rather than creditors, so the issuing corporation does not have the same requirement to make dividend distributions to preferred stockholders. Thus, preferred stock is generally referred to as a "hybrid" security, since it has elements similar to both fixed income securities (i.e., a stated periodic payments) and equity securities (i.e., shareholders are considered owners of the issuing company rather than creditors).

Convertible preferred stocks (and convertible corporate bonds) are also considered hybrid securities since they have both equity and fixed income characteristics. A convertible security whether a preferred stock or a corporate bond, generally includes a provision that allow the security to be exchanged for a given number of common stock shares in the issuing corporation. The holder of a convertible security essentially owns both the preferred stock (or the corporate bond) and an option to exchange the preferred stock (or corporate bond) for shares of common stock in the company. Thus, at times the convertible security may behave more like the issuing company's common stock than it does the issuing company's preferred stock (or corporate bonds), depending upon how close the common stock's market price is to the designated conversion price of the convertible security.

FOREIGN STOCK

Investing in companies located anywhere outside of its investors' country of residence is known as foreign investing. In theory, foreign stocks offer considerable diversification benefits because they tend to be affected by dissimilar economic factors than the U.S. markets. Thus, the zigs and zags in return of foreign stocks do not always correspond with those of the U.S. stocks. This occurs despite the reality that the world's economies are becoming more interdependent. The fact is the U.S. no longer makes up even half of the world market capitalization of all equities. According to Professor

TABLE 11.9
Randomness of Returns

	2003	2004	2005	2006	2007	2008	2009	2010	2011	2012
Highest Return	56%	26%	35%	33%	40%	−37%	79%	19%	2%	18%
	39%	21%	14%	27%	12%	−43%	32%	15%	−12%	17%
Lowest Return	29%	11%	5%	16%	5%	−53%	26%	8%	−18%	16%

S&P 500 Index
MSCI Emerging Markets Index (gross dividends)
MSCI EAFE Index (gross dividends)

Source: Center of Research in Security Prices (CRSP).

Note: Indexes are unmanaged baskets of securities that investors cannot directly invest in. Past performance is no guarantee of future results.

Jeremy J. Siegel (*CFA Institute Conference Proceedings Quarterly* (09/07)), by 2050 the United States will account for only 17% of the world's market capitalization. The year-by-year returns of foreign markets and the U.S. vary widely as seen in Table 11.9.

Diversification between international markets not only reduces many risks but also offers potential to augment returns as one country's economy may grow faster than the other. Many pundits have argued that international diversification did not assist investors during the global financial crisis of 2008–2009. This is true as international markets followed the U.S. markets down. However, the longer term benefits of foreign stock diversification are evident. Based on the data since 1972, investing outside of the U.S. has resulted in higher returns, though coupled with a small increase in volatility. The graph below demonstrates that an allocation of a hypothetical portfolio of 75% domestic stocks and 25% international stocks delivered a higher return with lower risk than an investment in either market alone.

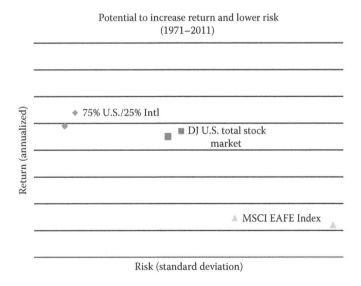

Potential to increase return and lower risk
(1971–2011)

Source: Vanguard Group, Valley Forge, Pennsylvania.

However, many U.S. investors still tend to have substantial U.S. exposure, with an average allocation according to Morningstar a mere 11% in foreign stocks. One area of foreign investing that a medical professional should consider is emerging markets. Emerging markets are economies or markets that are just entering the global arena. For example, the World Bank classifies emerging markets as economies beneath the upper-middle-income threshold. Because of highly focused political, economic, and financial risks, investing in individual emerging market countries can be particularly risky. However, because individual emerging markets are comparatively uncorrelated, the hazard of investing across all countries is much reduced. In addition, the distinctive development patterns of emerging markets add to diversification. The correlations between developed foreign markets (such as Germany and Japan) and emerging markets have averaged 0.65 since 1985. Emerging markets have also delivered higher average returns. According to Vanguard, from 1985 through 2011 emerging markets offered an average annual return of 13.1% with an standard volatility (measured by standard deviation) of 24.4%, versus average annual returns for developed foreign markets over the same period of 9.2% with an standard volatility of 17.8%. For a medical professional, adding emerging market stocks can potentially increase return over extended time periods.

SUMMING UP EQUITIES

Equity investments represent actual ownership in the issuing company. While being an owner in a company allows investors to participate in its upside, equity owners' interests are generally secondary to the interests of the corporation's creditors. In other words, shareholders only have a stake in the corporation's profits after accounting for expenses (including interest paid to bondholders) and taxes. Likewise, under a bankruptcy or liquidation scenario, shareholders generally only have rights to any assets remaining after all of the corporation's liabilities have been met. Although stocks come in many different flavors, the important thing for medical professionals to keep in mind when investing in equity securities is that stock prices generally reflect investors' expectations regarding the stock's future prospects. Medical professionals should understand that dividends account for a large part of an investor's total return and should not be discounted. Foreign stocks, including emerging markets, add substantial diversification effects to a portfolio. Foreign stocks can also add to return while potentially reducing total portfolio risk.

ALTERNATIVE INVESTMENT CLASSES

Beyond stocks and bonds, there are several distinct types of investments that may be referred to as alternative investments. Alternative investments (AIs) to stocks and bonds include real estate, private equity/venture capital, derivative securities, commodities, arts/collectibles, and so on. While such investments often have features that differentiate them from the equity and fixed income securities that are central to most modern portfolio construction approaches, alternative investments can also be boiled down to their basic expected cash flows. As a result, the evaluation of alternative investments involves fundamentally similar concepts to the basics discussed for stocks and bonds earlier.

REAL ESTATE

The most common alternative investment and often the single largest investment made by most individuals is real estate, since the family home is considered a key portion of wealth. Whether considering the family home, an office building, or a rental property, the evaluation of a real estate investment involves an assessment of the rents that may be received from those occupying the property. Likewise, the value of real estate may be measured by the value of the property's assets less its liabilities. Many real estate investors consider their real estate holdings to be similar to a fixed income security in that the income from the investment tends to be relatively stable over time. However, the true nature of a real estate investment is more akin to equities. First, the income earned on a real estate investment must be considered on an after-expense basis, since the property owner is responsible for maintenance, property management, taxes, debt servicing, etc. Secondly, while long-term leases may dampen the uncertainty of the rents received by the property owner, both rental amounts and occupancy rates may be variable for a particular real estate investment. Occupancy rate can be thought of as either the number of units rented in a multiple unit property such as an apartment or office building, or as the number of days/weeks of rental income achieved in a year for such property as vacation homes or hotels. Thus, like an equity security, the income from real estate is a net of expense number that may be quite variable, depending upon factors related to the demand for the property.

When considering real estate from an asset value basis, the similarity between real estate and equity investments becomes even more apparent. Specifically, there is no preset par value or maturity date for a real estate investment anchoring its market value. Instead, the value of the real estate holding is driven by the supply and demand for land at a particular location, the building and other fixed property on the land and the potential future cash flows achievable from the property less all liabilities, including any potential environmental concerns. Thus, the value of a real estate holding may fluctuate with economic cycles, demographics, inflation/deflation cycles, local business conditions, and so on.

REAL ESTATE INVESTMENT TRUSTS (REITs)

In general, two characteristics of real estate as an alternative asset class are a deficiency in liquidity and a lack of direct comparability across properties. The lack of liquidity comes from the fact that the real estate market is a negotiated market with individual transactions that typically occur infrequently. REITs were developed in part, to help offer greater liquidity to real estate investors. REITs are generally traded on organized stock exchanges, thus providing investors a mechanism for buying and selling real estate related investments in an efficient manner. Likewise, REITs generally allow investors to acquire diversified exposure to real estate securities, since REITs generally invest in multiple underlying properties.

REITs essentially are a hybrid investment. The investment category maintains aspects of both fixed income investments (with their reliable interest) and equities (ability to appreciate in value). REITs produce a regular stream of cash, primarily by collecting rents from the numerous tenants occupying the properties they manage. By law, REITs must pay out at least 90% of their taxable income annually as dividends to shareholders. This high dividend payout requirement means a majority share of REIT investment returns come from dividends. This amalgamation of characteristics has historically provided REIT investors with greater higher total returns than many other investments. According to National Association of Real Estate Investment Trusts (NAREIT), REIT total return performance over the past 20 years has outstripped the performance of the S&P 500 Index, the Barclays U.S. Aggregate Bond Index, and even the rate of inflation. REITs thus provide significant return benefits for medical professionals. Additionally, the correlation of REITS over the 20-year period from the end of 1991 to year-end 2011 demonstrated REITs maintained a low to moderate correlation with large-cap, small-cap, international stocks, as well as the U.S. and international bonds. For example, large-cap equities and equity REITs were only 56% correlated in the same period. This indicates REITs also provide solid diversification benefits. A key portfolio advantage of REIT diversification is the potential to increase long-term returns without taking on additional risk. NAREIT has found that reallocating 10% of a diversified 60/40 portfolio to equity REITs would have improved annual returns by 0.5% per year on average from 1991 to 2011. That could add up to thousands of dollars of additional gains for a medical professional over 20 years without any additional risk.

PRIVATE EQUITY/VENTURE CAPITAL

Similar to the equity securities discussed earlier, private equity and venture capital investments typically involve ownership of shares in a company and represent title to a portion of the company's future earnings. However, private equity is an equity interest in a company or venture whose stock is not yet traded on a stock exchange. Venture capital is typically a special case of private equity in which the investment is in a company or venture that has little financial history or is embarking on a high-risk/high-potential reward business strategy.

Like real estate, private equity and venture capital investments generally share a general lack of liquidity and a lack of comparability across different individual investments. The lack of liquidity comes from the fact that private equity and venture capital investments are typically not tradable on a stock exchange until the company has an IPO. The lack of comparability is due to the fact that most private equity and venture capital investments are the result of direct negotiation between the investor/venture capitalist and the existing owners of the company/venture. With widely divergent terms and provisions across different investments, it is difficult to make general claims regarding the characteristics of private equity and venture capital investments.

DERIVATIVES

A derivative security is a security whose value is derived from one or more underlying securities. Derivatives can range from securities as simple as a stripped bond or pooled mortgage security to extremely complex securities customized for a particular investor's risk management needs. Even though derivative securities in some contexts can be a key source of volatility in the financial markets, these securities may be useful tools in the portfolio management process. Likewise, just as the basic asset classes discussed previously may be separated into a series of expected cash flows, any given derivative security may be understood as a series of date or event contingent cash flows.

Two basic derivative securities created from more traditional fixed income securities are pooled mortgage securities and strips. A stripped security represents either principal or interest payments from some underlying fixed income security. As an example, a principal-only Treasury strip represents the face value payment of a U.S. Treasury bond, while an income-only Treasury strip represents the right to the coupon payments of a particular U.S. Treasury bond. A pooled mortgage security is a derivative security that represents ownership in a collection of mortgages. An interesting feature of a pooled mortgage security is the principal paydown, with shares of the pooled mortgage security returned at face value as mortgages are refinanced and/or repaid. Refinancing and prepayment of mortgages tend to happen when the original mortgage rate is above currently available rates, so pooled mortgages with higher coupon rates will tend to have the greatest prepayment risk.

Puts and Calls

Two equity-related derivative securities are puts and calls. Puts and calls fall under the general category of options, because each offers the holder the right to sell or purchase a security at a predefined price over a predetermined period. A put represents the right to sell a security at a particular price within a specific period of time, while a call represents the right to buy at a particular price over a given time period. An option is exercised when an investor invokes his/her right to buy or sell as provided for with the option. A European option is an option that is only exercisable at its maturity date, while an American option may be exercised at or before its maturity date. If the price of a stock falls below (rises above) the put (call) price within the term of the option, then the option is said to be in the money and the holder is likely to exercise the option and sell (buy) the stock from the writer of the option at its strike price.

- *Example:* A party writes (i.e., sells) a 6-month American put on Microsoft at a strike price of $35, which gives the buyer of the put the right to sell the put writer a certain number of shares of Microsoft stock at $35 anytime over the next 6 months. If the buyer of the put already owns shares of Microsoft stock, then the put effectively limits the put buyer's downside in Microsoft to the put's strike price in exchange for the premium paid on the put. This transaction is known as a protective put or portfolio insurance, since the buyer of the put may sell the shares of Microsoft at $35 in the event that the stock's price falls below that level. If, on the other hand, Microsoft's stock price remains above $35 for the full 6 months, then it is likely that the buyer of the put would let the option expire worthless, since the buyer could sell Microsoft for more in the open market than by exercising the option.

- *Example:* A party that writes a 6-month American call on Microsoft at $50 gives the buyer of the call the right to buy a specific number of shares of Microsoft stock for $50 anytime over the next 6 months. If the seller of the call already owns shares of Microsoft stock, then the call effectively limits the call seller's upside in Microsoft to the call's strike price in exchange for the premium received from the buyer of the call. This transaction is considered a covered call, since the seller of the call already owns the shares of Microsoft that may be purchased at $50 if Microsoft's price rises above that level. If, on the other hand, Microsoft remains below $50 for the full period, then the buyer of the option is better off buying Microsoft directly in the equity markets rather than exercising the option and it (the option) is likely to expire worthless.

FUTURES

A future represents the purchase of a particular investment at a predetermined date. Futures are traded on a wide range of investments (e.g., baskets of stocks, interest rates, currencies and commodities) and are useful tools for controlling the risk of cash flow timing for those that wish to lock in a particular price for a security. Likewise, they also provide some insight as to the expected future price in the market of the security. The key difference between futures and options is that futures obligate both parties to make the agreed upon transaction, whereas options give the option holder the right, but not the requirement, to make the transaction.

Futures are typically traded on an organized exchange, such as the Chicago Board of Trade (e.g., interest rate and stock index futures) or the Chicago Mercantile Exchange (e.g., foreign exchange and stock futures). The design of the contract traded on an exchange typically includes a predefined contract size and delivery month. Also, futures transactions generally require maintaining a margin deposit (i.e., a fraction of the trade value held in reserve to help ensure the final settlement at the contract settlement date) and the recognition of gains and losses on a daily basis with movements in contract prices. The pricing of a futures contract is based upon the price of the underlying security (e.g., the S&P 500 Index price), the opportunity cost of cash (e.g., current borrowing rates), and any distributions expected from the security over the period (e.g., dividends). A "no arbitrage" pricing formula, in which an investor could not earn a risk-free profit from selling the security and buying the future or vice-a-versa, is as follows:

$$F = S\left[1 + \frac{rt}{360}\right] - D_t$$

In this formula, F is the futures price, S is the current security price, r is the current interest rate for the period of the futures contract, t is the period of the contract, and D_t is the distributions over the period.

One of the key uses of futures contracts is to hedge an underlying exposure in a portfolio that may be a source of unwanted risk. As an example, an investor may wish to own a particular foreign company's stock (e.g., a European stock), but avoid the risk of an adverse movement in the local currency of the stock (e.g., the Euro) versus the dollar. By using a futures contract, the investor may be able to lock in a future exchange rate of the currency and limit the risk of a fall in the spot price of the currency adversely affecting the value of the investment. In our example, any gain in the futures transaction will offset the unrealized loss in the stock that relates to a drop in the Euro exchange rate. The price of a foreign exchange futures contract may be defined as follows:

$$F = \frac{S\left[1 + \frac{r_1 t}{360}\right]}{\left[1 + \frac{r_2 t}{360}\right]}$$

In this case, r_1 represents the domestic interest rate and r_2 represents the foreign interest rate, while S is the spot price for the currency.

While the formula above represents the price expected under a "no arbitrage" condition in which there is "parity" between the spot price and the futures price, it is important to remember that futures are traded on exchanges. Therefore, futures are influenced by supply and demand factors that may impact their price over any period. That is, if there are not enough buyers to offset the supply created by sellers of a futures contract, then deviations from the "no arbitrage" price may be sustained. It is such dislocations caused by periods of low liquidity that can cause futures contract mispricing and imperfect hedges.

Therefore, most derivative securities may be best understood as a series of cash flows contingent upon the price of underlying assets at specific dates and/or events. While derivatives may be useful to satisfy a particular investor's needs, these securities often have clear risks that should be considered and understood by a prudent investor. Thus, derivatives may be an important tool to manage the risk of failing to achieve a specific goal for an investor, but are not typically considered a separate asset class having a central place in most modern portfolio construction approaches.

COMMODITIES

A commodity is a standardized asset that is typically used as an input for production of one or more products. Almost any raw material or product that has very consistent characteristics irrespective of the producer (i.e., little to no differentiation between producers) may be considered a commodity. Examples of commodities that are traded broadly in the financial markets include food products, such as wheat and pork bellies, and metals, such as gold and aluminum. In most cases, the trading of commodities is done through futures.

Commodities do not have ongoing cash payments associated with them. Instead, a commodity's value is a result of supply and demand for the asset as a consumable or as an input for other goods. Thus, while some investors use commodity futures as a hedge to offset changes in the value of the commodity between now and the date the commodity is needed by the investor, others will make commodity investments based upon a belief that the supply/demand relationship will change in their favor. In the latter case, commodities represent a knowledge-based market in which an investor must believe that he/she has a better perspective on the future price of the commodity than other speculators. Consequently, if an investor does not have superior information regarding the future supply and demand for the commodity, then commodity investments become generally less attractive as compared to investments providing ongoing cash payments.

COLLECTIBLES

So far, the focus of the discussion on investments has been on securities representing legal title to an underlying stream of cash payments. However, many medical professionals have a broad range of investments that are typically not securities and rarely provide entitlement to specific cash flows. One example is *collectibles*, which are durable real property expected to store value for the owner. The term collectible may represent such items as artwork, jewelry, sports memorabilia, stamps, and wine.

While a detailed discussion of the wide variety of collectibles markets is outside the scope of this chapter, there are common characteristics of collectibles as an investment. First, the value of a collectible generally rests entirely in the eye of the beholder. Since there is typically no cash flows associated with a collectible, unless the collector charges at the door for a look at their collection, the value of the collectible is only what another collector is willing to pay for that particular item. Also, while there are some collectibles that may be considered standardized across individual pieces in terms of quality and other defining characteristics, collectible investments are generally unique. As a result, there is typically not an active market with prices established on a regular basis for most collectibles in a manner similar to the stock and bond markets.

In total, the lack of ongoing cash payments from a collectible and the general noncomparability of items result in the collectibles market being more of a knowledge-based market than most of the investments discussed previously. Since the value of a collectible is limited to the amount that another collector is willing to pay for the item, a knowledgeable investor may be able to benefit from the lack of information of another investor. By the same token, if an investor does not have superior information regarding the value of a collectible, then the basic lack of economic fundamentals behind a return assumption for such investments makes collectibles generally less attractive as compared to investments providing ongoing cash payments.

CURRENCIES AND CRYPTOCURRENCIES

Medical professionals might not know rupees from ringgits, but any investor should consider the benefits of currency investing. Buying currencies allow for a hedge against the U.S. dollar and also permit for an investor to take advantage of major movements of foreign currencies for profit. Today it is easier than ever to invest in currencies through mutual funds or exchange traded funds. The U.S. investors are impacted by foreign currency fluctuations through international stock and bond exposure. The advantage of investing in currencies is the investment generally has limited correlation with other real or liquid assets. Medical professionals can initiate the process of currency investing by starting a forex account. In many instances, an account can be opened with minimal investment. One caveat is the tax consequences, as currency-based profits are taxed as ordinary income rather than the more favorable capital gains rate.

Litecoin and *Bitcoin* is an open source, peer-to-peer payment network and digital currency. The latter was pioneered in 2009 by pseudonymous developer "Satoshi Nakamoto." Bitcoin has been called a cryptocurrency because it utilizes public-key cryptography for protection. Users send payments by broadcasting digitally signed messages that reassign ownership of bitcoins. A decentralized network of specialized computers verifies and timestamps all transactions using a proof-of-work system. The operators of these computers, known as "miners," are satisfied with transaction fees and newly minted bitcoins. Commercial use of Bitcoin, illicit or otherwise, is currently diminutive compared to its use by speculators, which has led to extreme price volatility. Companies and merchants have an enticement to recognize the currency because transaction fees are lower than the 2–3% classically imposed by the major credit card companies like Visa®. Given the fact that Bitcoin is a new currency with extreme volatility, medical professionals should be very cautious with any potential investment; especially after Autumn Radtke, the CEO, died under mysterious circumstances at her home in Singapore last year.

Nevertheless, as virtual currency Bitcoin gradually becomes a mainstream phenomenon, the firm *Coinbase* is trying to make it easy to use. Founded by a former Goldman Sachs currency trader named Fred Ehrsam, the company is attempting to build "the PayPal for Bitcoin." Coinbase is trying to make the cryptocurrency accessible to the everyday consumer and merchant, and has raised $30 million from high profile venture capitalists like Andreessen Horowitz, making it the top-funded Bitcoin startup. And, physicians like San Francisco's Paul Abramson MD, of *My Doctor Medical Group,* accept Bitcoins, finding that doing so is simple (http://mydoctorsf.com).

A related start-up named *Clinkle* is a mobile payment firm. Founded by Lucas Duplan in 2011, the company began as a small group of students. In 2013 it raised $25 million in what became Silicone Valley's largest seed funding round. Clinkle released an app for download on Google Play and the iTunes Store. The current versions have very limited functionality and only allow users to join a waitlist. Future products include a mobile app that serves as an online wallet linked to existing credit cards or bank accounts, and an app used high-frequency sound to send payments between devices. This product will also provide merchants with information about their customers for the purpose of targeted sales promotion.

And most recently, in an attempt to jumpstart the country's flagging economy with an Iceland-specific variant of Bitcoin called Auroracoin, every Icelandic citizen received an allotment of them to an unknown future.

CROWD-FUNDING

Start-ups and small businesses may soon be able to sell ownership stakes in their companies by soliciting investors over the Internet under a proposal advanced by the Securities and Exchange Commission (SEC). The plan would set rules for equity Crowd-Funding which would spur growth by easing financing for companies when mandated in the 2012 Jumpstart Our Business Startups Act. (JOBSA) The rules may boost the nascent Crowd-Funding movement that demonstrates progress in advancing a backlog of regulations required by the JOBS Act and Dodd-Frank law. Firms include: KickStarter, RockHub, CrowdFunder, PeerBackers, AngelList, and others.

For example, businesses using Crowd-Funding could raise no more than $5000 a year from someone whose income or net worth is less than $100,000. Investors with income or net worth greater than $100,000 could contribute as much as 10% of their annual income or net worth, to a maximum of $100,000 in 1 year. Crowd-Funding wouldn't be open to public companies, non-U.S. companies, or those that have no specific business plan. A company using equity Crowd-Funding would be limited to raising a maximum of $1 million per year. Companies raising less than $100,000 would have to disclose financial statements and income-tax returns for the most recent fiscal year. A company seeking to raise more than $500,000 would have to provide audited financial statements. Companies raising more than $100,000 but less than $500,000 would need to provide financial statements reviewed by an independent public accountant.

PEER-TO-PEER LENDING (P2PL)

Similar to private equity or venture capital, peer-to-peer lending (aka person-to-person lending), peer-to-peer investing, and social lending is the practice of lending money to unrelated individuals without the benefit a traditional financial intermediary like a bank or financial institution. P2P lending takes place online using various platforms and credit checking tools. It has been in existence for about a decade. Here are some important characteristics:

- P2PL offers a chance to get a lower interest rate than a bank, and gives investors a chance to receive higher returns. Of course, more rewards means more risk.
- The two largest P2PL companies are Prosper.com and LendingClub.com. Prosper is older, Lending Club is bigger. Prosper allows bidding on the interest rates you are willing to provide a loan. Lending Club sets the rates.
- Initial returns on Prosper were disappointing because default rates were high; today it is better. For loans originating in the last 6 months of 2009, both Lending Club and Prosper have a default rate (including currently late loans) of about 13.5%. Using loans from that same time period, Prosper had overall returns of 8.3% and Lending Club had returns of 4.3%.
- Since avoiding defaults is an important part of P2PL, investors should buy many lots of notes—for as little as $25 each—which make it relatively easy to achieve broad diversification.

- Compared to buying index funds and rebalancing once a year, P2PL is more time-consuming as you must pick the loans to invest in individually. Filtering through the offered loans is time-consuming, but can be rewarding. Some investors sell off their notes at a discount once the borrower goes late on a payment for instance, or just because they need their money out of the investment before the term is up.
- No matter how closely watched, there will be a drag on returns from the cash in your portfolio. It takes time to choose loans acceptable and then for them to be approved. Just as with a mutual fund, this will lower your returns, perhaps as much as 1%.
- One of the real benefits of P2PL is a low correlation with other investments, as it is different than other asset classes and ought to perform differently from equity and fixed income investments.

OVERHEARD IN THE ADVISOR'S LOUNGE: ARE THERE TOO MANY ASSET CLASSES?

Some financial analysts believe that the focus on asset classes may have gone too far as physicians and other investors have sought to "overoptimize" their portfolios. In fact, our colleague David Loeper, CEO of Wealthcare Capital Management, explained this concept as follows:

> Where things have really got off track has been the insistence on breaking asset classes into sub-classes by style, market capitalization, etc. The unpredictability of all the inputs into our optimizers, even over long periods of time, has been ignored. We have attempted to take efficient portfolios of stocks, bonds and cash and make them even more efficient by breaking the unpredictable asset classes into even less predictable sub-classes. This has all been done into the pursuit of "efficiency" as the proposal was validated by the Brinson & Beebower study, which purports to find that over 90% of the investment return variance is explained by asset allocation. The risk that you produce inefficient portfolios INCREASES if you increase the number of "asset classes" for which you must forecast not only the risk and returns but also each asset class' correlation to the others.

The creation of "new" asset classes and subclasses by wholesalers (product purveyors) seems to be driven not by solid research, as this article suggests, but rather by other motivations.

Wholesalers have always existed to convince financial analysts and advisors that they have the one negatively correlated asset class that is missing in our portfolios that we must have to achieve maximum Alpha (excess risk-adjusted return). The "asset classes" of alternative investments and packaged real estate products come to mind.

Recent studies by credible market academics such as Roger Ibbotson cast doubt on the Brinson, Hood, and Beebower article from 1986 that as much as 90% of the variation in returns is caused by the specific asset allocation mix. Nonetheless, in my experience there is no doubt that MOST of the variation in return is caused by the simple allocation mix of stocks versus bonds/cash in the portfolio.

So if true, the results of optimizer and portfolio efficiency are based on the accuracy of the inputs and NOT THE NUMBER OF THE INPUTS.

Lon Jefferies, MBA, CFP®
www.NetWorthAdvice.com

INVESTMENT VEHICLES

To this point, the chapter has covered fundamentally distinct asset classes or broad security types. In general, medical professionals are able to access these securities either directly with a brokerage account or through a separate account manager buying securities for them on a discretionary basis.

However, many physician investors who are building their own investment portfolio (ME, Inc), or are working with a financial advisor, will have a host of different investment vehicles (e.g., mutual funds or variable annuities) available, which provide indirect exposure to the basic security types discussed above. When one of these investment vehicles is considered for investment, it is important for the medical professional to understand the characteristics of that vehicle, its cost structure, and the cash flows and valuations represented by the underlying investments of the vehicle.

SEPARATE ACCOUNT MANAGEMENT

Separate account management offers medical professionals customized personal money management services. In the typical separate account structure, a money manager invests the individual's assets in stocks and bonds (as opposed to mutual funds providing exposure to specific asset classes) on a discretionary basis. For healthcare providers with significant investment assets (e.g., $100,000), a separately managed portfolio can be customized to reflect their tax situation, social investment guidelines, and cash flow needs. An additional benefit of the separate account management structure is that a client's portfolio may be positioned over time as opportunities arise, rather than forcing stocks into the portfolio without regard to current conditions. Although separate account management generally offers a higher degree of customization than mutual funds, fees for separate account management are generally consistent with mutual funds fees, especially given that separate account managers may discount their fees for larger portfolios.

MUTUAL FUNDS

Mutual funds are one of the most common investment vehicles available. A mutual fund is an investment company registered with the Securities and Exchange Commission (SEC) under the Investment Company Act of 1940 investing in securities in a manner consistent with the fund's prospectus on behalf of its shareholders. In other words, a mutual fund represents (equity) ownership of a company that is regulated by the SEC and makes investments based upon the terms outlined in its prospectus. Mutual funds generally provide investors diversified exposure to the securities markets at lower investment amounts than separate account management. In fact, the minimum investment in many mutual funds is as low as $2000. Thus, by pooling assets from multiple investors in an investment vehicle managed toward a broad goal such as capital growth (as opposed to a customized goal unique to each investor), mutual funds are able to offer investors access to areas of the financial markets that they would not otherwise be able to gain due to minimum investment restrictions.

The prospectus is a legal document describing the objectives, guidelines, restrictions, and disclosures of the investment company. A key reason why mutual fund advertisements end with a statement similar to "read the prospectus carefully before you invest" is that this document governs the management decisions made for shareholders. Typically, the prospectus will provide the investment manager of the mutual fund wide latitude in the types of securities that may be purchased in the mutual fund. A fund that focuses on domestic equity investments may have flexibility to allocate significant portions of assets to foreign stocks, bonds, derivatives, and so on. Thus, while mutual funds are often separated in databases and by the media into categories reflecting the basic type of investments their managers may focus on, these broad categories may fail to capture the broad flexibility and wide array of investments in any one of the funds within a category.

Mutual Fund Types

There are currently more than 10,000 mutual funds, as reported by CDA/Wisenberger, the leading provider of mutual fund information services to financial professionals. Two basic types of mutual funds are open-end and closed-end.

Closed Funds

A closed-end mutual fund that is traded in the stock market like as any other equity security, with buy and sell prices established by supply and demand for the security. Thus, in contrast to an open-end fund, a closed-end fund may possibly trade at a substantial discount, which means at a price below its NAV, or even at a premium, which means a price above its NAV.

Open Funds

An open-end mutual fund is a mutual fund that accepts new investors and allows investors to sell the fund at a specific price determined by the investor's prorated share of the market value of the fund. That price, known as net asset value or NAV, represents the market value of the mutual fund's portfolio less any accrued liabilities (e.g., management fees). The NAV is calculated once a day and governs all transactions until the next closing price.

The following general criteria may be used to help select a domestic open-end fund:

1. Review the fund's track record back since inception, especially reviewing results in the bear stock market of 2008.
2. Examine the total fees charged by reading the prospectus.
3. Examine risk-adjusted performance relative to the appropriate index benchmark.

The debate about fund fees is often perplexing to the medical profession. Load (commission based) funds are not necessarily bad, and no-load (noncommission based) funds are not necessarily good. In fact, one might even argue that there is no such thing as a no-load (expense) fund, since all have fees associated with them, disguised under various terms. These include management fees, advisory fees, 12b-1 fees, redemption fees, low load fees, diminishing (vanishing) loads, operating expenses, marketing, sales and advertising fees, and so on. As a general rule, the aggregate fee for a mutual fund should probably not exceed about half percent for a domestic bond fund, 1% for a domestic stock fund, 1.5% for an international fund, and about 2% for an emerging market fund. The lower the fees, the more money a medical professional will keep in his or her pocket. There are generally three types of open-ended mutual fund class shares:

1. Class A is a front-loaded fund that offers break points for volume discounts. The more money invested, the lower the load. It is not wise to invest in a front load fund if you plan to cash out within a couple of years. For a true long-term investor however, it might be smarter to use Class A funds, since your costs are spread out over the number of year you hold the fund. These funds are sold with a commission (load) by brokers. A medical professional can also buy these funds without the upfront commission through discount brokerage firms like Schwab, Fidelity, and TD Ameritrade.
2. Class B fund, or back-end load shares have an exit fee associated with them that usually diminishes after 5 or 7 years. They typically have higher annual yearly operating fees than Class A shares, but are reduced after the seventh year surrender penalty has elapsed. A medical professional can also buy these funds without the upfront commission through discount brokerage firms like Schwab, Fidelity, and TD Ameritrade.
3. Class C fund, or level load shares do not have an initial sales charge, but may have higher 12b-1 or operating expense fees, on a deferred basis, as well as a deferred sales charge depending on the date of redemption. A medical professional can also buy these funds without the upfront commission through discount brokerage firms like Schwab, Fidelity, and TD Ameritrade.

Closed-end funds trade on the stock exchanges, much like a stock. One item of note for a medical professional is the annual fees charged by closed-end funds. For closed-end funds, the average expense ratio is 1.39% for a domestic stock fund, 1.95% for a foreign stock fund, and 1.19% for a bond fund according to the December 2000 Morningstar Closed End Fund database. While sales charges do not apply to closed-end funds, there are transactions costs such as brokerage commissions that apply to the purchase/sale of a closed-end fund.

Other sources of mutual fund information and evaluation:

No-Load Mutual Fund Investor
Sheldon Jacobs
www.noloadfundinvestor.com

Morningstar Mutual Funds
225 West Wacker Drive
Chicago, Illinois 60608
800-735-0700
www.morningstar.com

Value Line Mutual Fund Survey
220 E. 42nd. Street
New York, NY 10017
800-535-8760
www.valueline.com

Free Edgar
Corporate 10-K reports, filed annually with the SEC, are available at:
www.freeEdgar.com, as well as from: www.edgar-online.com and: www.sec-gov.com.

These databases will tell you fascinating tidbits about company financial statements, investments, executive perks and other corporate shenanigans, before you invest money in them. For example, Apple Computer nearly halved its finished goods inventory to $16 million, from $30 million, in the last quarter of Y 2000, while it took a charge of $90 million or so it could buy the late CEO, Steve Jobs, an airplane.

EXCHANGE TRADED FUNDS (ETFs)

ETFs or tracking stocks are essentially index funds that are traded on an organized stock exchange. ETFs provide investors with broad exposure to economic sectors, market indices, including foreign stock markets. Examples of common ETFs include Spiders (SPY—tracking the S&P 500), Diamonds (DIA—tracking the Dow Jones Industrial Average), and Cubes (QQQ—tracking the NASDAQ 100). Beyond their diversification benefits, ETFs also allow investors the opportunity to take advantage of intra-day price fluctuation in various indices since the shares are traded just like individual stocks on the major exchange markets. In contrast, an open-end index mutual fund can only be traded at one price (i.e., NAV) determined at the end of the day. Furthermore, the fact that ETFs are traded on an organized exchange means that investors can short the shares (i.e., bet that the relevant index will go down), buy the securities on margin, and enter market, limit, and/or stop orders. ETFs typically have low expense ratios given the passive investment approach used in managing the underlying securities. A passive investment approach is the same as indexing. There are currently 1439 ETFs on the three primary stock exchanges as of 3/31/2013. Assets have now reached a record level of $1.47 trillion in assets. The primary advantages to ETFs are

- *Cost effectiveness*: The average total expense ratio for ETFs globally is a mere 0.31% on an annualized basis.

- *Diversification*: Total exposure to an entire index or benchmark.
- *Flexibility*: Trade and settle like stocks, with intraday pricing and trading, place stop and limit orders, increments of one share and go long or short like a stock.
- *Transparency*: Typically the full list of holdings is published daily.

ETFs also provide a primary method for an investor to practice passive investing, through index funds. "Indexing" is a passive form of management that has been triumphant in outperforming many actively managed mutual funds over the preceding 30 years. While the most popular index funds track the S&P 500 stock index, a number of other index funds focus on less popular benchmarks. This includes the Russell 2000 Index (small companies), the Dow Jones Wilshire 5000 Index (total stock market), the MSCI EAFE Index (foreign stocks in Europe, Australasia, Far East) and the Barclays Capital Aggregate Bond Index (total bond market). The principal advantage to such an approach is the lower management expense ratio on an index fund. Also, a majority of mutual funds fail to beat broad indexes, such as the S&P 500. The thinking behind index funds has much academic essence to it. A theory known as Efficient Market Hypothesis (EMH) also follows what is known as the "random walk" thesis. The random price action of the stock markets was first discovered by a French broker Jules Regnault in 1863. It was further highlighted in a 1900 PhD thesis, "The Theory of Speculation" by Louis Bachelier. What is today known as the formal "efficient-market hypothesis" was developed by Professor Eugene Fama at the University of Chicago Booth School of Business. Professor Fama published his Ph.D. thesis in the early 1960s that examined in detail this random walk process. In 1975, John Bogle of Vanguard took the position that "if you can't beat 'em, join 'em" and created the first low-cost mutual fund that mirrored the S&P 500 index. This was the first true "index" fund.

It has been a successful launch for Mr. Bogle. Since he started the first index fund in 1975, anywhere from 50–80% of active mutual funds get beat by the market in any given year. The chief raison d'être for this fact is the higher costs that mutual funds charge on an annual basis. A fund's total return each year is the total return of the portfolio minus the fees an investor pays for management and fund expenses. If an active mutual fund charges 2%, then an investor must outperform the market by that amount just to be even. The advantage of index funds, especially through the ETF vehicle, is the low absolute costs. An average nonindex fund has an expense ratio of around 1.5%, whereas many ETF index funds have an expense ratio of around 0.2%. The explanation the costs are lower in an index fund occurs because the fund is not actively managed. A medical professional should always realize that investing in an index fund doesn't guarantee no loss of money. You will in fact lose money in a poor stock market. But given the fact that index funds do outperform most actively managed mutual funds, any investor should give consideration for at least part of their portfolio residing in a low cost option.

DRIP Programs

For those with either smaller accounts or wish to avoid the costs associated with mutual funds or ETFs, a medical professional might consider various dividend reinvestment plans (DRIPs) to purchases shares cheaply and easily. You may find a list of all companies that offer DRIP programs at www.dripdatabase.com or you may also consider online brokerage companies that funnel your funds at www.sharebuilder.com or www.buyandhold.com. These companies will allow you to invest as little as $20 per months in stocks. If you invest $20, and select a stock that sells for $10, you will get about 2 shares, minus a tiny commission. If you select a company that sells for $60, you'll receive a third of a share. In this manner, virtually any health care professional can afford to automatically invest, and re-invest, $25–50 per month in the stock market without annual operating or trading fees. Since not all companies offer dividends, or DRIP programs, another potential advantage of these two companies is the fact that they also allow the purchase of non-DRIP companies, such as Visa, Microsoft, and Yahoo!

VARIABLE ANNUITIES

Another common investment vehicle representing a commingled interest in an underlying portfolio of securities is the variable annuity. A variable annuity is an insurance company investment product representing ownership in both the net asset value of an investment portfolio and certain insurance provisions, such as a guarantee of original investment in the event of death. Variable annuities are one of several different types of insurance company-based commingled investment products, including variable life, variable universal life, and so on.

One key feature of insurance products is that taxation on the capital gains and income generated in the underlying investment portfolio typically does not pass through to the investor until liquidation of the investor's shares in the insurance product. Thus, while a mutual fund must pass on capital gains and income to its investors through a periodic dividend, the growth from income and capital gains may occur in a tax-deferred manner for a variable annuity investor. On the other hand, variable annuities have insurance costs that tend to increase their expense ratio significantly versus a similar mutual fund. Typically, there is a crossover point where the benefits of tax-deferral overcome the added insurance costs of a variable annuity versus a similar mutual fund. However, this needs to be assessed on a case-by-case basis given an investor's tax rate as well as a fund's expected turnover rate, expense ratio differential, and range of potential future returns. Also, like some mutual funds, many variable annuities will have significant front-end or back-end sales charges, which add to the cost of the investment vehicle.

BANKS

A third provider of investment vehicles is a bank. While many banks have mutual funds registered with the SEC, a bank may also develop commingled funds under the banking regulations. The two most prevalent types of bank-maintained funds are the collective fund, which is a commingled fund for IRS qualified retirement plans, and the common fund, which is a pooled fund for nonqualified plans or individual investors.

In essence, bank-maintained commingled funds are trusts over which the sponsoring bank has discretionary management responsibility. Nonmutual fund pools sponsored by banks are generally pass-through entities in which the investor owns a prorated share of the underlying securities in the portfolio of the fund. In the case of collective funds, this pass-through feature has the added benefit of making the banking institution a fiduciary under the Employee Retirement Securities Act (ERISA 1974) for the investment decisions being made on behalf of each individual plan. While a common or collective fund may have a standardized fee schedule deducted from the portfolio like an expense ratio, these funds often have individually negotiated fees on a client-by-client basis and should be evaluated on a case-by-case basis accordingly.

INVESTMENT TRUSTS AND LIMITED PARTNERSHIPS

A final category of investment vehicles includes limited partnerships and investment trusts. These commingled funds are not considered mutual funds, insurance funds or bank-maintained funds from a regulatory oversight point-of-view. Instead, these vehicles represent a specific contractual relationship between the investor and the management company. A unit investment trust (UIT) represents proportional ownership of a generally static portfolio of securities. The securities underlying the UIT are typically fixed income securities, with maturity of the securities resulting in liquidation of the trust and a return of principal to the investor. Generally, there is a management fee deducted from the UIT on an annual basis.

In a limited partnership, the investor is a partner providing financial backing and having a liability equal to their original investment. In contrast, a general partner has responsibility for management of the entity and broader personal liability for the endeavor. Examples of limited partnerships as investment vehicles providing access to a pool of securities or property include oil and gas partnerships, real estate partnerships and hedge funds.

HEDGE FUNDS

A hedge fund in the United States is generally a limited partnership providing a limited number of qualified investors with access to general partner investment decisions with little restriction in the type of investments or use of leverage. While the flexibility available to a hedge fund from a regulatory standpoint implies a high degree of potential risk, there is a wide range of investment philosophies, strategies, security types, and objectives captured under the broad title of hedge fund. Thus, generalizations regarding the characteristics of hedge funds are even less appropriate than with mutual funds, and evaluation of the investment characteristics and merits of a hedge fund strategy must be on a case-by-case basis. Likewise, the cost structure of a hedge fund often includes a base management fee to the general partner plus a performance-based fee or percentage of the profits, and must be evaluated on a case-by-case basis.

Several different investment vehicles operate under the oversight of varying regulatory bodies which provide access to an investment-managers' discretionary decisions. While each approach generally represents ownership of an underlying pool of securities, there is usually a great deal of flexibility for the manager to deviate from a specific asset class or investment approach. Also, the fee structure of each vehicle can vary greatly and be quite large once distribution fees and sales charges are taken into account. Thus, it is important for a medical professional to remember the following:

- Evaluate the features and costs of an investment vehicle carefully
- Consider the cash flows and valuations of the securities that the manager or management approach will focus on as if the investments were being made directly
- Above all, read the prospectus or agreement carefully before making an investment

ONLINE TRADING PLATFORMS

Active trading in the financial markets requires specialized software that rises above the web-based platforms used for many online brokers. Conventional web design technology is effective for trading decisions that do not require split-second execution, but these sites make it nearly impossible to day trade. However, many online brokers also offer more robust trading platforms to complement their investment services. These platforms require separate installation like any other piece of software, and can turn a good computer into a comprehensive—and fast—tool for analyzing and trading any financial vehicle. Stocks, bonds, and foreign exchange are among the most popular instruments traded using these platforms. Some of the platforms are free for account holders, but most charge a monthly subscription.

E*TRADE PRO

E*Trade was one of the first major brokerage firms, and its active investment and trading services are used worldwide. The platform set an early standard in active trading and remains one of the most robust tools available.

THINKORSWIM

This trading platform has led the industry in active trading of financial derivatives, including stock options and futures. While the platform offers standard trading tools for stocks, it includes several exclusive features for options that are not available in other systems.

MARKET DELTA

A segment of the trading population looks at special indicators that transcend traditional chart models. A close, intricate analysis of trading volume and statistical price distributions informs these traders more than other popular tools. Market Delta software is a premium-trading platform based around Market Profile and "footprint" charting methods.

FOREX PLATFORMS

FOREX (foreign exchange) has ignited strong interest from traders, businesses, physician-investors, and individuals all over the world. FOREX enables traders to buy and sell foreign currencies. These platforms process trades rapidly and produce charts (FOREX.com; GFTFOREX.com, MultiCharts system, FX Trading Station and AVATrade.com among others).

STATISTICAL PLATFORMS

Physicians, investors, finance, and insurance agents are bombarded with a barrage of numbers and figures, all of which must be considered in order to maintain economic vitality. Software and other computational aids can assist in statistical analyses for several data sets and, in the process, will expedite a good deal of the work. Many statistical tools also retain data; such a function reduces statistical redundancy. Here are a few leading platforms.

Derivative Solutions

The International Association of Financial Engineers (IAFE) lists several online tools for analyzing various sets of monetary data, though several of them are geared specifically toward financial data. For example, "Derivative Solutions" provides rigorous analytical information, which is consistently applied to all fixed-income financial measurements. And, "Fact Set," a Derivative Solutions database, provides global data regarding debt-driven markets to a user base of top asset, investment, insurance, and hedge fund managers.

ForeTrade

The IAFE also endorses ForeTrade, an international-financial-market data aggregator, provides data to traders using cutting-edge nonlinear analysis techniques. One new tool is the "Genetic Pattern Finder" which uses technology inspired by artificial intelligence to detect and analyze patterns in financial data, and designed around "Trade Station;" a discretionary trading technique.

Rosella DB

Risk management is of paramount importance for the medical and healthcare sectors. With the goal of analyzing the most risk-oriented data, Rosella DB offers a predictive knowledge and data-mining tool to aid in analyzing the most data and factors to quote premiums and fees.

American Association of Insurance Services (AAIS) Tools

The AAIS has several actuarial and statistical reporting services; including custom coverage and endorsements analysis, including integration of pertinent research to bolster their credibility. AAIS also calculates and projects an insurer's profits, losses, and assists in interpreting data.

Estimize

Estimize is an open financial estimates platform that facilitates the aggregation of fundamental estimates from independent, buy-side, and sell-side analysts, along with those of private investors and students. By sourcing estimates from a diverse community of individuals, Estimize provides both a more accurate and more representative view of expectations compared to sell-side only data sets that suffer from several severe biases.

OVERHEARD IN THE DOCTOR'S LOUNGE:
CONSUMER REPORTS NOT AVAILABLE

You can spot comparison shoppers a few aisles away at any retail store. They are the ones carrying articles from *Consumer Reports*, badgering the salesperson with a million and one questions. People who manage money well are usually big fans of comparison shopping. If comparison shopping is important before choosing a new refrigerator or lawn mower, it is even more essential before choosing an investment advisor (IA). Unfortunately, there is no easily available consumer's report on advisors. Even more frustrating, those selling financial products often have incentives not to be forthcoming with the information that is crucial for comparing advisors.

One aspect of shopping for an investment advisor is to know what questions to ask. One common mistake is to focus on investment returns. Shoppers may ask for the average recent returns of the advisor's portfolios or may want to know whether the advisor's returns beat the market averages. There are several problems with focusing on returns.

First, the numbers mean nothing without also knowing how much risk the advisor took to produce the return. It is like someone on a diet focusing only on fat grams without regard to total calories. Consuming ten soft drinks in a day may give you zero fat grams, but you could easily exceed your daily calorie limit before eating one bit of food. Second, any unscrupulous advisor can put together a portfolio consisting of the hottest investment classes over the past 10 years and show you how fantastically they did. Third, whether or not an advisor beats the market is overrated. Why? A whopping 97% of all mutual fund managers do not generate an "average return" over 20 years. Just finding an advisor who has done so means you found someone in the top 3%. Fourth, some financial advisors may show you a phenomenal track record for the short term (under 10 years). Since wise investing focuses on the long term, beating the averages over a short term is not necessarily significant.

If so many games can be played around returns, what questions should a savvy comparison shopper ask? Focus on one word: transparency. You want to find out if the returns, costs, and risk (standard deviation) of your portfolio will be clearly displayed and contrasted against appropriate benchmarks. Here is how to accomplish that goal.

Most advisors have model portfolios. Ask them to show you the standard deviation and the expense ratio of their model over 5 and 10 years. Ask them to contrast the return of the portfolio against a similar benchmark. For example, if the portfolio has the U.S. stocks, the U.S. bonds, and foreign stocks, have them compare it to a benchmark of indexes proportionate to those asset classes.

Next, either ask the advisor to run a similar analysis on your existing portfolio or have one done independently. You may even have done better than the advisor's model. Ask the advisor to disclose all fees in addition to the expense ratios charged by mutual fund or subaccount managers. You need to find out how the advisor is paid and how much. Ask whether there are any wrap fees, transaction costs, administrative fees, mortality fees, redemption fees, annual 12b(1) fees, surrender charges, or up-front sales charges.

Do not be surprised if you get a bit of resistance when you ask for all this information. Brokerage firms, life insurance companies, and many commission-based advisors do not have much incentive to give you this data and may not even be able to. If you do not get clear disclosure on fees and costs, keep asking. If you persist and still do not get understandable answers, you may need to do more comparison shopping before you choose an advisor.

By Rick Kahler, MS, CFP®
www.KahlerFinancial.com

ASSESSMENT

Effective investment management requires proper diversification of assets to manage risk and maximize the likelihood of reaching your goals. However, the traditional approach for doing so focuses on investment portfolio results alone, or perhaps your personal residence. But it often ignores your greatest asset or the ability to continue earning income as the fruits of your medical professional labor ("human capital").

Just as with financial capital, the value of any human capital will rise and fall over time. However, the reality is that human capital for some medical specialists is far more volatile than others. Other careers like working for the government, or being a tenured professor, produce human capital that exhibits "bond-like" risk and return characteristics, while more corporate and/or entrepreneurial positions are stock-like (including the fact that they may be outright correlated to the economic cycle and stock market returns).

IS YOUR CAREER AN ASSET CLASS?

Accordingly, effective diversification of your entire household balance sheet may entail using financial capital to counterbalance against the risks of human capital; in other words, those with stock-like careers should own more bonds, while those with bond-like careers can afford to own more stocks. Similarly, decisions about savings should recognize that sometimes, investing in human capital can actually produce a greater Return on Investment (ROI) than saving (even better than buying stocks in a Roth IRA for the long run)!

So, the next time you consider a financial planning decision, remember to consider whether your medical career and human capital behave more like a stock, or a bond!

CONCLUSION

This chapter reviewed a wide range of investment categories and alternative ideas for the physician-investor and medical professional. Various security selection strategies, and online trading platforms, were also reviewed.

COLLABORATE

Discuss this chapter online with others at www.MedicalExecutivePost.com

ACKNOWLEDGMENT

To Christopher Cummings, CFA, CFP® of Manning-Napier Investment Advisors, New York.

FURTHER READING

Bernstein, W: *The Four Pillars of Investing: Lessons for Building a Winning Portfolio*. McGraw-Hill, New York, 2013.

Bogle, J: *The Little Book of Common Sense Investing: The Only Way to Guarantee Your Fair Share of Stock Market Returns*. Wiley, New York, 2007.

Carlson, CB: *The Little Book of Big Dividends: A Safe Formula for Guaranteed Returns (Little Books—Big Profits)*. Little Books, New York, 2010.

Cohen, M, Malburg, C and Forbes, S: *Making Money in the New Fixed Income Landscape*. Wiley, New York, 2013.

Coons, J and Cummings, C: Investing basic for physicians. In, Marcinko DE (editor): *Financial Planning for Physicians*. Jones and Bartlett, Sudbury, MA, 2007.

Ferri, R: *The ETF Book: All You Need to Know about Exchange-Traded Funds*. McGraw-Hill, New York, 2009.

Geske, RL and Delianedis, G: The Components of Corporate Credit Spreads: Default, Recovery, Taxes, Jumps, Liquidity, and Market Factors; UCLA Anderson Working Paper; NO. 22-01, December 2001.

Houweling, P, Mentink, A and Vorst, T: Comparing possible proxies of corporate bond liquidity. *Journal of Banking and Finance 29*, 1331–1358, 2005.

Huang, J-Z and Huang, M: How Much of the Corporate-Treasury Yield Spread Is Due to Credit Risk? NYU Working Paper No; FIN-02-04, October 2002.

Israelsen, C: How Market Timing affects your portfolio. *Financial Planning*, March 25, 2014.

Kozhemiakin, A: The risk premium of corporate bonds. *The Journal of Portfolio Management*, 33, 101–109, 2007.

Loughran, T: Book-to-market across firm size, exchange, and seasonality: Is there an effect? *Journal of Financial and Quantitative Analysis* 32, 249–268, 1997.

Malkiel, BG: *A Random Walk Down Wall Street: The Time-Tested Strategy for Successful Investing*. 10th edition. Norton, New York, 2012.

Mayo, H: *Investments: An Introduction*. Cengage Learning, New York, 2010.

12 Asset Protection and Planning Principles
What Is at Risk—How to Protect It

J. Christopher Miller

CONTENTS

This chapter demonstrates how avoiding risk and handling your assets in certain ways can minimize your chances of losing assets to creditors. Asset protection receives attention from medical professionals in all spheres who have accumulated wealth. Some have conservatively built their nest eggs with careful savings over decades of work, some are healthcare entrepreneurs, and others have seen their fortunes rise and fall with the economy. The real-estate bubble and the Great Recession of the past decade have taught many doctors and nurses a difficult lesson that highlighted the vulnerability we all face in safeguarding the earnings for which we have worked so hard.

INTRODUCTION

The first step in constructing a solid asset protection plan is to assemble an experienced attorney and professional advisory team that can be trusted to stay current on the swift changes in this area. Together, you will be able to plan and execute a course of action customized to your needs and objectives.

GETTING STARTED

Strong asset protection substantially depends on timing. The sooner you act to protect your assets, the greater the odds of your success. Many asset protection strategies construct barriers between assets and creditors, and if these barriers are built when creditors are closing in, courts will not respect them. If, on the other hand, you use the asset protection tools described in this chapter when your financial outlook is healthy, the tools can be an effective barrier between your wealth and the reach of future creditors.

APPRECIATING THE RISKS

Physicians and medical professionals share a unique disadvantage when it comes to asset protection. They are constantly haunted by the prospect of being sued for malpractice. Most of them have solid malpractice insurance coverage in force, but if that pool runs dry, the courts may look to the professional individually to compensate patients for injuries suffered while under the professional's care. Malpractice insurance itself may not be sufficient to completely protect a physician against professional liability claims. As verdicts increase in size, policy limits may become inadequate. Likewise, insurance companies have a strong incentive to deny coverage by arguing that a claim falls outside the scope of coverage. Preparing for these possibilities will leave you much more financially sound than if you had not planned ahead.

Aside from the professional risks you take merely by agreeing to examine and treat a patient, dangers to your assets surround you. As discomforting as it may sound, your practice partners, your family, and even your neighbors are in fact potential adversaries. Unfortunately, your position as a medical professional in today's society subjects you to elevated risks of a nasty lawsuit if you are negligent in your personal conduct.

An accident while driving to the hospital in response to a call, or a simple slip-and-fall incident on your home's sidewalk, will more likely find its way into a courtroom because plaintiffs (and their lawyers) perceive you as a deep pocket.

On a more personal level, there may come a time when your marriage fails, and you are faced with equitably dividing property between you and your spouse. Asset protection strategies act differently in the context of a divorce, and family-oriented claims need to be treated differently in the scope of creating a plan. In the event that a claim arises from outside your professional activities, or if you find yourself swallowed by consumer debts, several asset protection methods will help you to prevent your assets from slipping away.

OVERHEARD IN THE DOCTOR'S LOUNGE: ON ASSET PROTECTION FOR MEDICAL PRACTITIONERS

A doctor sipping coffee at the water cooler recently opined that asset protection was only for super specialists, or the very wealthy, and probably less applicable to physicians in the era of the PP-ACA.

I replied that if you practice medicine and you have any savings at all, then you should learn about asset protection. Even a modest nest egg is worth protecting. The experience of being a defendant in a serious medical malpractice case is very stressful for the average physician. While the odds are low that a doctor will face a judgment in excess of the insurance policy limits, the fear of this outcome is a major contributor to litigation stress. Remember, the fear of losing one's life savings is behind some very cloudy thinking in the lawsuit settlement negotiation process.

So, if you work on protecting your assets now, you will have one less thing to worry about in the future if [when] you become a defendant.

Douglas Segan, MD, JD
(Physician and Attorney)

ASSET PROTECTION TOOLS

GOOD RECORDKEEPING

The best defense against any claim is a complete and accurate record of the facts. In particular, medical malpractice claims will frequently be stalled or thwarted by a consistent written or electronic (eHRs) description of the symptoms you observe and the treatments you prescribe. Extensive record keeping will not only help to formulate a defense against a claim, but it will also (and perhaps more importantly) create the appearance that you are careful and highly competent in all of your affairs. Members of a jury may not be able to discern whether the medical judgments you made in a particular case were good or bad, as they do not have the years of education and training that you do. Jurors can, however, sense whether your practice is organized and professional. If your records are thorough and consistent, jurors will assume that you dedicate as much attention to the substantive aspects of your work as you do to the tedium of recordkeeping. If you are active in the management of your office, you should keep track of its operations and establish logs for your employees to complete as they perform their daily tasks. Not all information, however, ought to be written down. Keep your written records to the facts you have observed and leave your speculations for department meetings.

INSURANCE

The next line of defense against creditors having an adverse effect on your net worth is insurance. Insurance is the easiest way to avoid risk because you are paying someone else to pool your risk with the risks of hundreds or thousands of others. Insurance carriers derive their profit from estimating and managing that risk and then paying only a few claims from among their many policyholders. As frustrating as they can sometimes be, they do provide a valuable service to the society.

The best piece of advice anyone can share with someone about to purchase an insurance policy is to compare insurance policies before signing up. Just as you should comparison shop for a new car, you should ask your agent to present you with the offerings of multiple carriers and take the time to discuss with him/her the gaps and exclusions that might be addressed with riders or additional policies. Rates for comparable policies vary widely, and policies may differ significantly in the size and scope of coverage they offer. Research the attributes of a policy, such as its deductible and the extent of its exclusions. Find out whether the insurance carrier is financially secure and whether its investments are liquid. Deciding which combination is right for you demands careful consideration and a trusted advisor.

Malpractice Insurance

With respect to the scope of malpractice coverage, many liability insurance policies will deny coverage if an intentional tort is alleged. A tort is an injury inflicted by one person on another, and an intentional tort is when the person intends to do an act that the law decides is wrong, even if the person does not intend to injure the victim. One example of an intentional tort is intentional infliction of emotional distress, which doctors may need to defend against if they misdiagnose a patient while having a financial interest in the treatment of the diagnosis. Battery is another intentional tort with which doctors are often charged. *Battery* can be defined as any injurious contact without consent.

The necessity of obtaining informed consent from each patient is becoming increasingly important as a defense against such claims. Intentional torts are different from torts of negligence, which are usually covered under most liability insurance policies. Negligence claims arise out of mistakes usually attributable to carelessness. Make sure your insurance policy extends to intentional torts to prevent these kinds of cases from being denied coverage by your insurance company.

Life Insurance and Disability Insurance

The most valuable asset of most physicians is not their homes or their stock portfolios, rather, it is their future income potential. You can protect against its loss by ensuring that its full value is replaced if you are unable to continue working into the future. Life and disability insurance are the tools used to protect this value. An easily overlooked factor to consider when buying life insurance is the amount of outstanding debt you have. Be sure that the proceeds will satisfy any obligations you have assumed, such as the mortgage on your home or continued payments on automobiles or boats, as well as enough money to satisfy the known future expenses such as a child's college education or wedding, and to support your spouse and children until they can find other sources of income. In some cases, you may need to plan for a spouse's retirement. If you are an insurable candidate, think twice before turning down additional coverage, because sometime later, you might lose that status and be unable to add to your insurance posture.

General Liability Insurance

When consulting with an insurance agent, inquire about "umbrella" general liability policies. These policies protect you from a plaintiff adopting a shotgun approach to litigation, because the general liability insurer bears a burden to defend covered claims as well as to indemnify against losses. That is, the insurance carrier pays the legal fees and expenses that build up while the claim is being litigated. Because of this duty, consider the stress and money you would save in finding good representation in addition to the possible damage awards when considering the purchase of an umbrella policy.

Natural Disaster Insurance

Finally, protect against the loss of accumulated assets by insuring them against the wrath of Mother Nature. Most homeowners' policies do not cover damages arising from floods or earthquakes. If a home, or any other real property such as a vacation home or beach condo, is in an area subject to floods or earthquakes, consider the value of purchasing insurance that covers such catastrophes. Take the time to review your homeowners' policy, making sure that it will repair or replace your roof if damaged by hail, and will apply in the event of high winds, rather than only in tornadoes. The key to the maintenance of any type of insurance is to anticipate all the possible calamities, and then to decide whether you can afford to lose the assets exposed to these calamities.

LAYERED ORGANIZATIONS

Practice Format

The format and corporate structure of your healthcare practice is another way to limit personal liability and protect your assets. The most successful means of reducing the risk from your professional conduct is the creation of a layered organization. Your practice should operate through an entity (or set of entities) that limits the liability of its owners. A series of subsidiary organizations operating under a parent entity may limit your personal liability after a colleague suffers liability in a claim, or if the practice is found liable for a breach of contract.

Traditionally, layering of a physician's business structure involved the use of a professional corporation governing an office whose stockholders were either the physicians themselves or other professional corporations embodying each practicing physician. Nowadays, new and different forms of business entities do not require the time-consuming formalities associated with a corporation, but they still benefit from statutory limits on the liability of their owners. Such entities include limited liability companies (LLCs) and limited liability partnerships (LLPs). Layering these types of organizations on top of one another can provide the same protection from claims by creditors without incurring the double-income taxation of more traditional corporations. Many entity types are designed to make asset protection easier, although sorting through the alphabet soup created by these new entity types and deciding which one to use can be difficult.

A Comparison of Business Entity Types

Corporation

Generally speaking, a corporation consists of one or more shareholders that appoint one or more directors, who in turn manage the corporation and its actions. Shareholders suffer a loss for the liabilities of the corporation only to the extent that they have value in their shares. More specifically, the shareholders' personal risks are limited by the interest they have in the corporation, which equals the investment they made when buying or subscribing for the shares, plus any corporate earnings that have not yet been distributed as dividends. Except for special circumstances discussed later in this section, personal assets of each shareholder are not at risk when a corporation suffers losses or is presented with a liability. For this reason, many professional corporations make annual or more frequent distributions to their owners of most of the earnings gained by the corporation, leaving only enough assets in the corporation to cover its outstanding known debts and enough capital to weather cash flow fluctuations.

Limited Liability Company

A limited liability company (commonly known as an LLC) is very similar to a corporation in its role as a barrier between the personal assets of its owners and its liabilities. An LLC can also be owned entirely by one person, by a parent entity, or by more than one person, which makes it a convenient format for a medical practice. LLCs also offer increased flexibility for tax planning and management purposes. Certain single-member LLCs can be entities that are disregarded for tax purposes, but in many states, still provide a layer of insulation between the owner's assets and the LLC's operational debts. Florida is a notable exception to this rule because it allows creditors to treat assets of a wholly owned LLC as if there is no liability shield.

You can think of an LLC as a hybrid or cross-over entity using the best parts of both corporation law and partnership law to build a separate type of business. Instead of shareholders, an LLC is owned by all members who can have the same rights and responsibilities or, if you choose, the members can be split into managers and nonmanagers. The managing members of an LLC have the right to make decisions on behalf of the business and have a say in its operations, but they have no additional liability like they would in a general partnership or in a limited partnership.

Limited Liability Partnership

An LLP is much like an LLC, except that as a form of partnership, there must be more than one partner. You would likely use an LLP instead of an LLC in a situation where you want cohesiveness among several people or bodies, but want to minimize subjecting each partner to the risks carried by other partners. An LLP has several advantages over a general partnership because, as its name suggests, the liability of each of the partners is limited to the value of the partners' interests in the partnership. That is, a partner in an LLP would not risk personal assets to the same degree as a partner in a general partnership. In a general partnership, any liabilities that the partnership incurs flow back to the partners, and each partner is jointly and severally liable for these general partnership debts.

The difference between an LLP and a limited partnership (LP) is rather subtle. Both types of entities are improvements over a general partnership from an asset protection standpoint in that not every partner puts the partner's assets on the line when partnership liabilities arise. The difference between the two is that in an LP, there must be at least one general partner who risks paying for liabilities of the LP beyond the general partner's interest in the partnership. In other words, the general partner exposes personal assets to creditors of the partnership. In an LLP, every partner can absorb the benefit of limited liability, but every partner must be given management authority.

Limited Liability Limited Partnership

The last type of entity is a limited liability limited partnership, sometimes called a "Triple-LP." These entities are harder to form, and less common. Their rarity makes them hard to deal with as banks may refuse to lend to them, and both judges and jurors may view the entity as a type used only by someone trying too hard to avoid liability rather than conducting an operating business. The mere sound of the name makes it suspect in the eyes of too many people, and for that reason, the author discourages their use when it is also possible to build a two-layer organization with an LP and an LLC. The LLC can serve as the general partner of the LP, and this accomplishes the same level of protection and additional flexibility without sounding quite so defensive as a limited liability limited partnership, or LLLP.

BUSINESS ENTITY TYPES AND THEIR IDENTIFIERS

- General partnership
- Limited partnership (LP)
- Corporation (Inc. or Corp.)
- Limited liability company (LLC)
- Limited liability partnership (LLP)
- Professional corporation (PC)
- Professional limited liability company (PLLC)
- Limited liability limited partnership (LLLP)

An Ideal Approach

A modern structure of a practice might be an LLP in which several LLCs are general partners. The LLP would be the umbrella organization in which all the practice's operations take place. Each of the general partner LLCs might be wholly owned and managed by an individual practicing medical professional, and each general partner LLC would have a voice in the management of the LLP. Each of the LLCs and the physicians owning them would also be insulated from liability arising from the acts or omissions of the other physicians in the practice, whether such harms were intentional or not.

In this hypothetical organization, the LLP would be the practice's umbrella and would be at the forefront of litigation proceedings. It would also be the primary operational entity to which patients remit payments and would pay staff members. The LLP would then distribute its profits and the physician's negotiated compensation to the various LLCs. The LLCs would employ the physicians who were part of the practice, and then pass along the earnings received from the LLP to the doctors individually. To be effective in insulating the LLCs, the LLP would need to make distributions of its profits promptly and regularly, so that these profits are not exposed to the claims of plaintiffs. Also, the operational entity would not own the building in which the office is housed. Instead, a holding company of some form would be created, and a lease signed between the holding company and the LLP would help to prevent the building from exposure to seizure by creditors. The operating LLP cannot be merely a phantom. It must have some working capital of its own to be respected as a litigable party. It must also have its own incidents of business, such as a checking account and letterhead, and the functional differences between the LLP, the facilities-holding company, and the LLCs should be respected in practice to ensure the success of the shields created by layering the organization.

The benefit of layering an organization derives from the fact that courts treat corporations, LLPs, and LLCs as individual legal entities. Certain claims against the entity must first exhaust the assets of the entity before attaching the assets of the entity's owners. In summation, it is a good idea to minimize the value of assets held by the businesses conducting the operations of your practice, but not allow those quantities to be so small as to make reasonable the argument that the LLP is merely a shell that carries no weight.

As stated above, the owners of LLPs and LLCs, as opposed to partners in a general partnership, will not be liable for more than their investment and their share of the profits unless a claimant can pierce the veil of the entity. Although this rule, like any summary of the law, has several exceptions in cases where there are egregious facts, courts now allow plaintiffs and creditors to pierce the veil only when the alternative would sanction fraud or promote injustice, or when the entity and its owners have comingled their assets, which leads to the conclusion that they have perfectly aligned interests. This lumping of an entity and its owners into the same category is called an "alter-ego" theory. In other words, treating each part of the layered organization as a separately functioning entity gives it separate personalities and makes it more difficult for plaintiffs to reach the assets of the owners. Since the owners of the LLP in the sample model are LLCs, plaintiffs would need to pierce two veils and show two alignments of interest before getting to the assets of the physicians themselves.

Layering an organization, however, does not protect an individual from direct *tort liability* if the individual is negligent or has committed a fraud. In cases of potential professional tort liability, such as a malpractice claim, the professional is personally liable for any claims arising from his or her negligent conduct. Layering a business organization will not protect you against medical malpractice claims or other tortuous wrongdoing. The layering of a business organization is instead meant to prevent claims based on contract and vicarious claims against colleagues' negligent or intentional acts (i.e., harassment, violence, or discrimination claims) from reaching the personal assets of a physician. For these sources of liability, treating each layer as serving a different function in the business, and dealing with each entity as a separate business has proven to be effective at protecting the assets of the owners of the business.

QUALIFIED RETIREMENT PLANS

Current tax laws encourage both employers and employees to create and regularly contribute to retirement plans for use at a later stage in life. Qualified retirement plans may be set up by individuals in the form of an individual retirement account (IRA), or in employer-sponsored plans meeting the requirements of Internal Revenue Code section ("I.R.C") 401(k), 403(b) from which 401(k) plans get their name.

In general, employer-sponsored qualified retirement plan assets are protected from the claims of creditors under the provisions of the Employee Retirement Income and Security Act (ERISA). Thus, it makes for good long-term planning to contribute as much as possible to retirement plans created by your employer during your career. Under ERISA, contributions made to a qualified retirement plan are treated as being withheld from the employee, or not paid to them, so that they cannot be subject to any claims against the employee. Although the employee holds the promise of future payments from the plan assets, he or she may not make use of those funds or have any of the other benefits of the current ownership of those funds. Because of the restricted nature of the employees' access to plan assets, the creditors of the employees are likewise prevented from seizing those assets while they are in the plan.

The general rule for IRAs is not the same as the rule applied to employer-sponsored plans. Contrary to popular belief and to the surprise of many, IRAs are *not* protected under ERISA, and thus may be exposed to creditors' claims unless state law provides creditor protection. The good news is that the laws of many states protect IRAs from creditors' claims in a manner similar to the way ERISA shields employer plans from creditors. For example, in the State of Georgia, IRAs are exempted from the claims of creditors by statute, and in the event of bankruptcy, IRAs are not considered available assets for liquidation.

Claims for alimony and child support, however, are given an exception to this rule, proving once again that no single tool of asset protection should be relied upon exclusively. Additionally, several states consider the value of an employee's retirement plan contributions when deciding how to split the assets of a couple during a divorce. Because of the variety of rules applied by different states, and the speed with which these rules change in this field, you should consult with an expert in the area of deferred compensation before relying heavily on retirement plans for protection of your assets.

Another factor in making the most out of a retirement plan is having a robust succession of designated beneficiaries. If a spouse or child is named as a beneficiary, then that nonprobate transfer at your death entitles the beneficiary to the funds built up in the plan without exposure to the creditors of the employee or his or her estate. Without a designated beneficiary, however, IRA assets do flow into and through a decedent's estate, which is a pool of resources used by an executor or personal representative to pay any debts left behind before distribution to the beneficiaries. Consult with the plan administrator to establish a structured retirement plan providing the most protection for the retirement assets, but not negatively impacting the ability to enjoy these assets when they become available.

The theory supporting the protective value of retirement assets is that the nominal owner does not actually own the assets. In most cases, a brokerage or investment company will serve as a custodian of the IRA for the investor, holding the account for the benefit of that investor, and agreeing to comply with the complex rules governing the administration of retirement accounts. The benefits are not permanent; however, in that once a person has reached retirement age (currently 59½), the custodial relationship does not give the custodian sufficient power to withhold assets from the investor if the investor wishes to dissolve or "cash out" the IRA. This right of immediate access to the funds may give creditors the right to demand the same access, again depending on the relevant state law. It not only allows creditors to seize the assets held in a custodial IRA, but it also imposes adverse tax consequences on the investor because of the early termination of the IRA.

A relatively new development in this area is the enactment of the Roth IRA. A Roth IRA is an IRA in which the participant receives no income tax deduction for a contribution to the Roth IRA. That sounds bad, but the trade-offs can easily make it worthwhile. In addition to its principal and income-growing tax exempt, the distributions to a participant from a Roth IRA are tax free. In many states, the ability of the Roth IRA to escape the claims of creditors is treated just as a traditional IRA, especially when a flurry of legislative activity overruled a renegade court ruling that a Roth IRA was accessible to a judgment creditor because Roth IRAs were not specifically mentioned in the statute providing protection from seizure.

Joint versus Separate Ownership of Assets

Do you remember when Andy DuFresne confronts the chief guard of his prison in *The Shawshank Redemption* and tells him to divert an inherited sum of money into his wife's name? Even 65 years after the 1949 setting of that conversation, a common means of protecting assets from the reach of creditors is to transfer property into a spouse's name. Assuming that the spouse is also not at substantial risk of being the target of lawsuits because of the spouse's profession or lifestyle, it is an effective means of accomplishing that goal. Creditors with valid judgments against an individual may only attach and seize those assets owned by that individual. Anything worth doing is worth doing right, however, and there are several pointers to structuring asset ownership in a way that maximizes its protective value.

A small number of states, such as Hawaii, Pennsylvania, and Florida, have statutes that automatically protect property jointly owned by spouses from creditors of either spouse, but often not from creditors of both spouses together. Property that benefits from this characterization is held in as a "tenancy by the entirety," and prevents only one spouse from transferring away property that the married couple obtained together. Again, variation in state law determines just how beneficial the formation of a "tenancy by the entirety" can be from an asset protection standpoint. This protection comes from a public interest in the preservation of marital assets, such that one spouse's indiscretion may not harm the position of the other spouse. The most significant limits to the advantage provided by the tenancies of the entirety are first, that the creditors with claims against both spouses may seize such jointly held property, and second, that upon the first death between the spouses, the property flows directly to the surviving spouse alone, who then no longer has the benefit of the creditor protection. Moreover, in April of 2002, the U.S. Supreme Court sharply curtailed the benefit provided by tenancies by the entirety by ruling that it does not shield an asset from the federal authorities, even if the tax liability was incurred only by one spouse.[*]

Some states in the South and West are community property states, which are similar to, but not the same as, tenancy by the entirety. Under the community property theory, all property acquired by either spouse during the residency in that state (or in some states, prior to or during the residency), will be considered jointly owned property even if titled to an individual spouse. Merely by moving to one of these community property states, a person can automatically shift assets, thus reducing the quantity of assets subject to the creditors of the wealthier spouse.

Community property and land owned as tenants-by-the-entirety is different from a third type of ownership called joint tenancy with rights of survivorship, sometimes abbreviated as "JTWROS." JTWROS may ease some burdens associated with probating a decedent's estate, but this form of ownership is not ideal when viewed through the asset protection prism. An alternative is to hold assets in the name of one spouse or the other, or as "tenants-in-common." Tenancy-in-common is best described as a situation in which each spouse owns a one-half undivided share in the property, but does not have the automatic right to full ownership at the death of the other spouse. Three advantages flow from this form of ownership:

- *Neither spouse owns the property exclusively* A creditor seizing the interest of one spouse would not have a valuable asset because it could not evict the remaining spouse; so, creditors will attack these assets only as a last resort to satisfy their claims. However, a lien recorded against either fractional interest would have to be satisfied upon its sale, so that the net proceeds would be reduced by the amount of the lien. For this reason, tenancy-in-common is only a temporary means of protecting an asset from an adverse judgment, and not quite the same as fully separate ownership. This flaw is one reason why many estate planners recommend the funding of property into the name of a spouse or family member less vulnerable to adverse judgments.

---

[*] See United States v. Craft, 535 U.S. 274 (April 17, 2002).

- *If either spouse were to die, only half of the property would be subject to estate tax*   Ownership of property as tenants-in-common helps in the estate-planning arena by facilitating the process of equalizing the assets held by each spouse. Changes made during 2010 and 2013 to the estate tax laws have pushed the federal estate tax exemption above $5 million; so, fewer individuals (<½ of 1% of the general public by some estimates) will realize an actual tax savings from such planning. Even more appealing is that surviving spouses can now claim the unused exemption left behind by a deceased spouse. Estate tax concerns are now playing a much smaller role in recommending how spouses own their property.
- *A dying spouse has the ability to control how his or her interest is distributed*   In many simple wills, all property of a spouse is given by bequest to the surviving spouse. Such a bequest could include partial ownership interests in real estate. If the surviving spouse is concerned about asset protection, this additional property would not be beneficial because it would easily be sacrificed to the survivor's creditors. One way of avoiding this result is to build an estate plan in which each spouse bequeaths the partial interest owned by that spouse to a trust. At the first death between two spouses, the trust will hold the partial ownership interest for the benefit of the surviving spouse. The trust holding the partial residence interest preserves the deterrent faced by creditors of the surviving spouse because seizure of the surviving spouse's interest would not terminate the spouse's right to use the land provided for in the trust.

A different set of rules applies to property held jointly by medical professionals who are not married to each other. If property is owned jointly among siblings or business associates instead of a business entity, the owners should make sure that the deed names them as tenants-in-common. Otherwise, each successive death among the owners will shift the ownership to the survivors, and leave the family of the deceased owner with no lasting value from the owner's investment into the property and its improvements.

Assets should be held in a way that protects them from creditors for the long term. The form of asset holdings should thus be a significant part of the discussions held with professional advisors, so that the protection lasts beyond your death or that of your spouse. Structure the protected assets so that they do not flow back to you if your spouse should pass away. In this manner, integrated asset protection, estate planning, and financial planning unite to protect the family's interests by extending the benefits of creditor protection for the long term.

FORMS OF JOINT OWNERSHIP

- Tenancy by the entirety
- Tenancy in common
- Community property
- Joint tenancy with rights of survivorship (JTWROS)

GIFTING

One easy asset protection tool you can use to ensure that your children inherit your legacy is to begin giving assets to them early, before your future creditors claim them. Gifting should be used much more frequently than it is, but the obvious disadvantage of gifting property to children is that the donor no longer has the use of or control over the property. More emphatically, you must commit to the permanent loss of the property; so, you must be absolutely sure that you will not ever need the gifted assets. This risk is especially significant when planning for future possibilities of creditor invasion.

Gifting is an effective protection against creditors, and a number of different methods are available to affect this intent, without always subjecting the assets to the whims of descendants not ready to handle money. First, small outright gifts to multiple beneficiaries may be made annually. This has the effect of reducing the quantity of assets subject to creditors' claims, but it also entrusts the donee receiving those gifts with control over those assets. Some recipients of gifts given to them are not appreciative of the work that went into earning the gifted property; so, while gifting is an effective asset protection strategy when timed properly, it sometimes has an unwanted impact on the family dynamics.

Gifts made to any individual other than a donor's spouse are subject to gift taxation if they exceed $14,000 in a calendar year. Amounts <$14,000 are exempted from gift tax under I.R.C. § 2503(b), also known as the annual exclusion. Spouses may combine their exclusions to provide up to $28,000 in benefits to their children or other beneficiaries, but it is important to consult with a tax professional before making sizable gifts.

One alternative to outright gifting is to gift property in trust. This option involves giving your property to a trustee, who holds the property for the benefit of a beneficiary other than the donor. The trustee bears a fiduciary duty to obey the instructions set forth in the document establishing the trust, otherwise known as the trust instrument or trust agreement. The transfer of property into a nongrantor, or third-party trust is still considered a gift for tax and property ownership purposes, but the trust instrument may include spendthrift provisions, which prohibit the trustee from distributing assets to certain beneficiaries except for specific uses and at particular times. The vital point here is that the trust separates creditors of both the donor and the beneficiary from the assets.

SPENDTHRIFT TRUSTS

Despite a handful of exceptions discussed near the end of this chapter, retaining control or the benefit of assets held in a trust you create and fund means that state and tax law treat the gift as illusory and will ignore the creation of the trust, allowing your creditors to reach the property. Control of a trust is determined by several factors, including the power to exchange trust assets and the ability to withdraw money.

If the reality of the situation is that the trust was created merely as a smoke screen, and the assets are still within your reach, courts in most jurisdictions will reach through the formalities and treat the property as held solely in the donor's hands.

If that is the case, then how can a trust be considered an asset protection tool? The protection found in a spendthrift trust lies in your sacrifice of such rights in favor of third parties, such as your spouse and children. Suppose that after your death, a trust you create instructs the trustee to hold assets for the benefit of your spouse or children, and distribute assets to them only at the trustee's discretion to meet the actual needs of your children. If the trust has good language preventing the beneficiaries from ordering the trustee to withdraw those assets from the trust, those assets will for the most part be inaccessible to the claims of any creditors of your children. Once a child has the right to request those assets from the trustee, however, that spendthrift protection falls away, and the trust assets become a part of the child's assets in a debtor–creditor dispute.

SAMPLE SPENDTHRIFT LANGUAGE

No interest in this trust shall be subject to the beneficiary's liabilities or creditor claims, assignment, or anticipation. If the trustee shall determine that a beneficiary would not benefit as greatly from any outright distribution of trust income or principal because of the availability of the distribution to the beneficiary's creditors, the trustee shall instead expend those amounts for the benefit of the beneficiary. This direction is intended to enable the trustee to give the beneficiary the maximum possible benefit and enjoyment of all of the trust income and principal to which the beneficiary is entitled.

A gift in trust can be made without saddling the beneficiary with the responsibility of managing the money wisely, and the beneficiary may still gain the benefits of the appreciation and income derived from the gift. The gift in trust is most useful when beneficiaries are too young to effectively manage the assets, or perhaps too immature to invest the money wisely. To educate the beneficiaries in money management, trust provisions often allow the income and principal of the trust to be distributed to the beneficiaries in stages. These stages are often delayed until the beneficiaries have reached adulthood, and are intended to ease the transition from the beneficiary to the owner. While you would like your children or grandchildren to turn a gift into something more valuable, trial and error plays a significant role in money management. Giving incremental gifts to the beneficiaries over time creates the opportunity for beneficiaries to learn the lessons of finance with smaller quantities of money, preserving the remainder of the trust property for a later distribution. Long-term asset protection means more than just protection from creditors. It means protecting the beneficiaries from themselves as well.

In addition to the stages of distribution, many trusts give the trustee the power to distribute assets to beneficiaries or on behalf of beneficiaries for specific purposes. In this way, a trust that delays distribution of money until after a child reaches the age of 25 may still pay for the beneficiary's college and postgraduate education. The trustee may also be allowed to pay for specific events such as weddings and home purchases. This power must be discretionary, however, to preserve the asset protection features of the trust, and the beneficiary may refuse the distributed proceeds, though such an occurrence is extremely rare.

If a creditor can point to gifts made just prior to the effective date of the creditor's judgment, the creditor may be able to persuade a court to forcibly return the gifted property to the ownership of the donor and subject it to the claims of the creditors.

COMPLEX ASSET PROTECTION TOOLS

The following methods of asset protection are significantly more sophisticated than those described above, and will often require a substantial investment of time and money. They are also much more effective at sheltering large quantities of assets from creditors. A working knowledge of their availability will help you know to what degree you might wish to carry out your asset protection efforts.

Complex asset protection tools are aimed at deterrence rather than bulletproof shelter. They make the seizure of assets more difficult than it would otherwise be, and make those assets less attractive to creditors. Although asset protection specialists now practice each method with regular frequency, there are exceptions to almost every rule. Your likelihood of success depends in a large part on the factual circumstances surrounding the inception of your asset protection plan. The primary object should be to steer clear of transfers that could be characterized as fraudulent conveyances. You should discuss the following ideas at length with your advisory team before making any moves with respect to these tools.

AVOIDING FRAUDULENT CONVEYANCES

As a general rule, courts respect the efforts of people to preserve and foster the growth of their assets. Courts balk, however, if such efforts seem fraudulent, or are taken when there is potential liability to creditors or plaintiffs. The courts then label such efforts unethical, void, or even criminal. If you skipped to this part of the chapter because you see trouble on the horizon or are already involved in litigation, it is too late to act. A rescue attempt using the suggestions in this chapter will not patch existing problems. Despite your best intentions, you could be committing a fraud.

Fraudulent conveyances are transfers made by a debtor with the intent to hinder, delay, or defraud creditors. In the absence of concrete evidence of intent, such as a "smoking gun" memorandum, or the availability of testimony, courts look to a number of factors in deciding whether a debtor has the requisite intent. Among these factors are familial relationships between the debtor and the person receiving the conveyance, the timing of the transfer in relation to a creditor's threats of collection or litigation, and whether the debtor received fair value in exchange for the transfer.

There is no bright-line rule to help determine whether a conveyance will be deemed fraudulent because courts use such factors and arbitrarily weigh them to decide the existence of intent. This makes predicting the outcome of any particular fraudulent conveyance case almost impossible. There does, however, seem to be a spectrum along which some landmarks may be plotted. For instance, a physician with a thriving practice, a happy marriage, and a healthy financial balance sheet will not likely be charged with fraudulent conveyance, even if he or she does not receive full value in exchange for a transfer. On the other hand, a defendant in the midst of litigation making a transfer that leaves him or her without sufficient assets to pay a reasonable estimate of the damages will probably be accused of making a fraudulent conveyance.

One of the key factors in determining the fraudulent nature of a conveyance is whether the transfer leaves the transferor either unable to pay his or her debts or with fewer assets than potential liabilities. In other words, if a transfer makes a person insolvent, or if the person is already insolvent, the transfer will likely be ruled by a fraudulent conveyance. Thus, a doctor with a $7 million net worth who has recently become liable for a claim worth $3 million ought not to convey any amount close to $4 million at the risk of being punished for conveying the property fraudulently.

The punishment for a debtor found to have made a fraudulent conveyance is harsh. Creditors' remedies vary from state to state, but creditors are often given the option of voiding the transfer and taking back any property that was given. The debtor, however, may not undo the transfer in the same way. Additionally, the debtor will likely be forced to pay all of the creditor's expenses incurred in revoking the fraudulent conveyance. This rule of law leaves more power in the hands of creditors, and makes it wiser to avoid making fraudulent conveyances at all costs rather than risk the potential for punishment.

RELOCATION

Relocation to another state that has passed debtor-friendly laws is a drastic step, but nevertheless a popular one. Some of the friendlier states include Florida, Arizona, and Nevada. These states have enacted laws that create special rights of ownership for debtors when creditors attempt to collect on judgments. Several states make joint ownership of property between spouses into an effective asset protection device.

Another debtor-friendly rule of law pertains to a debtor's ownership of the cash value of life insurance. Some life insurance policies accrue a cash surrender value, against which the policy-holder may withdraw an advance on the death benefit payable, or for which the policyholder may exchange the policy. The cash surrender value turns the insurance policy into a liquid asset, which creditors could seize and then exchange for money. Florida and some other states offer their residents protection against creditors for the cash value of life insurance policies by declaring the surrender value exempt from garnishment upon an adverse judgment. This convenient legal feature makes the purchase of selected life insurance policies an even more attractive asset protection tool because creditors will choose not to seize the policy in an effort to recover the debt.

HOMESTEAD EXEMPTION

Florida also offers a generous homestead exemption. A homestead exemption is an asset protection shelter created by the statute that prevents one parcel of real estate and its improvements from being attached and levied upon by creditors. By investing money in luxurious homes on large tracts of land in rural areas of Florida, many wealthy individuals are prudently protecting their estates from the reach of creditors.

EXAMPLE 12.1

Dr. David Mackenzie, a Florida resident and domiciliary, invests $4 million of his earned cash into a home with acreage in Florida. The home fully qualifies for the homestead exemption. If Dr. Mackenzie later declares bankruptcy, his home will be exempt from the liquidation of his assets. After the liquidation, all of his debts will be discharged by the bankruptcy court. Although Dr. Mackenzie may have lost his nonexempt assets, he will still own a $4 million asset free and clear of outstanding creditors, with which he may rebuild his accustomed lifestyle.

Another effective use of the homestead exemption is to backstop an incorrect form of jointly owned property. Although tenancies by the entirety and joint tenancies with rights of survivorship automatically leave the surviving spouse with the full ownership of property, the surviving spouse often may use the homestead exemption to preserve a primary residence against creditors' claims.

IRREVOCABLE LIFE INSURANCE TRUSTS

An irrevocable life insurance trust (ILIT) is a specialized trust instrument designed primarily to reduce estate taxes or to enable a client with significant nonliquid assets an opportunity to generate liquidity to pay estate taxes or other obligations without increasing the total estate tax liability. The client creating an ILIT transfers to the ILIT a preexisting life insurance policy on his or her life, or enough money to pay the premiums on a new life insurance policy. If the client survives 3 years beyond the contribution of an existing policy to the trust, or if the policy is a purchased by a trust, the proceeds of the insurance policy payable on the client's death will not constitute a part of his or her taxable estate. An ILIT is also helpful in protecting the cash value of policies from creditors in states where the cash value of life insurance is not protected from creditors' claims.

The primary drawback of the ILIT is that you cannot change the terms of the trust after it is signed, such as the lineup of the trustees or the list of beneficiaries. The second drawback is that money spent on the premiums is not returnable to the creator of the trust, and the proceeds of the insurance policy owned by the trust must flow into the trust at the death of the person on whose life the policy was purchased. Even though the ILIT is not revocable, it may nevertheless be drafted with great flexibility. For example, terms such as "grantor's spouse" may be broadly defined as "the person to whom Grantor is married at the time of Grantor's death." As with any irrevocable document, care must go into its structure and textual references so that the document will have relevance and utility long after its creation.

ILITs also provide creditor protection to beneficiaries because the trust assets are not necessarily immediately available to them. If the ILIT is properly drafted, creditors will not be able to capitalize on an influx of money to the beneficiaries, as they would if the insurance proceeds were paid directly to the beneficiaries. Rather, as with spendthrift trusts created by a third party, the ILIT will serve as a barrier between creditors and beneficiaries, ensuring that the proceeds are spent for the benefit of the beneficiaries, rather than being ceded to their creditors. In favorable comparison to retirement assets, the ILIT can even protect a beneficiary from prioritized claimants, such as a beneficiary's former spouse.

Moreover, an irrevocable trust may prove to be a much more palatable alternative than a prenuptial agreement from the beneficiary's standpoint, particularly in a first-marriage situation. In this regard, ILITs and other irrevocable trusts provide creditor protection in a number of ways to both the creator and the beneficiaries.

FAMILY-LIMITED PARTNERSHIPS

Family-limited partnerships (FLPs) are business entities specializing in the management and prudent investment of family assets. They are used for the same reasons that professional business offices use layered organizations. As with other complex asset protection tools, FLPs do not necessarily make it impossible for a creditor to access an asset, but they instead place obstacles between some claims of creditors and the valuable assets of the family. An FLP will often keep potential claims against individuals from endangering the assets held by the partnership by deterring creditors from pursuing the assets. A family LP is a business, and must be treated as a separate functioning entity, or the partnership will not be respected by the courts, and the protections it offers will be unavailable. The creation and proper funding of an FLP are highly technical maneuvers with serious income tax and estate tax implications, and the timing of your transfers of property is critical to the success of this planning technique.

FLLCs

A modern alternative to the FLP, allowed in a growing number of jurisdictions, is a family-limited liability company. With respect to the family LLC's asset protection capabilities, the structure of an LLC is similar enough to that of a partnership to indicate that creditors will not wish to seize interests in the LLC.

FLPs are different from general partnerships in that some, but not all, of the partners are insulated from liability for losses of the partnership. In a general partnership, all the partners share liability for losses of the partnership. In a limited partnership, at least one partner is appointed as a general partner, and that general partner is fully liable for losses of the partnership. In exchange for this disadvantageous position, the general partner has the power to manage the assets of the partnership.

Limited partners are passive owners and have very limited powers under the laws of most states. Additionally, limited partnerships are almost always governed by an agreement among the partners containing provisions that further limit the rights of the limited partners. One caveat must be raised, however, about the characterization of general partners as opposed to limited partners. If limited partners are proven to be making decisions about the operations of the partnership, limited partners may be treated as general partners, and may be forced to share the liability for losses with the general partner.

In a typical LP agreement, a limited partner may have the power to assign, or transfer, all or part of the economic value of his or her partnership interest to another person with the prior consent of the general partner. The person receiving that assigned interest, called an "assignee," often receives the right to receive the distributions that would otherwise have been delivered to the transferor, but the assignee does not become a limited partner. As a result, the assignee is unable to exert much power within the partnership or redeem his interest in exchange for partnership assets. Even worse for the assignee, the tax attributes of a family LP often require that the assignee pays income tax on a share of the limited partnership's income. Unless distributions are issued to the assignee by the general partner, the assignee will actually experience a negative cash flow upon gaining possession of the LP interest.

Forming an FLP requires a significant amount of advance planning and legal advice. FLPs are not appropriate for all situations, and the Internal Revenue Service (IRS) has in recent years devoted increased attention to the practice. If successful, however, an FLP can be used to discount the value of assets, and thus reduce estate tax liabilities, as well as provide a formidable barrier to the reach of creditors.

EXAMPLE 12.2

Dr. Jack and Dr. Jill each contributes assets to form a family limited partnership, and in exchange, each receives a limited partnership interest. Jack and Jill also form an LLC to serve as a third partner, which will act as the general partner, and thus the lightning rod for any partnership liability. Jack and Jill then assign portions of their limited partnership interests to their three lovely children, Peter, Paul, and Mary, who each become limited partners in the family limited partnership.

Creditors of the limited partners are not able to force their way into the partnership in the capacity of a limited partner. Instead, courts will allow creditors to step into the shoes of a limited partner, or assignee, by means of a charging order. A charging order gives the creditor an assignment interest similar to that of any other assignee. However, it is only an economic interest in the distributions of the partnership. The creditor (or for that matter, any other assignee) does not have any right to immediate payment because distributions are determined by the general partner according to the terms of the partnership agreement, or by statute.

FLPs are particularly effective in some states, such as Georgia, because a creditor levying on the partnership interest does not have the power to force dissolution of the partnership. In some other states, a limited partner (as opposed to an assignee) may have the ability to force the partnership to exchange its interest in the partnership for a pro rata share of the partnership assets by requesting redemption. Thus, choosing the appropriate jurisdiction in which to form the family LP is very important.

Another disadvantage faced by the creditor seeking to take over a partnership interest from a limited partner (or an assignee) is that the general partner has the ability to make or withhold distributions of cash to the creditor. Since partners are taxed on income realized by the partnership, regardless of whether that income is actually distributed to partners, the general partner's control over distributions places the creditor in peril of realizing income without receiving any cash with which to pay the tax generated by his share of the FLP's income.

Finally, the partnership agreement may provide that the existing partners have a right to purchase the assigned partnership interest from the creditor (or assignee) at the fair market value of the partnership interest. Since the fair market value of an assigned partnership interest is usually less than the value of that partner's percentage share of the partnership's assets, the creditor may be forced to settle for less than the value it had expected to realize from the assigned partnership interest. These significant drawbacks to the remedy of a charging order usually deter creditors from attempts to become an assignee of a partnership interest. Instead, creditors will often negotiate a reduced payment schedule or turn to other nonexempt assets of the debtor.

FLPs are also very useful in segregating separate property from marital property in the context of a divorce. If a spouse enters the marriage with a partnership interest, that partnership interest will usually not be blended into the marital estate for purposes of dividing property in a divorce. This attribute enables newlyweds to shelter family assets without the awkwardness of negotiating a prenuptial agreement.

When properly constructed and implemented, FLPs have the potential to significantly reduce the taxable estate of the partners contributing assets. It is vital that only an experienced practitioner well versed in the statutes and case law surrounding FLPs implements the FLP.

Asset Protection Trusts

The transfer of assets to a specifically designed asset protection trust is a technique designed to deter creditors from seeking assets by putting these assets in a trust governed by laws that both protect the trust from certain claims of creditors and still permit the creator of the trust to receive discretionary distributions of principal and income from the trust. Laws that permit this type of trust exist in selected foreign countries and a growing number of states, starting with Alaska and Delaware. Before then, all states followed the common law rule against creditor protection through self-settled trusts. In other words, until very recently, trusts in which the trust creator was a controller of the assets or a beneficiary of its resources could be accessed by creditors of the trust creator. These states passed such laws with the intent to attract investment capital, and as a result, imposed certain restrictions on the trustee and the investments made with the trust assets.

The difference between the asset protection trusts discussed in this section and the spendthrift trusts introduced above is that specialized asset protection trusts may provide creditor protection benefits to the person who contributed the assets to the trust without forbidding the trustee from distributing trust assets back to the creator of the trust. Generally speaking, asset protection trusts have at least four common elements:

- The trustee is independent, meaning someone other than a relative, partner, or employee.
- A high level of discretion is given to the trustee so that distributions are made only when the trustee decides it is appropriate.
- A spendthrift provision preventing the beneficiary of the trust from assigning or conveying the beneficiary's interest in the trust for his or her own benefit.
- An irrevocability clause that keeps the trust creator from making changes to the trust or unwinding it under pressure from a court or creditors.

An asset protection trust generally provides that a trustee has exclusive control over the trust management, and also that the trustee be permitted to distribute or withhold the trust income and principal, at the trustee's sole discretion, provided that the trustee follows the instructions contained in the trust instrument. Often, the trustee is advised, but not directed, through the language in the trust not to distribute assets when the grantor or beneficiary is insolvent or involved in collection proceedings. This type of provision, called an "anti-duress clause" shelters the trust proceeds from exposure to the creditors during the time when creditor protection is needed most.

The most important requirement of the asset protection trust is that it must be established in a jurisdiction with laws that provide that judgments against the trust's grantor will not be enforced against the trust assets. In 1997, Delaware and Alaska each established laws providing some protection for certain trusts established in those states, and states such as Nevada, Missouri, Ohio, South Dakota, Tennessee, Rhode Island, Virginia, and Wyoming have jumped on the bandwagon since then.

In addition to the states that now permit self-settled trusts to offer some sort of creditor protection, offshore jurisdictions such as the Cook Islands, the Cayman Islands, and the Bahamas offer exotic asset protection alternatives. Such offshore alternatives have advantages and disadvantages when compared with domestic trusts and are addressed separately.

Domestic Asset Protection Trusts

Domestic asset protection trusts (DAPTs) are created by transferring property to a trustee under a trust instrument that includes very narrow instructions for returning property to the trust creator, and will be interpreted under the laws of a state that allow such trusts. The states enacting DAPT laws have shrewdly drafted those statutes to maximize the in-state benefit realizable from the trusts. In Alaska, for example, the trust merits protection only if it is closely connected to Alaska, in that both a trustee and some trust assets are located there, as well as several other requirements contained in the statute. If all these requirements are met, the Alaska courts will assert jurisdiction over lawsuits attempting to seize the property, and the courts will apply Alaska law.

Alaska law validates and will enforce trusts that give a trustee the power to distribute assets, at the trustee's exclusive discretion, to a person who transferred property into the trust. The Alaska statute furthermore refuses to permit judgments of any creditor to impact property that was placed in a qualifying trust, unless one of the several exceptions applies. Among the exceptions are fraudulent conveyances and trusts requiring the trustee to distribute assets to the grantor. Additionally, the law forbids most suits alleging that a transfer into the trust was fraudulent unless these suits are brought within 4 years of the transfer into the trust. This means that a qualifying trust properly funded at least 4 years before the grantor faces potential liability stands a good chance of being protected under the Alaska statute because a creditor may not raise the argument that the transfer into the trust was a fraudulent conveyance.

Delaware's statute regarding asset protection trusts is very similar to the law in Alaska. Delaware also requires that a trust must be closely connected with the state of Delaware before extending its influence to the assets held by that trust, but once qualified, the trust may provide both optional distributions to the grantor creating the trust, and trustee discretion in making these distributions. The 4-year rule against lawsuits alleging fraudulent conveyance is carried over as well, but the statutes are not identical in their requirements. Delaware, for example, provides a more extensive list of rights that trust creators may retain without allowing creditor access. All jurisdictions permitting a DAPT, however, allow the trust create to be a potential distributee of income and principal of the trust at the discretion of the trustee. The two pioneer states in this field, Delaware and Alaska, also differ in the way they treat claims among family members, such as judgments for child support and alimony. Finally, each transfer into an Alaska DAPT must be accompanied by an affidavit of the transferor establishing his or her solvency after the transfer. On the contrary, Delaware does not require such an affidavit before honoring the trust. The choice between selecting Delaware law, Alaska law, or another more recently enacting jurisdiction, for the establishment of DAPT is one that must be made with great care.

Nevada and South Dakota are currently viewed as the states with the most debtor-friendly DAPT laws. This is because the statute of limitations barring claims against the transfer of property into the trust is only 2 years, or one-half of the 4-year window set forth in Alaska and Delaware. Furthermore, the Nevada statute provides no exception for divorcing spouses to attach DAPT property or for claims of unpaid alimony and child support to breach the trust protection. Nevada and South Dakota are also jurisdictions following Delaware's lead in not requiring a transferor's affidavit of solvency when transfers are made to the trust.

If an attorney successfully drafts a trust that may be interpreted only under the laws of a jurisdiction with an asset protection trust statute in effect, several advantages fall to the grantor. For example, the laws regarding trusts in several DAPT-friendly states allow trusts to last indefinitely, whereas in most other jurisdictions, a trust's lifetime is limited. In addition, few of those states apply an income tax to income realized by trusts. Thus, it may be possible to escape state income tax on trust income by creating a trust to which only the law of the trust *situs* applies.

Despite these elements, the creator of a DAPT runs the risk that a court will object to the constitutionality of the statutes that make them possible, leaving the grantor with a trust vulnerable to the claims of its creditors. Several academic arguments have been raised that the statutes allowing self-settled asset protection trusts violate the full faith and credit clause of the U.S. Constitution, which requires states to enforce judgments of sister states. To date, the Supreme Court has yet to rule on these issues, so that the validity of these statutes is neither certain nor implausible.

Another source of concern is that the supremacy clause enables federal bankruptcy courts to overrule the statutory language of the states, and reach into asset protection trusts to satisfy creditors in a bankruptcy proceeding. The bankruptcy laws were substantially rewritten in 2005 so that fraudulent transfers may be unwound by a bankruptcy trustee up to 10 years after the transfer.[*]

One recent example of when a DAPT was ruled ineffective using the new rules is in the case *In re Huber.*[†] In that case, a set of unpleasant facts were used by the bankruptcy trustee to persuade a bankruptcy judge that Alaska law did not apply to a trust that purportedly claimed to take advantage of the Alaska creditor protection statutes. Relying on the State of Washington's public policy against self-settled spendthrift trusts, the opinion treated all the assets of the trust as part of the bankruptcy estate available for the trustee to distribute to creditors. In *Huber*, the bankruptcy trustee was able to show that the transfers into the DAPT occurred at the same time that creditors were closing in, and used correspondence of the trust creator and his attorneys to demonstrate that the trusts were set up with the intent of hindering the access of creditors to the trust assets. This "fraudulent conveyance" treatment underscores why the timing of asset protection planning is so critical to its success.

---

[*] 11 U.S.C. 548(e) (2005).
[†] Waldron v. Huber (*In re*: Huber), Bankr. W.D.Wa Adv. No. 12-04171, May 17, 2013 (opinion available at http://goo.gl/1TPMn).

An earlier example of an Alaska DAPT failing to accomplish the goal of shielding trust property from inclusion in the bankruptcy estate is found *In re Mortensen*.[*] In that estate, the trust creator tried drafting the trust on his own, and funded the trust with property after he had burned through most of his liquid assets in dealing with a divorce and several years of low income. Even though Mr Mortensen claimed that he was solvent at the time of the trust creation and transfer, the bankruptcy court found evidence to the contrary and ruled that the transfer was fraudulent and fell within the 10-year window of his bankruptcy filing. The court then allowed the trustee to access and liquidate the trust property for the benefit of the estate's creditors.

Despite these warning tales, it is generally believed among lawyers practicing in the area that when DAPTs are set up well ahead of creditor threats and when a person is solvent, they present the opportunity for individuals to transfer property to a trustee subject to the laws of the United States. This provides a level of comfort for people that would not be available to creators of offshore trusts. DAPTs furthermore are generally less expensive to create and maintain than foreign asset protection trusts. A medical professional interested in creating one of these trusts should adopt a cautious approach, and be ready to initiate a backup plan in the event that the trusts are invalidated or disrespected.

Foreign Asset Protection Trusts

Offshore trusts are trusts established under the laws of a foreign jurisdiction, with foreign trustees, and using assets transferred outside the United States. The laws of the United States thus do not apply to the administration of those trusts, and the assets within offshore trusts are not subject to the jurisdiction of any U.S. court. Although the foreign venue may make it more difficult to pursue claims against trustees who mismanage money, the difficulty in pursuing claims is also faced by creditors, who must fight a legal battle in a foreign land to reach the assets of the trust. That can be very expensive, not just because the creditor will need to hire lawyers who can practice there, but because the procedural laws of these jurisdictions make it very difficult to sue. Some jurisdictions require that a sizable bond must be posted before a suit may be filed. Once in court, the rules of law in the foreign nation also apply to the trust, and several popular nations follow a rule of law allowing much more protection from creditors than would be available in the United States. Trusts created that provide the grantor with benefits at the discretion of the trustee are often insulated from creditors' attempts to seize them. Many jurisdictions do not enforce the fraudulent conveyance doctrine. A few nations even bestow upon the grantor some control over the size and timing of distributions by enforcing anti-duress provisions. These provisions in an offshore trust advise the trustee to follow the directions of the grantor when the grantor is giving directions using his independent free will. If a court or a creditor is forcing the grantor to ask the trustee for money, however, the trustee has the power to refuse to comply with the request.

Tactics such as the use of anti-duress provisions inspire disfavor by the U.S. courts no longer having jurisdiction over the assets. In a ruling by the Ninth Circuit Court of Appeals in California, Denyse and Michael Anderson were held in contempt of court and sentenced to time in jail, because they did not prove that their assets held in an offshore trust were impossible to reach.[†] That court stopped short of declaring the trust invalid, but its hostility to the trust's creation may be reflective of how other courts might view offshore trusts. Although the Andersons served a sentence for angering the court, the U.S. courts' inability to assert jurisdiction made it impossible for the creditor to access the assets. Ultimately, the asset protection device succeeded. Now that the contempt sentence has been served, and the Andersons are back to their usual shenanigans, it is arguable that the benefits were worth the price paid. On the other hand, however, any assets that may later be repatriated

---

[*] Battley v. Mortensen (*In re*: Mortensen), Bankr. D. Alaska, Adv. No. 09-90036, May 26, 2011 (opinion available at http://goo.gl/7gWjA).

[†] *See* Federal Trade Commission v. Affordable Media, L.L.C., 179 F.3d 1228 (9th Cir. 1999).

to the United States will be subject to creditors' claims immediately upon arrival. The outcome in *Anderson* is therefore a mixed blessing.

Several asset protection specialists point to the extreme facts of the *Anderson* case, and dismiss the notion that offshore trusts are a dangerous strategy. The Andersons were found guilty of managing a Ponzi-type pyramid scheme, and the court was attempting to recover the proceeds for the investors. Such facts would not arise in a case of medical malpractice, for example, because the patient would not have been the traceable source of the full amount of the damages.

Another demonstration of disfavor-given offshore trusts was decided by a bankruptcy court in the case *In re Stephan Jay Lawrence.** Mr Lawrence was an options trader who had moved several million dollars into an offshore trust just before a $20 million award was granted against him. When he later attempted to have the debt discharged in a bankruptcy proceeding, the bankruptcy court refused to grant the discharge because it viewed Mr Lawrence as undeserving. In Mr Lawrence's case, the asset protection trust effectively protected his assets, but the court ruled that he could not protect his assets under foreign law and protect himself under the U.S. law as well, because that was not consistent with the spirit of the bankruptcy code. The court then ordered Mr Lawrence to repatriate the assets in the offshore trust. In rehearing the case a year later, the same bankruptcy court held Mr Lawrence in civil contempt of court and sentenced him with heavy daily fines and incarceration.† The court refused to believe Mr Lawrence's testimony that he did not have the power to comply with the order. It specifically denied Mr Lawrence the argument that compliance was impossible because, said the court, Mr Lawrence himself had created the impossibility. On appeal, both the District Court and the Eleventh Circuit Court of Appeals affirmed the decision of the bankruptcy court, and reasoned that the actions of Mr Lawrence were entirely voluntary, and denied him the benefits of a true discharge available to most debtors in bankruptcy.‡ Refusing to give up, Mr Lawrence filed a lawsuit against the bankruptcy trustee from his prison cell, but the District Court and the Court of Appeals have dismissed those claims.§

The common thread in cases such as *Anderson* and *Lawrence* is the courts' hostility to transfers they determine to be fraudulent conveyances. Without the taint of fraud, the creation of an offshore trust would stand a greater chance of being supported.

Offshore trusts were once used to hide assets from the IRS, such that the income they generated would avoid tax, although all foreign income of the U.S. citizens is, and always has been, part of their taxable income. In response to this fraud, the IRS now requires that each offshore trust created by a U.S. citizen must be registered, and provide continuous reporting to the U.S. government. This requirement substantially increases the cost of creating and maintaining an offshore trust.

Both domestic and foreign jurisdictions giving shelter to trust assets against creditors' claims provide an opportunity to place sizable quantities of assets into a trust, while still having the potential to receive the funds at the discretion of the trustee. The asset protection trust is a very effective tool against creditors, notwithstanding the court rulings that have frowned on them so.

ASSET PROTECTION TRUSTS AND DIVORCE

One area in which asset protection trusts are not typically successful is in the context of a divorce. In an equitable division of marital property, courts will frequently rule that assets placed into an asset protection trust are marital assets and subject to the jurisdiction of the court. The court will then shortchange the spouse contributing to the asset protection trust, or order that spouse to terminate the trust and split the income and principal with the divorcing spouse. Two recent examples of the

---

* 227 B.R. 907 (Bankr. S.D. Fla. 1998).
† *See In re* Stephan Jay Lawrence, 238 B.R. 498 (Bankr. S.D. Fla. 1999).
‡ See Lawrence v. Goldberg, 279 F.3d 1294 (11th Cir. 2002).
§ See Lawrence v. Goldberg, 573 F.3d 1265 (11th Cir. 2009).

latter type of ruling in New York have created the precedent that asset protection trusts are ineffective against spouses in a divorce. In most other contexts, however, the asset protection trust remains a viable solution to the challenges of creating an asset protection strategy.

TIMING IS EVERYTHING

It merits repeating: timing is everything! Each method of asset protection introduced in this chapter works best if completed before danger of creditors appears on the horizon. Advance planning is key to the success of an asset protection strategy, and the ideas were intended to inspire the current action, rather than provide an escape route for medical professionals already nearing financial difficulty. Much like the diversification of assets in an investment portfolio, the methods are frequently used in concert with one another as redundant strategies to ensure effectiveness. Sanguine asset protection planners will employ several of them collectively because all of them provide a unique approach to the challenge of asset protection. The tools in this chapter are also qualified with the intent that they must be used with the consultation and advisement of professionals, since there are loopholes and pitfalls that make asset protection into a legal and financial planning subspecialty itself.

The complex forms of asset protection are primarily used because they require creditors to expend additional time, effort, and money, and in this way are often more effective than the simple ones and used frequently by physicians and couples of high net worth. Implemented properly and at the proper time, complex asset protection tools have proven to be highly effective at sheltering millions of dollars from the hands of creditors and plaintiffs, to the betterment of the people who use them wisely.

OVERHEARD IN THE ADVISOR'S LOUNGE: ON ASSET PROTECTION FOR PHYSICIAN ENTREPRENEURS

Once upon a time, I had a lot of practicing physicians as clients. Now, the only physicians I have as clients are those entrepreneurs who invented some product and have a royalty stream, or who made a lot of money selling their practice. HMOs and large corporate practices have driven down the compensation being paid to most physicians to where they can no longer afford my services.

This is a dramatic turnaround in only about the last decade. Truth is, most physicians can't afford the sophisticated asset protection structures which work very well, and are now designed to give effective protection to upwards of at least $10 million dollars in net assets.

Instead, today physicians are often burned when placed into "cheapie" trusts, limited partnerships, or the like. Physicians also seem to be particularly susceptible to losing their money to offshore trust and investment schemes. Many would be much better off with umbrella liability policies or litigation expense policies than the structures they have now.

Jay D. Adkisson, JD
(Riser Adkisson LLP)

CONCLUSION

This chapter demonstrated how to reduce and avoid risk, and handle assets to minimize the chances of losing them to creditors; regardless of how they are acquired. If used early when your financial outlook is healthy, they can be an effective barrier between your wealth and the reach of future creditors.

COLLABORATE

Discuss this chapter online with others at www.MedicalExecutivePost.com.

FURTHER READING

Adkisson, J and Riser, C: *Asset Protection*. McGraw-Hill, New York, 2006.

Gassman, AS: *Creditor Protection for Florida Physicians: A Comprehensive Handbook for Physicians and Their Advisors*. Haddon Hall Publishing, New York, 2012.

Gassman, AS and Markham, MC: *Gassman and Markham on Florida and Federal Asset Protection Law*. Haddon Hall Publishing, New York, 2013.

Korn, DJ: Are your HNW client covered? *Financial Planning*. New York, March 12, 2014.

Miller, C: Asset protection for physicians. In Marcinko, DE (ed.), *Financial Planning for Physicians*. Jones and Bartlett, Sudbury, MA, 2007.

Presser, H: *Asset Protection Secrets*. Brookline Press, LLC, Boston, 2013.

Taylor, CC: *Asset Protection Made Easy: How to Become Invincible to Lawsuits, Save Thousands in Taxes, and Set Up a Successful Estate Plan*. Mount Lanai Publishing, Vista, CA, 2011.

Section III

For Mid-Career Practitioners

Doctors, like most people, tend to experience financial losses more intensely than gains, and evaluate investing and other risks in isolation. Much, like they do in clinical practice.

Similarly, risky technology investments, initial public offerings (IPOs), exorbitant portfolio "wrap" account fees and asset management percentages are often hawked by high-priced financial advisors (FAs) and stock brokers selling loaded mutual funds, costly hedge and market-neutral funds, alternative investments (AIs), and even real estate. So, it is not only important to review these modern topics and considerations in Section III, but traditional retirement planning, as well.

In life's journey, from birth to death, the stage is being set for the emerging medical practitioner to assume the mantle of mature, successful, and affluent physician-investor; self-educating, monitoring, and perhaps even relying more on self-wits or ME Inc, rather than paid advisors.

After all, we believe the analogy of collaborate financial planning and client-centered advice is akin to the new concept of collaborative medicine and the patient-centered care movements.

In other words: *Omnia pro medicus cluentis*, or "all for the doctor client."

13 Investment Banking, Securities Markets, and Margin Accounts
Fundamental Trading and Operational Principles

David Edward Marcinko and Timothy J. McIntosh

CONTENTS

There are several different kinds of banks. A general understanding of these concepts is suggested for any medical professional prior to launching a self-directed (ME, Inc.), or even a guided investment strategy or wealth-building portfolio effort with an FA, stock broker or wealth manager, and so on. This operational and trading information is usually not included in a text on financial planning, until now.

DEFINITION OF RETAIL BANK

A retail bank is a typical small mass-market financial institution in which individual customers use local branches, usually of larger commercial banks. Services offered include savings and checking accounts, mortgages, personal loans, debit/credit cards, and certificates of deposit (CDs).

DEFINITION OF COMMERCIAL BANK

A commercial bank is a financial institution that provides services, such as accepting deposits, giving business loans and auto loans, mortgage lending, and basic investment products such as savings accounts and certificates of deposit. The traditional commercial bank is a brick and mortar institution with tellers, safe deposit boxes, vaults, and ATMs. However, some commercial banks do not have any physical branches and require consumers to complete all transactions by phone or Internet. In exchange, they generally pay higher interest rates on investments and deposits, and charge lower fees.

DEFINITION OF INVESTMENT BANK

Investment banking activities are different than those of retail and commercial banking and include underwriting securities, acting as an intermediary between an issuer of securities and the investing public, facilitating mergers and other corporate reorganizations, and also acting as a broker for institutional clients.

INVESTMENT BANKING AND SECURITIES UNDERWRITING

New economy corporate events of the past several years have provided many financial signs and symptoms that indicate a creeping securitization of the for-profit healthcare industrial complex. Similarly, fixed income medical investors should understand how Federal and State regulations impact upon personal and public debt needs. So, without investment banking firms it would be almost impossible for private industry, medical corporations, and government to raise needed capital or for doctors to understand the securities business for their own personal investing needs.

INTRODUCTION

When a corporation such as a mobile-health company or similar entity needs to raise capital for growth or expansion, there are two methods: debt or equity. If raising equity is used, the corporation can market securities directly to the public by contacting its current stockholders and asking them to purchase the new securities in a rights offering by advertising or by hiring salespeople. Although this last example is somewhat exaggerated, it illustrates that there is a cost to selling new securities, which may be considerable if the firm itself undertakes the task. For this reason, most corporations employ help in marketing new securities by using the services of investment bankers who sell new securities to the general public. Although the investment banking is an exciting and vital industry, the many Securities Exchange Commission (SEC) rules regulating it are not.

FUNDAMENTALS OF THE INVESTMENT BANKING INDUSTRY

Investment bankers are not really bankers at all. The fact that the word banker appears in the name is partially responsible for the false impressions that exist in the medical community regarding the functions they perform. For example, they are not permitted to accept deposits, provide checking accounts, or perform other activities normally construed to be commercial banking activities. An investment bank is simply a firm that specializes in helping other corporations obtain money they need under the most advantageous terms possible.

When it comes to the actual process of having securities issued, the corporation approaches an investment banking firm, either directly, or through a competitive selection process and asks it to act as adviser and distributor. Investment bankers, or under writers, as they are sometimes called, are middlemen in the capital markets for corporate securities.

The corporation requiring the funds discusses the amount, type of security to be issued, price and other features of the security, as well as the cost to issuing the securities. All of these factors are negotiated in a process known as negotiated underwriting. If mutually acceptable terms are reached, the investment banking firm will be the middle man through which the securities are sold to the general public. Since such firms have many customers, they are able to sell new securities, without the costly search that individual corporations may require to sell its own security. Thus, although the firm in need of additional capital must pay for the service, it is usually able to raise the additional capital at less expense through the use of an investment banker, than by selling the securities itself.

The agreement between the investment banker and the corporation may be one of two types. The investment bank may agree to purchase, or underwrite, the entire issue of securities and to re-offer them to the general public. This is known as a *firm commitment*. When an investment banker agrees to underwrite such a sale; it agrees to supply the corporation with a specified amount of money. The firm buys the securities with the intention to resell them. If it fails to sell the securities, the investment banker must still pay the agreed upon sum. Thus, the risk of selling rests with the underwriter and not with the company issuing the securities.

The alternative agreement is a best effort agreement in which the investment banker makes his best effort to sell the securities acting on behalf of the issuer, but does not guarantee a specified amount of money will be raised.

When a corporation raises new capital through a public offering of stock, one might inquire where the stock comes from. The only source the corporation has is authorized, but previously un-issued stock. Anytime authorized, but previously un-issued stock (new stock) is issued to the public, it is known as a primary offering. If it's the very first time the corporation is making the offering, it's also known as the *Initial Public Offering* (IPO). Anytime there is a primary offering of stock, the issuing corporation is raising additional equity capital.

A *secondary offering*, or distribution, on the other hand, is defined as an offering of a large block of outstanding stock. Most frequently, a secondary offering is the sale of a large block of stock owned by one or more stockholders. It is stock that has previously been issued and is now being re-sold by investors. Another case would be when a corporation re-sells its treasury stock.

Prior to any further discussions of investment banking, there are several industry terms to be defined. For example, an *agent* buys or sells securities for the account and risk of another party and charges a commission. In the securities business, the terms *broker* and agent are used synonymously. This is not true of the insurance industry. On the other hand, a *principal* is one who acts as a dealer rather than an agent or broker. A dealer buys and sells for his own account. Finally, the *dealer* makes money by buying at one price and selling at a higher price. Thus, it is easy to understand how an investment banking firm earns money handling a best efforts offering; they make a commission on every share they sell.

THE SECURITIES ACT OF 1933 (ACT OF FULL DISCLOSURE)

When a corporation makes a public offering of its stock, it is bound by the provisions of the Securities Act of 1933, which is also known as the Act of Full Disclosure. The primary requirement of the Act is that the corporation must file a registration statement (full disclosure) with the Securities and Exchange Commission (SEC), containing some of the following items:

- Description of the business entity raising the money
- Biographical data regarding officers and directors of the issuer
- Listing of share holdings of officers, directors, and holders of more than 10% of the issuer's securities (insiders)
- Financial statements including a breakdown of existing capitalization (existing debt and equity structure)
- Intended use of offering proceeds
- Legal proceedings involving the issuer, such as suits, antitrust actions, or strikes

Acting in its capacity as an adviser to the corporation, the investment banking firm fills out the registration statement for the SEC. It then takes the SEC a period of time to review the information in the registration statement. This is the "cooling off period" and the issue is said to be "in registration" during this time. When the Act was written in 1933, Congress thought that 20 days would be enough time from the filing date, until the effective date the sale of securities was permitted.

In reality, it frequently takes much longer than 20 days for the SEC to complete its review. But, regardless of how long it lasts, it's known as the *cooling off period*. At the end of the cooling off period, the SEC will either accept the issue or they will send a letter back to the issuer, and the underwriter, explaining that there is incomplete information in the registration statement. This letter is known as a *deficiency letter*. It will postpone the effectiveness of the registration statement until the deficiency is remedied. Even if initially or eventually approved, an effective registration does not mean that the SEC has approved the issue.

For example, the following well-known disclaimer statement written in bold red ink, is required to be placed in capital letters on the front cover page of every prospectus:

THESE SECURITIES HAVE NOT BEEN APPROVED OR DISAPPROVED BY THE SECURITIES AND EXCHANGE COMMISSION NOR HAS THE COMMISSION PASSED UPON THE ACCURACY OR ADEQUACY OF THIS PROSPECTUS. ANY REPRESENTATION TO THE CONTRARY IS A CRIMINAL OFFENSE.

During the cooling off period, the investment bank tries to create interest in the market place for the issue. In order to do that, it distributes a *preliminary prospectus,* more commonly known as a "*red herring.*" It is known as a red herring because of the red lettering on the front page. The statement on the very top with the date is printed in red as well as the statements on the left-hand margin of the preliminary prospectus.

The cost of printing the red herring is borne by the investment bank, since they are trying to market it. The red herring includes information from the registration statement that will be most helpful for potential medical investors trying to make a decision. It describes the company and the securities to be issued; includes the firm's financial statements; its current activities; the regulatory bodies to which it is subject; the nature of its competition; the management of the corporation; and what the expected proceeds will be used for. Two very important items missing from the red herring are the *public offering price* and the *effective date* of the issue, as neither are known for certain at this point in time.

The public offering price is generally determined on the date that the securities become effective for sale (effective date). Waiting until the last minute enables the investment bankers to price the new issue in line with current market conditions. Since the investment banker uses the red herring to try to create interest in the market place, stock brokers (registered representatives with a Series # 7 general securities license) will send copies of the red herring to their clients for whom they feel the issue is a suitable investment. The SEC is very strict on what can be said about an issue, in registration. In fact, during the *pre-filing period* (the time when the negotiations are going on between the issuer and the underwriter), absolutely nothing can be said about it to anyone.

For example, if the regulators find out that your stock broker discussed with you (the potential investor) the fact that his firm was negotiating with an issuer for a possible public offering, he could be fined, or jailed. During the cooling off period (the time when the red herring is being distributed), nothing may be sent to you; not a research report, nor a recommendation from another firm, or even the sales literature. The only thing you are permitted to receive is the red herring. The red herring is used to acquaint prospects with essential information about the offering. If you are interested in purchasing the security, then you will receive an "*indication of interest,*" but you can still not make a purchase or send money. No sales may be made until the effective date; all that can be used to generate interest is the red herring.

Tombstone Advertising and the Prospectus

Despite the above SEC restriction, some idea of potential demand for a new issue can be gauged and have a bearing on pricing decisions. For example, as CEO of a medical instrument company, or interested investor, would you rather see a great deal of interest in a potential new issue or not very much interest? There is, however, one kind of advertisement that the underwriter can publish during the cooling off period. It's known as a *tombstone ad.* The ad makes it clear that it is only an announcement and does not constitute an offer to sell or solicit the issue, and that such an offering can only be made by prospectus. SEC Rule 134 of the 1933 Act itself, refers to a tombstone ad as "communication not deemed a prospectus" because it makes reference to the prospectus in the ad. Tombstones have received their name because of the sparse nature of details found in them. However, the most popular use of the *tombstone ad* is to announce the effectiveness of a new issue, after it has been successfully issued. This promotes the success of both the underwriter as well as the company.

Since distributing securities involves potential liability to the investment bank, it will do everything possible to protect itself. So, near the end of the cooling off period, a meeting is held between the underwriter and the corporation. It is known as a *due diligence meeting.* At this meeting they both discuss amendments that are going to be necessary to make the registration statement complete and accurate. The corporate officers *and* the underwriters sign the final registration statement. They have civil liability for damages that result from omissions of material facts or misstatements of fact. They also have criminal liability if the distribution is done by use of fraudulent, manipulative, or deceptive means. Due diligence takes on a whole new meaning when incarceration from a half-hearted underwriting effort; can occur. The investment bank strives to ensure that there have been no material changes to the issuer or the terms of the issue since the registration statement was filed.

Again, as a physician, how would you feel if you were an investment banker raising capital for a new pharmaceutical company that had developed a drug product that was highly marketable? But on the day after the issue was effective, there was a major news story indicating that the company was being sued for patent infringement? What effect do you think that would have on the market price of this new issue? It would probably plunge. How could this situation have been prevented? The due diligence meeting is more than a cocktail party or a gathering in a smoke-filled room. Otherwise, the company would require specially trained people to do a patent search, lessening the likelihood of this scenario. At the due diligence meeting work is done on the preparation of the final prospectus, but the investment bank does not set the public offering price or the effective date at this meeting. The SEC will eventually set the effective date for the registration and it is on that date that the final offering price will be determined.

Once the SEC sets the effective date, sales may be executed and money can be accepted by the investment bank. It is at this time that the *final prospectus,* similar to the red herring but *without* the red ink and *with* the missing numbers, is issued. A prospectus is an abbreviated form of the registration statement, distributed to purchasers, on and after the effective date of the registration. It is *not* the same as the registration statement. A typical registration statement consists of papers that stand more than a foot high; rarely does a prospectus go beyond 40 or 50 pages. All purchasers will receive a final prospectus and then it becomes permissible for the underwriter to provide sales literature.

In addition to the requirement that a prospectus must be delivered to a purchaser of new issues no later than with confirmation of the trade, there are two other requirements which physicians, medical professionals, and healthcare executive investors should know.

90-day: When an issuer has an *initial* public offering *(IPO),* there is generally a lack of publicly available material relating to the operations of that issuer. Because of this, the SEC requires that all members of the underwriting group make available a prospectus on an IPO for a period of 90 days after the effective date.

40-day: Once an issuer has gone public, there are a number of routine filings that must be made with the SEC so there is publicly available information regarding the financial condition of that issuer. Since additional information is now available, the SEC requires that, on all issues other than IPOs, any member of the underwriting group must make available a prospectus for a period of *40 days* after the effective date.

In the event that the investment bankers misgauged the marketplace, and the issue moves quite slowly, it is possible that information contained in the prospectus would be rendered obsolete by the SEC. Specifically, the SEC requires that any prospectus used more than 9 months after the effective date, may not have any financial information more than 16 months old. It can however, be amended or stickered, with updated information, as needed.

SYNDICATION AMONG UNDERWRITERS

Because the investment banking firm may be underwriting (distributing) a rather large dollar amount of securities, to spread its risk exposure it may form a group made up of other investment bankers or underwriters, known as a *syndicate*. The syndicate is headed by a *syndicate manager,* or *lead underwriter*, and it is his job to decide whether to participate in the offering. If so, the managing underwriter will sign a nonbinding agreement called a *letter of intent.*

If all has gone well and the market place is sufficiently interested in the security, and the SEC has been satisfied with respect to the registration statement, it is time for all parties to the offering to formalize their relationships with a contract including the basic understandings reflected in the letter of intent. Three principal underwriting contracts are involved in the usual public offering, each serving a distinct purpose. These are the Agreement Among Underwriters, Underwriting Agreement, and the Dealer Agreement.

In the *Agreement Among Underwriters (AAU),* the underwriters committing to a portion of the issue, enter into an agreement establishing the nature and terms of their relationship with each other. It designates the syndicate manager to act on their behalf, particularly to enter into an Underwriting Agreement with the issuer, and to conduct the offering on behalf of each of them. The AAU will designate the managing underwriter's compensation *(management fee)* for managing the offering.

The authority to manage the offering includes the authority to agree with the issuer as to the public offering price, decide when to commence the offering, modify the offering price and selling commission, control all advertising, and control the timing and effectiveness of the registration statement by quickly responding to deficiency letters. Each underwriter agrees to purchase a portion of the underwritten securities, which is known as each underwriter's *allotment* (allocation). It is normally signed severally, but not jointly, meaning each underwriter is obligated to sell his allocation but bears no financial obligation for any unsold allotment of another underwriter. This is referred to as a divided account or a *Western account*. Much less frequently, an undivided or *Eastern account,* will be used. Each underwriter is responsible for unsold allotments of others based upon a proportionate share of the offering.

The above comments referred to firm commitment underwriting. Another type of underwriting commitment is known as best efforts underwriting. Under the terms of *best-efforts* underwriting, the underwriters make no commitment to buy or sell the issue; they simply do the best they can, acting as an agent for the issuer and having no liability to the issuer if none of the securities are sold. There is no syndicate formed with a best efforts underwriting. The investment bankers form a selling group, with each member doing his best to sell his allotment. Two variations of a best efforts underwriting are: the all-or-none, and the mini-max (part-or-none) underwriting. Under the provisions of an all-or-none offering, unless all of the shares can be distributed within a specified period of time, the offering will terminate and no subscriptions or orders will be accepted or filled. Under mini-max, unless a set minimum amount is sold, the offering will be terminated.

SEC Rule 15c2-4 requires the underwriter to set up an escrow account for any money received before the closing date, in the event that it is necessary to return the money to prospective purchasers. If the "minimum" or "all" the contingencies are met, the monies in escrow go to the issuer with the underwriters retaining their appropriate compensation. In order to make sure that investors are properly protected, the escrow account must be maintained at a bank for the benefit of the investors until every appropriate event or contingency has occurred. Then, the funds are properly returned to the investors. If the money is to be placed into an interest bearing account, it must have a maturity date no later than the closing date of the offering, or the account must be redeemable at face with no prepayment penalty as regards principal.

UNDERWRITER COMPENSATION HIERARCHY

As we have seen, in a firm commitment the underwriter buys the entire issue from the issuer and then attempts to resell it to the public. The price at which the syndicate offers the securities to the public is known as the public offering price. It is the price printed on the front page of the prospectus. However, the managing underwriter pays the issuer a lower price than this for the securities. The difference between that lower price and the public offering price is known as the spread or underwriting discount. Everyone involved in the sale of a new issue is compensated by receiving part of the spread. The amount of the spread is the subject of negotiations between the issuer and the managing underwriter, but usually is within a range established by similar transactions between comparable issuers and underwriters. The spread is also subject to NASD/FINRA review and approval before sales may commence. The spread is broken down by the underwriters so that a portion of it is paid to the managing underwriter for finding and packaging the issue and managing the offering (usually called the manager's fee); and a portion is retained by each underwriter (called the underwriting or syndicate allowance) to compensate the syndicate members for their expenses, use of money, and assuming the risk of the underwriting. The remaining portion is allocated to the selling group and is called selling concession. It is often useful to remember the compensation hierarchy pecking order in the following way:

- Spread (syndicate manager)
- Underwriters allowance (syndicate members)
- Selling concession (selling group members)
- Re-allowance (any other firm)

While the above deals with corporate equity, the only other significant item with respect to corporate debt is the Trust Indenture Act of 1939. This Federal law applies to public issues of debt securities in excess of $5,000,000. The thrust of this act is to require an indenture with an independent trustee (usually a bank or trust company) who will report to the holders of the debt securities on a regular basis.

Successful marketing of a new issue is a marriage between somewhat alien factors: compliance and numerous federal, state, and self-regulatory rules and statutes, along with finely honed and profit-motivated sales techniques. It's not too hard to see that there could be a real, or apparent, conflict of interest here. Most successful investment bankers have built their excellent reputations upon their ability to properly balance these two objectives consistently, year after year.

NEW ISSUE STABILIZATION

Some issues move very well, like traditional blue chips stocks (i.e., Walgreens). Some are dogs, like smaller dot.com companies (iixl.com). Then, there are issues that were former darlings, but are now ice cold; like PPMCs (i.e., Phycor) and Internet stocks (i.e., Dr. Koop). How far can an underwriting manager go in nudging along an issue that's not selling well? SEC rules do permit a certain amount of help by the manager, even if this takes on the appearance of price fixing. This help is called stabilizing the issue. Simply put, if shortly after a new offering begins, supply exceeds demand, there will be downward pressure on the price. But the law requires that all purchasers of the new issue pay the official offering price on the prospectus. If public holders of the stock become willing to bail out and accept a low selling price, the investor looking to buy will find he is able to buy stock of the issuer cheaper in the open market than buying it new from the syndicate members.

To prevent such a decline in the price of a security during a public offering, SEC rules permit the manager to offer to buy shares in the open market at a bid price at, or just below, the official offering price of the new issue. This is referred to as stabilizing and his bid price is called the stabilizing bid. There is always the risk in a firm commitment underwriting that the underwriters will have difficulty selling the new issue. What they can't sell, they're "stuck" with. That's where the term "sticky issue" comes from. As a potential investor in a new issue, be aware that the best way to get an issue to sell is to increase the compensation to the sales force (i.e., your stock broker *aka* "financial advisor").

Another choice is through *stabilization*. Stabilizing is a permitted form of market manipulation which tends to protect underwriters against loss. It allows the underwriting syndicate (usually through the efforts of the syndicate manager) to stabilize (peg or fix) the secondary market trading price in a new issue at the published public offering price. It works something like this.

When a new issue is selling slowly, some of the investors who initially purchased, may be dissatisfied with the performance of the stock (if it is selling slowly and the underwriters have plenty to sell at the public offering price, this is anything but a hot issue and the security price will not have risen). This dissatisfaction with performance leads to these investors desiring to sell the securities they have just purchased. If the underwriters are unable to sell at the public offering price, certainly an individual investor will have to take less when bailing out. As market makers begin to trade the stock in the secondary market, they would only be able to compete with the underwriters by offering the stock at a lower price than the public offering price. This would make it difficult (if not impossible) for the underwriters to distribute the remaining new shares.

To prevent this from happening, the managing underwriter (who is usually the one to assume the role of stabilizing underwriter), agrees to purchase back any of the new shares at or just slightly below the public offering price. That is a higher price than any market maker could, in all practicality, bid for the shares. When the shares are repurchased by the stabilizing underwriter, it is as if the initial trade was annulled and never took place so that these new shares are now placed back into the distribution and are sold as new shares at the public offering price. SEC rules do, however, require disclosure of this practice. Therefore, no syndicate manager may engage in stabilizing unless the following phrase appears in bold print on the inside front cover page of the prospectus:

IN CONNECTION WITH THIS OFFERING, THE UNDERWRITERS MAY OVER ALLOT OR EFFECT TRANSACTIONS WHICH STABILIZE OR MAINTAIN THE MARKET PRICE OF (XYZ COMPANY) AT A LEVEL ABOVE THAT WHICH MIGHT OTHERWISE PREVAIL IN THE OPEN MARKET. SUCH TRANSACTIONS MAY BE EFFECTED ON (NYSE) STABILIZING, IF COMMENCED, MAY BE DISCONTINUED AT ANY TIME.

Of course, it would be manipulation and, therefore, a violation of law if this "price-pegging" activity continued after the entire new issue was sold out. This activity costs the syndicate manager money which is recouped by levying a syndicate penalty bid against those members of the syndicate whose clients turn shares in on a stabilizing bid.

One way to avoid stabilization is to over allot to each of the syndicate members. This is the same concept as "over booking" that's done by the airlines. Most airlines typically sell 5–10% more seats than the airplane has knowing that there will be last minute cancelations and no shows. This tends to ensure that the plan will fly full. In the same manner, managing underwriters frequently over allot an additional 10% to each of their syndicate members so that last minute cancelations should still leave the syndicate with sell orders for 100% of the issue. If there are no "drop outs," one of two things may happen:

1. The issuer will issue the additional shares (which results in it raising more money).
2. The issuer will not issue the additional shares and the syndicate will have to go short. Any losses suffered by the syndicate through taking of this short position are shared proportionately by the syndicate members.

Now, what if market conditions and the fervor surrounding a new issue, like e-commerce company Ariba in 1999, remain so that the issue doesn't cool down during the cooling off period? Such hot issues are a mixed blessing to be sure. On the one hand, the issue is a sure sell-out. On the other, just how many healthcare investors are going to be told by brokers that additional shares cannot be obtained? Furthermore, the SEC and the FINRA/NASD are vigorous in their scrutiny of proper distribution channels for hot issues. Just what is a "proper" distribution? It can be summed up in one sentence. Member firms have an obligation to make a "bona fide" public distribution of all the shares at the public offering price. The key to this rule lies within the definition of bona fide public distribution.

Municipal Underwriting

While the underwriting procedures for corporate bonds are almost identical to corporate stock, there are significant differences in the underwriting of municipal securities. Municipal securities are exempt from the registration filing requirements or the Securities Act of 1933. A state or local government, in the issuance of municipal securities, is not required to register the offering with the SEC, so there is no filing of a registration statement and there is no prospectus which would otherwise have to be given to investors.

There are two main methods of financing when it comes to municipal securities. One method is known as *negotiated*. In the case of a negotiated sale, the municipality looking to borrow money would approach an investment bank and negotiate the terms of the offering directly with the firm. This is really not very different from the above equity discussions.

The other type of municipal underwriting is known as *competitive bidding*. Under the terms of competitive bidding an issuer announces that it wishes to borrow money and is looking for syndicates to submit competitive bids. The issue will then be sold to the syndicate which submits the best bid, resulting in the municipality having the lowest net interest cost (lowest expense to the issuer).

If the issue is to be done by a competitive bid, the municipality will use a Notice of Sale to announce that fact. The notice of sale will generally include most or all of the following information:

- Date, time, and place. This does not mean when the bonds will be sold to the public, but when the issue will be awarded (sold) to the syndicate issuing the bid.
- Description of the issue and the manner in which the bid is to be made (sealed bid or oral).
- Type of bond (general obligation, revenue, etc.)
- Semi-annual interest payment dates and the denominations in which the bonds will be printed.
- Amount of good faith deposit required, if any.
- Name of the law firm providing the legal opinion and where to acquire a bid form.
- The basis upon which the bid will be awarded, generally the lowest net interest cost.

Since municipal securities are not registered with the SEC, the municipality must hire a law firm in order to make sure that they are issuing the securities in compliance with all state, local, and federal laws. This is known as the bond attorney, or independent bond counsel. Some functions are included below:

1. Establishes the exemption from federal income tax by verifying requirements for the exemption.
2. Determines proper authority for the bond issuance.
3. Identifies and monitors proper issuance procedures.
4. Examines the physical bond certificates to make sure that they are proper.
5. Issues the debt and a legal opinion, since municipal bonds are the only securities that require an opinion.
6. Does not prepare the official statement.

When medical or other investors purchase new issue municipal securities from syndicate or selling group members, there is no prospectus to be delivered to investors, but there is a document which is provided to purchasers very similar in nature to a prospectus. It is known as an *Official Statement*. The Official Statement contains all of the information an investor needs to make a prudent decision regarding a proposed municipal bond purchase.

The formation of a municipal underwriting syndicate is very similar to that for a corporate issue. When there is a negotiated underwriting, an *Agreement Among Underwriters* (AAU) is used. When the issue is a competitive bid, the agreement is known as a Syndicate Letter. In the syndicate letter, the managing underwriter details all of the underwriting agreements among members of the syndicate. *Eastern* (undivided) and *Western* (divided) accounts are also used, but there are several different types of orders in a municipal underwriting. The traditional types of orders, in priority order, are

Pre-Sale Order: Made before the syndicate actually offers the bonds. They have first priority over any other orders.

Syndicate (Group Net) Order: Made once the offering is under way at the public offering price. The purchase is credited to each syndicate member in proportion to its allotment. An institutional buyer will frequently purchase "group net," since many of the firms in the syndicate may consider this buyer to be their client and he wishes to please all of them.

Designated Order: Sales made to medical investors (usually healthcare institutions) at the public offering price where the investor designates which member or members of the syndicate are to be given credit.

Member Orders: Purchased by members of the syndicate at the take-down price (spread). The syndicate member keeps the full take down if the bonds are sold to investors, or earns the take down less the concession if the sale is made to a member of the selling group. Should the offering be over-subscribed, and the demand for the new bonds exceeds the supply, the first orders to be filled are the pre-sale orders. Those are followed by the syndicate (sometimes called group net) orders, the designated orders, and the last orders filled are the member's.

Finally, be aware that the term *bond scale*, which is a listing of coupon rates, maturity dates, and yield or price at which the syndicate is re-offering the bonds to the public. The scale is usually found in the center of a tombstone ad and on the front cover of the official statement. One of the reasons why the word "scale" is used is, that like the scale on a piano, it normally goes up. A regular or positive scale is one in which the yield to maturity is lowest on the near term maturities and highest on the long term maturities. This is also known as a positive yield curve, since the longer the maturity, the higher the yield. In times of very tight money, such as in 1980–1981, one might find a bond offering with a negative scale. A negative (sometimes called inverted) scale is just the opposite of a positive one, where yields on the short-term maturities are higher than those on the long-term maturities.

UNDERWRITING GOVERNMENT ISSUES

The underwriting of U.S. Government securities is the largest underwriting market in the world, but issues a bit differently. For example, there is no such thing as a negotiated underwriting on a U.S. Government security. All offerings of the Treasury are sold by auction. The auction is conducted by the Federal Reserve Bank of New York in accordance with a published schedule. Unfortunately, they are not open to the public, just primary dealers. A bank or investment dealer is appointed by the president of the Federal Reserve Bank of New York and are the only entities authorized to buy and sell government securities in direct dealings with the FED. One becomes a primary dealer through qualifications of reputation, underwriting capacity, and adequacy of staff and facilities.

Currently, 13- and 26-week treasury bills are offered every week on Mondays, while 52-week bills are auctioned once a month. Treasury notes and bonds are auctioned much less frequently. Those dealers wishing to acquire a particular Treasury security enter bids on a yield basis rather than at a specific price. This method is sometimes called a Dutch auction. As a practical matter, about a week or so before the proposed auction, the Treasury announces the following four items: amount, maturity date, nominal or coupon rate anticipated, and the minimum denominations available (except for T bills which don't have interest coupons and always carry a minimum denomination of $10,000).

Can the individual medical professional purchase newly issued Treasuries? Yes! Rather than turning in a competitive bid as the primary dealer does, the individual will turn in a noncompetitive bid. Competitive bidding with governments is similar to the other competitive bidding discussed above. The underwriter turning in the lowest bid wins. Due to the enormous size of Treasury offerings it is extremely rare that the lowest bidder is able to take the entire issue. That being the case, the Treasury moves to the next best and the next best bidders until most of the issue is taken. There is always a small portion left over for the noncompetitive bidders. Noncompetitive bids may only be made in amounts of $1 million or less. All noncompetitive bids are automatically filled at the average yield of the competitive bids which have been accepted.

Underwriting State Issues (Blue Sky Registration)

Unlike Federal issues, there are three types of State registration that are important for the medical professional to know:

Notification: This is the simplest form of registration and is used by an issuer who has been in continuous operation for at least the previous three years. Most, but not all, states permit registration by notification.

Coordination: This occurs when an issuer wishes to coordinate a Federal registration under the Securities Act of 1933 with Blue Sky registration in one or more states. Under most circumstances, the Blue Sky registration automatically becomes effective when the Federal registration statement becomes effective.

Qualification: Any security may be registered in a state by qualification, but is most commonly used by those issuers who are unable to use notification or coordination. Registration by Qualification becomes effective when so ordered by the State Administrator.

Exempt Securities

There are many securities which are exempt from the Act of 1933 registration and prospectus requirements. They include

- The U.S. Government and Federal Agency issues.
- Municipal, State issues, and commercial paper with a maturity not in excess of 270 days.
- Intra-state offerings (Rule 147) because they are blue-sky chartered within the state.
- Small Public offerings (Regulation A) if the value of the securities issued does not exceed $5,000,000 in any 12-month period. An issuer using the Regulation A exemption does not make the normal filings with the SEC in Washington. Instead, they file a simplified disclosure document with their SEC Regional Office, known as an Offering Statement. It must be file at least 10 business days prior to the initial offering of the securities. No securities may be sold unless issuer has furnished an offering circular (full disclosure document) to the purchaser at least 48 h prior to the mailing of confirmation of the sale, and, if not completed within 9 months from the date of the offering circular, a revised circular must be filed. Every 6 months, issuers must file a report with the SEC of sales made under the Regulation A exemption until the offering is completed.
- Traditional insurance policies are considered to be securities and are exempt, as are fixed annuities. However, some of the newer forms of life insurance, like variable life, as well

as variable annuities, have investment characteristics and, therefore are not exempt from registration.
• Commercial paper and banker's acceptances (9 month or shorter maturity) since they are money market instruments.

THE PRIVATE PLACEMENT (REGULATION D) SECURITIES EXEMPTION

Since the Securities Act of 1933 requires disclosure of all public offerings (other than the exemptions just described), it should make sense that any securities offering not offered to the public would also be exempt. The Act provides a registration exemption for private placements, known as Regulation D.

Since one of the stated purposes of the Act of 1933 is to prevent fraud on the sale of new public issues, an issue which has only a limited possibility of injuring the public may be granted an exemption from registration. The SEC just doesn't have the time to look at everything so they exempt offerings which do not constitute a "public offering." Strict adherence to the provisions of the law, however, is expected and is scrutinized by the SEC. This exemption provision of the Act lies within Regulation D.

Regulation D describes the type and number of investors who may purchase the issue, the dollar limitations on the issue, the manner of sale, and the limited disclosure requirements. Bear in mind at all times that from the issuer's viewpoint, the principal justification for doing a private, rather than public offering, is to save time and money, not to evade the law. Remember, it is just as illegal to use fraud to sell a Regulation D issue as it is in a public issue. However, if done correctly, a Regulation D can save time and money, and six separate rules (501–506).

Rule 501: Accredited investors are defined as: corporations and partnerships with net worth of $5,000,000 not formed for the purpose of making the investment; corporate or partnership "insiders"; individuals and medical professionals with a net worth (individual or joint) in excess of $1,000,000; individuals with income in excess of $200,000 (or joint income of $300,000) in each of the last two years, with a reasonable expectation of having income in excess of $200,000 (joint income of $300,000) in the year of purchase; and any entity 100% owned by accredited investors.

Rule 502: The violations of aggregation and integration are defined:

Aggregation: Sales of securities in violation of the dollar limitations imposed under Rules 504 and 505 (506 has no dollar limitations).

Integration: Sales of securities to a large number of nonaccredited investors, in violation of the "purchaser limitations" set forth in Rules 505 and 506 (504 has no "purchaser limitations").

Rule 503: Sets forth notification requirements. An issuer will be considered in violation of Regulation D, and therefore subject to Federal penalties, if a Form D is not filed within 15 days after the Regulation D offering commences.

Rule 504: Enables a nonreporting company to raise up to $1,000,000 in a 12-month period without undergoing the time land expense of an SEC registration. Any number of accredited and nonaccredited investors may purchase a 504 issue.

Rule 505: Enables corporations to raise up to $5,000,000 in a 12-month period without a registration. The "purchaser limitation" rule does apply here. It states that the number of nonaccredited investors cannot exceed 35. Obviously, we would have few problems if only medical investors in private placements were accredited investors, but that is not always the case. Since we are limited to a maximum of 35 nonaccredited investors, how we count the purchasers becomes an important consideration. The SEC states that if a husband and wife each purchase securities in a private placement for their own accounts, they count as one nonaccredited investor, not two. It would also be true that if these securities were purchased in UGMA accounts for their dependent children, we would still be counting only one nonaccredited investor. In the case of a partnership, it depends upon the purpose of the partnership. If the partnership was formed solely to make this investment, then each of the partners counts as an individual accredited or nonaccredited investor based upon their own personal status, but if the partnership served some other purpose, such as a law firm, then it would only count as one purchaser.

Rule 506: Differs from 505 in two significant ways. The dollar limit is waived and the issuer must take steps to assure itself that, if sales are to be made to nonaccredited investors, those investors meet tests of investment "sophistication."

Generally speaking, this means that either the individual nonaccredited investor has investment savvy and experience with this kind of offering, or he is represented by someone who has the requisite sophistication. This representative, normally a financial professional, such as an investment advisor, accountant, or attorney, is referred to in the securities business as a *Purchaser Representative*.

Regulation D further states that no public advertising or solicitation of any kind is permitted. A tombstone ad may be used to advertise the completion of a private placement, not to announce the availability of the issue. As a practical matter, however, whether required by the SEC or not, a Private Offering Memorandum for a limited partnership, for example, is normally prepared and furnished so that all investors receive disclosure upon which to base an investment judgment.

If any of the provisions of the Securities Act of 1933 are violated by an issuer, underwriter, or investor, this is known as "statutory underwriting" of underwriting securities in violation of statute. One who violates the Act is known as a statutory underwriter. One all too common example of this occurs when a purchaser of a Regulation D offering offers his unregistered securities for re-sale in violation of SEC Rule 144, an explanation of which is given below:

In simple English, SEC Rule 144 was created so that certain re-sales of already-existing securities could be made without having to file a complete registration statement with the SEC. The time and money involved in having to file such a registration is usually so prohibitive as to make it uneconomical for the individual seller. What kinds of re-sales are covered by Rule 144 and are important to the medical investor? Let's first define a few terms.

Restricted Securities: Are unregistered Securities purchased by an investor in a private placement. It is also called Letter Securities or Legend Securities referring to the fact that purchasers must sign an "Investment Letter" attesting to their understanding of the restrictions upon re-sale and to the "Legend" placed upon the certificates indicating restriction upon resale.

Control Person: A corporate director, officer, greater than 10% voting stockholder, or the spouse of any of the preceding, are loosely referred to as Insiders or Affiliates due to their unique status within the issuer.

Control Stock: Stock held by a control person. What makes it control stock is who owns it, not so much how they acquired it.

Nonaffiliate: An investor who is not a control person and has no other affiliation with the issuer other than as an owner of securities.

Rule 144 says that restricted securities cannot be offered for re-sale by any owner without first filing a registration statement with the SEC:

1. Unless the securities have been held in a fully paid-for status for at least two years
2. Unless a notice of Sale is filed with the SEC at the time of sale and demonstrating compliance with Rule 144
3. Unless small certain quantities apply

SHELF REGISTRATION

A relatively new method of registration under the Securities Act of 1933 is known as shelf registration. Under this rule, an issuer may register any amount of securities that, at the time the registration statement becomes effective, is reasonably expected to be offered and sold within two years of the initial effective date of the registration. Once registered, the securities may be sold continuously or periodically within 2 years without any waiting period for a registration to clear issuers generally like shelf registration because of the flexibility it gives them to take advantage of changing market conditions. In addition, the legal, accounting, and printing costs involved in issuance are reduced, since a single registration statement suffices for multiple offerings within the 2-year period. In effect, what the issuer does is register securities that will meet its financing needs for the next 2 years. It issues what it needs at the current time, and puts the balance on the shelf to be taken off the shelf as needed.

SECURITIES MARKETS

The purchase of common stock in an IPO (initial public offering) is facilitated through the use of members an investment bank underwriting syndicate or selling group. This is known as the *primary market* and the proceeds of sale go directly to the issuing company. Six months later however, if a doctor wants to sell his shares, this would be accomplished in the *secondary market*. The term secondary market refers to trading in outstanding issues as the proceeds do not go to the issuer, but to the current owner of the securities, such as the physician investor.

Therefore, the secondary market provides liquidity to doctors who acquired securities in the primary market. After a doctor has acquired securities in the primary market, he wants to be able to sell the securities at some point in the future in order to acquire other securities, buy a house, or go on a vacation. Such a sale takes place in the secondary market. The medical investor's ability to convert the asset (securities) into cash is heavily dependent upon the secondary market. All investors would be hesitant to acquire new securities if they felt they would not subsequently have the ability to sell the securities quickly at a fair price in the secondary market.

SECURITIES ACT OF 1934

Every trade of stocks and bonds that is not a purchase of a new issue is a trade that takes place in the secondary market. The market place for secondary trading is the stock exchanges and the over-the-counter (OTC) market, and is governed by the *Securities Act of 1934,* which actually created the *Securities and Exchange Commission (SEC)* and outlines the powers of the SEC to interpret, supervise, and enforce the securities laws of the United States. The Act of 34 is very broad and governs the sales of securities, including the regulation of securities markets exchanges, OTC markets, broker/dealers, their employees, the conduct of secondary markets, the extension of credit in the purchase and sale of securities, and the conduct of corporate insiders (officers and directors and holders of more than 10% of the outstanding stock). The Act also prohibits fraud and manipulative and deceptive activities in securities transactions.

THE STOCK EXCHANGES

A stock exchange is a private association of brokers. The main purpose of an exchange is to provide a central meeting place for its member brokers. This central meeting place is called the floor. It is on the floor that the members trade in securities. It is important to remember that a stock exchange itself does not own any of the securities that are traded on its floor. Nor does it buy or sell any of the securities traded on the exchange. Instead, the securities are owned by member firms, customers, or perhaps, by the exchange member firm itself.

It is also important to remember that a stock exchange does not establish or fix the price at which any security is traded on the exchange. The price is determined in a free and open auction type of trading. It depends on the supply and demand relationship of that security at a particular time. In other words, if sellers of a stock are offering to sell more shares of that stock than buyers want to buy, the price of that stock will tend to go down. On the other hand, if buyers want to buy more shares of a stock than the sellers are offering to sell, the price of that stock will tend to go higher because of the strong demand.

Any discussion of stock exchanges has to focus on the New York Stock Exchange (NYSE), which is by far the largest and most important of the exchanges. There are two exchanges referred to as national stock exchanges, the NYSE and the American Stock Exchange (AMEX). In addition to these two national exchanges, there are several regional stock exchanges including the Philadelphia Exchange, the Chicago Exchange (formerly Midwest), the Pacific Exchange, the Boston Exchange, and the Cincinnati Exchange. Stocks that are traded on an exchange are referred to as *listed stocks*. The term "listed on an exchange" means that the issue is eligible for trading on the floor of the exchange.

How does a stock become listed? The issuing company, having decided that they wish the prestige and broad visibility of being listed on the NYSE, applies to the exchange for listing. A critical condition for listing is that the issuer agrees to solicit proxies from those common stock shareholders unable to attend shareholder meetings. Once the securities have been accepted for listing (trading) on an exchange, the issuer must continue to meet certain requirements which are not quite as stringent as the original listing requirements, and may be de-listed if the firm ceases to solicit proxies on its existing voting stock, or meet other minimal requirements.

Physically, the exchange brings together buyers and sellers on a trading floor. The NYSE floor is larger than several football fields and is divided into 19 trading posts. Eighteen of the posts are horseshoe or U-shaped stations 100 square feet in area. The 19th post (post number 30) is in the northwest corner and really isn't a post at all; it's just an area where the inactive stocks trade.

THE SPECIALIST

Specialists are experts in trading one or more specific stocks at their particular post on the exchange floor. Their activity is vital to the maintenance of a free and continuous market in the specific issues they represent. They are responsible for conducting the auction at the post. Everyone interested in buying the stock calls out a price and the shares go to the highest bidder. The buyers compete, but there is only one seller. Unlike the usual auction market, the auction on the floor of the exchange is a two-way auction with some brokers seeking to buy at the lowest possible price for their doctor clients and other brokers trying to sell at the highest possible price for their doctor clients. When two brokers, one representing a buyer and one a seller, agree on a price, a sale is made. The specialist functions in a dual capacity as a dealer and as a broker. As a dealer or principal, he buys and sells for his own account with risk to maintain a fair and orderly market in the stocks in which he specializes.

For example, if a commission broker approaches the specialist at the post with a buy or sell order, and there are no other brokers in the crowd that are currently interested in buying or selling the stock, the specialist will buy the stock from that commission broker (if it's a sell order) for his own account or sell the stock from his inventory (if it's a buy order). Perhaps, he may even be able to fill the order from his specialist's book.

SPECIALIST'S BOOK

This is done by using the specialist's book of buy orders (bids), marked on the left-hand page, or sell orders (offers) on the right. There is a book for each stock in which the specialist specializes. The pages are ruled and are usually printed with fractional stock points at regular intervals to permit easy insertion of orders. The orders are entered in the book by the specialist according to price and in the sequence in which they are received at the post. He notes the number of shares, putting down 1 for 100 shares, 2 for 200 shares, and so on. He also notes the name of the member firm placing the order and if the order is *Good Till Cancelled* (GTC), or not. When orders are executed, they are executed in the same order recorded in the book at that particular price.

The specialist's book also keeps track of all orders "away from the market" (limit orders and stop orders) in his book. The book is organized with all buy orders on the left-hand side of the page and all sell orders on the right-hand side. In the absence of bids and offers from the "trading crowd" on the floor, the specialist can quote the best available market for the security by announcing the highest bid and the lowest offer (ask). The best bid is always the highest buy limit order on his book and the best offer (ask) is always the lowest sell limit on his book. In addition to quoting the best price, he will also give the "size of the market" which is determined by the number of shares being bid for and offered at the respective best bid and best ask prices. The quote is price and size. When asked to quote the market for a security, the specialist disregards any stop orders on his book since those orders do not become activated until triggered by another trade. One thing to remember is that since most doctors place stop orders to hedge (protect) against a price movement adverse to their interests, most stop orders are entered with the fervent wish that they never be executed.

On stop and limit orders placed below the market, the specialist is required to reduce the price of those orders on the ex-dividend (ex-split, ex-rights) date. The two critical things to remember are: what types of orders are reduced and by how much? The specialist will reduce all GTC (open) buy limit and sell stop orders on an ex-date. The acronym BLISS where the BL equals buy limit and the SS equals sell stop; may be used as a memory aid. The only time either of these orders will not be reduced is if the medical client turned in DNR (do not reduce) instructions. The price of the order is then reduced by enough to equal or exceed the amount of the dividend.

If we go back to the example approaching the specialist to buy or sell stock and there is no one in the "crowd," the specialist will first give the commission broker a quote from his book. That quote will be the highest bid price (the highest priced limit order to buy on his books) and the best asked price (the lowest priced sell limit on his books). If the commission broker is willing to buy at the lowest ask or offering price on the specialist's book, then a trade will take place; if the commission broker is looking to sell and is willing to accept the highest bid price on the specialist's book then, again, a trade will take place. It is the responsibility of the specialist to maintain an orderly market and to keep the spread between the bid and asked prices as narrow as possible. If the spread between bid and asked is too wide to generate market activity, the specialist will act on his own account.

If the specialist is presented with sell orders at the post and he has no buyers, he must bid at least 1/8 of a point higher than the best bid on his books. If he has buyers and no sellers, then he must offer stock from his inventory at a price at least, 1/8 of a point below the lowest offer on his book. Why? It's because the specialist cannot "compete" with public orders and if his bid matched a customer's bid or his offer matched a customer's offering or ask price, he would be considered to be "competing." Since the specialist is required to bid higher and ask lower than the best public orders on his book, the spread is narrowed. That is why it is said that the specialist acts in a dual capacity, as a dealer and as a broker. When buying and selling for his own account, he is acting as a dealer. The specialist acts as a broker when he executes limit orders left with him by commission brokers. When these limit orders are executed out of the specialist's book (the doctor's limit price is reached), the specialist uses a priority, parity, and precedence system, as to which order is executed first. These rules, like most others, are designed to give preference to the general public, not to members of the exchange, on a first come first served basis.

WALKING THROUGH A TRADE

To see how the transactions are actually handled on the floor of an exchange, let us assume that an order to buy 100 shares of General Electric has been given by a customer to the registered representative of a member firm in Atlanta. The order is a market order (an order to buy at the lowest possible price at the time the order reaches the floor of the exchange). This order is telephoned by direct wire or computer to the New York office of the member firm, which in turn telephones its order to its clerk on the floor of the exchange.

Each member firm has at least one member of the exchange representing them and making trades on the floor. Each one of these members is assigned a number for identification. When the floor clerk receives the order to purchase the General Electric, he causes his member call number to appear on three large boards situated so that one is always in view. These boards are constantly watched by brokers so that they will know when they are wanted at the phone, since there's too much noise on the floor to use a paging system. Seeing his number on the board, the broker hurries to his telephone station or cell phone and receives the order to buy 100 shares of G.E. "at the market." Acting as a commission broker, he immediately goes to the post where G.E. is traded and asks "how's G.E.?," of the specialist.

ORDER AND POSITION TYPES

At this point, it is important to understand the different types of orders and positions that can be used to buy and sell securities from the specialist.

Market Order: A market order is an order to be executed at the best possible price at the time the order reaches the floor. Market orders are the most common of all orders. The greatest advantage of the market order is speed. The doctor specifies no price in this type of order, he merely orders his broker to sell or buy at the best possible price, regardless of what it may be. The best possible price on a buy is the lowest possible price. The best possible price on a sell is the highest possible price. In other words, if a medical professional customer is buying, he logically wants to pay as little as possible, but he is not going to quibble over price. He wants the stock now, whatever it takes to get it. If he's a seller, the doctor client wants to receive as much as possible, but will not quibble, he wants out, and will take what he can get, right now. No other type of order can be executed so rapidly. Some market orders are executed in less than one minute from the time the broker phones in the order. Because the investor has specified no price, a market order will always be executed. The doctor is literally saying, "I will pay whatever it takes, or accept whatever is offered."

Limit Order: The chief characteristic of a limit order is that the doctor decides in advance on a price at which he decides to trade. He believes that his price is one that will be reached in the market in reasonable time. He is willing to wait to do business until he has obtained his price even at the risk his order may not be executed either in the near future or at all. In the execution of a limit order, the broker is to execute it at the limit price or better. Better means that a limit order to buy is executed at the customer's price limit or lower, in a limit order to sell at price limit or higher. If the broker can obtain a more favorable price for his doctor customer than the one specified, he is required to do so.

Order Length: Now, even though the doctor has given his price limit, we need to know the length of effectiveness of the order. Is the order good for today only? If so, it is a day order, it automatically expires at the end of the day. Alternatively, the doctor may enter an open or, "good until canceled" order. This type of order is used when the doctor believes that the fluctuations in the market price of the stock in which he's interested will be large enough in the future that they will cause the market price to either fall to, or rise to, his desired price, that is, his limit price. He is reasonably sure of his judgment and is in no hurry to have/his order executed. He knows what he wants to pay or receive and is willing to wait for an indefinite period.

Years ago, such orders were carried for long periods of time without being reconfirmed. This was very unsatisfactory for all parties concerned. A doctor would frequently forget his order existed and, if the price ever reached his limit and the order was executed, the resulting trade might not be one he wished to make. To avoid the problem, open (GTC) orders must be reconfirmed by the doctor customer each six months. Does that mean six months after the order is entered?...No! The exchange has appointed the last business day of April and the last business day of October as the two dates per year when all open orders must be reconfirmed.

Example: Dr. Smith wants to buy 100 shares of XYZ. The price has been fluctuating between 50 and 55. He places a limit order to buy at 51, although the current market price is 54. Limit orders to buy (buy limit orders) are always placed below the current market. To do otherwise makes no sense. It is possible that, within a reasonable time, the price will drop to 51 and his broker can purchase the stock for him at that price. If the broker can purchase the stock at less that 51, that would certainly be fine with the doctor customer since he wants to pay no more than 51. A sell limit order works in reverse and is always placed above the current market price.

Example: Dr. Smith wants to sell 100 shares of XYZ stock. The order is 54. A sell limit order is place at 56. Sell limit orders are always placed above the market price. As soon as the pride rises to 56, if it ever does, the broker will execute it at 56 or higher. In no case will it be executed at less than 56.

The advantage of the limit order is that the doctor has a chance to buy at less or to sell at more than the current market price prevailing when he placed the order. He assumes that the market price will become more favorable in the future than it is at the time the order is placed. The word "chance" is important. There is also the "chance" that the order will not be executed at all. The doctor just mentioned, who wanted to buy at 51, may never get his order filled since the price may not fall that low. If he wanted to sell at 56, the order may also not ever be executed since it might not rise that high during the time period the order is in effect.

Stop Orders: A very important type of order is the stop order, frequently called a stop-loss order. There are two distinct types of stop orders. One is the stop order to sell, called a sell stop, and the other is a stop order to buy, called a buy stop. Either type might be thought of as a suspended market order; it goes into effect only if the stock reaches or passes through a certain price.

The fact that the market price reaches or goes through the specified stop price does not mean the broker will obtain execution at the exact stop price. It merely means that the order becomes a market order and will be executed at the best possible price thereafter. The price specified on a stop order bears a relationship to the current market price exactly opposite to that on a limit order. Whereas a sell limit is placed at a price above the current market, a sell stop is placed at a price below the current market. Similarly, while a buy limit is placed at a price below the current market, a buy stop is placed at a price above the current market. Why would a doctor investor use a stop order?

There are two established uses for stop orders. One of them might be called *protective;* the other might be called *preventive.*

Protective: This order protects a doctors' existing profit on a stock currently owned. For example, a doctor purchases a stock at 60. It rises to 70. He has made a paper profit of $10 per share. He realizes that the market may reverse itself. He therefore gives his broker a stop order to sell at 67. If the reversal does occur and the price drops to 67 or less, the order immediately becomes a market order. The stock is disposed of at the best possible price. This may be exactly 67, or it may be slightly above or below that figure. Why?... Because what happened at 67 was that his order became a market order; the price he actually received was dependent upon the next activity in the market. Let us suppose that the sale was made at 66 1/2. The doctor customer made a gross profit of 6 1/2 points per share on his original purchase. Without the stop order, the stock may have dropped considerably below that before the customer could have placed a market order and his profit might have been less or, in fact, he might have even sold at a loss.

Preventive: A doctor purchases 100 shares of a stock at 30. He obviously anticipates that the price of the stock will rise in the near future (why else would he buy?). However, he realizes that his judgment may be faulty. He therefore, at the time of purchase, places a sell stop order at a price somewhat below his purchase price, for example, at 28. As yet, he has made neither profit nor loss; he's merely acting to prevent a loss that might follow if he made the wrong bet and the stock does fall in price. If the stock does drop, the doctor knows that once it gets as low as 28, a market order will be turned in for him and, therefore, he will lose only 2 points or thereabout. It might have been much more had he not used the sell stop.

MISCELLANEOUS ORDERS AND POSITIONS

Beside market, limit and stop orders, there are some other miscellaneous orders for the ME, Inc physician or guided investor, to know.

A *stop limit order* is a stop order that, once triggered or activated, becomes a *limit* order. Realize that it is possible for a stop limit to be triggered and not executed, as the limit price specified by the doctor may not be available.

In addition, there are *all or none* and *fill* or *kill orders*, and even though both require the entire order to be filled, there are distinct differences. An all or none (AON) is an order in which the broker is directed to fill the entire order or none of it.

A fill or kill (FOK) is an order either to buy or to sell a security in which the broker is directed to attempt to fill the entire amount of the order immediately and in full, or that it be canceled.

The difference between an all or none and a fill or kill order is that with an all or none order, immediate execution is not required, while immediate execution is a critical component of the fill or kill. Because of the immediacy requirement, FOK orders are never found on the specialist's book. Another difference is that AON orders are only permitted for bonds, not stocks, while FOK orders may be used for either.

Also, there exists an immediate or cancel order (IOC), which is an order to buy or sell a security in which the broker is directed to attempt to fill immediately as much of the order as possible and cancel any part remaining. This type of order differs from a fill-or-kill order which requires the entire order to be filled. An IOC order will permit a partial fill. Because of the immediacy requirement, IOC orders are never found on the specialist's book.

Long and Short Positions

A long buy position means that shares are for sale from a market makers inventory or owned by the medical investor outright. Market makers take long positions when customers and other firms wish to sell, and they take short positions when customers and other firms want to buy in quantities larger than the market maker's inventory. By always being ready, willing, and able to handle orders in this way, market makers assure the investing public of a ready market in the securities in which they are interested. When a security can be bought and sold at firm prices very quickly and easily the security is said to have a high degree of liquidity, also known as marketability.

A short position investor seeks to make a profit by participating in the market price decline of a security.

Now, let's see how these terms, long and short, apply to transactions by medical investors (rather than market makers) in the securities markets.

When a doctor buys any security—he is said to be taking a long position in that security. This means the investor is an owner of the security. Why does a doctor take a long position in a security?

Well, receiving dividend income to make a profit from an increase in the market price is one reason. Once the security has risen sufficiently in price to satisfy the investor's profit needs, the investor will liquidate his long position or sell his stock. This would officially be known as a long sale of stock, though few people in the securities business use the label "long sale." This is the manner in which the above investor had made a profit is the traditional method used: buy low, sell high.

Let's look at an actual investment in General Motors to investigate this principle further. A medical investor has taken a long position in 100 shares of General Motors stock at a price of $70 per share. This means that the manner in which he can do that is by placing a market order which will be executed at the best "available market price at the time," or by the placing of a buy limit order with a limit price of $70 per share. The investor firmly believes, on the basis of reports that he has read about the automobile industry and General Motors specifically, that at $70 a share, General Motors is a real bargain. He believes that based on its current level of performance it should be selling for a price of between $80 and $85 per share, but the doctor investor has a dilemma. He feels certain that the price is going to rise, but he cannot watch his computer, or call his broker, every hour of every day. The reason he can't watch is because patients have to be seen in the office. The only people who watch a computer screen all day are those in the offices of brokerage firms (stock broker registered representatives), and doctor day traders, among others.

In the above example, with a sell limit order, if the doctor investor was willing to settle for a profit of $12 per share, what order would he place at this time? If you said, "sell at $82 good until canceled," you are correct. Why GTC rather than a day order? Because our doctor investor knows that General Motors is probably not going to rise from $70 to $82 in one day. If he had placed an order to sell at $82 without the GTC qualification, his order would have been canceled at the end of this trading day. He would have had to reenter the order each morning until he got an execution at 82. Marking the order GTC (or open) relieves him of any need to replace the order every morning. Several weeks later, when General Motors has reached $82 per share in the market, his order to sell at 82 is executed. The medical investor has bought at 70 and sold at 82 and realized a $12 per share profit for his efforts.

Let's suppose that the medical investor, who has just established a $12 per share profit, has evaluated the performance of General Motors common stock by looking at the market performance over a period of many years. Let's further assume that the investor has found by evaluating the market price statistics of General Motors that the pattern of movement of General Motors is cyclical. By cyclical, we mean that it moves up and down according to a regular pattern of behavior.

Let's say the investor has observed that in the past, General Motors had repeated a pattern of moving from prices in the $60 per share range as a low, to a high of approximately $90 per share. Furthermore, our investor has observed that this pattern of performance takes approximately 10–12 months to do a full cycle; that is, it moves from about 60 to about 90 and back to about 60 within a period of roughly 12 months. If this pattern repeats itself continually, the investor would be well advised to buy the stock at prices in the low to mid-60s, hold onto it until it moves well into the 80s, and then sell his long position at a profit. However, what this means is that our investor is going to be invested in General Motors only 6 months of each year. That is, he will invest when the price is low and, usually within half a year, it will reach its high before turning around and going back to its low again. How can the doctor-investor make a profit not only on the rise in price of General Motors in the first 6 months of the cycle, but on the fall in price of General Motors in the second half of the cycle? One technique that is available is the use of the short sale.

The Short Sale

If a doctor investor feels that GM is at its peak of $90 per share, he may borrow 100 shares from his brokerage firm and sell the 100 shares of borrowed GM at $90. This is selling stock that is not owned and is known as a short sale. The transaction ends when the doctor returns the borrowed securities at a lower price and pockets the difference as a profit. In this case, the doctor investor has sold high, and bought low.

Odd Lots

Most of the thousands of buy and sell orders executed on a typical day on the NYSE are in 100 share or multi-100 share lots. These are called round lots. Some of the inactive stocks traded at post 30, the non-horseshoe-shaped post in the northwest corner of the exchange, are traded in 70 share round lots due to their inactivity. So, while a round lot is normally 700 shares, there are cases where it could be 10 shares. Any trade for less than a round lot is known as an odd lot. The execution of odd lot orders is somewhat different than round lots and needs explanation.

When a stock broker receives an odd lot order from one of his doctor customers, the order is processed in the same manner as any other order. However, when it gets to the floor, the commission broker knows that this is an order that will not be part of the regular auction market. He takes the order to the specialist in that stock and leaves the order with the specialist. One of the clerks assisting the specialist records the order and waits for the next auction to occur in that particular stock. As soon as a round lot trade occurs in that particular stock as a result of an auction at the post, which may occur seconds later, minutes later, or maybe not until the next day, the clerk makes a record of the trade price.

Every odd lot order that has been received since the last round lot trade, whether an order to buy or sell, is then executed at the just noted round lot price, the price at which the next round lot traded after receipt of the customer's odd lot order, plus or minus the specialist's "cut." Just like everything else he does, the specialist doesn't work for nothing. Generally, he will add 1/8 of a point to the price per share of every odd lot buy order and reduce the proceeds of each odd lot sale order by 1/8 per share. This is the compensation he earns for the effort of breaking round lots into odd lots. Remember, odd lots are never auctioned but, there can be no odd lot trade unless a round lot trades after receipt of the odd lot order.

OTC Markets

Securities are bought and sold every day by medical investors who never meet each other. The market impersonally enables transfer (or sale) of securities from individuals who are selling to those who are buying. These trades may occur on an organized exchange such as the New York Stock Exchange, or a decentralized dealer-to-dealer market, which is called the over-the-counter (OTC). Any transaction that does not take place on the floor of an exchange, takes place OTC.

The OTC market is a national negotiated market, without a central market place, without a trading floor, composed of a network of thousands of brokers and dealers who make securities transactions for themselves and their customers. Professional buyers and sellers seek each other out electronically and by telephone and negotiate prices on the most favorable basis that can be achieved. Often, these negotiations are accomplished in a matter of seconds; there is no auction procedure comparable to that on the floor of an exchange.

The OTC market is by far the largest market in terms of numbers of securities issues traded. There are over 30,000 issues on which regular quotations are published OTC; while there are less than 4000 stocks listed on all securities exchanges. There are frequently days when the reported volume of OTC trades exceeds that of the NYSE. What really is the OTC market? Is it where securities of inferior quality trade? Here is a list to remember of the types of securities traded exclusively OTC:

- All government bonds
- All municipal bonds
- All mutual funds
- All new issues (primary distributions)
- All variable annuities
- All tax shelter programs
- All equipment trust certificates

Of course, the OTC market is also where all of the "unseasoned" issues are traded and most of them are quite speculative, but there certainly are many high-quality issues available OTC. Now, let's take a look at how this OTC market works.

MARKET MAKER

Whereas, the "main player" on the exchange is the specialist, his OTC counterpart, in terms of importance, is the market maker. In the OTC market, many securities firms act as dealers by creating and maintaining markets in selected securities. Dealers act as principals in a securities transaction and buy and sell securities for their own account and risk. Since they do not act as agents or brokers but instead as principals or dealers in securities transactions, they do not receive any commission for their services but instead buy at one price and sell at a higher price making a profit from "mark-up" on the security price. A dealer is said to have a position in a stock when he purchases and holds a security in his inventory. The dealer of course takes a risk that the market price of the security he holds may decline in value. This is how dealers make money; they buy wholesale and sell it retail, and the medical professional or other investor pays retail.

The OTC market bears little resemblance to the one of the mid-60s. The major difference has been the electronic technological advances as embodied by the NASDAQ system. NASDAQ stands for National Association of Securities Dealers Automated Quotation system. Back in 1966, if you wanted to find out who was the market maker in the particular security you would go to a brightly colored stack of papers called the pink sheets, containing a listing, alphabetically, of OTC stocks and underneath each issue is listed the name of one or more market makers, securities firms willing to trade that stock. After each firm name is the firm's telephone number and a "bid and ask price," that is, an approximate price representing what the dealer is asking for the stock and is bidding for the stock.

Back 50 years ago, the only way of locating a market maker was by using the pink sheets, while O-T-C traded corporate bonds are quoted on yellow sheets. Under certain conditions, it could take a good deal of effort to try to get the best deal. Today, with the computer that sits on doctor's desks, or smart phone, you can push a few buttons and instantaneously see the best bid and the best offer that exists right now on over 4000 of the most active OTC stocks. Not only that, you can pull up the names of every market maker in that particular stock and the actual (firm) quotes on those securities right now.

ELECTRONIC SOURCES OF SECURITIES INFORMATION

Level 1 service, available on the stock broker's desk top, provides price information only on the highest bid and the lowest offer (the inside market). No market makers are identified, and since this is an inside quote, it may not be used by the registered representative (stock broker) for giving firm quotes.

Level 2 service provides a doctor subscriber with price information and quotation sizes of all participating registered market makers. When a trader, or medical investor, looks at his computer screen on Level 2, he sees who's making a market, their firm bid-or-ask, and the size of the market. One can get firm calls from Level 2 information.

Level 3 takes it one step further; and allows registered market makers to enter bid and ask prices (quotes) and quotation sizes into the NASDAQ system and to report their trades. This is the level of service maintained by market makers.

THIRD MARKET

In most cases, a market maker of a stock in the NASDAQ system must report his trade in 90 seconds, but there is another circumstance in which the trade must be reported. This is called the third market, and is defined as transactions in exchange listed securities in the OTC market. For example, even though IBM is listed on the NYSE, an OTC market marking firm can acquire the IBM stock and begin to make a market for it just like an OTC stock. All of these trades are considered the third market, and are reported to the Consolidated Quotation System (CQS) within 90 s of the trade.

FOURTH MARKET

The fourth market is defined as private transactions made directly between large medical investors, institutions such as banks, mutual funds, and insurance companies, without the use of a securities firm. In other words, fourth market trading is usually one institution swapping securities in its portfolio with another large institution. From the stock broker's viewpoint, there is one problem with the fourth market. Since no broker/dealer is involved, no registered representative is involved and there is no commission to be earned. These trades are reported on a system called *Instinet*. This is advantageous to larger medical foundations or institutional investors.

BROKERAGE ACCOUNTS, MARGIN, AND DEBT

Most medical professionals execute orders and buy securities for cash. This occurs either through a stock broker, telephone order, computerized online trade or the rapid fire buy/sell momentum of day trading. Regardless, since cash is used, this brokerage account is known as a *cash account*. Now, we will explore the use of credit to buy securities. This process, called buying on margin, is done in a *margin account*, and is allowed through an SEC ruling known as Regulation T.

REGULATION T

Regulation T, of the Securities Exchange Act of 1934, defined the two basic types of accounts: cash and margin. A cash account is one in which the medical professional agrees to pay the full purchase price of his trade within three full business days of the trade date. The trade date is the day on which the buy order was executed, either on an exchange, or OTC. Regulation T requires a broker/dealer to cancel the trade if payment is not made on time.

If the doctor client has made a partial payment but owes more than $1000 by the end of the 3rd business day, the unpaid portion will be sold off. If, however, only $1000 or less is owed, the broker/dealer is permitted to use its own best judgment as to whether to give the doctor client more time to come up with the amount owed.

If a doctor client feels his reasons for not paying on time are exceptional, a request can be made by the broker/dealer for an extension of the 3-business-day time limit. Only three organizations can approve such an extension: a national securities exchange, the National Association of Securities Dealers (NASD)—Financial Industry Regulatory Authority (FINRA), or a Federal Reserve Bank.

If a doctor client violates Regulation T, his broker/dealer will cancel the trade or liquidate the unpaid portion, and his cash account will be *frozen* for 90 *calendar days*. This means that if the doctor wishes to purchase additional securities in his cash account during the next 90 days, he must pay for the trade in full *in advance*. An easy way to remember the rule is: in a frozen cash account, cold cash up front is required for new purchases. Interestingly, margin accounts are never frozen, only cash accounts.

Regulation T Percentage (Credit)

The use of credit to finance securities transactions is governed by Regulation T of the Securities Exchange Act of 1934. Regulation T empowers the *Federal Reserve Board* to establish standards by which such transactions may take place. These standards include margin ability (which securities may be purchased on credit), and the applicable percentage of down payment required from the doctor when financing such a transaction. This percentage is commonly referred to as the Regulation T percentage, or just Regulation T.

Although Regulation T is 50% today, and has been since January 1974, the following examples will assume a Regulation T of 60% (unless otherwise stated), strictly for the purposes of clarity since using 50% can sometimes become confusing when discussing the 50% down payment versus the other 50%, which is the loan value.

MARGIN TERMS AND DEFINITIONS

1. A *Margin Account* is opened for the purposes of engaging in securities transactions using credit extended by the brokerage firm.
2. *Hypothecation* is the pledging of securities as collateral for a margin loan. Before a brokerage firm can lend any money whatsoever, the law requires the loan to be secured or collateralized. The doctor desiring the loan hypothecates the stock in order to obtain the financing in the margin account.
3. *Rehypothecation* is a brokerage firm's pledge of a doctor's securities to secure loans from a bank. These loans help the brokerage industry to afford to carry margin accounts for their doctor clients. Legally, the maximum dollar amount of a security that may be rehypothecated for carrying a margin account is 140% of the loan.
4. *Street Name Registration* occurs so a broker may be in a position to liquidate the loan collateral quickly, since the securities are registered in the name of the brokerage firm, or its nominee.
5. *Beneficial Owner* represents the healthcare professional whose securities are registered in street name remains the actual owner of all benefits of ownership, such as dividends or interest, capital appreciation, voting rights, preemptive rights, and, of course, the right to sellout the position and liquidate the account in whole or in part. Remember, though, the securities are actually in the name of the brokerage firm.
6. *Commingling* is an abuse that occurs when a brokerage firm mixes, or combines, its own securities with those of its clients to obtain loans and other benefits that go beyond what is fair and reasonable according to the law. This is an illegal practice.
7. *Debit Balance* is the amount of the loan from the brokerage firm, to the doctor, to finance the purchase of margin able securities.

Now let's learn the mechanics of the loan by working a problem from the inception of physician-client Dr. William D. Smith's margin purchase through the effects of market fluctuations on the account's status.

INITIAL MARGIN CALL AND EQUITY

Let's suppose that Dr. Smith purchases 100 shares of Microsoft stock, at $100 per share, in a margin account, with Regulation T at 60%. To calculate the initial margin call, use the formula: Regulation T times purchase price or, $60\% \times \$10,000 = \$6000$. A phrase to clearly express equity in a margin account is: "what you own, minus what you owe, is your equity."

Note, since the doctor is required to put up $6000, the broker is lending the other $4000, or 40%, of the purchase price. This 40% figure is known as the loan value of the account and represents the maximum loan the broker is permitted to extend to Dr. Smith based upon current market value. This percentage and the Regulation T% will always add up to 100%.

SECURITIES IN LIEU OF CASH

An initial margin call may also be met with securities, in lieu of cash. Since a stock broker (registered representative) is permitted to loan 40% of the current market value (CMV) of their securities

(Regulation T at 60%), Dr. Smith can deposit into his margin account stock he owns outright, obtain a loan of 40% of CMV, and utilize that loan to meet a margin call on a purchase.

For instance, in the initial example in which Dr. Smith purchased $10,000 worth of Microsoft stock, the margin call could have been satisfied with $15,000 worth of fully-paid-for margin able stock in lieu of cash: 60%/40% × $10,000 = $15,000.

In other words, the $10,000 purchase would require a cash deposit of 60% or $6000. Since Dr. Smith is not going to put up cash, he must deposit marginable securities with a loan value of $6000. The broker/dealer will loan him the $6000, if he will deposit $15,000 of paid for securities. Again, here's how he does it: $6000 = 40%/$15,000

EXCESS EQUITY (SMA) AND BUYING POWER

Let's look at what happens should Microsoft stock appreciate in value. Suppose the stock rises in price from $100 to $120 per share, or to $12,000. The main thing to keep in mind is that while the market value of the shares changes continuously in the marketplace, Dr. Smith's original loan from the broker does not change. The debit balance remains constant. An analogy that may be helpful is that homeowner Dr. Smith's mortgage does not change when there is a rise in the value of his property.

Note that since the debit does not change, the equity increased exactly $2000, the same as the amount of increase in the CMV ($12,000–$10,000). Any change in market value (either up or down) causes a dollar for dollar change in equity. When securities purchased in a margin account increase in value, we have a situation called excess equity. Let's examine this concept further by looking at the example after its appreciation to the new CMV of $12,000.

Your broker is permitted to give loans of 40% of the CMV of Microsoft, with Regulation T at 60%. Thus, the amount that could be loaned to Dr. Smith, on securities which are now worth $12,000, is $4800. (40% times $12,000). However, the doctor has only borrowed $4000 to this point in time. Therefore, there is an $800 ($4800–$4000) amount that represents additional borrowing power available to Dr. Smith if, and when, he wishes to utilize it. This $800 is called excess equity, also referred to as SMA, which is the Special Memorandum Account that brokers use to record excess equity. Dr. Smith has three distinct choices regarding excess equity.

1. First, he could borrow it in cash and remove it from the account. In this case, the doctor requests that the cashier forward a check for $800. When this is done, the doctor's new debit balance is $4800, because he is, in fact, borrowing the money. It may be easier to understand SMA, if you consider the initials to stand for, Second Mortgage Account. In the same way that an increase in the market value of a home makes it possible to obtain a second mortgage (the lender is willing to loan money on the higher collateral value), an increase in the market value of an account gives more collateral which translates into more loan value or SMA. But, just as taking out a second mortgage (or home equity loan) on your home increases total indebtedness (your first and second mortgages) removing your SMA increases your debit balance.

2. Second, he could use it to buy more Microsoft stock. In this case, Dr. Smith may make an additional purchase in his margin account and utilize the excess equity to "offset" his Regulation T down payment requirement on the new purchase. For example, he could make a $12,000 new purchase and be required to deposit only $6400, instead of the $7200 that would have been required under Regulation T had there been no excess equity in the account.

3. Third, he could reserve the right to do either 1, or 2, at a later time. Now let's compute the exact amount of securities he can buy without putting up any new money, using only excess equity to meet the call, with the formula

EXCESS EQUITY/REGULATION T = $800/60\% = \$1333.33$, called *BUYING POWER*.

This means that if Dr. Smith were to place an order to buy exactly \$1333.33 worth of Microsoft stock on margin, he would not have to put up a penny out of his own pocket. To verify, compute the normal Regulation T margin call on a \$1333.33 purchase: $60\% \times \$1333.33 = \$800$. This "call" for \$800 would be "met" by instructing his broker that he wishes to use the excess equity of \$800 in his account for that purpose.

The easiest way to remember the formula for buying power is by using the expression SMA/RT. In this case, SMA/RT means SMA divided by the Regulation T%, by remembering the expression, "it's SMART to use your buying power." In this case, Dr. Smith chooses to wait until a later time to utilize his excess equity and his buying power. To this end, brokerage firms normally make a written record of the amount of the excess equity at the time it is created by a rise in CMV. In this way, it is reserved for future use.

From an accounting point of view, the broker will make a written entry in the Special Memorandum Account (SMA). Among other things, this special account is used to record these additional loan amounts that result due to market value increases. What do you think happens when a cash dividend is received on stock held in a margin account? Dr. Smith has the option of taking the dividend out of the account or leaving the money in. If he chooses the latter, from a bookkeeping standpoint, the cash is used to reduce the debit balance and the SMA is increased by that amount.

Once the excess equity amount has been entered into the SMA, it remains there until used, even if the market turns down subsequently. This is done primarily to encourage additional transactions, by Dr. Smith, even if he didn't wish to act at the precise moment the excess equity comes into existence. Remember this important statement about SMA: You only lose it, if you use it! Excess equity has been given many names in Wall Street jargon. Among them are: equity excess, margin excess, Regulation T excess, SMA, or additional loan value.

Restricted Accounts

Let's now take a look at what happens in a margin account when CMV declines. In the following examples, Regulation T of 50% is used. Assume a purchase of 100 Microsoft shares at \$80, followed by a decline in CMV to \$70. Note as before, the debit balance is constant and the equity changed exactly \$1000, the same amount the CMV changed downward.

Initial CMV	CMV after Decline
CMV \$8000	CMV \$7000
(−) Debit \$4000	(−) \$4000
Equity \$4000	**Equity \$3000**

A margin account in which the equity has fallen below the Regulation T percentage is called a Restricted Margin Account. Therefore, the account is restricted since it has less than \$3500 equity and the equity percentage is 43% (\$3000/\$7000), rather than 50% (\$3500/\$7000). What are the consequences of a restricted account on subsequent purchases, and sales?

Purchases—A doctor wishing to buy additional securities in a restricted account will find there are no restrictions on the ability to do so. He is only required to deposit the Regulation T percentage on each new purchase, just as in a nonrestricted account.

Sales—A doctor wishing to liquidate some of his holdings in a restricted margin account will find that the Retention Rule of the Federal Reserve comes into play. The Retention Rule requires the brokerage firm to retain 50% of the sale proceeds and use this retention to reduce the client's debit balance. The other 50% is made available to the client to do with as he so chooses. He may take it in cash, buy more stock, or leave it in the account for future use.

For instance, in the above example, suppose Dr. Smith sells 10 of his 100 Microsoft shares, at the CMV of $70 per share. What transpires?

Liquidation proceeds = 10 × $70 = $700
Retention by broker = 50% × $700 = $350
Available to Dr. Smith = $700 − $350 = $350

Failure to Meet a Margin Call

If a medical professional doesn't meet an initial margin call under Regulation T in an existing margin account, the firm is required to sell off securities in the account in an amount equal to twice the margin call, assuming Regulation T is 50%. However, the account would not be frozen, since only a cash account can be frozen.

Withdrawal of Distributions in a Restricted Account

In a restricted account, it is the usual industry practice that all dividends and interest received are automatically taken out of the margin account, and put into the SMA (Special Memorandum Account) on the day received. For example, if dividends of $200 were received into the account, the debit balance would be reduced by $200 and the SMA increased by that same $200.

SAME DAY SUBSTITUTIONS

This term refers to the netting of a purchase and sale of different securities in a doctor's restricted margin account, on the same day. A determination of any margin call due, or proceeds due a doctor, is done by the brokerage firm at the end of the day.

Example: If, in a restricted margin account, Dr. Jones makes a same day substitution by selling $5000 of Lucent stock, and then purchases $6000 of Cisco systems, with Regulation T at 60%, the required margin deposit would be $600. The net trade in this case is a buy of $1000. The Regulation T on a buy of $1000 is 60% of that, or $600.

SALES IN A NONRESTRICTED ACCOUNT

If a doctor's equity is equal to the Regulation T percentage, a sale of securities in her account releases proceeds equal to the Regulation T percentage.

For example:
$10,000 CMV Sell $1000 worth of securities
−$4000 Debit $1000 × 60% = $600 to Dr. Jones
$6000 Equity (60% = Regulation T) $1000 × 40% = $400 to pay down debit balance.

MINIMUM MAINTENANCE REQUIREMENTS (LONG CASH ACCOUNT)

What happens if the market continues to decline, say to $50 per share? Again, keep in mind that the debit balance remains constant, as the market value changes. Then, $5000 CMV − $4000 debit = $1000 equity. Again as before, the doctor's equity has changed by the exact amount of the change in CMV (a $3000 decline in the market = a $3000 decline in equity). And suppose the market continued to decline to a point below $40 per share. In what position would that put the brokerage firm? It would be holding collateral worth less than $4000 on a loan of $4000 which is an intolerable situation for any lender! In fact, to prevent this from occurring, the SROs created a rule that requires a client to maintain at all times equity of at least 25% of the market value of the securities in his margin account. This is known as the minimum maintenance requirement.

To better understand maintenance, let's look again at the above account with the $1000 equity and the $5000 CMV. The NYSE/FINRA minimum equity requirement of this account is 25% of $5000 or $1250. Therefore, there is a deficiency of $250 ($1250–$1000) in this account.

An account with equity below the NYSE/FIWRA minimum maintenance requirement is called an under-margined account. NYSE/FINRA rules insist that if equity drops below 25% it must be brought back up to 25% immediately. Note that there is no requirement to bring the equity back to a point higher than the minimum 25% level. The doctor in this example will be issued a maintenance margin call in the amount of the $250 deficiency. The $250 is used by the firm to reduce the debit balance.

Note that before the maintenance call was satisfied, the equity percentage was 20% ($1000/$5000). After the call was satisfied, the equity percentage rose to 25% ($1250/$5000); the minimum equity percentage allowed under this SRO rule.

Example: Suppose a doctor wanted to know how low his account market value could fall before the account would be at the maintenance level. Can he determine the minimum market value down to which an account may drop without incurring a maintenance call? Yes—multiply the doctor's debit balance by 4/3.

In the example we have been using, the doctor's debit balance is $4000. We can immediately compute the market value down to which the account may drop as follows:

$4/3 \times$ Debit = maintenance level
$4/3 \times \$4000 = \$5333.33$

This means, if the stock drops from $80 per share to $53.33 per share, the equity in the account will have fallen to the NYSE minimum level of 25%. ($5333.33 CMV – $4000 debit = $1333.33).

NYSE/FINRA Minimum Credit Requirements

These rules stipulate that no brokerage firm may arrange for any credit to any client whose margin account does not have equity of at least $2000. The principal application of this rule is to initial transactions in newly opened margin accounts, however, it does apply at all times.

Example: A doctor buys 100 shares, at $15, in a new margin account. His margin call is $1500.
Rationale: $2000 would be too much to require as it exceeds the total purchase price. However, a loan to the doctor isn't allowed to be extended until, and unless, the account has equity of $2000. The trade is simply paid in full –100% of the purchase price is the margin call.
Example: A doctor buys 200 shares, at $15, in a new margin account (assume Regulation T = 60%). His margin call is $2000.
Rational: Regulation T 60% would be $1800 (60% × $3000). Since this would be $200 shy of the minimum equity level of $2000, the call is the $2000 minimum equity.
Example: A doctor buys 300 shares, at $15, in a new margin account. (assume Regulation T = 60%) His margin call is $2700.
Rationale: The account will have equity of $2700 (60% × $4500), which is more than the $2000 minimum. Therefore, the Regulation T initial requirement prevails.

The important points to remember about minimum credit requirements are

1. You are not called upon to pay more than the purchase price.
2. You cannot be granted a loan until the account has an equity of at least $2000.
3. If a decline in the market value of an existing account puts the equity below $2000, there is no requirement to bring the equity back up to $2000.

4. You may not withdraw money or securities from the account, if in doing so, you either
   a. Bring the equity below $2000
   b. Bring the equity below the maintenance level

These are the only times SMA may not be withdrawn from an account.

The Short Sale

Selling short is engaged in by medical professionals who anticipate a market decline. By selling borrowed property (shares of stock) at the current market value, the doctor expects to return the borrowed property (shares of the same issuer bought in the marketplace) to the lender, normally the investor's brokerage firm, when the market price is lower, thus profiting from the drop in price.

Essentially, this is the buy low and sell high philosophy. However, when executing a short sale, one is selling high initially then buying low later to "cover," or close out the deal by buying low and selling high in the reverse order.

Bear in mind that the short seller is borrowing property, not money. However, due to the high degree of risk inherent in short selling, it is permitted only in a margin account. A Regulation T call is required as a show of good faith, a way the client demonstrates the financial wherewithal to buy back the property. Let's look at a short sale transaction and the subsequent effects of market fluctuations on equity, as we did previously with buying on margin (long margin).

Credit Balance and Equity

A doctor shorts (sells short) 100 shares at $100 per share with Regulation T at 60%. The margin account would be credited with the proceeds of the sale, though the doctor has no access to these monies at this point in the deal. The account should also be credited with the doctor's required Regulation T margin call. Therefore, the credit balance in a doctor's margin account is the sum of the proceeds of the short sale, plus the Regulation T margin call. This number will not change regardless of future market fluctuations. The credit balance in a short margin account is a constant.

What does change with market fluctuations?

1. The cost of buying back the borrowed property to cover the short sale
2. The equity in the account

Equity in a short margin account is computed as follows:

Credit of $16,000 – CMV $10,000 equals $6000 equity.

Now, let's evaluate the effect of appreciation in the market price.

If the stock rises to $120 per share, then the credit of $16,000 – CMV $2000, equals $4000 equity.

Remember, the credit balance does not change when CMV fluctuates. The equity in this account is no longer Regulation T.

Let's determine the amount by which the account is restricted (remember, any margin account with equity below Regulation T is restricted). Or, $60\% \times \$12,000 = \$7200 - \$4000 = \$3200$

Also, it should be clear that the equity percentage of this account is less than 60%, by the formula:

Equity/CMV = $4000/$12,000 = 33.33%

This is the basic principle of the short sale: as the market price of the shorted stock increases, the equity decreases. The reverse is also true: as the price declines, the equity rises. Remember, short sellers are anticipating a market decline. Also, when buying long or selling short, any change in market value causes a dollar for dollar change in equity.

Minimum Maintenance Requirements (Short)

If the market continues to appreciate to $160 per share, the equity drops to zero. Suppose that the market price rose to its theoretical maximum, or infinity? The doctor's loss would be infinite. Remember, the maximum potential loss on a short sale is unlimited!

To protect against such an occurrence, industry Self-Regulatory Organizations (SROs) developed rules regarding the minimum equity that must be maintained in a margin account. The minimum maintenance in a short account is equity of 30% of CMV. Note that this is higher than the 25% figure for long margin accounts due to the nature of extreme risk of loss in the short sale.

Given that the CMV has risen to $160 per share ($16,000 total CMV), the minimum equity required to be maintained under SRO rules is 30% × CMV or $4800 equity. The doctor would receive a $4800 maintenance call to bring his equity from -0- to the $4800 minimum.

Remember, as in (cash) long accounts, there is no requirement to bring a margin account up to Regulation T equity. The maintenance equity is the percentage up to which the account must be brought when and if equity drops below the 25% or 30% levels.

Excess Equity (SMA) and Buying Power

We have seen what market appreciation does to a short seller. Let's evaluate the effects of market depreciation in value. If the decline goes to $85 per share, then $16,000 credit—CMV $8500 = $7500 equity. Again, market fluctuations don't affect credit balance. The equity in the account is now higher than Regulation T, and SMA (excess equity) has just been created.

And, as before, excess equity (SMA) can be used to buy more securities. Couldn't it also be used as the Regulation T down payment on another sale? Yes, this is another use of SMA that is called shorting power or "selling power." The formula for buying power as well as shorting power is exactly the same: Remember, it's SMA/RT to use buying power.

In this case, $2400/60% = $4000 of buying (shorting) power after the decline to $85, the doctor could buy long or sell short another $4000 worth of stock and use his SMA to meet his 60% ($2400) Regulation T Margin call. Recall that the margin call for a short sale is the same as for a long purchase.

Cheap Stock Rule

The SROs created a set of special maintenance rules in short margin accounts to protect against unreasonable risk in low-priced issues. These rules are appropriately labeled the "cheap stock" rules.

At all times, a doctor must maintain equity in a short margin account of the greater of the following:

1. 30% of the CMV (SRO minimum maintenance requirement)
2. $2000 (SRO minimum credit requirement)
3. Equity as required under the rules below

The cheap stock rules are as follows:

Stock Price	Minimum Maintained Equity
0–$2.50 per share	$2.50 per share
$2.50–$5.00 per share	100% of per share price
$5.00 per share and up	$5.00 per share

Example: A doctor shorts 1000 shares of a $1.50 per share stock. How much must he deposit initially and how much must be maintained in the account?

First, since Regulation T won't come into play until equity hits $2000 the SRO minimum credit requirement of $2000 should come into play. However, since this is a cheap stock, we determine if the requirements of those special rules require more than $2000. They do, and require a minimum be maintained in this short margin account of at least $2.50 per share sold short (1000 shares at $2.50 each = $2500 minimum that needs to be in this account at all times to comply with SRO rules).

Furthermore, if the market begins to rise, the cheap stock rules would require that at all times the amount of money in the account be at least 100% of the price per share until the stock hits $5. For example, if the stock rose to $4 per share, the doctor would have to have $4000 in the account to carry the position (1000 shares times 100% of CMV, $4 per share in this case).

Options Trading

Stock options are contracts that obligate medical investors to either buy or sell a stock at a specific price, by a specific date. For example, a put option is a bet on falling prices. Let's suppose Dr. Jane Smith holds a put option on XYZ stock, with a $50 exercise price, and the stock falls to $45. The value of the put rises in the options market because it lets her sell a $50 share, which is above the market price. A call option, on the other hand, is a bet on rising prices. Again, Dr. Smith holds a call option on XYZ stock with an exercise price of $50. If the share rises to $55, the value of the option increases since she may buy for $50, a stock now worth $55.

In 1999, Charles Schwab, the biggest on-line brokerage executed more than 30 million option trades. Due to this demand, Schwab launched other complex services, such as the on-line simultaneous buying and selling of options. Also crowding the options field, are new upstart on-line brokerages, such as: Interactive Brokers, Preferred Capital Markets Technology, and CyberCorp. They provide powerful software which will allow options in the future to trade as effortlessly and efficiently as stocks.

In mid-2000 the Reuters Group PLC Instinet Corporation, the electronic network most widely used by institutional investors, opened an Internet brokerage aimed at consumers, including healthcare practitioners. Instinet will let retail clients place orders alongside institutions, and will offer access to charts, news, and research. Thus, artificially empowering the individual investor, as well as again tempting the compulsive prone addict.

**OVERHEARD IN THE DOCTOR'S LOUNGE: ON
PROJECTING PP-ACA WINNERS AND LOSERS**

The first trading session following the election on Wednesday, November 7, 2012, gave us some clues on how different sectors of the health care market may be affected by the PP-ACA, as President Obama's election win confirmed that health reform marches forward. "Mr Market" will speak.

For those that may be unaware, "Mr Market" was Benjamin Graham's term for the stock market in explaining fluctuations. Graham is the father of value investing and Warren Buffet's most influential mentor. According to Graham, Mr Market is emotionally unstable but doesn't mind being slighted. If Mr Market's quotes are ignored, he will be back again tomorrow with a new quote.

So, the point is that successful investors do not place themselves in emotional whirlwinds often created by the market. This first post-election trading session was one such a whirlwind. Large groups of people (such as those that voted with their pocketbook in this telling stock market session) are smarter than an elite few, or so goes the premise of James Surowiecki's Wisdom of the Crowds.

Now, what did we learn from the combined investing public wisdom about the future of healthcare companies profitability with ACA?

David K. Luke MIM, MS-PFS, CMP™
(Net Worth Advice)
Salt Lake City, Utah

FUTURE PROGNOSTICATIONS?

Keep in mind the overall market was down 2.4% on November 7, 2012, as measured by both the Dow Jones Industrial Average and the Standard & Poor 500. The biggest concern of the day was investor worry about the so-called "fiscal cliff" and the debate over billions in spending and tax increases. Considering the total market on November 7, health care stocks performed as a group better than the averages, but Mr Market definitely parsed health care stocks by sector from "great" to "dreadful" based on the implications of impending health care reform:

Great
Hospital Stocks

- Health Management Associates (HMA) +7.3%
- HCA Holdings Inc. (HCA) +9.4%
- Community Health Systems Inc. (CYH) +6.0%
- Tenet Healthcare Corp. (THC) +9.6%

Yes, there were stocks that went up stridently on the big down day. Not surprisingly, hospital stocks are expected to benefit from the estimated 30 million Americans lined-up for the insurance coverage that began in 2014, increasing profits and decreasing bad debts.

Medicaid HMOs

- Molina Healthcare Inc. (MOH) +4.6%
- Centene Corp. (CNC) +10.1%
- WellCare Health Plans Inc. (WCG) +4.4%

Health insurers that typically focus heavily on Medicaid are up in line with ACA provisions to expand care for the poor. Mr Market tips his hat to Centene Corporation, which has been successful in procuring multiline coverage contracts with States including long-term care, vision, dental, behavioral health, CHIP, and disability.

Good
Drug Wholesalers

- McKesson (MCK) +1.3%
- Cardinal Health (CAH) +.5%
- AmerisourceBergen (ABC) +1.0%

Growth in prescription drug spending means increased revenues for the drug wholesalers, so the ACA should ultimately be a positive for this group. But, because a majority of wholesaler profits come from generic drugs, and because wholesalers are indirectly affected by changes in pharmacies, pricing pressures will keep the wholesalers in check.

Fair
Pharmacy Benefit Managers

- Express Scripts (ESRX) −0.4%
- CVS Caremark Corp (CVS) −0.4%

As an intermediary between the payer and everyone else in the healthcare system, PBMs process prescriptions for groups such as insurance companies and corporations and use their large size to drive down prices. These companies, incentivized to cut costs, are thought to benefit greatly from ACA and expanded prescription drug insurance plans.

Generic Pharmaceuticals
- Teva Pharmaceutical Industries Ltd ADR (TEVA) −0.7%
- Mylan Inc (MYL) −0.8%
- Dr. Reddy's Labs (RDY) −0.6%

Healthcare reform is good for generic drugs with anticipated increased dispensing of drugs in general. With more funds spent on Medicaid, the ACA will certainly be generic oriented and should fare better than the name-brand drugs. Pricing pressures are expected over the longer term however.

Testing Laboratories
- Quest Diagnostics (DGX) −1.5%
- Laboratory Corp of America (LH) −1.9%

More patients than you would think would mean more medical tests. In a recent survey, physicians attributed 34% of overall healthcare costs to defensive medicine (think diagnostic blood tests/invasive biopsies, etc.). The ACA may curb this expensive part of medicine and appears to have very negative implications going forward as Labs will have intense pressure to reduce rates. However, these larger labs held up better than the market averages suggesting that lab work isn't going away with ACA.

Big Pharmaceutical Companies
- Pfizer Inc. (PFE) −2.2%
- GlaxoSmithKline PLC (GSK) −0.8%
- Eli Lily & Co. (LLY) −1.2%

The name-brand large Pharmaceutical companies agreed to rebate Uncle Sam on Medicaid purchases and must give the elderly discounts. But, there will be a lot more of us taking drugs, too.

These four health care sectors are ranked as "fair" considering that broader stock market averages were down 2.4% for the day and Mr Market was kinder to this group with only a slight negative. Likewise, it appears that he is anointing this group as a benefactor of upcoming reforms.

Not Good

Medical Device Companies

- Medtronic Inc. (MDT) −3.0%
- Stryker Corporation (SYK) −1.6%
- Boston Scientific Corp. (BSX) −3.6%
- Zimmer Holdings Inc. (ZMH) −1.8%

The 2.3% excise tax on revenue of medical-device companies is looking more inevitable, in spite of industry lobbying group efforts.

Dreadful

Medicare Part D Companies

- Humana Inc. (HUM) −7.9%
- WellPoint (WLP) −5.5%
- Cigna Corp. (CI) −0.7%

Even though managed-care companies should gain millions of new customers thanks to the ACA, profit margins are expected to decline significantly. Mr Market went easy on Cigna, perhaps because of the company's focus on self-insured large employers.

Currently it is unclear how the increased revenue generated from more patients will affect the increased margins to the various sectors of the healthcare market. Also, too much weight should not be placed on this one day action by the market. One thing is clear however, and that is how Mr Market and the market at large feels at first blush towards the ACA based on the November 7, 2012, trading of these respective stocks. But, what happens going forward is anyone's guess …. How have these positions faired today?

So remember; Mr Market is temperamental and can change his mind anytime! Buyer-beware!

DAY TRADING AND THE INTERNET

Since most people, including medical professions, initially lose at day trading, they give up and decide not to do it anymore. As there is a minimum amount of money, about $25,000–50,000 of trading capital needed to start, this loss is a powerful de-motivator. Still, scared by Mark O. Barton, the murderous day trader in Atlanta more than a decade ago, the NASD-FINRA and NYSE have recently proposed new rules for those who engage in questionable day trading activities. One proposal would provide that a minimum equity of $25,000 be maintained at all times, versus the current $2000 for other margin accounts. If the amount fell below the new threshold, no further trading would be permitted until the threshold was maintained.

Still, Internet day trading has become an investment bubble of late, suggesting that something lighter than air can pop and disappear in an instant. This has occurred despite the fact that most lay and healthcare professionals that engage in such activities do not appreciate even the basic rules of margin and debt, as reviewed herein. History is filled with examples: from the tulip mania of 1630 Holland and the British South Sea Bubble of the 1700s to the Florida land boom of the roaring 1920s and the Great Crash of 1929 and to the collapse of Japan's stock and real estate market in early 1990s. To this list, one might now add day Internet trading during the bull markets of 1999–2000 and 2011–2014.

HIGH-FREQUENCY TRADERS AND THE MARKET

Is the U.S. stock market rigged with elite traders buying access to a high-speed network (600 orders per second for a single stock) that allows them to figure out what you've just ordered, order it first, then raise the price before your order is complete? Well, it may be, according to Michael Lewis, author of a new book about High-Frequency Trading (HFT) called *Flash Boys*. And this form of "front running" is completely legal. So, you decide.

Nevertheless, to counter HFT trading, IEX may be the first equity trading venue owned exclusively by a consortium of buy-side investors, including mutual funds, hedge funds, and family offices. Dedicated to institutionalizing fairness in the markets, IEX is reported to provide a more balanced marketplace by simplified market structure design and cutting-edge technology. IEX aims to offer a fair-access platform to any qualified broker dealer. IEX is driven by a team of cross-industry experts with backgrounds spanning market venues, electronic trading, and broker-dealers. http://www.iextrading.com/

CONCLUSION

A general review of investment banking, securities markets, and margin accounts was presented in this chapter. Such vital information is rarely included in a text of this type.

COLLABORATE

Discuss this chapter online with others at www.MedicalExecutivePost.com.

ACKNOWLEDGMENTS

To James Nash of the Investment Training Institute in Tucker, Georgia, and Jeff Kuest, CFA, CFP®, founder and managing principal of Counterpoint Capital Advisers, Lake Oswego, Oregon.

FURTHER READING

Atkinson, W and Crawford, AJ: On-line investing raises questions about suitability. *Wall Street Journal*, November, 28, 1999.

Farrell, C: *Day Trade On-line*. John Wiley & Sons, New York, 1999.

Fleuriet, M: *Investment Banking Explained: An Insider's Guide to the Industry*. McGraw-Hill, New York, 2008.

Friedfertig, M: *Electronic Day Trader's Secretes*. McGraw-Hill, New York, 1999.

Gibowicz, P: *Quick Seven*. Edward Fleur Financial Education Corporation, New York, 1999.

Gibowicz, P: *Registered Representative (Study Program, Volume I)*. Edward Fleur Financial Education Corporation, New York, 2000.

Gibowicz, P: *Registered Representative (Study Program, Volume II)*. Edward Fleur Financial Education Corporation, New York, 1998.

Kadlec, CW: *Dow 100,000: Fact or Fiction*. New York Institute of Finance, New York, 1999.

Kaufmann, PJ *Trading Systems and Methods*. Wiley Finance, New York, 2013.

Khalife, D: *The Best Book on Investment Banking Careers*. Create a Space Independent Publishing, New York, 2012.

Lewis, M: *Flash Boys: A Wall Street Revolt*. W. W. Norton & Company, New York, 2014.

Nash, J: Margin. In: Nash, J: *International Training Institute Manual*. International Training Institute Press, Atlanta, 2002.

Nash, J: Securities markets. In: Nash, J: *International Training Institute Manual*. International Training Institute Press, Atlanta, 2000.

Nassar, DS: *How to Get Started in Electronic Day Trading*. McGraw-Hill, New York, 1999.

Rosenbaum, J, Pearl, J and Perella, JR: *Investment Banking: Valuation, Leveraged Buyouts, and Mergers & Acquisitions*. Wiley Finance, New York, 2013.

Surowieck, J: *The Wisdom of Crowds*. Amazon Digital Services, Anchor Press, New York, 2013.

14 Hedge Funds
Wall Street Personified

Michael J. Burry

CONTENTS

The investment profession has come a long way since the door-to-door stock salesmen of the 1920s sold a willing public on worthless stock certificates. The stock market crash of 1929 and the ensuing Great Depression of the 1930s forever changed the way investment operations are run. A bewildering array of laws and regulations sprung up, all geared to protecting the individual investor from fraud. These laws also set out specific guidelines on what types of investment can be marketed to the general public—and allowed for the creation of a set of investment products specifically not marketed to the general public.

For all practical purposes, these early mid-twentieth-century lawmakers specifically exempted from the definition of "general public," those investors that meet certain minimum net worth guidelines. The lawmakers decided that wealth brings the sophistication required to evaluate, either independently or together with the wise counsel, investment options that fall outside the mainstream. Not surprisingly, an investment industry catering to such wealthy individuals such as doctors, healthcare professionals, and qualifying institutions has sprung up.

INTRODUCTION

Nevertheless, many investors—even those who meet the net worth guidelines—are surprised to learn that there exists a $500–$999 billion, or more, alternative investment industry that is not generally marketed to the public. Such alternative investments have also been known as hedge funds or private investment funds. Unlike mutual funds, these alternative investments can be structured in a wide variety of ways. Because of the very same regulations discussed above, these funds cannot be advertised, but they are far from illegal or illicit.

In fact, physicians were among the most significant early investors in one of the last century's most successful hedge funds. Mr Warren Buffett, Chairman of Berkshire Hathaway, Inc. and a legendary investor, got his start in 1957 running the Buffett Partnership, an alternative investment fund not open to the general public. Mr Buffett's first public appearance as a money manager was before a group of physicians in Omaha, Nebraska. Eleven decided to put some money with him. A few of these original investors followed him into Berkshire Hathaway, which is now among the most highly valued companies in the world.

The alternative investment, or hedge, funds of today are similar to the original Buffett Partnership in many ways. This chapter will introduce and explain this industry, as well as the pertinent historical, structural, legal, tax, and operating issues of which potential investors should be aware.

HISTORY

The original hedge fund was an investment partnership started by A.W. Jones in 1949. A financial writer prior to starting his investment management career, Mr Jones is widely credited as being the prototypical hedge fund manager. His style of investment, in fact, gave the hedge fund its name— although Mr. Jones himself called his fund a "hedged fund." Mr. Jones attempted to "hedge," or protect, his investment partnership against market swings by selling short overvalued securities while at the same time buying undervalued securities. Leverage was an integral part of the strategy. Other managers followed in Mr Jones' footsteps, and the hedge fund industry was born.

In those early days, the hedge fund industry was defined by the types of investment operations undertaken—selling short securities, making liberal use of leverage, engaging in arbitrage, and otherwise attempting to limit one's exposure to market swings. Today, the hedge fund industry is defined more by the structure of the investment fund and the type of manager compensation employed.

The changing definition is largely a sign of the times. In 1949, the United States was in a unique state. With the memory of the Great Depression still massively influencing common wisdom on stocks, the postwar euphoria sparked an interest in the securities markets not seen in several decades. Perhaps it is not so surprising that at such a time a particularly reflective financial writer such as A.W. Jones would start an investment operation featuring, most prominently, the protection against market swings rather than participation in them.

Apart from a few significant hiccups—1972–1973, 1987, and 2006–2007 being the most prominent—the U.S. stock markets have been on quite a roll for quite a long time now. So, today, hedge funds come in all flavors—many are not hedged at all. Instead, the concept of a private investment fund structured as a partnership, with performance incentive compensation for the manager, has come to dominate the mindscape when hedge funds are discussed. Hence, we now have a term in "hedge fund" that is not always accurate in its description of the underlying activity. In fact, several recent events have contributed to an even more distorted general understanding of hedge funds.

During 1998, both the high-profile long-term capital management crisis and the spectacular currency losses experienced by the George Soros organization contributed to a drastic reversal of fortune in the court of public opinion for hedge funds. Most hedge fund managers, who spend much of their time attempting to limit risk in one way or another, were appalled in the manner with which the press used the highest-profile cases to vilify the industry as dangerous risk takers. At one point during late 1998, hedge funds were even blamed in the lay press for the currency collapses of several developing nations; whether this was even possible got short thrift in the press.

Needless to say, more than a few managers have decided they did not much appreciate being painted with the same "hedge fund" brush. Alternative investment fund, private investment fund, and several other terms have been promoted but inadequately adopted. As the memory of 1998 and 2007 fades, "hedge fund" may once again become a term embraced by all private investment managers.

Investors should be aware, however, that several different terms defining the same basic structure might be used. Investors should therefore become familiar with the structure of such funds, independent of the label. The Securities Exchange Commission (SEC) calls such funds "privately offered investment companies" and the Internal Revenue Service calls them "securities partnerships." For the purposes of this chapter, they will be referred to as simply "hedge funds."

ELIGIBILITY

Not just anyone is eligible to invest in hedge funds. Unlike mutual funds, where a check written generally results in an investment made, hedge fund managers typically give themselves wide latitude to reject potential investors on a variety of grounds, and not uncommonly do so. Indeed, hedge funds may impose nearly any legal means to exclude investors. Aside from the vagaries of various managers, however, there are certain laws that guide the admittance of investors into hedge funds and which cannot be violated.

In general, only accredited investors are eligible to invest in hedge funds, or participate in any private offering for that matter. To qualify as an accredited investor, as defined under Rule 501 of Regulation D promulgated under the Securities Act of 1933, an individual must be a natural person whose individual net worth, or joint net worth together with that person's spouse, exceeds $1,000,000. Alternatively, under the same rule, an accredited investor is a natural person who had an individual income in excess of $200,000 in each of the two most recent years or joint income with that person's spouse in excess of $300,000 in each of those years and has a reasonable expectation of reaching the same income level in the current year.

A manager may be required to register as an investment adviser either with the SEC or with one or more states. If so, there is a good chance that in addition to meeting the accredited investor definition, an individual must either have a net worth of >$1,500,000 or invest $750,000 with the manager to become eligible to invest in the manager's fund. Equity in an individual's home does count toward these criteria. If a manager is registered as an investment adviser and does not impose these additional criteria, the manager may not be able to charge fees linked to the performance of the investment.

In general, each hedge fund manager has the option of allowing up to 35 nonaccredited investors into his or her fund. This option is generally reserved only for close family or friends, and it is typically neither economical nor advisable for a manager to allow nonaccredited investors into his or her fund.

Very large hedge funds, which are really a separate category from small hedge funds and will be discussed in more detail below, may impose a higher standard on potential investors, that of the "qualified purchaser." Qualified purchasers include any trust, natural person, or family-controlled entity owning $5 million or more in investments net of liabilities. Note that this requirement is at least five times more stringent than that which is imposed on investors in smaller funds. For very large funds, however, this is not a matter of choice but rather one of law.

Because of these laws and various eligibility requirements, potential investors in hedge funds should expect, in many cases, to fill out an eligibility questionnaire (often called an "accredited investor questionnaire" or a "pre-qualification worksheet") prior to even receiving basic information with which to evaluate the investment. Common data requested include a certification that certain standards of net worth or income are met, employment information, income history and composition, and investment experience or skill level. Often, potential investors will be asked to sign the document testifying as to the truth of the representations made in the questionnaire. A hedge fund manager will use these data not only to ensure that a potential investor meets the necessary legal standards, but also to enable the manager to act responsibly in deciding whether to make an official offer to the potential investor.

STRUCTURE

Investment Vehicle

In the United States, hedge funds are structured as either a limited partnership or a limited liability company. When used as a fund, a limited partnership is a legal entity consisting of one or more general partners and one or more limited partners. The portfolio manager is usually positioned as the general partner, and investors become limited partners. A limited liability company, when used as a fund, is a legal entity composed of one or more managing members and one or more nonmanaging members. The portfolio manager takes the managing member role and investors become nonmanaging members. A limited liability company can elect to be taxed either as a partnership or as a corporation. Hedge funds structured as limited liability companies will typically elect partnership status for tax purposes. Hence, from an operating and tax standpoint, both limited partnerships and limited liability companies look much the same to both potential investors and the Internal Revenue Service (IRS).

Traditionally, hedge funds have been limited partnerships. More recently, however, some law firms have begun to advise their clients to form their funds as limited liability companies rather than general partnerships because the managing member of a limited liability company cannot generally be held responsible for liabilities of the limited liability company. The general partner in a partnership has no such protection from the liabilities of the partnership. Limited liability companies are relatively new, but as case law supporting the limited liability of the manager matures, managers are likely to use the limited liability format more frequently when forming hedge funds.

Portfolio Manager

The managing member or general partner working as the portfolio manager for the limited liability company or limited partnership, respectively, may itself be a limited liability company, a corporation (including a subchapter S Corporation), a limited partnership, a sole proprietorship, or just about any other type of entity. There is no rule that says the portfolio manager must be an individual natural person, although traditionally—before the era of frivolous tort—this was the case. Recently, the trend is for more and more managers to organize as limited liability companies.

Generally speaking, no matter the organizational structure of the portfolio manager, a single individual functions as the captain of the ship, so to speak. In nearly all cases, this person has established a reputation of investment skill through any of a variety of endeavors. The traditional route is for a portfolio manager within a financial services firm of some repute to split off and form a hedge fund. Potential investors should expect hedge fund managers today to come from a wide variety of backgrounds, not one of which should be automatically viewed as particularly favorable over another.

Fund Size

The vast majority of hedge funds are <$100–250 million in size, but they can range into the billions of dollars in size. For several practical reasons having to do with brokerage functions, funds holding under $2–5 million in assets under management (AUM) are extremely rare.

Several factors conspire to limit the size of most hedge funds. The most important factor is the desire of hedge fund managers to avoid registering the hedge fund under the Investment Company Act of 1940. To avoid such registration, which would seriously limit the types of trading and investment activities hedge funds could undertake, most hedge funds limit the number of investors to 100 beneficial security holders or less. Contrast this relatively small number of investors to the tens of thousands of investors who may participate in a typical large mutual fund. Sixty-five of these 100 investors must be accredited investors, while there is a provision for up to 35 nonaccredited investors to participate in the typical hedge fund. For these funds, the size of the fund is also limited by the inability or lack of desire of the fund manager to attract large numbers of the biggest clients.

If a fund wishes to accept more than 100 investors, there is an option under a different law. In 1996, the National Securities Markets Improvement Act increased the number of investors that may be allowed, without subjecting the hedge fund to registration under the Investment Company Act of 1940, to 500. However, to accept up to 500 investors, a fund must require that all post-1996 investors meet stringent "qualified purchaser" provisions. A "qualified purchaser" is any trust, natural person, or family-controlled entity owning at least $5 million in investments net of all liabilities. This is a much higher bar than the $1 million net worth requirement required for investors in funds wishing to keep 100 or fewer investors. The net effect, therefore, is to create two categories of funds: the very large hedge fund families that cannot only attract the highest net worth clients and institutions, but also accept 5 times as many of them, and those smaller funds that accept lower net worth clients, and only one-fifth as many of them.

The size of the fund affects the costs of the fund, the services that investors can expect, and the types of investments a fund can make.

Costs

The very large funds accepting only qualified purchasers need a good amount of office space, marketing, research, and administrative staff, and will have higher overhead in general. This higher overhead will be spread over a larger asset base, however, so that the effect on the expense ratio experienced by investors is uncertain. Managers not seeking out these 500 qualified purchasers may run their smaller funds out of a single office, or even out of a bedroom. But even relatively small fixed costs can lead to a high expense ratio if the fund is too small.

Services

Potential investors in the larger funds may expect a slick-marketing program. Those investors in smaller funds may find the marketing to be a bit rough around the edges. Indeed, when it comes to printed materials, potential investors may be struck as to the difference between a print shop prize on one hand and a color ink-jet nightmare on the other. It is important for potential investors to look through the glamorous glitz—or the marketing morass, as the case may be—and examine the underlying qualities of the investment and the manager. While taking care not to mistake an everyday-starving artist for a Picasso, potential investors should understand that it is not a stretch to expect that a rumpled portfolio manager working out of a bedroom with no staff support may in fact be the perfect manager. A certain group of Omaha physicians circa 1960 would have done well to go with just such a manager—by the name of Mr Warren Buffett.

Investments

Finally, on the subject of size, potential investors should understand that very large funds generally must make very large investments. The hot $50 million retail stock may be off-limits to a $5 billion behemoth. Generally speaking, as funds surpass several hundred million dollars in AUM, fund managers find that the more illiquid securities become impractical to trade. How this affects returns depends on the style of the manager.

Minimums

Relative to more familiar mutual funds, hedge funds generally require a larger minimum initial investment to open and to maintain an account. These minimums vary widely. Smaller funds may require as little as $50,000 to open an account, while other larger funds may require much more than $1,000,000. Fund managers often give themselves the flexibility to waive minimums. When doing so, fund managers are generally counting on a larger investment at a future date. This practice is more common with newer funds, and potential investors should not expect more mature or successful funds to waive minimums.

Hedge funds may require investors to add to their investment at a later date. Investors failing to do so may not be able to maintain a place in the fund. This occurs because as hedge funds grow, there is pressure to increase the average size of a capital account in the fund. Fund managers will show broad variability in how such pressures are handled, and this is one reason that potential investors should inquire as to how large the manager expects the fund to grow.

FEE STRUCTURES

The hedge fund fee structure is relatively unique, and requires an understanding of several concepts. A famous example may help, with definitions to follow.

EXAMPLE 14.1

Mr Warren Buffett, as manager of the Buffett Partnership, took a 0- and -25 fee structure, with a 6% hurdle rate. What this means is that he charged no asset management fee and earned not a cent unless he exceeded a 6% annual rate of return. Once that 6% return was met, Mr Buffett took 25% of the profits over and above 6%. He did not use a crawlback provision, nor did he set a high water mark. Below, we will examine these features.

Asset Management Fee

The asset management fee is fairly easy to grasp. The manager is allocated a percentage of AUM. Typically, this fee is 1% of AUM, although a manager may charge no asset management fee or charge a higher asset management fee. The asset management fee may be deducted on nearly any schedule, but typically, the fee is deducted on a quarterly or annual basis. The fee may be calculated based on the beginning, ending, or average account size. Typically, the fee is calculated or accrued based on ending the capital account size.

EXAMPLE 14.2

As an internist, you have placed $100,000 with a hedge fund manager who charges a 1% asset management fee. Every 3 months, the manager deducts 0.25% of AUM. After the first 3 months, your capital account has grown to $104,000. The manager deducts $260 for the asset management fee.

Some states place restrictions on how high an asset management fee can get before it is considered unreasonable, and hence illegal. In California, for example, an asset management fee above 3% is considered unreasonable. In general, the department of corporations in each state will be able to provide guidelines on this matter. Typically, the asset management fee ranges from 0% to 2%, a range that is generally considered reasonable in the United States.

The asset management fee was originally conceived as a method for reimbursing the manager for the manager's out-of-pocket expenses incurred on the fund's behalf. Historically, such expenses would be reimbursed by the fund as the manager incurred them. As managers found themselves managing larger and more complex funds—as well as managing multiple funds—they found it easier to just estimate these expenses and charge them all at once as a fixed annual or quarterly fee. In this manner, the concept of the annual asset management fee was born.

Today, especially in the case of the larger funds, the asset management fee is increasingly viewed not only as reimbursement for fund expenses incurred by the manager, but also as an income stream for the manager. For example, a $500 million fund with a 1% asset management fee allows the manager to earn $5 million in annual fees just for showing up to work. This amount is likely much greater than the out-of-pocket expenses incurred by the manager on behalf of the fund.

Among hedge funds today, a 1% asset management fee is considered standard, but in rare cases, potential investors will find a fund that charges no fee and instead charges "expenses off the top." In such cases, the fund manager is trying to get back to the historical intent of the asset management fee: not as an income stream, but rather as simple reimbursement for expenses incurred. The benefits of such an arrangement are variable. Small funds will often find that reimbursable expenses routinely run higher than 1% of AUM, while larger funds will find that they run much lower. Hence, investors in large funds with an "expenses off the top" arrangement are getting a break on the asset management fees, while investors in small funds with such an arrangement are possibly paying more for such reimbursable expenses than they would with a simple 1% asset management fee. Since most fund managers plan on growing the fund size significantly, very few choose to charge "expenses off the top" rather than an annual asset management fee—most of them look forward to that substantial and virtually guaranteed income stream.

Fund managers who choose to charge "expenses off the top" certainly may run a high-expense fund, but there is generally great incentive for such fund managers to actually limit expenses. "Off the top" means that expenses are deducted before the performance incentive fee, discussed below, is calculated. In other words, expenses eat right into the performance that determines the whole of the income for the manager, who has forgone an annual management fee. Just as a physician will seek to minimize expenses within the office—within reason and without harming patient care—it follows that rational fund managers who choose this "expenses off the top" arrangement in lieu of an annual fee will seek to minimize those expenses without harming the total performance.

Fund managers charging an annual asset management fee may charge certain expenses, such as accounting fees, back to the fund over and above the annual asset management fee. As well, managers who charge "expenses off the top" in lieu of an asset management fee vary widely in the types of expenses included. Therefore, potential investors should review the offering documents carefully to fully assess the character and magnitude of the asset management expenses to which investors are exposed.

Performance/Incentive Compensation

A hallmark of hedge funds is the participation of the manager in the profits of the fund. Not every hedge fund manager charges an asset management fee, but nearly every hedge fund manager charges some sort of fee linked to fund performance. A typical arrangement is for a manager to receive 20% of the total profits, but the performance fee arrangements are limited only by the imagination of the hedge fund manager and are not generally negotiable. The goal of this compensation scheme is to give hedge fund managers more of an incentive to earn excess profits for the investors in the fund.

It must be acknowledged, however, that performance compensation provides tremendous reward for high performance, while providing virtually no direct penalty for lousy performance. To be sure, if a hedge fund manager consistently performs poorly, he or she will lose business. Nevertheless, the frequent pairing of an asset management fee to a performance fee—typically a 1% asset management fee paired to a 20% performance incentive—can provide especially large hedge funds with a guaranteed 1% income stream, a large upside due to the 20% performance incentive, and essentially no direct short-term incentive to avoid risk.

Hence, while performance incentives are the rule in the hedge fund industry, potential investors should be aware of the potential for hedge fund managers to accept undue risks, primarily via the use of leverage, in pursuit of outsized returns. Indeed, in the hands of a greed-driven manager with little sense of integrity or fiduciary caution, the performance fee compensation arrangement can become deleterious to the financial health of the fund's investors. Managers who are registered investment advisers are required to disclose this sort of risk to potential investors, and in any case, most hedge fund managers are risk averse. Nevertheless, this characteristic of hedge funds requires potential investors to develop a solid understanding of the investment policies of the hedge fund manager under consideration.

Hurdle Rate

Hedge funds may feature a hurdle rate as part of the calculation of the fund manager's performance incentive compensation. Also known as a "benchmark," the hurdle rate is the amount, expressed in percentage points, an investor's capital account must appreciate before the account becomes subject to a performance incentive fee. Potential medical investors should view the hurdle rate as a form of protection in context with other features of the fee arrangement.

The hurdle rate, which benchmarks a single year's performance, may be considered mutually exclusive of any other year, or the hurdle rate may compound each year. The former case is more common. In the latter case, a portfolio manager failing to attain a hurdle rate in the first year will find the effective hurdle rate considerably higher during the second year.

Once a fund manager attains the hurdle rate for an investor, the medical investor's capital account may be charged a performance incentive fee only on the performance above and beyond the hurdle rate. Alternatively, the account may be charged a performance fee for the entire level of performance, including the performance required to attain the hurdle rate. Other variations on the use of the hurdle rate exist, and are limited only by the contract signed between the fund manager and the investor. The hurdle rate is not generally a negotiating point, however.

EXAMPLE 14.3

A fund charges a performance fee with a 6% hurdle rate, calculated in a mutually exclusive manner. Dr. Lanouette, a radiologist investor places $100,000 with the fund. The first year's performance is 5%. The investor therefore owes no performance fee during the first year because the portfolio manager did not attain the hurdle rate. During year two, the portfolio manager guides the fund to a 7% return. Since the hurdle rate is mutually exclusive of any other year, the portfolio manager has attained the 6% hurdle rate and is entitled to a performance fee.

High-Water Mark

Some funds feature a high-water mark provision, also known as a "loss-carryforward" provision. As with the hurdle rate, potential investors should consider the high-water mark as a form of protection. A high-water mark is an amount equal to the greatest value of an investor's capital account, adjusted for contributions and withdrawals. The high-water mark ensures that the hedge fund manager charges a performance incentive fee only on the amount of appreciation over and above the high-water mark set at the time the performance fee was last charged. The current trend is for newer funds to feature this high-water mark, while older, larger funds may not feature it.

EXAMPLE 14.4

A fund charges a 20% performance fee with a high-water mark but no hurdle rate. Dr. Butala, a dentist investor contributes $100,000 to the fund. During the first year, the hedge fund manager grows that capital account to $110,000 and charges a 20% performance fee, or $2000. The ending capital account balance and high-water mark is therefore $108,000. During year two, the account falls back to $100,000, but the high-water mark remains $108,000. During year three, for the manager to charge a performance fee, the manager must grow the capital account to a level above $108,000.

Claw-Back Provision

Rarely, a fund may provide investors with a claw-back provision. This term, borrowed from the venture capital fund world, result in a refund to the investor of all or part of a previously charged performance fee if a certain level of performance is not attained in subsequent years. Such refunds in the face of poor or inadequate performance may not be legal in some states or under certain authorities.

EXPENSES

Hedge funds vary widely in the manner with which they expose investors to the expenses of the fund. The fairness of such exposure can be summed up in a figure called the expense ratio. The expense ratio is defined as fund expenses divided by AUM. In general, hedge funds respond very well to economies of scale. Hence, as fund AUM increases, expense ratios tend to decline. Investors must be aware of both the organizational costs of a fund and the expected ongoing costs that the fund manager expects the fund to bear. Fund managers generally have leeway to absorb costs if the expense ratio gets too high, although investors should never count on fund managers to do so. The expense ratio should always be considered in context with the size of the asset management fee.

Organization Costs

When a would-be hedge fund manager decides to set up a hedge fund, the manager incurs start-up costs. The cost to start a hedge fund typically ranges from $25,000 to $150,000 or more, and it is a common practice for the fund, once capitalized with investor money, to reimburse the manager for these expenses. The reimbursement typically covers legal costs to create the fund and write the fund-offering documents, accounting consulting costs in connection with preparation of the fund, and document printing costs. Whether the reimbursement will include all the expenses or just the expenses up to a given level is up to the manager. Such information can be found in the offering documents. This reimbursement cost is capitalized by the fund and amortized over 12 months. Therefore, this cost is borne by the investors who invest during the first 12 months of the fund's existence. This is one reason new funds tend to have higher expense ratios during their first year relative to subsequent years.

Ongoing Costs

The agreement developed by the hedge fund manager and agreed to by the investor is what determines which costs will be borne by the fund, and hence its investors. With rare exceptions, trading commissions are borne by the fund investors. Also with rare exceptions, the fund is responsible for bearing its own bookkeeping and accounting costs. The most expensive component of these costs is generally the annual audit. If the fund is charged an annual asset management fee, these bookkeeping and accounting costs may or may not be limited by the amount of the asset management fee.

With regard to other costs, there is great variability between funds. One fund manager may operate out of a bedroom with nothing but a subscription to the *Wall Street Journal*, and charge none of his or her costs to the fund. Another fund manager may rent high-end office space and a Bloomberg terminal, fly all over the country recruiting clients, hire expensive analysts, and charge a good portion if not the entire amount of these costs to the fund. Potential investors would do well to be very clear as to what sort of cost culture the hedge fund manager embraces, and how much of this cost culture he or she expects the fund's investors to bear. These matters should be detailed in the fund-offering documents and may need to be clarified directly with the hedge fund manager or representative.

Reporting

During the days of the Buffett Partnership, Mr Warren Buffett forbade his clients from asking questions and only reported to his clients once per year. Times change. As the hedge fund industry has grown in size, hedge fund managers have begun to compete for customers by offering more liberal disclosure and more frequent, detailed reporting; secure website and smartphone applications, and so on. In some cases, intraday real-time Internet updates are even available. This would have been unforeseeable—or at least unthinkable—a few years ago. Nevertheless, when it comes to reporting, investors will never mistake the hedge fund industry for the mutual fund industry. At least not yet.

The typical hedge fund will send out monthly or quarterly reports detailing capital account balances. With quarterly reports, hedge fund investors can generally expect a brief letter from the portfolio manager updating investors on various issues. Hedge fund managers continue to have tremendous flexibility in how they schedule their reporting, however, and investors should expect great variability among managers on this front.

Since hedge funds are generally taxed as partnerships, an investor in a hedge fund should expect to receive a Schedule K-1, completed with all the appropriate information, in a timely manner following the annual audit in the first quarter of the subsequent fiscal year.

In summary, hedge fund investors can expect the following materials: monthly, quarterly, or annual statements of capital account balances; monthly, quarterly, or annual letters from the portfolio manager; and an annual Schedule K-1. In many cases, the fund manager also forwards to investors a marketing data sheet or brochure summarizing various data regarding the performance of the fund.

The Internet has changed the daily life of millions of Americans, and the hedge fund industry is responding. There is a nascent trend toward greater use of the Internet and e-mail for reporting functions, and it may be expected that this trend will only gain steam going forward. Certainly, cost-conscious managers will be among the first to jump on this trend, as printing costs are among the costs managers and funds face. Because of the wide variability between hedge fund managers, any given portfolio manager may have quite sound reasons for resisting the trend to increased detail and frequency in reporting. Potential investors, alone or in conjunction with their adviser, must assess these reasons in this context.

Liquidity

Hedge funds are not as liquid as stocks or mutual funds because of the potential increased expense of frequent openings and closings of the fund as well as the potential disruption to the fund strategy are simply too great. Indeed, the costs of opening and closing an entity such as a hedge fund—which is really a business that invests in securities—are quite significant. It is simply cheaper and entails less administrative burden to open and close the fund on a monthly or quarterly basis. Also, many hedge funds gain their largest advantage over mutual funds by seizing the opportunity to enter into concentrated, undervalued, and illiquid investments that mutual funds generally must shun. Such investments require a stable pool of capital in the fund. This factor contributes to the reduced liquidity of most hedge funds.

One mechanism that contributes to the illiquidity of many hedge funds is the lockup. A lockup restricts a new investor from withdrawing all or part of the investor's investment before a certain amount of time elapses. The common lock-up periods are for 1 year, but there are many variations to suit both the manager and the strategy.

Industry Players

Hedge funds are part of an industry catering to high net worth individuals and institutions, and it may not be surprising that hedge funds do not act alone in this endeavor. In fact, behind every hedge fund, there is a cast of supporting players without whom hedge funds would have a difficult time operating.

Prime Broker

With rare exceptions, every hedge fund manager hires one prime broker to act as the fund's custodian and to reconcile and clear all the hedge fund's trades. Despite having one prime broker, a hedge fund manager, in executing trades for the fund, may use any number of brokers. By doing so, the manager can use a broker with one specialty to execute one type of trade, but then can use another broker with another specialty to execute a different type of trade. The manager therefore accesses the best of breed qualities of various brokers—as well as their research and investment-banking functions—and all the data are funneled through a single "prime" broker at the end of the day, thereby simplifying reporting.

Prime brokers do much more than just collate trades. Prime brokers may provide favored hedge fund managers with data feeds, technology, office space, computer equipment, software, research, and any number of other items that make it easier for the portfolio manager to do his or her primary job. As well, each manager is generally provided with a virtual back-office staff of individuals who cater to that manager's needs.

The standard institutional rate for commissions on stock trades is $0.05/share. It should not be a surprise that, given the level of service institutional brokers provide, the trades are not executed for $8/trade. Because of the volume of trades and the special needs of various manager techniques, a regular retail broker is generally not equipped to handle most hedge fund managers' needs. If a manager decides to do without a prime broker, the fund must maintain separate records and reconcile transactions for each and every broker the fund uses.

Nearly every major investment bank has a prime brokerage arm catering to hedge fund managers. By and large, it should not be much of a concern to potential investors which of these prime brokers the hedge fund manager chooses, as the differences for the investor in a hedge fund are not terribly great.

Administrator

Smaller funds, and even some larger funds, may find that outsourcing the paperwork and bookkeeping functions of a hedge fund is the way to go. Fund administration firms can often be hired for less than the cost of an office staff—and without the entire human resources headache that goes along with the hiring of a staff. Such firms vary in the services offered. The range is from simple services such as monthly bookkeeping to full service: bookkeeping, interfacing with lawyers and accountants, marketing, printing and mailing client reports, website development, and so on. These administrators will often charge a portion of AUM, so that the cost is borne by the fund.

Offshore funds are required to have an offshore administrator if the fund manager is actually working in the United States. These offshore administrators perform the added function of providing an offshore place of business for the fund and hence enabling the fund to qualify as an offshore fund.

Independent Representative

If a hedge fund manager has registered as an investment adviser either with a state or with the SEC, the manager will find some incentive to avoid being deemed by the regulatory authorities to have custody of client funds. If the manager is deemed to have custody of client funds, then the manager faces an increased administrative burden as well as higher capital adequacy requirements.

To avoid the custody issue, a registered investment adviser can rely on a series of no-action letters issued by the SEC. Several of these letters make it clear that an independent representative must stand between the manager and access to client funds. Hence, when a manager wants to send an invoice to the fund for services rendered or expenses incurred on behalf of the fund, the invoice must first go through an independent representative. This independent representative must review the agreements between the fund manager and the fund clients, compare the agreements to the amounts listed on the invoice, and issue a statement as to the validity of the invoice. Only then can the custodian, who is usually the prime broker, disburse a payment to the hedge fund manager.

SEC no-action letters covering the identity of an independent representative are somewhat complex and beyond the scope of this chapter. The independent representative is most commonly an accountant or bookkeeper, although there is no requirement that the representative must be a certified public accountant (CPA). The independent representative cannot be the accountant in the employment of the manager or the fund. It is not uncommon to see the fund administrator act as an independent representative.

Law Firm

Every fund manager and fund has a law firm. In fact, it is the law firm that is responsible for most of the start-up expense associated with a fund. Once the organization of the fund is completed, the ongoing legal costs decrease considerably. Ongoing legal costs are *sporadic* and usually minor in nature. The law firm may help in the preparation of the Regulation D filing that fund managers must make each time they accept new investors. As well, the law firm will assist the manager in compliance issues related to the "blue sky" laws of each state in which the manager solicits interests in the fund. The quality of the law firm will be reflected in the quality of the offering documents and agreements that potential investors receive. Potential investors may want to have a lawyer of their own to review these documents.

Accountant

The accountant is an integral part of every hedge fund. The inflow and outflow of capital, often complex trades, multitude of investors, and numerous other issues all make the job of a hedge fund accountant a tough one. A fund using an administrator who performs monthly bookkeeping will minimize the burden, and hence the expense of, the accountant.

The accountant will perform the year-end audit for the fund and complete the Schedule K-1 for investors. Hence, while an accountancy firm for a hedge fund need not be a household name, it is important that the firm must be of sound repute. At a minimum, the accountant should be a CPA.

Taxes

Hedge funds have a potentially large edge over mutual funds when it comes to the subject of fairness in taxation. In fact, the tax structure of hedge funds may be one reason that some of the highest net worth—and most heavily taxed—individuals in our society gravitate toward the hedge fund structure rather than that of mutual funds. As has been discussed, hedge funds are generally either limited partnerships or limited liability companies electing partnership status for tax purposes. From the viewpoint of the IRS, therefore, most hedge funds look very much the same: they are all "securities partnerships."

Partnership accounting is a subject not easily digested—and very much worthy of its own book for those with a deep interest. The nutshell is that investors in a partnership will find that the tax gains and liabilities of their investment in the fund, with little limitation, flow through the partnership directly to their own income tax returns each and every year. A fund investor will therefore be taxed on all realized gains of the fund—including dividend income, interest income, and both short-term and long-term capital gains. The fund investor is not taxed on unrealized gains. If the investor's capital account in the fund has a loss for a given year, the loss flows through to the investor and will offset other realized capital gains for the year as well as up to $3000 in ordinary income, with the balance of the loss carried into subsequent years. A favorable result of this tax treatment is that new hedge fund investors cannot be subject to taxes on gains earned prior to the investor joining the fund, as can often happen with mutual funds.

When drafting the fund documents, most portfolio managers set the fiscal year equivalent to the calendar year ending on December 31st. If a fund adopts a fiscal year different than the calendar year, then most of its investors will have fiscal years different than that of the fund. The partnership then must make enhanced tax payments or deposits on behalf of its partners.

The hedge fund manager, who is either a general partner or managing member, is typically endowed with the power to make tax elections on behalf of the fund in the course of the normal fund operations. Two types of elections stand out as noteworthy.

A §754 election increases the cost basis of securities the fund carries by the amount of unrealized appreciation paid to a withdrawing investor. If the fund does not elect §754, then the fund typically allows the manager to allocate an amount of the fund's taxable realized gains to a withdrawing investor in an amount equal to the unrealized appreciation in the withdrawing investor's capital account. The withdrawing investor's unrealized gains are then allocated to the remaining investors. This is called "directing gains." The net effect is that both §754 and directed gains help the fund manager to maneuver to avoid hitting the investors who choose to stay with the fund with a tax liability simply because another member chooses to withdraw.

HEDGE FUND STRATEGIES

TOOLS OF THE TRADE

When a hedge fund manager hedges a portfolio by taking positions that counterbalance the risk in other positions, the manager generally uses a combination of leverage, short selling, and/or arbitrage. These terms should be well understood before potential investors attempt to understand the various fund strategy categories.

Leverage

Hedge fund managers who use leverage are borrowing money or securities. The theory is that the investment returns on the borrowed assets will exceed the costs of borrowing those assets. There are many different ways to use leverage, some of which arguably diminish risk.

Short Selling

When a manager sells a security that the manager does not own, he or she is short selling, or "shorting" that security. The manager's broker enables this action by borrowing the security to be sold short from another customer of the same brokerage firm who may hold the security. When the manager buys back the security (also known as "covering" the short), the security is returned to the lender. If the security falls in value, the manager makes money. If the security rises in value, the manager loses money. One may think of the goal of short selling as selling high prior to buying low. The opposite of a short strategy is a long strategy, or buying and holding stocks in hopes of price appreciation.

Arbitrage

When a hedge fund manager buys one security while simultaneously selling short another security to profit from a discrepancy in the relative prices of the two securities, the manager is engaging in arbitrage. Several varieties of arbitrage exist.

EXAMPLE 14.5

Risk arbitrage. Company A announces that it will acquire Company B, and that the deal will close in 2 months. The terms of the deal are one share of Company A common stock for every single outstanding share of Company B stock. Because of deal uncertainties, timing, and an ever-changing Company A stock price, Company B stock may move to trade at just below the price of Company A stock. Arbitrageurs may sell short Company A stock while simultaneously purchasing an equivalent amount of Company B stock, thereby attempting to lock in the price discrepancy as a profit.

CATEGORIES

Hedge funds, as described in this chapter, are today defined as a group by their structure and fee arrangements. However, the group is far from being homogeneous. Indeed, hedge funds may generally pursue any legal means to earn a satisfactory return on investment; so, it is no surprise that funds vary tremendously in their investment styles. Several themes recur, however, and the potential investor will generally find that most hedge funds fall into one of the several broad categories of investment style.

Macro

Perhaps, the most flamboyant of the hedge fund strategies, macro hedge fund managers look at the world political and economic landscape and take leveraged positions in financial instruments that reflect how they believe these worldly events and trends will affect the financial markets. Macro funds tend to be large, and the offering documents give the manager wide latitude to pursue nearly any legal means around the globe to make money.

Equity

Generally, equity hedge fund managers use traditional fundamental and technical analysis techniques to take long and/or short positions in common stocks. There are several subtypes of equity hedge funds. The traditional equity hedge manager takes long positions in stocks and counterbalances the long positions with short positions in other stocks. The relative mix of long and short positions can vary with the manager's view on the market's direction, and leverage is often an integral part of maximizing the returns of such a strategy. Funds that tend to favor long positions may be called "long bias" funds while those that favor short positions have been termed "short bias" funds. Some equity hedge funds may focus exclusively on short selling.

Other equity hedge fund managers may decide to short stocks either not at all or only occasionally. Such fund managers may even structure the fund as a 100% long equity fund, with no hedge, leverage, or short-selling features. Because of the organizational, regulatory, and fee arrangements discussed elsewhere in this chapter, this type of fund is still considered a hedge fund.

Equity hedge funds may feature certain traditional styles, such as growth, aggressive growth, or value, may focus on certain industries or sectors, or may focus on certain market capitalization ranges, such as small cap or large cap.

Arbitrage

Arbitrage, previously defined, comes in many flavors, and there is a hedge fund type to take advantage of every one of them. A few are discussed here.

- *Fixed income arbitrage* involves taking long positions in certain fixed income instruments, such as bonds, and simultaneously taking short positions in other fixed income instruments to profit from a temporary deviation from the normal historical relative value or price differential between the instruments involved. Leverage is a prominent feature in such funds.
- *Statistical arbitrage* involves taking offsetting long and short equity positions in equal amounts. This 50–50 split is mathematically designed to remove all general market risk from the portfolio. Returns theoretically entirely depend on the ability of the manager to pick overvalued and undervalued stocks. As a result, statistical arbitrage is also often called equity market neutral (see Chapter 15).
- *Convertible arbitrage* involves taking long positions in convertible bonds while simultaneously shorting the stock into which the bond converts. This is a highly specialized type of fund designed to produce steady low-risk returns.
- *Merger arbitrage* involves investing in the securities of companies being acquired or undergoing a merger. Typically, the stock of the company being acquired is bought while the acquirer's stock is sold short. This type of arbitrage is often called "risk" arbitrage because merger arbitrage managers profit from their ability to correctly judge the probabilities and risks associated with the outcome of a merger or acquisition.

Event Driven

Event-driven hedge fund managers look to take advantage of the price distortions that occur in the securities of companies undergoing restructurings. Financial engineering, spin-offs, bankruptcy, mergers, and acquisitions—all these activities tend to create new or otherwise inefficiently priced securities. As with equity and arbitrage funds, event-driven funds come in a variety of subtypes. As with arbitrage funds, event-driven funds tend to correlate poorly with the overall market direction.

- *Distressed securities* fund managers examine those securities of companies undergoing severe financial or operational stress. Often, these companies have filed bankruptcy. Fund managers will take positions in undervalued securities of these companies and hold them until the completion of the necessary restructuring. The expectation is that full value will be realized once the company emerges from its restructuring. Sometimes known as "vulture investors," these fund managers generally do not sit on the sidelines but rather become quite aggressive during the long restructuring process to ensure a favorable outcome. Distressed securities funds, or vulture funds, are generally extremely illiquid, reflecting the illiquid nature of the investments the funds make.

- *Special situations* fund managers tend to look for the mispriced, undervalued securities that arise out of spin-offs, mergers, acquisitions, demutualizations, and various other corporate- restructuring activities. These managers tend to become involved only with bankrupt companies as they come out of bankruptcy. By applying special knowledge to these sorts of the often-misunderstood situations, the manager can buy securities below the true value and often estimate a time to the full realization of that value. Such managers focus on a timely catalyst for value realization in most investment positions.

Industry/Sector Focus

Hedge fund managers may have a special knowledge base in a certain industry or sector of the economy. Hence, it is not uncommon for these managers to apply this knowledge base very narrowly in the management of a hedge fund. Generally, sector funds concentrate on the faster- growing sectors, but every sector has its occasional bumps along the way. The unique aspect of hedge funds relative to mutual funds and other publicly offered investments is that sector hedge fund managers can use leverage, arbitrage, and short selling to profit continuously as the chosen sector goes through its cycles. Common stocks are typically the focus of sector fund managers, and hence, the sector fund is also another variety of equity fund.

Commodity Pools

Hedge funds run by commodity-trading advisors, or CTAs, may pool together investors who wish to invest in the commodities or future markets, but who do not have the time or expertise to do so individually. Regulated by the Commodity Futures Trading Commission, these funds are called commodity pools—the manager is called a commodity pool operator—and is subject to additional reporting, disclosure, and position limit rules. A fund of funds, defined later, that invest in commodity pools becomes subject to much the same rules. Unlike stocks, commodities future contracts are inherently highly leveraged instruments. They are also extremely volatile and generally not subject to very long-term, stable trends. Hence, commodities fund managers tend to use a combination of fundamental and technical factors to take advantage of relatively short-term swings in commodity prices. Investors in commodities hedge funds should not expect the fund to be tax efficient.

Emerging Markets

Emerging markets fund managers out of necessity invest in the local markets of the target countries. Hence, emerging markets funds are subject to only the barest of securities infrastructure. Short selling, arbitrage, and leverage are generally not practical. Emerging markets fund managers, therefore, act to exploit inefficient and chaotic markets by buying securities low and attempting to sell them high. Since the inefficiencies can be tremendous, massive profit potential is possible even without leverage. Nevertheless, hedging or diversifying an emerging markets portfolio is extremely difficult. In addition to currency risk, emerging markets investors face the risk of geopolitical events that can devalue nearly all emerging markets assets simultaneously. Information may become distorted as it flows out of the emerging market. For all these reasons, emerging markets funds typically require a physical presence in the chosen markets. Potential investors need to know that the manager undertakes a first-hand investigative process to discover and to confirm the information that goes into valuing securities.

Options

Hedge funds may exclusively focus on the trading of options. Like futures, options are inherently leveraged instruments, and there are myriad techniques for trading them. While some managers focus on options arbitrage—the exploitation of price differences between related options—many others apply a broad definition to the trading of options and have the freedom to use mostly any available option strategy to profit. Like commodity funds, option funds have little likelihood of being tax efficient.

Fund of Funds

A fund of funds is a hedge fund that invests in a portfolio of two or more hedge funds. This unique structure allows investors to diversify across strategies, markets, and managers while only dealing with one fund manager. Moreover, some investors might not be able to afford to access certain hedge fund managers who impose high minimum initial investments or huge net worth require-ments. A fund of funds, which is an institution with a substantial block of capital at its disposal, can access these more exclusive managers.

The fee structure of the fund of funds is a significant issue. The typical fund of funds manager charges an asset management fee. The fund of funds typically must pay an asset management fee and a performance incentive—a share of profits—to the hedge funds in which it invests. Therefore, an investor in a fund of funds will typically pay an asset management fee twice and a performance incentive fee once. If the manager of the fund of funds also charges a performance incentive, then the investor is double charged for both performance incentive and asset management fees.

INVESTIGATING HEDGE FUNDS

It is not well understood how or why hedge fund investors pick one hedge fund over another. The reasons people give are as varied as the people giving them. For the potential investor in hedge funds, perhaps the most important concept to keep in mind is that hedge funds do not by themselves make a financial plan. Investors should approach investing in hedge funds as if they are trying to fill in the missing pieces of a much more comprehensive investment strategy. Hedge funds generally have a narrow focus, and while no one fund makes a portfolio, one fund may make a great fit as part of a larger portfolio of assets.

Investors are therefore asked to take an inventory of current and future assets and liabilities. Risk tolerance should be considered in context with the need for growth, preservation of capital, and/or current income. The degree to which one's current portfolio of assets is meeting these needs will largely determine what sort of hedge fund or funds may make a perfect fit. So, while it is beyond the scope of this chapter, the first step to investing in hedge funds is to formulate a financial plan.

Once the needs of a financial plan are determined, the search for the right hedge fund or funds begins. The natural inclination is to first look for numbers. However, no mass-market print publi-cation detailing the performance of hedge funds exists. In fact, the initial search for information may be a bit frustrating. The truth is, hedge funds are neither mysterious nor sinister—they simply cannot advertise or solicit the public. As a result, hedge funds, while a thoroughly viable option for accredited investors, are not as easy to investigate as mutual funds or stocks.

Potential investors should not be deterred, however. What exists here is a tremendous infor-mation chasm between potential hedge fund investors and hedge fund managers. If an interested accredited investor could signal to all hedge fund managers this interest, the investor's answering machine would be full within hours. If one wishes to invest in a hedge fund, therefore, one only needs to transmit this information in a proper and effective manner. In fact, many hedge fund managers privately complain about how difficult it is to find high net worth individuals and family offices. So, the two parties—hedge fund managers and potential investors—simply need to make contact. Several businesses exist to assist in this endeavor, and it is important to understand the function as well as the incentives of each.

INVESTMENT ADVISERS

An investment adviser is generally registered with either the SEC or the state in which the adviser does business. The task of an investment adviser is to help clients find and maintain an appropriate mix of investments. A good adviser will almost certainly be able to expound upon and assist entry into a wide variety of financial instruments, including hedge funds.

Investment advisers operate under different structures, however. Some have a relationship with a broker, or are directly employed by a broker, and are under some financial incentive to generate commissions for the broker. This may lead to a bias favoring the broker's products, or at least requiring his stable of portfolio managers to use the broker for trades. Fee-only advisers operate under an improved system, but even fee-only advisers may have relationships with brokers or other institutions that introduce some bias into the advice given to clients.

The tremendous upside to engaging an investment adviser or financial planner is that such entities or individuals are likely to have first-hand knowledge of the financial plan into which the hedge funds are supposed to fit. Investors must simply realize that an investment adviser may or may not be the most knowledgeable person about the hedge fund industry. An independent, trusted investment adviser familiar with the hedge fund landscape and willing to operate on a fee-only basis—whereby the adviser charges only a percentage of AUM—would be the ideal candidate. There may be some difficulty in finding one such as this. Here, no examples are provided, as endorsements on these matters are quite hazardous.

THIRD-PARTY MARKETERS

Third-party marketers are hired by the hedge funds themselves to recruit investors. These businesses have two functions: build a list of every known institution and high net worth individual, and sell the fund to that list. Phone calls, personal meetings, and the like are the mode of operation. The fees, which the hedge fund pays, vary widely. Individuals can also contact these firms with the intention of finding hedge funds, but they are likely to get a fairly one-sided story.

CONSULTANTS

Consultants are to clients what third-party marketers are to hedge funds. Consultants are generally independent operations that do not have discretion over client funds but rather simply sell information to the potential investor for either a percentage of assets or an hourly fee. The distinguishing feature of consultants is access to a proprietary database of information, either developed internally or bought, that guides the consultants in their advice. The better consultants will have interviewed the managers that they recommend and hence will be able to provide information that goes beyond numbers and biographies. Consultants vary widely in terms of services offered and fees charged, and minimum account sizes may be expected. The line between the consultant and investment adviser is often a blurry one.

WORD OF MOUTH

By law and by tradition, the hedge fund industry is an intensely personal business. In the case of many smaller and mid-size hedge funds, it is a commonplace for investors to speak or meet directly with the portfolio manager. The portfolio manager may even be the only person with whom investors interact. Many managers do not participate in the databases or hire third-party marketers and are below the radar of the consultants and investment advisers. In such cases, the primary mode of attracting investors is word of mouth. Some managers simply believe there is a very good likelihood that the first 25 accredited investors probably have another 25 accredited friends, and that solid performance will induce word-of-mouth marketing. With most hedge funds legally restricted to holding a total of 100 investor slots, a fund with an outperforming manager—often the smaller, most nimble funds can rack up the niftiest returns—can fill up very quickly without ever participating in the hedge fund information industry.

The implication for the potential hedge fund investor is that there is a decent chance a trusted friend or business associate already invests in hedge funds. Potential hedge fund investors should treat these people as solid resources. Common sense of course should prevail, but a candid and detailed assessment of various hedge fund managers from these resources may be both free and at least as trustworthy as other third-party advisers and information sources.

TRANSPARENCY

As the potential investor peruses the various entities standing ready and willing to assist in a hedge fund manager search, the investor will notice the concept of transparency as a recurring theme in the marketing materials and websites of these businesses. Transparency refers to the ability to look directly into a hedge fund's portfolio and see the various investments the manager has made. Without fail, consultants, investment advisers, and the Internet hedge fund portals will tout the virtues of transparency. There are several features to this praise that potential investors should understand.

If a business purports to present information or recommendations to an investor regarding hedge fund choice, it stands to reason that the business is generally limited to covering those hedge funds that offer partial or complete transparency. For instance, daily net asset values are not possible without transparency. By declaring transparency the gold standard, the hedge fund information industry—an industry with growing influence—persuades more hedge fund managers to embrace transparency. As a result, of course, these hedge fund managers in turn become profit sources for the hedge fund information industry.

Such influences must be considered within the context of the current trend toward more transparency in the hedge fund industry. To be sure, a hedge fund manager who insists on zero transparency is bucking an industry trend, but the manager may also have very good reasons for this choice. It bears noting that Warren Buffett not only failed to notify his investors of his Buffett Partnership portfolio selections, but also forbade his investors from even asking a single question! Such lack of transparency allowed Buffett to buy large amounts of American Express at a time when both stock and company were widely ridiculed, only to reap large profits later. Some managers indeed argue that if transparency reigns, the hedge fund industry will lose a significant differentiating factor setting it apart from the mutual fund industry.

At the same time, many investors will find a great degree of comfort in transparency. A prudent view may be that transparency is not a litmus test but rather a feature to be considered along with many other features of hedge funds.

OVERHEARD IN THE DOCTOR'S LOUNGE: IS MALTA A HEDGE FUND HAVEN?

Malta has quietly leveraged the rising tide of the financial transparency imperative to attract hedge funds.

There was a time when the quaint island sought to play on the traditional terrain, offering anonymity and a 'laissez-faire regulatory regime' not to mention very low taxes, as in no capital gains taxes and no taxes on dividends; all while English speaking and USD currency denominated.

While many leading domiciles for offshore hedge funds remain in the Caribbean—notably the Cayman Islands, the British Virgin Islands, Bermuda, and the Bahamas—the island of Malta is drawing attention, especially from European funds.

Dr. David E. Marcinko, FACFAS, MBA, CMP™
(www.CertifiedMedicalPlanner.org)

HOW TO INVEST

Once an investor has found the right hedge fund and received preliminary approval from a hedge fund manager, the investor will receive the offering documents in the mail. Increasingly, the documents may be delivered via e-mail or the Internet. Hedge funds vary widely in strategy, but the offering procedures are fairly standard. In the offering packet, the investor will receive the following items.

COVER LETTER

The cover letter will often detail how to proceed in order to invest, and may contain wiring instructions or other payment directions. The letter will also specify when the next investment period commences. Since most funds do not accept investors everyday, the investment period typically begins on the first day of the next month or the next quarter.

PAYMENT INSTRUCTIONS

Either in the investment contract, in the cover letter, or on a separate piece of paper, the potential investor will find wiring instructions and/or instructions for investing by check. Given the sums of money generally involved, wiring is nearly always the preferred method for making an investment. Money received by the fund prior to the beginning of the investment period will generally be held in a contribution account, and the investor typically will not earn interest or otherwise see capital appreciation of the capital account until the investment period starts.

FUND AGREEMENTS

Depending on whether the fund is a limited liability company or a limited partnership, the investor will receive either an operating agreement or a limited partnership agreement, respectively. These documents describe the legal agreement between the fund manager and the fund investors. If the fund is a limited liability company, the document signed by the investor is a subscription agreement linked by reference to the operating agreement. The subscription agreement may be a physically separate document, however.

PRIVATE PLACEMENT MEMORANDUM

Also called an offering memo, the private placement memorandum is the document that is used to actually offer an interest in the fund to prospective investors. This memorandum contains a summary and detail of the various disclosures, rules, and restrictions of which both the fund manager and the fund investors must be aware. This document also discloses the relationships between the fund manager and various other entities, which may include associated investment advisory companies. It is very important that the potential investor understands all the business relationships of the manager of the fund. This document should be ground zero for investors investigating a fund.

PART II OF FORM ADV

If the fund manager is also a registered investment adviser, the fund manager must provide potential investors with either a copy of the current Part II of Form ADV on the file with the appropriate regulatory body or a brochure covering all the same information. Form ADV is the document that managers use to register as investment advisers, and Part II is the portion of that document that discloses all business relationships, fee structures, business activities, and other information deemed necessary by the SEC. Many managers strive to avoid registering as investment advisers; so, this document is not a part of all offering document packets.

AFTER THE INVESTMENT

Stock investors often talk about the investment thesis—the reason or reasons that they took a stock position in the first place. If the thesis is no longer valid, these investors feel that it becomes time to exit the position. Hedge fund investors are dealing with less liquid investments, but the same logic should apply. In this case, however, there are two investment theses to monitor: the reason for the investment in the hedge fund in the first place, and the style or strategy of the hedge fund manager. It is important to stay on top of what the manager is doing and not to be overly mesmerized or disenchanted with short-term returns. If the manager does not practice transparency, then the information in the monthly or quarterly letters becomes even more valuable. There are several factors that may conspire to change either a manager's style or the effectiveness of that style over time. These and other factors ought to affect whether the investor's reason for investment with the manager still holds.

Size of Fund

Many hedge funds thrive on the pricing inefficiencies brought about by the illiquidity of the securities in which they invest. It is possible and even probable that there comes a point where the size of the fund in terms of AUM becomes so large as to make the strategy impractical. If the manager charges an asset management fee with an eye to using some of that fee as a reliable income stream, the manager may have some motivation to let the fund grow to a maximum size, with associated diminishing returns. Quite simply, some funds should stay small.

Another aspect of increasing fund size is a possible decrease in the motivation of the manager. An upstart manager may be hot to trot to get wealthy and sees the fund as the means to this end. An established and highly successful manager with scores of pension accounts may make millions each year from the asset management fee alone, regardless of performance.

Strategy Obsolescence

The very strategy upon which a hedge fund manager relies—especially in complex derivative security and arbitrage funds—may become moot as success of the strategy attracts capital that drives nearly all pricing inefficiency out of the market.

Lure of Leverage

Hedge fund managers may start out wary of the risks in a tremendous amount of leverage, but may eventually succumb to the lure of the outsized returns that leverage can provide. Even funds that refuse transparency as it relates to portfolio positions will generally provide monthly or quarterly information on the leverage in the portfolio. The amount of leverage—essentially dictated by the type of strategy employed—may be less important than the trend in the amount of leverage used. A steadily increasing amount of leverage bears watching and may warrant explanation.

Style Drift

This may occur when a portfolio manager is essentially an individual, but also when the portfolio manager is an institution, success can breed style drift. Consistency in investment over long periods of time is a rare trait and leads many leading pension fund investors to cite the "lifespan" of a manager as the reason for the decline of many funds over time.

Deception

There is no room in the hedge fund industry for deception, misrepresentation, or fraud. Investors should very seriously consider withdrawing funds from a manager that demonstrates the capacity for fraud or deceit either before or after an investment is made. The slightest inconsistency in reports, letters, or conversation should be the cause for alarm and should require both clarification and satisfactory resolution. Honest mistakes may indeed crop up—tax issues are notorious for tripping up hedge fund managers, most of whom are generally just attempting to regurgitate facts told to them by their accountants—but investors should be extremely diligent in monitoring such inaccuracies. There are many honest hedge funds vying for investor capital, and there is no need to stay with a dubious one.

MANAGER'S CHARACTER

Some like to say that people never really change. Well, some have never seen people become filthy rich. Successful hedge fund managers certainly may change—personality, ego, and character. If an investor has a personal relationship with a portfolio manager, it may pay to monitor subtle changes in that manager's lifestyle or professional demeanor. Berkshire Hathaway chairman Warren Buffett is known for keeping essentially the same lifestyle and professional demeanor since he started his Buffett Partnership back in 1957. Perhaps, it is not surprising that he has perhaps the most stunning long-term investment record ever recorded.

SPECIAL QUESTIONS AND ISSUES

1. The fund manager I am considering is a registered investment adviser. What does this mean?

   If the fund manager is an entity, then any individual you deal with will be a registered investment adviser representative. If the fund manager is an individual, then that individual is a registered investment adviser. In either case, the designation implies that several steps have been taken.

   To become a registered investment adviser, an individual must register for and pass the Series 65 Uniform Investment Adviser Law Exam, a 3-h, 130-question computer-based exam administered by the North American Securities Administrators Association. Topics covered include economics and analysis, investment vehicles, investment recommendations and strategies, and ethics and legal guidelines. A passing score is 70% or higher.

   Once an individual has passed the Series 65, s/he must then apply via Form ADV to become a registered investment adviser. This application is made to either a state authority or to the SEC, depending on the adviser's AUM. If AUM exceed $30 million, then the adviser must register with the SEC. Form ADV consists of two parts. Part I provides general information to the regulatory authority. Part II is designed to be distributed to potential clients and includes disclosure of a decent amount of information about the adviser. If the manager is a registered investment adviser, then you should expect to receive as part of the offering documentation either a current copy of Part II of the adviser's Form ADV or a brochure that contains all the current information in Part II of Form ADV.

   In addition to filing Form ADV and paying a small fee, the registered investment adviser becomes subject to extra administrative/regulatory burden as well as capital adequacy requirements that state the adviser must maintain certain net worth levels.

   By and large, because of the extra administrative burden as well as restrictions on certain activities, hedge fund managers attempt to avoid registering as investment advisers. Whether such managers can or cannot avoid such registration is largely dependent on the state in which the manager operates. In California, for instance, hedge fund managers must register as investment advisers. In New York, such registration is not necessary. Not surprisingly, hedge fund managers located in California are rare, while they are quite plentiful in New York.

2. The hedge fund manager I am considering also runs a mutual fund. Why?

The mutual fund business is a fundamentally different business than that of hedge funds. Mutual funds are marketed aggressively to the general public and are managed for a flat fee. Performance incentive fees of the hedge fund variety are not allowed within the mutual fund structure. Confident portfolio managers may feel that getting a "piece of the action" is much more lucrative, and might find the performance incentive fee structure of hedge funds attractive.

Since mutual funds are aggressively marketed, it is not uncommon that a portfolio manager develops quite a name for him or herself. High net worth individuals and institutions might start asking this manager to manage some private investment accounts on the side—in the hope that with a smaller account the manager could achieve outsized returns. In some cases, the portfolio manager might just leave the mutual fund altogether and start up a hedge fund business. In other cases, the portfolio manager stays at the mutual fund post while simultaneously opening up a hedge fund.

This practice, while neither frowned upon nor thought to be unethical, does raise some questions for the potential investor. Namely, when a very good investment idea arises, to which fund does the portfolio manager allocate the idea first? On the one hand, the marketing of the mutual fund is dependent on good performance. On the other, the manager knows that there is potentially more personal and direct participation in the profit potential of the hedge fund.

3. Can my practice's retirement plan invest in a hedge fund? The plan is a small self-directed pension plan with profit-sharing features.

Such a pension fund falls under a category called self-directed "plan" assets. Among the rules are that each participant in the plan counts toward the 100 investor maximum under which most hedge funds operate, that each plan participant be a fully accredited investor, and that the hedge fund keeps investments such as pension plans and other funds covered under Employment Retirement Income Security Act of 1974 (ERISA) to <25% of total AUM. These factors will conspire to make it difficult for most small-office, self-directed pension plans to qualify for admittance into a hedge fund.

4. Can I invest my individual retirement account (IRA) in a hedge fund?

This is up to the manager, but there is no legal restriction on a hedge fund accepting IRA assets. IRA accounts are not well suited for funds that make extensive use of leverage, however. In such cases, the fund is likely to generate significant amounts of unrelated business-taxable income (UBTI)—profits of the fund attributable to the use of leverage. The holder of an IRA account must pay taxes on UBTI, even if the UBTI was generated in an IRA account.

As has been mentioned before, today's hedge funds may or may not use leverage. Many hedge funds are not hedged at all, but rather are just specialized versions of regular long-stock portfolios. If such funds do not use much leverage, IRA investors will not encounter much difficulty with UBTI and should not hesitate in considering these funds.

In considering whether to accept IRA money, hedge fund managers must consider several factors. If the only type of retirement money accepted by the hedge funds is IRA money, then the manager has no limit on how much retirement money the fund can accept. If, however, there are other types of retirement money invested in the fund, such as pension funds, IRA money will be counted toward a total of 25% of fund assets that can be invested in retirement accounts before the fund becomes subject to the ERISA. Funds subject to ERISA regulations face a heavy administrative burden and more restrictions than most fund managers like.

IRA distributions from a hedge fund are subject to the standard 20% withholding unless the funds are directly rolled over to other qualified plans.

5. The hedge fund manager I am considering also runs an offshore fund under a "master feeder" arrangement. What does this mean? In which fund should I invest?

The master feeder arrangement is a two-tiered investment structure whereby investors invest in the feeder fund. The feeder fund in turn invests in the master fund. The master fund is therefore the one that is actually investing in securities. There may be multiple feeder funds under one master fund. Feeder funds under the same master can differ drastically in terms of fees charged, minimums required, types of investors, and many other features—but the investment style will be the same because only the master actually invests in the market.

A master feeder structure is a very popular arrangement because it allows a portfolio manager to pool both onshore and offshore assets into one investment vehicle (the master fund) that allocates gains and losses in an asset-based, proportional manner back to the onshore and offshore investors. All investors, both offshore and onshore, get the same return. In this manner, the portfolio manager, despite offering more than one fund with different characteristics to different populations, is not faced with the dilemma of which fund to favor with the best investment ideas.

A manager may offer an offshore fund because there is demand for that manager's skill, either abroad where investors may wish to preserve anonymity, or more commonly, where investors simply do not wish to become entangled with the U.S. tax code. American citizens should generally avoid the offshore fund, since American citizens are taxed on their allocated share of offshore corporation profits whether or not a distribution occurs. Therefore, there is no benefit for most American taxpayers investing in an offshore fund.

Tax-exempt institutions, such as medical foundations, in the United States may have reason to consider an offshore hedge fund, however. Domestic tax-exempt organizations are generally not subject to UBTI—the portion of hedge fund income that comes about as a result of the use of leverage—when investing with an offshore corporation. If the same tax-exempt organization was to invest in a domestic fund, and if UBTI was generated, then the organization would have to pay taxes on that UBTI. Most domestic hedge funds generate UBTI.

6. My investment advisory firm (or bank, or brokerage firm) is offering me an "alternative investment program." Is this a hedge fund?

If the investor is being asked to invest in a limited partnership or limited liability company vehicle similar to that which is described elsewhere in this chapter, yes. These institutions have recently begun to home grow hedge funds and market them to their high net worth clientele. All the same principles and features of hedge funds discussed in this chapter should apply.

7. My broker is telling me about a wrap-fee program involving a hedge fund manager. Why do I need my broker? Can I just go directly to the hedge fund manager?

Yes, you can, but you may find a different fee arrangement when you reach the hedge fund manager, and you may be participating in an unethical transaction. When hedge fund managers set up separate accounts for wrap-fee clients, they agree to take a set fee in exchange for managing this money. They also enter into agreements with one or more brokers to help market this aspect of their money management business. A portion of the wrap fee you pay goes to the broker, and a portion goes to the manager. Incentive compensation is not generally used.

When approached directly, hedge fund managers will typically offer only the hedge fund, complete with incentive compensation and pooled investment features. However, if the hedge fund manager is willing to set up a separate account, it is possible that the investor will find the set fee much less than what he or she would have paid in a wrap-fee account through a broker. However, the very large caveat to all this is that the ethics of a hedge fund manager who steals clients from brokers with whom he has a marketing relationship ought to be called into question. And when it comes to hedge funds, the ethics of the manager are of paramount importance.

8. I want to invest with a manager who has the skills to "hedge" a portfolio, but I do not wish to mix my money with a bunch of other investors as in a hedge fund. Can I hire hedge fund managers to manage my account separately?

Some hedge fund managers do take the time to recruit and manage separate accounts, with or without the help of referring brokers. However, before long, the administrative burden of managing so many separate accounts can become quite significant. Hence, the minimums for such separate accounts are generally much higher than if one was to invest in the manager's hedge fund. The best feature of these separate accounts is that potentially every aspect of the investment account, including fees, is negotiable. Other features include greater transparency and increased liquidity, since separately managed accounts can often be shut down on short notice. Investors must be aware, however, that for practical purposes, the portfolio manager generally will buy and sell the same securities in the separately managed accounts that the portfolio manager buys and sells in the hedge fund; yet, the expenses incurred by the investor will likely be higher.

CONCLUSION

Modern hedge funds are still like the original Buffett Partnership in many ways. This chapter introduced and explained the industry, as well as pertinent historical, structural, legal, tax, and operating issues of which all potential physician investors should be aware.

COLLABORATE

Discuss this chapter online with others at www.MedicalExecutivePost.com.

ACKNOWLEDGMENT

To Ken Eaton, CFP®, CFA of Stepp & Rothwell Inc., Overland Park, Kansas.

FURTHER READING

Klein, R: Hedge funds: In: *Investment and Portfolio Strategies for the Institutional Investor*. Edited by Jess Ledrman. McGraw-Hill Companies, New York, 1996.

Seykota, E: *The Hedge Fund Market Wizards*. Wiley, New York, 2012.

Wilson, RC: *The Hedge Fund Book*. John Wiley, New York, 2010.

Yu, JS: *From Zero to Sixty on Hedge Funds and Private Equity 3.0: What They Do, How They Do It, and Why They Do the Mysterious Things They Do*. Amazon Kindle edition, New York, 2014.

Zask, E: *About Hedge Funds by Ezra Zask*. McGraw-Hill Companies, New York, 2013.

WEBSITES

Alternative Investment Management Association, an educational forum for investors interested in hedge funds and other alternative investment options. www.aima.org

Hedge Fund Research is a research and consulting firm specializing in alternative investments. www.HFR.com

Hedgeworld is a website dedicated to alternative investing. www.hedgeworld.com

15 Market Neutral Funds
Demystifying the Strategy

Dimitri A. Sogoloff

CONTENTS

It's hard to believe that just 40 years ago, physician investors had only two primary asset classes from which to choose: the U.S. equities and the U.S. bonds. Today, the marketplace offers a daunting array of investment choices. Rapid market globalization, technology advancements, and investor sophistication have spawned a host of new asset classes, from the mundane to the mysterious. Even neophyte medical investors can now buy and sell international equities, emerging market debt, mortgage securities, commodities, derivatives, indexes, and currencies, offering infinitely more opportunities to make, or lose, money.

Amidst this ongoing proliferation, a unique asset class has emerged, one that is complex, nontraditional, and not easily understood like stocks or bonds. It does, however, offer one invaluable advantage; its returns are virtually uncorrelated with any other asset class. When this asset class is introduced into a traditional investment portfolio, a wonderful thing can occur; the risk-return profile of the overall portfolio improves dramatically. This is known as a market-neutral strategy.

INTRODUCTION

The reason few medical professionals have heard of market-neutral strategies is that most of them are offered by private investment partnerships otherwise known as hedge funds. To the uninitiated, "hedge fund" means risky, volatile, or speculative. With a market-neutral strategy however, just the opposite is true. Funds utilizing market-neutral strategies typically emphasize the disciplined use of investment and risk control processes. As a result, they have consistently generated returns that display both low volatility and a low correlation with traditional equity or fixed income markets.

DEFINITION OF MARKET-NEUTRALITY

All market-neutral funds share a common objective: to achieve positive returns regardless of market direction. Of course, they are not without risk; these funds can and do lose money. But a key to their performance is that it is independent of the behavior of the markets at large, and this feature can add tremendous value to the rest of a portfolio.

A typical market-neutral strategy focuses on the spread relationship between related securities, which is what makes them virtually independent of underlying debt or equity markets. When two related securities are mispriced in relation to one another, the disparity will eventually disappear as the result of some external event. This event is called *convergence* and may take the form of a bond maturity, completion of a merger, option exercise, or simply a market recognizing the inefficiency and eliminating it through supply and demand.

HERE'S HOW IT MIGHT WORK

When two emerging technology companies announce a merger, there is an intended future convergence, when the shares of both companies will converge and become one. At the time of the announcement, there is typically a trading spread between two shares. A shrewd trader, seeing the probability of the successful merger, will simultaneously buy the relatively cheaper share and sell short the relatively more expensive share, thus locking in the future gain.

Another example of convergence would be the relationship between a convertible bond and its underlying stock. At the time of convergence, such as bond maturity, the two securities will be at parity. However, the market forces of supply and demand make the bond underpriced relative to the underlying stock. This mispricing will disappear upon convergence, so simultaneously buying the convertible bond and selling short an equivalent amount of underlying stock, locks in the relative spread between the two.

Yet, another example would be two bonds of the same company—one junior and one senior. For various reasons, the senior bond may become cheaper relative to the junior bond and thus display a temporary inefficiency that would disappear once arbitrageurs bought the cheaper bond and sold the more expensive bond.

While these examples involve different types of securities, scenarios, and market factors, they are all examples of a market-neutral strategy. Locking a spread between two related securities and waiting for the convergence to take place is a great way to make money without ever taking a view on the direction of the market. How large are these spreads, you may ask? Typically, they are tiny. The markets are not quite fully efficient, but they are efficient enough to not allow large price discrepancies to occur.

In order to make a meaningful profit, a market-neutral fund manager needs sophisticated technology to help identify opportunities, the agility to rapidly seize those opportunities, and have adequate financing resources to conduct hundreds of transactions annually.

DESCRIPTION OF STRATEGIES

The universe of market-neutral strategies is vast, spanning virtually every asset class, country, and market sector. The spectrum varies in risk from highly volatile to ultra conservative. Some market-neutral strategies are more volatile than risky low-cap equity strategies, while others offer better stability than U.S. Treasuries. One unifying factor across this vast ocean of seemingly disparate strategies is that they all attempt to take advantage of a relative mispricing between various securities, and all offer a high degree of "market neutrality," that is, a low correlation with underlying markets.

CONVERTIBLE ARBITRAGE

Convertible arbitrage is the oldest market-neutral strategy. Designed to capitalize on the relative mispricing between a convertible security (e.g., convertible bond or preferred stock) and the underlying equity, convertible arbitrage was employed as early as the 1950s. Since then, convertible arbitrage has evolved into a sophisticated, model-intensive strategy, designed to capture the difference between the income earned by a convertible security (which is held long) and the dividend of the underlying stock (which is sold short). The resulting net positive income of the hedged position is independent of any market fluctuations. The trick is to assemble a portfolio wherein the long and short positions, responding to equity fluctuations, interest rate shifts, credit spreads, and other market events offset each other.

Hedge Fund Research (HFR) New York offers the following description of the strategy:

> Convertible Arbitrage involves taking long positions in convertible securities and hedging those positions by selling short the underlying common stock. A manager will, in an effort to capitalize on relative pricing inefficiencies, purchase long positions in convertible securities, generally convertible bonds, convertible preferred stock or warrants, and hedge a portion of the equity risk by selling short the underlying common stock. Timing may be linked to a specific event relative to the underlying company, or a belief that a relative mispricing exists between the corresponding securities. Convertible securities and warrants are priced as a function of the price of the underlying stock, expected future volatility of returns, risk free interest rates, call provisions, supply and demand for specific issues and, in the case of convertible bonds, the issue-specific corporate/Treasury yield spread. Thus, there is ample room for relative mis-valuations.

Because a large part of this strategy's gain is generated by cash flow, it is a relatively low-risk strategy.

FIXED-INCOME ARBITRAGE

Fixed-income arbitrage managers seek to exploit pricing inefficiencies across global markets. Examples of these anomalies would be arbitrage between similar bonds of the same company, pricing inefficiencies of asset-backed securities and yield curve arbitrage (price differentials between government bonds of different maturities). Because the prices of fixed-income instruments are based on interest rates, expected cash flows, credit spreads, and related factors, fixed-income arbitrageurs use sophisticated quantitative models to identify pricing discrepancies. Similarly to convertible arbitrageurs, fixed-income arbitrageurs rely on investors less sophisticated than themselves to misprice a complex security.

EQUITY MARKET-NEUTRAL ARBITRAGE

This strategy attempts to offset equity risk by holding long and short equity positions. Ideally, these positions are related to each other, as in holding a basket of S&P500 stocks and selling S&P500 futures against the basket. If the manager, presumably through stock-picking skill, is able to assemble a basket cheaper than the index, a market-neutral gain will be realized.

A related strategy is identifying a closed-end mutual fund trading at a significant discount to its net asset value. Purchasing shares of the fund gains access to a portfolio of securities valued significantly higher. In order to capture this mispricing, one needs only to sell short every holding in the fund's portfolio and then force (by means of a proxy fight, perhaps) conversion of the fund from a closed-end to an open-end (creating convergence). Sounds easy, right?

In considering equity market-neutral, one must be careful to differentiate between true market-neutral strategies (where long and short positions are related) and the recently popular long/short equity strategies. In a long/short strategy, the manager is essentially a stock-picker, hopefully purchasing stocks expected to go up, and selling short stocks expected to depreciate. While the dollar value of long and short positions may be equivalent, there is often little relationship between the two, and the risk of both bets going the wrong way is always present.

MERGER ARBITRAGE (A.K.A. RISK ARBITRAGE)

Merger arbitrage, while a subset of a larger strategy called event-driven arbitrage,[*] represents a sufficient portion of the market-neutral universe to warrant separate discussion.

Merger arbitrage earned a bad reputation in the 1980s when Ivan Boesky and others like him came to regard insider trading as a valid investment strategy. That notwithstanding, merger arbitrage is a respected strategy and when executed properly, can be highly profitable. It bets on the outcomes of mergers, takeovers, and other corporate events involving two stocks which may become one.

A classic example is acquisition of SDL Inc. (SDLI) by JDS Uniphase Corp (JDSU). On July 10, 2010, JDSU announced its intent to acquire SDLI by offering to exchange 3.8 shares of its own shares for one share of SDLI. At that time, the JDSU shares traded at $101 and SDLI at $320.5. It was apparent that there was almost 20% profit to be realized if the deal went through (3.8 JDSU shares at $101 are worth $383 while SDLI was worth just $320.5). This apparent mispricing reflected the market's expectation about the deal's outcome. Since the deal was subject to the approval of the U.S. Justice Department and shareholders, there was some doubt about its successful completion. Risk arbitrageurs who did their homework and properly estimated the probability of success bought shares of SDLI and simultaneously sold short shares of JDSU on a 3.8 to 1 ratio, thus locking in the future profit. Convergence took place about 8 months later, in February 2011, when the deal was finally approved and the two stocks began trading at exact parity, eliminating the mispricing, and allowing arbitrageurs to realize a profit.

HFR defines the strategy as follows:

> Merger Arbitrage, also known as risk arbitrage, involves investing in securities of companies that are the subject of some form of extraordinary corporate transaction, including acquisition or merger proposals, exchange offers, cash tender offers and leveraged buy-outs. These transactions will generally involve the exchange of securities for cash, other securities or a combination of cash and other securities. Typically, a manager purchases the stock of a company being acquired or merging with another company, and sells short the stock of the acquiring company. A manager engaged in merger arbitrage transactions will derive profit (or loss) by realizing the price differential between the price of the securities purchased and the value ultimately realized when the deal is consummated. The success of this strategy usually is dependent upon the proposed merger, tender offer or exchange offer being consummated.
>
> When a tender or exchange offer or a proposal for a merger is publicly announced, the offer price or the value of the securities of the acquiring company to be received is typically greater than the current market price of the securities of the target company. Normally, the stock of an acquisition target appreciates while the acquiring company's stock decreases in value. If a manager determines that it is probable that the transaction will be consummated, it may purchase shares of the target company and in most instances, sell short the stock of the acquiring company. Managers may employ the use of equity options as a low-risk alternative to the outright purchase or sale of common stock. Many managers will hedge against market risk by purchasing S&P put options or put option spreads.

---

[*] See § 23.03[E].

EVENT-DRIVEN ARBITRAGE

Funds often use event-driven arbitrage to augment their primary market-neutral strategy. Generally, any convergence which is produced by a future corporate event would fall into this category. According to HFR:

> Event-Driven investment strategies or "corporate life cycle investing" involves investments in opportunities created by significant transactional events, such as spin-offs, mergers and acquisitions, liquidations, reorganizations, bankruptcies, recapitalizations and share buybacks and other extraordinary corporate transactions. Event-Driven strategies involve attempting to predict the outcome of a particular transaction as well as the optimal time at which to commit capital to it. The uncertainty about the outcome of these events creates investment opportunities for managers who can correctly anticipate their outcomes. As such, Event-Driven trading embraces merger arbitrage, distressed securities and special situations investing. Event-Driven managers do not generally rely on market direction for results; however, major market declines, which would cause transactions to be repriced or break, may have a negative impact on the strategy.

Event-driven strategies are research-intensive, requiring a manager to do extensive fundamental research to assess the probability of a certain corporate event, and in some cases, to take an active role in determining the event's outcome.

RISK AND REWARD CHARACTERISTICS

To help understand market-neutral performance and risk, let's take a look at the distribution of returns of individual strategies and compare it to that of traditional asset classes (Table 15.1).

The most important observation about this chart is that the market-neutral funds exhibits considerably lower risk than most traditional asset classes.

While market-neutral strategies vary greatly and involve all types of securities, the risk-adjusted returns are amazingly stable across all strategies. The annualized volatility—a standard measure of performance risk—varies between 3.5% and 5%, comparable to a conservative fixed-income strategy.

Another interesting statistics is the correlation between market-neutral strategies and traditional asset classes (Table 15.2).

TABLE 15.1
Average Return/Volatility of Market Neutral Strategies and Select Traditional Asset Classes

Strategy	Average Return (%)	Annualized Volatility (%)
Convertible Arbitrage	11.95	3.57
Fixed Income Arbitrage	8.33	4.90
Equity Market-Neutral	11.62	4.95
Merger Arbitrage	13.29	3.51
Relative Value Arbitrage	15.69	4.31
Traditional Asset Classes		
S&P 500	12.62	13.72
MSCI World	8.57	13.05
High Grade U.S. Corp. Bonds[a]	7.26	3.73
World Government Bonds[b]	5.91	5.96

Source: Nicholas, J: Market neutral investing: Long/Short hedge fund strategies. Bloomberg, New York, 2004.

[a] Salomon Broad Investment Grade Index.
[b] Salomon World Government Bond Index.

TABLE 15.2

Correlation between Market Neutral Strategies and Traditional Asset Classes

Asset Class/Strategy	S&P500	MSCI World	Gov Bonds	Corp Bonds
Convertible Arbitrage	(0.082)	0.359	0.374	0.191
Equity Market Neutral	0.032	0.190	0.191	0.145
Relative Value Arbitrage	0.021	0.027	(0.021)	0.099
Fixed Income Arbitrage	(0.331)	(0.092)	(0.188)	(0.248)
Risk Arbitrage	(0.029)	0.331	0.368	0.040
S&P 500	1.000	0.242	0.106	0.497
MSCI World	0.242	1.000	0.852	0.213
World Government Bonds	0.106	0.852	1.000	0.301
U.S. High Grade Corp. Bonds	0.497	0.213	0.301	1.000

The correlation of all market neutral strategies to traditional assets is quite low, or negative in some cases. This suggests that these strategies would indeed play a useful role in the ultimate goal of efficient portfolio diversification.

To test the "market neutrality" of these strategies, we asked, "How well, on average, did these strategies perform during bad, as well as good, market months?" It turns out, in good times and bad, these strategies displayed consistent solid performance.

From 12/31/91, in months when S&P 500 was down, the average down month was 3.03%. Market-neutral strategies performed as follows:

Strategy	Average Monthly Return (%)
Convertible Arbitrage	+0.65
Fixed Income Arbitrage	+0.50
Equity Market-Neutral	+1.19
Merger Arbitrage	+0.88
Relative Value Arbitrage	+0.81

In months when S&P 500 was up, the average up month was +3.24%. Market-neutral strategies performed as follows:

Strategy	Average Monthly Return (%)
Convertible Arbitrage	+1.17
Fixed Income Arbitrage	+1.20
Equity Market-Neutral	+1.37
Merger Arbitrage	+0.60
Relative Value Arbitrage	+1.25

Clearly, a compelling picture emerges over the test of time. While these strategies, on average, underperform during good times, they show a positive average return during both good and bad markets.

INCLUSION OF MARKET-NEUTRAL IN A LONG-TERM INVESTMENT PORTFOLIO

A critical concern for any medical investor considering a foray into a new asset class is how it will alter the long-term risk/reward profile of the overall portfolio. To better understand this, we constructed several hypothetical portfolios consisting of traditional asset classes:

- The U.S. Treasuries (Salomon Treasury Index 10 yrs+)
- High-Grade Corporate Bonds (Salomon Broad Investment Grade Index)
- Speculative Grade Corporate Bonds (Salomon High Yield Index)
- The U.S. Blue chip equities (Dow Jones Industrial Average)
- The U.S. midcap equities (S&P400 Midcap Index)
- The U.S. small-cap equities (S&P600 Small-cap Index)

Portfolios varied in the level of risk from 100% U.S. Treasuries (least risky) to 100% small-cap equities (most risky), and are ranked from 1 to 10, 1 representing the least risky portfolio. Here, is a list of portfolios and the corresponding asset allocation traditional weights.

Portfolio	U.S. Treasuries (%)	U.S. High-Grade Corp Bonds (%)	U.S. Low-Grade Corp Bonds (%)	Large Cap Stocks (%)	Midcap Stocks (%)	Small-Cap Stocks (%)
1	50	50				
2		50	50			
3	10	30	50	40		
4		50		50		
5		10	10	50	30	
6			10	50	20	20
7			10	30	20	40
8				20	20	60
9					20	80
10						100

Each portfolio was analyzed on a risk/return basis using monthly return data since December 1991. The results are shown in Chart 15.1. Predictably, the least risky portfolio produced the smallest return, while the riskiest produced the highest return. This is perfectly understandable—you would expect to be compensated for taking a higher level of risk.

Five market-neutral strategies are also shown in Chart 15.1.

Clearly, the risk-return picture offered by market-neutral strategies is much more compelling (lower risk, higher return) than that offered by portfolios of traditional assets.

What happens if we introduce these market-neutral strategies into traditional portfolios? Let's take 20% of the traditional investments in our portfolio and reinvest them in market-neutral strategies (see Chart 15.2).

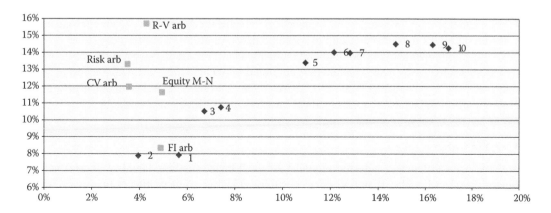

CHART 15.1   Risk/return characteristics of traditional portfolios versus market-neutral strategies.

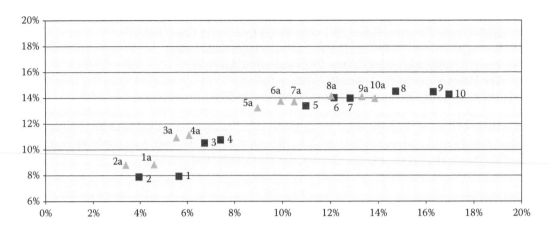

CHART 15.2   Result of inclusion of 20% of market-neutral strategies in traditional portfolios.

The change is dramatic: the new portfolios (denoted 1a through 10a) offer significantly less risk for the same return. The riskiest portfolio, for instance (number 10) offered 20% less risk for a similar return of a new portfolio containing market-neutral strategies (number 10a).

This is quite a difference. Everything else being equal, anyone would choose the new, "improved" portfolios over the traditional ones.

HOW TO INVEST

The mutual fund world does not offer a great choice of market neutral strategies. Currently, there are only a handful of mutual funds that label themselves market-neutral (AXA Rosenberg Market Neutral fund and Calamos Market Neutral fund are two examples). Mutual fund offerings are slim due to excessive regulations imposed by the SEC with respect to short selling and leverage, and consequently these funds lack flexibility in constructing truly hedged portfolios. The dearth of market-neutral offerings among mutual funds is offset by a vast array of choices in the hedge fund universe. Approximately 400 market-neutral funds, managing $60 billion, represent roughly 25% of all hedge funds. Therefore, further focus will relate to the hedge fund universe, rather than the limited number of market-neutral mutual funds.

Direct investing in a market-neutral hedge fund is restricted to qualifying individuals who must meet high net worth and/or income requirements, and institutional investors, such as corporations, qualifying pension plans, endowments, foundations, banks, insurance companies, and so on. This does not mean that retail investors cannot get access to hedge fund exposure. Various private banking institutions offer funds of funds with exposure to hedge funds.

Market-neutral funds are nontraditional investments. They are part of a larger subset of strategies known as alternative investments, and there is nothing traditional in the way doctors invest in them. Hedge funds are private partnerships, which gives them maximum flexibility in constructing and managing portfolios, but also requires medical investors to do a little extra work.

Lockup Periods

One of the main differences between mutual funds and hedge funds is liquidity. Market-neutral strategies have less liquidity than traditional portfolios. Quarterly redemption policies with 45- or 60-days notice are common. Many funds allow redemptions only once a year and some also have lock-up periods. In addition, few of these funds pay dividends or make distributions. These investments should be regarded strictly as long-term strategies.

MANAGERIAL RISKS

Success of a market-neutral strategy depends much less on the market direction than on the manager's skill in identifying arbitrage opportunities and capitalizing on them. Thus, there is significantly more risk with the manager than with the market. It's vital for investors to understand a manager's style and to monitor any deviations from it due to growth, personnel changes, bad decisions, or other factors.

FEES

If you are accustomed to mutual fund fees, brace yourself; market-neutral investing does not come cheap. Typical management fees range from 1% to 2% per year, plus a performance fee averaging 20% of net profits. Most managers have a "high watermark" provision; they cannot collect the performance fees until investors recoup any previous losses. Look for this provision in the funds' prospectus and avoid any fund that lacks it. Even with higher fees, market-neutral investing is superior to most traditional mutual fund investing on a risk-adjusted return basis.

TRANSPARENCY

Mutual funds report their positions to the public regularly. This is not the case with market-neutral hedge funds. Full transparency could jeopardize accumulation of a specific position. It also generates front running: buying or selling securities before the fund is able to do so. While you should not expect to see individual portfolio positions, many hedge fund managers do provide a certain level of transparency by indicating their geographical or sector exposures, level of leverage, and extent of hedging. It does take a bit of education to understand these numbers, but the effort is definitely worthwhile.

TAXATION

The issue of hedge fund taxation is quite complex and is often dependent on the fund and the personal situation of the investor. Advice from a competent accountant, specialized accountant, or tax attorney with relevant experience is worthwhile.

OVERHEARD IN THE DOCTOR'S LOUNGE: DOG NEARLY FETCHES PRESTIGIOUS FINANCIAL ADVISOR HONOR

According to money journalists Max Tailwagger and Allan Roth of MoneyWatch, the trade publication, *Medical Economics Magazine* ("advertising supplement") nearly listed a dog on its 2013 list of *Best Financial Advisors for Doctors*. Indeed, being listed as a top financial advisor in this publication would enhance any advisor's credibility as well as reach a high-income readership. For example, several advisors in the Financial Planning Association mention this prestigious award year after year. And, the NAPFA organization of fee-only financial planners has issued press releases when member advisors make this annual list. In fact, in 2008, it touted that 52/150 listed FAs were NAPFA members.

Yet, the dog is well-known in the financial advisory world, having allegedly received a plaque as one of *2009 America's Top Financial Planners* by the *Consumers' Research Council of America,* and has appeared in several books including *Pound Foolish* and *Money for Life.* The fee for Maxwell Tailwagger CFP® (a 5-year old Dachshund) was reported to be $750 with $1000 for a bold listing. Colorado Securities Commissioner Fred Joseph is reported to have said, "Once again, Max is gaining national notoriety for his astute, and almost super-human, abilities in the financial arena."

The only two qualifications for the listing were to pay the fee and not have a complaint against them. In 2009, James Putman, then the NAPFA chairman who touted his own *Medical Economics* award, was charged by the SEC for securities fraud. NAPFA spokesperson Laura Fisher allegedly opined that "NAPFA no longer promotes the Medical Economics Top Advisors for Doctors list. We felt promoting a list that included stock-brokers were inconsistent with NAPFA's mission to advance the fee-only profession." When an advisor name drops an honor to you, congratulate him and then ask how s/he achieved the award. Ask how many nominees versus award recipients there were. What were the criteria for selection and how were they nominated? Ask if they had to pay for the honor, and go online to check out the organization.

Then ask yourself this question: If your financial advisor is buying credibility, do you really want to trust your financial future to him or her?

D. Kellus Pruitt, DDS
(Fort Worth, Texas)
Source: http://www.cbsnews.com/news/dog-nearly-fetches-prestigious-financial-advisor-honor/.

ASSESSMENT

The bottom line is that investing in market-neutral funds is not a tax-planning exercise and it will not minimize your taxes. On the other hand, it should not generate any more or fewer taxes than if you invested in more traditional funds.

From the medical investor's perspective, the principal advantages of market-neutral investing are attractive risk-adjusted returns and enhanced diversification.

CONCLUSION

Many years of data indicate that market-neutral portfolios have produced risk-adjusted returns superior to traditional investments. In addition, the correlation between the returns of market-neutral funds and traditional asset classes has been historically negligible.

Adding exposure of market-neutral return strategies to the asset mix within a consistent, long-term investment program offers a medical investor the opportunity to improve overall returns, as well as achieving some protection against negative market movements.

COLLABORATE

Discuss this chapter online with others at www.MedicalExecutivePost.com.

ACKNOWLEDGMENT

To Ken Eaton, CFP®, CFA of Stepp & Rothwell Inc., Overland Park, Kansas.

FURTHER READING

Capocci, D: Neutrality of market funds. *Global Finance Journal*, 2006, 17, 309–333.
Carr, T: *Market-Neutral; Trading*. McGraw-Hill Companies, New York, 2013.
Klein, R: *Market Neutral, State of the Art Strategies for Every Market Environment*. McGraw-Hill Companies, New York, 1996.
Nicholas, J: M*arket Neutral Investing: Long/Short Hedge Fund Strategies*. Bloomberg, New York, 2004.
Travers, FJ: *Hedge Fund Analysis*. Wiley, New York, 2012.
Zigler, B: The perils of market-neutral funds. *Wealth Management*, March 25, 2014.

16 Real Estate Investing
Diversification beyond Paper Assets

Dennis Bethel

CONTENTS

Physicians have historically been heavy investors in paper assets such as stocks, bonds, and mutual funds. From 1982 to 2000, the United States saw the greatest bull market in history. However, the decade that followed left many with little to no portfolio growth. Tired of the volatility, unpredictability, and anemic long-term returns, many physicians have been searching for investments outside of the traditional paper asset financial advisory model. In their search for better investments, more and more physicians are turning to real estate. While high-quality real estate like commercial multifamily is a superior asset class, some have shied away from investing due to lack of information, insufficient experience, insufficient capital, and fears of management headaches.

INTRODUCTION

This chapter seeks to demystify the subject of real estate investing as well as provide an overview on the *What, Why, and How* of real estate. However, one thing must be made clear: There is a school of thought that claims a person's residence is a real estate investment. Many do not agree with this thinking and nothing mentioned in this chapter will refer to that. Financial planners are notorious for pushing this thinking. However, in states with high homestead exemptions, homes can be an asset protection tool. For the most part, a home is a place to live, raise a family, and make memories. If and when it is sold, it may or may not make money. Either way, it is not an investment.

COMMERCIAL REAL ESTATE

Two powerful reasons to invest in commercial real estate are illustrated in Figures 16.1 and 16.2.

First is the historical performance of real estate over the past 75 years. As can be seen in Figure 16.1, real estate has provided investors with more up years than down. By outpacing the other sectors of the market, real estate ultimately provides better returns with lower risk.

This leads to the second reason why everyone should have some part of their investment portfolio in real estate. In the following chart (see Figure 16.2), the vertical column measures the volatility of annual returns. With nearly a three-fold reduction in volatility, commercial real estate can be an attractive asset class for investing.

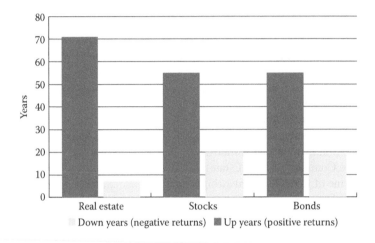

FIGURE 16.1 Up and down years for real estate, stocks, and bonds, 1934–2009. (From NCREIF, Bloomberg, Barclays, Lehman, RCG.)

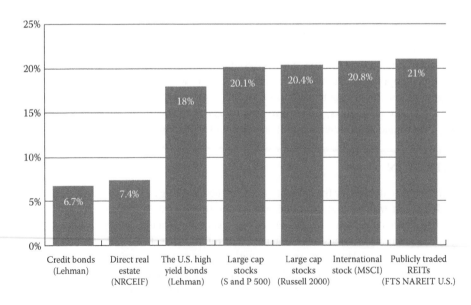

FIGURE 16.2 Risk level of direct real estate versus equities and publicly traded REITs. (From KBS Capital Market Group.)

WHY REAL ESTATE?

Real estate has many benefits that make it highly attractive.

- Principal Protection
- Current Income
- Principal Pay Down
- Appreciation
- Tax-Benefits
- Inflation Protection
- The Ability to Insure Against Loss
- Asset Protection
- Leverage

First and foremost is *principal protection*. One of the biggest reasons many people like commercial multifamily real estate, for example, is principal protection. Multifamily investments have the best risk-adjusted return (Sharpe-Ratio) of any real estate asset class and one of the lowest failure rates of any real estate investment. In fact, it is such a stable asset class that it comprises a significant portion of almost every AAA-rated insurance company's portfolio.

Next is *current income* or cash-flow. This is the monthly, quarterly, or annual cash coming in after expenses have been paid. Cash-flow is the income left over after subtracting operating expenses and any mortgage payments from gross operating income (collected rent). This net distributable income becomes yield for the investor.

Principal pay down is considered by many to be the safest of all wealth creation tools. Each and every month, the tenants of a property are paying down the mortgage. At the end of every year, the equity will grow regardless of rent growth, market conditions, and so on. Of course, the property needs to be leveraged in order to receive this benefit. Be careful not to overleverage the property. Instead, look to secure safer 60–75% loan-to-value (LTV) financing with attractive interest rates.

Appreciation is another way that the real estate investor grows his or her equity. Residential real estate (1–4 units) is primarily valued by the comparison or "comp" method of appraisal. In this method, the appraiser searches for recently sold properties of similar size, with similar amenities that are in close proximity to the subject property. By comparing the sales prices of those properties with the subject property, the appraiser can determine a value.

By comparison, commercial real estate valuation is determined by the money it generates. With these properties, net operating income (NOI) largely determines the value of the property. NOI is simply the net between gross income and all expenses (with the exception of debt service). If NOI goes up, then the property appreciates. Conversely, if NOI declines so does the value of the property. Unlike residential real estate, commercial real estate gives the investor the opportunity to force appreciation. To better understand this concept, look at the components of NOI. As previously stated, NOI is gross operating income minus operating expenses. Consequently, the owner of investment real estate can raise the value of his or her property by increasing income (raising rents, creating new income sources, or increasing retention) or by decreasing expenses. Successful commercial real estate investors do an excellent job-growing NOI to drive the appreciation of their properties.

While optimizing NOI helps with cash flow, its biggest advantage can be seen in appreciation. The formula for calculating the value of commercial real estate is as follows:

$$Property\ Value = NOI/Capitalization\ Rate\ (Cap\ Rate)$$

In the simplest of terms, the capitalization rate is the rate of return an investor would expect to receive if he or she paid all cash for the property. Given this definition, the higher the cap rate, the better it is for the buyer and the lower the cap rate, the better it is for the seller. Cap rates are market specific. The cap rate for an apartment building will be different in San Francisco than it will be in Dallas. By rearranging the above formula, the cap rate is calculated as follows:

$$\text{Cap Rate} = \text{NOI/Value}$$

To better illustrate how commercial real estate is valued based on this income approach, here is an example: There is a property in an 8% cap rate market that increases its annual net operating income from $200,000 a year to $300,000.

$$\text{Previous Value} = \$200,000/0.08 = \$2,500,000$$

$$\text{Current Value} = \$300,000/0.08 = \$3,750,000$$

By raising rents, decreasing expenses, and increasing renter retention, the astute property owner can maximize net operating income. As shown, doing so can be quite lucrative in the form of forced appreciation. As easy as this may look on paper, the truth is that whether a property appreciates in value and how quickly it does so is determined by a confluence of circumstances. These circumstances include buying the right property in the right market and using the right management strategies. Having or hiring the right knowledge and skill is critical in successful real estate investing. Keep in mind that the above formula works in the opposite direction and can lead to loss of value as well.

Another, often overlooked, but material financial benefit of real estate investing is the *tax benefits*. The two biggest drags on wealth accumulation are taxes and inflation. Real estate has some of the best tax advantages of any investment out there. Benefits such as

- Deduction of expenses including mortgage interest against the income
- Depreciation
- Accelerated depreciation
- Tax-free refinances
- 1031 exchanges
- Legacy wealth transfers on a stepped up basis

Any W-2 employee can tell you that they are taxed based on their gross income and that those taxes are taken out prior to receiving their check. Consequently, they pay their expenses with their after-tax net income. Real estate, similar to business, gets preferred tax treatment. The owners get their gross income and can deduct their expenses including mortgage interest before having to pay taxes on the net income that is left over.

In addition to a better tax framework (business vs. personal), real estate investors are given phantom or paper losses called depreciation that also gets subtracted against the actual income of the property. The theory behind depreciation goes something like this: If a person buys a physical asset, whether it is a computer for a business or a property as an investment, it will only have so much useful life before it will need to be replaced. Therefore, the IRS allows that person to write off or depreciate that asset over a given period of time. Currently, for residential real estate (1–4 units) that time is 27.5 years and for commercial real estate it is 39 years. They will not allow depreciation on the value of the land, so that must be taken out of the equation before calculating depreciation.

To better understand depreciation, take a look at these two examples. The first is a $300,000 residential rental triplex and the second is a $5,000,000 commercial office complex. For the purposes of this example, the value of the land is worth 20%.

$$\text{Depreciation} = \$300,000 - (\$300,000 \times 0.20) = \$240,000/27.5 \text{ years} = \$8727.27$$

$$\text{Depreciation} = \$5,000,000 - (\$5,000,000 \times 0.20) = \$4,000,000/39 \text{ years} = \$102,564.10$$

What this means is that for each year of ownership, the real estate investor is allowed to deduct the above amount ($8727 or $102,564) against his or her respective properties income in addition to the operating expenses. Depreciation is often called a "phantom" or paper loss, because this tax break is allowed to take place even when the property is making money and experiencing appreciation in value. Unlike the computer which has a short useful time frame, real estate lasts much longer and goes up in value over time. Think about it, if the above depreciation schedules were actually true for the useful life of real estate, then there would be no single family homes or other residential properties older than 27.5 years old. Also, these late 1980s homes would have gone down significantly in value from when they were first built. Given the current market values of an enormous supply of much older homes in this country, it should be crystal clear why depreciation is called a phantom loss.

After subtracting out the operating expenses and the depreciation, if there is still a taxable gain the IRS gives yet another tax reducing gift called accelerated depreciation. Accelerated depreciation is also known as cost-segregation. In this scenario, an owner can segregate all of the nonstructural elements of the property from the building itself. While the building still gets depreciated over the usual time frame, its contents get depreciated using an accelerated schedule of either 5, 7, or 15 years. This can create a much larger paper loss that is front-loaded in the earlier years of ownership as opposed to being spread out equally over a longer period of time. The time value of money for this benefit is significant.

Be aware that with the sale of the property, all depreciation that was taken will be recaptured creating a tax liability. To defer these taxes, many investors use what is called a 1031 exchange. A 1031 exchange allows the real estate investor to sell one property and exchange it for a like-kind property without having to pay tax. The tax is not erased, but it is deferred until the time that the investor either sells without doing a 1031 exchange or dies (Note, there are a few other wealth transfer and estate planning options to manage the 1031 tax burden in your lifetime, but they are advanced and beyond the scope of this chapter). Upon the death of a real estate owner, his or her heirs are allowed to inherit the property on a stepped-up basis. This erases the depreciation that was taken and resets the basis of the property to current market value at the time of inheritance. This is a huge wealth transfer benefit of owning real estate that can be used to manage legacy wealth through the years.

One last point about real estate, taxes, and refinances. Over time, equity can grow in property due to the effects of appreciation and principal pay down. Smart real estate investors do not like to let that equity sit doing nothing. These investors will look to accelerate their financial growth and increase the velocity of their money. To do this, they refinance their property and harvest the equity that they have built so that they can go out and buy another property. Fortunately, for these investors, refinances are tax-free. Keep in mind that refinances are not free of fees and that releveraging a property back to a higher loan-to-value is not without downsides. Nevertheless, professional real estate investors are quite adept at harvesting their equity to turn one property into two and then two properties into four growing their income and equity over time.

Another often misunderstood and significant benefit of real estate is *inflation protection* (resistance). Inflation is a silent tax that erodes the value of money over time. Given recent fiscal policy that saw the Federal Reserve produce round after round of quantitative easing, it is no surprise that many fear that inflationary times are coming. Thankfully, commercial real estate has a proven track record as a stable hedge against inflation (see Figure 16.3).

The ability to *insure* against loss is the sixth benefit of real estate. With real estate investing comes insurance against loss and liability. Just like other expenses, the tenants will provide the income to cover insurance costs. Insurance protects investors from natural and man-made disasters. With proper insurance, a property will be covered against loss, including rental loss, while the property is being rebuilt. In addition to the standard insurance as well as any prudent and or required add-ons, it is wise to carry general umbrella liability insurance as well.

For legal protection, business ownership structures like limited liability company's (LLC) can be used to hold real estate and therefore shelter the owner's other possessions and assets from legal claims. This provides for significant *asset protection*. Additionally, most investors will seek bank financing to purchase a property.

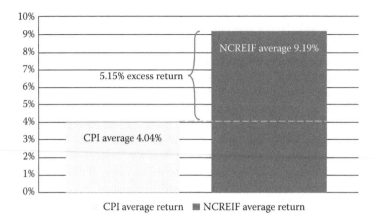

FIGURE 16.3 Direct real estate as an inflation hedge. (From NCREIF and the U.S. Bureau of Labor Statistics.)

With bank financing, investors are allowed to put a small fraction of the purchase price down while the bank provides the rest. What other investment can an investor put 10–30% of the purchase price down and get to control 100% of the entire investment? This use of bank financing is called *leverage*. Leverage can be a double edged sword; it magnifies profits on the upside, but can also compound losses on the downside. To minimize this risk, many larger commercial properties will qualify for nonrecourse lending. With this type of financing, banks secure the loan with the physical property and do not require any further guarantee from the owner. In other words, the owner's risk of loss is limited to his or her initial capital contribution.

On first blush, this may not sound significant. However, take a second look and see how significant the asset protection can be when leverage is combined with nonrecourse lending.

Consider two investments valued at $1 million each. The conventional way to cover that $1 million in stock would be for the investor to pay $1 million. However, the $1 million real estate asset can be purchased with 25% down or $250,000. Now consider the worst-case scenario in which both investments go belly up, losing their entire value.

In this scenario, the stock investor lost $1 million dollars. The real estate also lost $1 million, but the bank lost $750,000 while the investor only lost $250,000. This represents a 75% reduction in risk for the real estate investor.

THE WHAT OF REAL ESTATE INVESTING

With the knowledge of the many benefits of real estate investing, the next step is to know the available options. Before looking for properties, an investor needs to ask him/herself a couple of questions.

The first is whether to be an active or passive investor? Passive investors have no involvement in the operations of the property. They do their due diligence to find a good operator on the front end prior to investing and, if successful, reap the rewards of regular income and equity growth on the backend.

As the name implies, active investors are actively involved in the operations of real estate. Active investors can act as property managers, asset managers, or both. Property managers are involved in the day-to-day operations of the property. They collect rent, respond to complaints, arrange repairs, and numerous other duties that property management requires. Asset managers oversee the property manager. They also create the operating budget for the property, the plan for capital improvements, and the exit strategy.

As busy professionals, many physicians do not have the time, interest, or inclination to be actively involved with real estate. For those, passive investing is likely the better option. The key with passive investing is due diligence. Thorough investigation of both the asset and the asset manager is important prior to investing.

The second question, after deciding to be a passive or active investor, is whether to choose residential or commercial real estate? Residential real estate encompasses one to four units. These are single family homes, duplexes, triplexes, and quads. Due to the relatively low price of entry, most active real estate investors erroneously assume that residential real estate is their only option.

Commercial real estate is more diverse. In general, the broad categories of commercial real estate are

- Retail (big-box anchored centers, malls, neighborhood centers, etc.)
- Industrial (warehouses, distribution centers, etc.)
- Multifamily (apartment buildings five units and larger)
- Hospitality/Leisure (hotels, motels, resorts, etc.)
- Office (medical, single-tenant, multiuse, etc.)

OVERHEARD IN THE ADVISOR'S LOUNGE: REAL ESTATE AND PHYSICIANS

What I see in my accounting practice is that significant accumulation in younger physician portfolio growth is not happening as it once did. This is partially because confidence in the equity markets is still not what it was, and doctors are also looking for better solutions to support their reduced incomes.

For example, I see older doctors with about 25% of their wealth in the market and even in retirement years, do not rely much on that accumulation to live on. Of this 25%, about 80% is in their retirement plan, as tax breaks for funding are just too good to ignore.

What I do see is that about 50% of senior physician wealth is in rental real estate, both in a private residence that has a rental component, and mixed-use properties. It is this that provides a good portion of income in retirement.

So, could I add dialog about real estate as a long-term solution for retirement? Yes, as I believe a real estate concentration in the amount of 5% is optimal for a diversified portfolio, but in a very passive way through mutual or index funds that are invested in real estate holdings and not directly owning properties.

Today, as an option, we have the ability to take pension plan assets and transfer marketable securities for rental property to be held inside the plan collecting rents instead of dividends.

Real estate holdings never vary very much, tend to go up modestly, and have preferential tax treatment due to depreciation of the property against income.

Perry D'Alessio, CPA
(D'Alessio Tocci & Pell LLP)

THE HOW OF REAL ESTATE INVESTING

The previous two questions that were posed yield four different real estate investing options.

OPTION 1: ACTIVE RESIDENTIAL REAL ESTATE

Many real estate investors begin and end their career here. Most people know someone who has done this and as a consequence offers their stern admonition against managing "tenants and toilets."

While there is truth that active management of real estate is not suited for everyone, it can be lucrative when done skillfully.

These investors should pick a business strategy and work with a team to implement it, whether they are going to fix and flip distressed properties, focus on vacation rentals, deal exclusively with low-income government subsidized housing, provide student housing, senior housing, or some other strategy.

Due to the lack of economies of scale with residential real estate, the cash flow can be small and inconsistent. Often times, the real wealth building power of residential comes from appreciation or paying off the loan. For all of the frustrations that can come with residential real estate, the IRS does allow one incredible tax break. Under certain circumstances with very specific requirements, the active investor can qualify for real estate professional status. This allows depreciation from the rental properties to be taken against earned income and therefore reduce the owner's overall tax burden.

As mentioned, active residential real estate is the entry point for most beginning real estate investors. Many physicians know this and avoid real estate investing all together given their already busy lifestyles. What many do not know is that there are other options.

OPTION 2: PASSIVE RESIDENTIAL REAL ESTATE

For years, many investors would buy a property, hire a property manager, bury their head in the sand, and hope for good results. These investors felt like a property manager could insulate them from the headaches that come with being a landlord. Good property managers can definitely buffer some of the time commitment involved with residential real estate. However, be aware that a good residential property manager is hard to find. Most charge 8–10% of gross income for management. That means if you are renting your single family house for $800 a month, the manager makes $80. This small amount of money will not sustain their business or put food on the table. Consequently, residential property managers need to manage in bulk to make a decent living. That leaves them with little time to look after your property. Good residential managers do exist, but it is rare to find someone who will take care of the property as well as the investor would.

In recent years, several turn-key investment companies in various markets have sprung up to service the needs of passive residential investors. These companies all have slightly different models, but in general they secure below market properties for their clients, remodel those properties, obtain renters, and do the property management for their passive investor clients.

OPTION 3: ACTIVE COMMERCIAL REAL ESTATE

Small strip malls, office buildings, and multifamily properties are in the range of the individual physician investor. To secure larger buildings, most physicians will have to form partnerships with other investors. These multimillion dollar properties come with multimillion dollar down payments. Larger properties also come with more economies of scale that allow for better cash flow than residential real estate. Managing commercial property is serious business. It is highly recommended that a person becomes well educated before attempting to become an active commercial real estate investor.

Market and submarket analysis along with a sound business plan is just as crucial as picking a quality property that will provide ample cash flow and appreciation over time. Previous management experience is desirable and may make the difference when qualifying for commercial lending. Keep in mind that some physicians are already familiar with active commercial real estate. It is not uncommon to see groups of doctors come together to purchase and manage the building that houses their urgent care, free-standing radiology or surgery center, or medical office.

OPTION 4: PASSIVE COMMERCIAL REAL ESTATE

Realizing that the vast majority of medium and large commercial properties are owned by businesses and partnerships means that passive investing is commonplace in the commercial real estate space. This can be a very attractive option for the busy medical professional. Large partnerships formed to invest in commercial real estate are known as syndicates. There are numerous private real estate investment companies who specialize in various classes of commercial real estate and syndicate these types of deals.

These private real estate investment companies should have systems in place for acquisitions and operations. They should have a team that at a minimum will consist of a real estate attorney, an SEC attorney, CPA, real estate brokers, commercial real estate lender, and a property management company. They bring with them the expertise to manage the property and can qualify for an array of commercial lending including commercial banks, government sponsored entity (GSE), commercial mortgage-backed security (CMBS), and life insurance originations.

There is a range of ways these companies can take ownership:

- Limited Partnerships (LP)
- Limited Liability Companies (LLC)
- Delaware Statutory Trust (DST)
- Tenant in Common (TIC)

Limited partnerships and limited liability companies are the most common ownership structures used by private real estate investment companies. It is standard for the real estate company to be the general partner while the investors are limited partners. Delaware Statutory Trusts are gaining popularity in this space and largely replacing the old Tenant in Common structure. TICs have fallen out of favor due to the requirement that all investors must qualify on the loan.

When investing passively in commercial real estate through a private real estate investment firm, an investor is a fractional owner. Instead of whole ownership of the property, they own a percentage of the property based on their initial capital investment and the entire amount of the raise. It is important to remember that the real estate investment company will also take compensation for their services on this investment.

Each company has its own compensation structure, but typical fees include

- *Organization and Operations Fee or Acquisition Fee*—This is a one-time fee for developing the market, vetting the property manager, finding and evaluating the deal, negotiating and structuring the purchase, conducting due diligence, securing lending, and creating the partnership. It is compensation for the time, experience and expertise it takes to bring projects of this type to market. This fee varies between 1% and 5% of purchase price.
- *Asset Management Fee*—This is an ongoing fee for managing the property and partnership, creating and implementing the capital improvement plan, maintaining reporting and distributions to the partners, and planning for and implementing liquidity events. Some firms will charge 1% of the asset value annually while others take 2% of gross income annually for ongoing management.
- *Carried Interest/Equity Participation/Promote*—Private real estate investment firms will take a percentage of equity and or equity profit on any given deal. Typically, this participation comes in the range of 15–20%, but can be as high as 50%. This carried interest should be almost exclusively performance-based and is typically the largest benefit to the syndicator. This motivates your asset manager/syndicator to perform well.

Just as any wise investor would perform due diligence on a property prior to investing, strict due diligence should also be completed on any private real estate investment company prior to investing with them. How long have they been in business? What is their track record of performance? What is the background of the upper level management? Is there any pending legal action against them? Have they ever lost a project? Do they have references? Are their business/ethics framework aligned with the investor? These are just some of the questions that need to be answered before considering investments in this type of structure.

REITs: THE MARGARINE OF REAL ESTATE INVESTING

Just like real estate, butter has been around for thousands of years. Sometime in the 1800s someone decided that there was a need for something that looked like butter, tasted similar to butter, but was not butter. Along came margarine. Real estate investment trusts (REITs) are the margarine of the real estate investing world.

NAREIT, the National Association of Real Estate Investment Trusts, answers the question "What is a REIT?" in the following way:

> A REIT, or Real Estate Investment Trust, is a type of real estate company modeled after mutual funds. REITs were created by Congress in 1960 to give all Americans—not just the affluent—the opportunity to invest in income producing real estate in a manner similar to how many Americans invest in stocks and bonds through mutual funds. Income-producing real estate refers to land and the improvements on it—such as apartments, offices or hotels. REITs may invest in the properties themselves, generating income through the collection of rent or they may invest in mortgages or mortgage securities tied to the properties, helping to finance the properties and generating interest income.

While REITs typically own real estate, investors in REITs do not. REITs are paper assets that represent interest in a company that owns and operates income-producing properties. In essence they are real estate flavored stock. As such, REITs are generally highly correlated with the stock market.

When discussing REITs, you encounter the following terminology—public, private, traded, and nontraded. Public REITs can be designated as nontraded or traded depending on whether or not they are traded on a stock exchange. Since traded REITs are traded on the stock exchange, they enjoy a high degree of liquidity just like any other stock. Unfortunately, traded REITs tend to follow the economic cycles and can closely correlate with the stock market. This can lead to a higher degree of volatility than what is usually seen with physical real estate. Additionally, they do not afford the investor the tax-advantages that come with investments in physical real estate.

Private REITs and nontraded public REITs are not traded on an exchange. These are usually offered to accredited investors through broker-dealer networks. These REITs are illiquid and generally have high fees. They have been plagued with transparency issues as well as conflicts of interest. Valuation of this stock is difficult and can be misleading to the investor. Due diligence is very important as the quality of nontraded REITs can vary widely.

ASSESSMENT

According to Rick Kahler MS CFP®ChFC CCIM (www.KahlerFinancial.com) real estate is one of the largest asset classes in the world. The family home is the largest asset many middle-class Americans own. And, real estate makes up a significant portion of the net worth of many wealth accumulators. Directly owning real estate is not an investment for the faint of heart, the armchair investor, or the uneducated. Most wealth accumulators would do well to leave direct ownership of real estate to the pros and invest in real estate investment trusts (REITs) instead (personal communication).

Still, as we have seen, the lure of investing in a tangible asset like real estate is enticing for high-risk tolerant physician-investors who need a sense of control and interaction with their investments. If you are among them, here are a few guidelines that may keep you on a profitable path.

1. Do not attempt to purchase investment real estate without the help of a commercial real estate specialist who is a fiduciary bound to look out for your best interest. Engage a *Certified Commercial Investment Member* (CCIM) with years of training and experience in analyzing and acquiring investment real estate. To find a CCIM near you, go to http://www.ccim.com.

2. You will sign a disclosure agreement that will tell you who the Realtor represents. Be sure the Realtor you engage represents you and not the seller, both parties, or neither party.

3. Never trust the income and expense data provided by the seller's Realtor. While a seller represented by a CCIM will have a greater chance of supplying you with accurate data, most will significantly understate expenses and overstate the capitalization rate. Selling Realtors often understate the average annual cost of repairs and maintenance. I estimate this annual expense at 10%.

4. Another often understated expense is management. Many owners manage their own properties, so the selling broker does not include an estimate for management expenses. They should. Real estate does not manage itself, ever. You will either need to hire professional management or do your own management (always a scary proposition). Even if you do it yourself, you have an opportunity to cost your time, so you must include a management fee in the expenses. Most small residential apartments and single-family homes will pay 10% of their rents to a manager.

5. You must verify all the costs presented to you by the seller's Realtor. Demand copies of at least the last 3 and preferably 5 years of tax returns. Research items such as utility bills, property taxes, legal fees, insurance costs and repairs, maintenance costs, replacement reserves, tax preparation, and all management fees. As a rule of thumb, expenses will average 40% of rental income on average-aged properties where the tenants pay all utilities except water. Newer properties may have expenses as low as 35%, while older properties can be as high as 50%.

6. By subtracting the vacancy rate and stabilized expenses from the rent, you will find the net operating income. This is the income you will put in your pocket—assuming the property is paid for. By dividing the net operating income by the purchase price, you will find the return you will receive on your investment, called the capitalization or "cap" rate. In Rapid City South Dakota, for example, the cap rate tends to be 4% for single-family homes, 5–8% for duplexes to eight-plexes, and 8–12% for larger residential and commercial properties.

Yes, physician-investors and all of us can build wealth with real estate. You just need to educate yourself, work hard, start conservatively, think long term, and be prepared for lean years. This is not a quick or easy path to riches.

CONCLUSION

Real estate investing has several unique advantages that cannot be found in the same combination with other investments. Given this fact, it is no wonder that the majority of the Forbes 400 of wealthiest individuals either made or retained their wealth in real estate. Many physicians have avoided this superior asset class out of fear of management headaches. However, there are many different ways to make money in real estate and several of them do not require the investor to become a landlord.

For those whose portfolio is paper asset heavy, real estate can provide some needed diversification and stability. Investors who are looking for better yields without having to sacrifice growth should take a hard look at real estate. For those wanting to decrease their exposure to high volatility investments, real estate might be the way to go. Every physician should take a look at this asset class and see if it is right for them. Keep in mind that real estate can provide superior yield in the form of cash flow as well as longer term growth in the form of appreciation and principal pay down. Real estate is also highly tax-advantaged and can be an excellent hedge against inflation.

COLLABORATE

Discuss this chapter online with others at www.MedicalExecutivePost.com.

ACKNOWLEDGMENT

To Robin Bethel, licensed real estate agent, and CEO of the Bethel Investment Group.

FURTHER READING

Alcorn, R: *Dealmaker's Guide: Commercial Real Estate: Strategy and Practice for the Intelligent Investor.* Published by Golden Key Investments Ltd., Blacksburg, Virginia, 2005–2008.
Institutional Opportunities for Individual Investors (Web log post). 2010. Retrieved January, 23rd, 2014 from https://www.kbs-cmg.com.
National Council of Real Estate Fiduciaries. 2013. Retrieved January 23, 2014 from https://www.ncreif.org/property-index-returns.aspx.
What Is a REIT? (Web log post). (2014, January 23). Retrieved January 23, 2014 from http://www.reit.com/REIT101/WhatisaREIT.aspx.

17 Medical Practice as a New Asset Class?

Valuing the Quintessential Alternative Financial Investment

David Edward Marcinko

CONTENTS

As we have seen in the earlier chapters, the investment industry and modern portfolio theory (MPT) strive to make optimal "allocations" into different "asset classes," according to some defined risk tolerance level or efficient frontier. Equities, fixed income, property, private equity, emerging markets, and so on are all "asset classes," into which physician investors and mutual fund or portfolio managers will make an allocation of their total funds under the management. It is quite proper for them to do this as they seek to balance the risk and potential returns for their own; ME, Inc., or other clients' money. By creating a "new" asset class, this concept opens the door to significant capital flows, advisory, and management fees. Hence, the unrelenting innovation of Wall Street, and its commission-driven and fee-seeking mavens, is unending.

This concept may be illustrated using Social Security as an example. So, Wall Street opines, if you're not counting on Social Security benefits as a part of an overall asset allocation strategy, you may be missing out on bigger gains in a retirement portfolio. Those of this ilk say that retirement investors should consider the value of their Social Security as a portion of their fixed-income investments. Others believe it may be too risky.

Generally, adopting this strategy would mean shifting a big portion of investible assets out of bonds and into stocks and into the hands of money managers, stock brokers, and wealth managers for a fee, of course. This is akin to those financial advisors who rightly or wrongly goaded clients to not pay off a home mortgage and instead reposition the free cash flow into a rising, and then falling, market. Of course, there are detractors, as well as proponents of this emerging financial planning philosophy.

For example, Jack Bogle, founder of the Vanguard Group, often cites his penchant for basing one's asset allocation on age. (If you're 40 years old, you have 40% of your investments in fixed income and 60% in equities. By the time you're 60, you've got 60% in fixed income, 40% in equities).

So, let's consider Social Security, citing a physician with $300,000 in an investment portfolio, and capitalizing the stream of future payments. So, if the $300,000 is all in equity funds, even equity-index funds, and $300,000 is in Social Security, you are already at 50/50" fixed income versus equities. The next step is a conversation as this is the nexus of where Social Security meets risk management. So, how will the doctor feel when the market goes up and down? Some may believe the concept, but do not enjoy the inevitable, more fluctuating self-directed 401(k), or 403(b) plan. So, one must be comfortable with taking on a larger stock position. *Source*: Andrea Coombes; *MarketWatch*, September, 2013. http://money.msn.com/mutual-fund/social-security-as-part-of-your-portfolio

Other experts, such as Paul Merriman, opine that Social Security is not an asset class and the idea is fundamentally flawed and should not be a part of anyone's portfolio. Why? As classically defined, a portfolio is composed of financial assets. A financial asset is something that can be sold. Social Security cannot be bought and sold. Because of that, it has a market value of zero.

Therefore, since a medical practice can be bought or sold, the definitional decision is left up to the informed reader, modern physician, or financial enlightened advisor. *Source*: Paul Merriman, *MarketWatch*, November 2013.

INTRODUCTION

Physicians are entrepreneurial by nature, risk tolerant, and take great pride in the creation of their businesses. And, the current market and health economic pressures are motivating physicians to be proactive and to make informed decisions concerning the future of their businesses.

TRADITIONAL REASONS FOR A MEDICAL PRACTICE VALUATION

The decision to sell, buy, or merge a medical practice, while often financially driven, is inherently an emotional one for these impact investors who went into the profession largely because of a deep-seated zeal to help others.

Still, beyond impact-investing musings, there are other economic reasons for a practice valuation that include changes in ownership, determining insurance coverage for a practice buy–sell agreement or upon a physician-owner's death, organic growth meter, establishing stock options, or bringing in a new partner, and so on. Practice appraisals are also used for legal reasons such as divorce, bankruptcy, breach of contract, and minority shareholder complaints. In 2002, the Financial Accounting Standards Board (FASB) issued rules that required certain intangible assets to be valued, such as goodwill. This may be important for practices seeking start-up, service segmentation extensions, or operational funding. Some other reasons for a medical practice appraisal, and the considerations that go along with them, are discussed here.

ESTATE PLANNING

Medical practice valuation may be required for estate-planning purposes. For a decedent physician with a gross estate of more than the current in-place tax limits, his or her assets must be reported at fair market value on an estate tax return. If lifetime gifts of a medical practice business interest are made, it is generally wise to obtain an appraisal and attach it to the gift tax return.

Note that when a *"closely-held"* level of value (in contrast to *"freely traded,"* *"marketable,"* or *"publicly traded"* level) is sought, the valuation consultant may need to make adjustments to the results. There are inherent risks relative to the liquidity of investments in closely held, nonpublic companies (e.g., medical group practice) that are not relevant to the investment in companies whose shares are publicly traded (freely traded). Investors in closely held companies do not have the ability to dispose of an invested interest quickly if the situation is called for, and this relative lack of liquidity of ownership in a closely held company is accompanied by risks and costs associated with the selling of an interest-said company (i.e., locating a buyer, negotiation of terms, advisor/broker fees, risk of exposure to the market, etc.). Conversely, investors in the stock market are most often able to sell their interest in a publicly traded company within hours and receive cash proceeds in a few days. Accordingly, a discount may be applicable to the value of a closely held company due to the inherent illiquidity of the investment. Such a discount is commonly referred to as a *"discount for lack of marketability."*

Discount for lack of marketability is typically discussed in three categories: (1) transactions involving restricted stock of publicly traded companies; (2) private transactions of companies prior to their initial public offering (IPO); and (3) an analysis and comparison of the price-to-earnings (P/E) ratios of acquisitions of public and private companies respectively published in the *"Mergerstat Review Study."*

With a noncontrolling interest, in which the holder cannot solely authorize and cannot solely prevent corporate actions (in contrast to a controlling interest), a *"discount for lack of control,"* (DLOC), may be appropriate. In contrast, a control premium may be applicable to a controlling interest. A control premium is an increase to the pro rata share of the value of the business that reflects the impact on value inherent in the management and financial power that can be exercised by the holders of a control interest of the business (usually the majority holders). Conversely, a DLOC or minority discount is the reduction from the pro rata share of the value of the business as a whole that reflects the impact on value of the absence or diminution of control that can be exercised by the holders of a subject interest.

Several empirical studies have been done to attempt to quantify DLOC from its antithesis, control premiums. The studies include the Mergerstat Review Study, an annual series study of the premium paid by investors for controlling interest in publicly traded stock, and the Control Premium Study, a quarterly series study that compiles control premiums of publicly traded stocks by attempting to eliminate the possible distortion caused by speculation of a deal.[*]

Buy–Sell Agreements

The ideal situation is for physician partners to put in place a buy–sell agreement when practice relationships are amicable. This establishes the terms for departure before they are required, and is akin to a prenuptial agreement in the marriage contract. Disagreements most often occur when a doctor leaves the group, often acrimoniously. Business operations of the practice decline, employee and partner morale suffers, feuding factions develop spilling over into the office, and the practice begins to implode creating a downward valuation spiral. And so valuations should be done every 2–3 years, or as the economic circumstances of the practice change. Independence and credibility are provided, and emotional overtones are purged from the transaction.

Physician Partnership Disputes

Medical practice appraisals are often used in partnership disputes, such as breach-of-contract or departure issues. Obvious revenue declinations are not difficult to quantify. But, revenues may not immediately fall since certain Current Procedural Terminology (CPT®) code reimbursements may actually increase. Upon verification, however, lost business may be camouflaged as the number of procedures performed, or number of patients decrease after partner departure.

Divorce

Physicians getting divorced should get a practice appraisal, and either side may hire the appraiser, although occasionally the court will order an expert to provide a neutral valuation. Such valuations should be done in light of both court discovery rules and Internal Revenue Service (IRS) requirements for closely held businesses. Generally, this requires the consideration of eight elements:

---

[*] Published by FactSet Mergerstat, LLC. "FactSet Mergerstat Publications," FactSet Mergerstat, https://www.mergerstat.com/newsite/bookStore.asp (accessed 11/4/2009); Compiled by Mergerstat/Shannon Pratt's BV Resources. "Mergerstat/BVR Control Premium Study—Quantify Minority Discounts and Control Premiums," Business Valuation Market Data, http://www.bvmarketdata.com/defaulttextonly.asp?f=CPS%20Intro (accessed 11/4/2009).

- Practice specialty and operating history
- Economic and health-care industry condition
- Estimates of practice risks and future returns
- Book value and financial condition of the practice
- Practice future-earning capacity
- Physician bonuses, dividends, and distributions
- Intangible assets
- Comparable practice sales

Sometimes, the nonphysician spouse may desire a lifestyle analysis to evaluate the potential for underreported income, by a forensic accountant, or appraiser. A family law judge is often the final arbiter of different valuations, and because of varying state laws, there may be 50 different nuances of what the practice is really worth.

UNDERSTANDING VALUATION DEFINITIONS

According to the *Dictionary of Health Economics and Finance,* most practice valuations for mergers and acquisitions use *fair market value* as the standard term used to derive a reasonable value for the medical practice. This key definition of value is important, as it guides the appraiser's choice of methods to apply in determining the appropriate value. Fair market value means the appraiser will value your medical practice assuming an arm's-length transaction of "any willing buyer and any willing seller" scenario, and without synergies of a specific buyer.

Synergies common among the most likely hypothetical (any willing) buyers, however, are appropriately considered in valuing medical practices.

If you are selling your medical practice as a going-concern business, inclusive of all the medical practice's underlying assets, then you should understand the term *business enterprise.* The business enterprise of a medical practice equals the combined values of all practice assets (tangible and intangible) and the working capital of a continuing business. Stated another way, the business enterprise value is equal to the combined values of the owner's equity and long-term debt, also referred to as the invested capital of the operating business.

The value of the *Owner's Equity* of a medical practice equals the combined values of all practice assets (tangible and intangible), less all practice liabilities (booked and contingent). In essence, the equity value is the net worth of the business (after deducting debt). The business enterprise value is the total sum for the business including the owner's net worth, plus the long-term debt.

The business enterprise value and the owner's equity value definitions are relevant when you are contemplating a sale of your ongoing medical practice, inclusive of all medical practice assets. In transactions involving the sale of medical assets separate and apart from the ongoing business operations, other value definitions and methodologies will apply.

Many medical practices are acquired without working capital. The *working capital* of a medical practice equals the excess of current assets (cash, accounts receivable, supplies, inventory, prepaid expenses, etc.) over current liabilities (accounts payable, accrued liabilities, etc.). When working capital is not a part of the transaction, the business enterprise value is adjusted for the buyer's postacquisition buildup of practice receivables and the associated delay from the collection of these receivables.

WHAT MEDICAL PRACTICE ASSETS HAVE VALUE?

In the context of the valuation of medical professional practices, the typical focus of the classification of assets begins with determining the existence and quantifiability of assets. The tangible and intangible assets relevant to the valuation of a medical practice may include tangible (physical) assets and/or intangible assets, depicted below.

Medical practices can be valued in their entirety as an operating business, often referred to as the business enterprise. The business enterprise value includes all the underlying assets employed in the medical practice's business operations. The business enterprise analysis is the most cost-effective way of estimating practice value. Practice assets can also be valued apart from the operating business or in addition to the operating business. What assets can be acquired and the deal structure will determine whether there is a need to separately value the practice assets, or in addition to the business operations.

Medical practices are dependent on the highly specialized skills of the physician providers. With the exception of practices that own real estate, typically, the majority of practice value lies in intangible assets, or goodwill.

Keep in mind that goodwill is only one of the several intangible assets that may be found, not a "catch-all-moniker" for all intangible assets in the aggregate. This is in contrast to accounting and other definitions of goodwill (e.g., *The Goodwill Registry*, published by The Health Care Group) that consider all practice intangible assets as goodwill, and apparently relies on subtracting the tax basis-depreciated book value of tangible assets that happen to appear on the practice's balance sheet (in contrast to their economic fair market value) from the reported sale price, and then simply (and incorrectly) assuming that the residual amount of the sale price after that subtraction equals the value of "intangible assets" (which, as a term of convenience, it defines as "goodwill"), and ignores the very nature of how tangible and intangible assets coexist and relate to each other in the value of professional practices. Many valuation professionals consider goodwill to be the residual amount of intangible asset value that may exist after the separately identified, separately distinguishable, and separately appraised elements of intangible value have been determined.

Intangible assets that are sometimes considered as part of *goodwill and patient related* include custodial rights to medical charts and records; electronic medical records; patient recall lists; and both personal/professional and/or practice/commercial goodwill. The custody of medical charts, electronic medical records, and patient recall lists may be separately identified and quantified as a distinct intangible asset aside from goodwill; however, they are often considered together with goodwill as they create the background that supports the propensity for the continued patient–provider relationship, which constitutes goodwill.

In the event that the valuator determines the existence of intangible asset value in the practice and the existence of goodwill as one of the intangible assets existing, then, the next step is to identify, distinguish, disaggregate, and allocate the relevant portion of the existing goodwill to either "Professional/Personal Goodwill" or "Practice/Commercial Goodwill."

Professional/personal goodwill results from the charisma, knowledge, skill, and reputation of a specific practitioner and may include characteristics such as "(1) lacks transferability, (2) specialized knowledge, (3) personalized name, (4) inbound referrals, (5) personal reputation, (6) personal staff, (7) age, health, and work habits, and (8) knowledge of end user".[*] Since these attributes "go to the grave" with that specific individual physician and therefore can't be sold, they have no economic value and are not, as a practical matter, transferable.

Practice/commercial goodwill should be defined in a medical service enterprise that includes a practice component as "the propensity of patients (and the revenue stream thereof) to return to the practice in the future." Practice/commercial goodwill may include characteristics such as (1) number of offices, (2) business location, (3) multiple service providers, (4) enterprise staff, (5) systems and processes, (6) number of years in business, (7) outbound referrals, and (8) marketing.[†]

---

[*] In re Marriage of Alexander, 368 Ill.App.3d 192, 199 (2006).
[†] In re Marriage of Alexander, 368 Ill.App.3d 192, 199 (2006).

Defining the "Standard of Value"

At the outset of each valuation engagement, it is important to appropriately define and have all practices agree to the *Standard of Value,* which defines the type of value to be determined. In addition to fair market value, three other standards of value are often mentioned:

- *Investment value* focuses on the value to a specific physician buyer rather than the value to a hypothetical buyer. For example, let us examine the physician owner of an ambulatory surgery center (ASC) who is considering the acquisition of a competing ASC that operates in the same geographic market. The owner might calculate value based on the knowledge that the combination of the two ASCs will create economies of scale and less competition. This would result in greater profitability per dollar of revenue. Therefore, such a buyer, or else equal, may assess a greater value to the company than a buyer who would expect to operate the ASC in its current free-standing situation, without the expected cost saving and corresponding expectation of increased cash flow.
- *Intrinsic value* is similar to investment value; however, the practice is typically viewed in a stand-alone mode as a going concern. That is, the value is based on the expected cash flows of the practice based on its current operating configuration. However, changes in the operating policy, such as changing its financial structure can have an impact on its intrinsic value.
- *Premise of value* is an assumption further defining the standard of value to be used under which a valuation is conducted, and is determined at the outset of the valuation engagement. The premise of value defines the hypothetical terms of the sale and answers the question, "Value under what further defining circumstances?" (e.g., value-in-use as a going concern or value-in-exchange, ranging from orderly disposition and assemblage of the assets to forced liquidation, etc.). Two general concepts that relate to the consideration and selection of the premise of value are "value in use" the premise of value that assumes that the assets will continue to be used as part of an ongoing business enterprise, producing profits as a benefit of ownership of a going concern and "value in exchange" (an orderly disposition of a mass assemblage of the assets in place, but not as a going-concern enterprise).

HEALTH-CARE REGULATIONS: WHAT DOCTORS AND FINANCIAL ADVISORS NEED TO KNOW

Federal and state regulatory oversight is increasing. The trend of not-for-profit community hospital conversions into for-profit groups is generating business for appraisers, accountants, and attorneys to perform fairness opinions to calm community benefit fears. A number of industry regulations must be considered, regardless of the buyer's tax status, when organizations acquire or affiliate with physicians. These regulations include

- Medicare fraud and abuse legislation makes it a criminal offense to offer, pay, solicit, or receive payment for patient referrals for business covered by a federal health-care program, often referred to as antikickback.
- Anti-self-referral legislation (Stark I, II, and III) makes it illegal for physicians to refer Medicare patients for certain identified services if the physician or family holds an ownership interest in the business of the service provider. The legislation identifies health services such as lab work, radiology, magnetic resonance imaging, ultrasound, home health services, durable medical equipment (DME), computerized axial tomography, and hospital services.
- Section 501c(3) of the Internal Revenue Code makes it illegal for not-for-profit organizations to pay more than *or* receive less than the fair market value in physician and other transactions.

- An IRS payroll audit program of approximately 6000 companies (including tax-exempt organizations) that began in February 2010 scrutinizes executive compensation and determines how to regulate and penalize these tax-exempt entities that fail to meet fair market value for transactions.[*] The program is still in force today.
- Antitrust laws protect against combinations that may preclude market competition.

Valuation Regulations That Impact Practice Value

Both the practice buyer and seller need to understand how industry regulation impacts practice value and also have an appreciation for accepted appraisal definitions and methodologies used by qualified appraisers to estimate value. *The Uniform Standards of Professional Appraisal Practice (USPAP)* are promulgated standards, which provide the minimum requirements to which all professional appraisals must conform. USPAP requires the three recognized approaches to value (the income, market, and cost approaches) that must be considered to estimate value.

In the fall of 1994 and 1995, the IRS first issued training guidelines pertaining to the valuation of physician practices. These guidelines suggest that appraisers consider all three of the general approaches to valuation as required by the USPAP. Specifically, in transactions involving physician organizations, the IRS implied

1. The discounted cash flow (DCF) analysis is a relevant income approach.
2. The DCF analysis must be done on an "after-tax" basis regardless of the tax status of the prospective buyer.
3. Practice collections must be projected for the DCF based on reasonable and proper assumptions for the practice, market, and industry.
4. Physician compensation must be based on market rates consistent with age, experience, and productivity.

THE PRIVATE VALUATION PROCESS

Valuation of securities is, in essence, a prophecy as to the future and must be based on facts available at the required date of appraisal.

IRS Revenue Ruling 59-60

Closely held businesses, such as medical practices, clinics, and surgery and wound-care centers also produce economic benefits for their owners, but the value of these companies cannot be directly observed by activity in traded markets. And so, valuation professions estimate value by applying valuation theory. Among the wide array of sources of guidance with which business-valuation consultants should be familiar to conduct an accurate business valuation, the pronouncements of the IRS may be most widely cited. The IRS provides insights regarding its positions on business-valuation issues through various mediums: Internal Revenue Code, the Treasury Regulations to the Code, Technical Advice Memorandums, Private Letter Rulings, and various Revenue Rulings. RR 59-60 provides a general outline and review to "the approach, methods and factors to be considered in valuing shares of the capital stock of closely held corporations for estate tax and gift tax purposes."[†]

---

[*] "Enforcement Efforts Take Aim at Executive Compensation of Tax-Exempt Health Care Entities," by Candace L. Quinn and Jeffrey D. Mamorsky, 18 Health Law Reporter 1640, December 17, 2009; "Employment Tax Audits of Exempt Hospitals Could Turn Up Other Issues, Attorneys Warn," 18 Health Law Reporter 1653, December 24, 2009.

[†] "Valuations for Estate and Gift Tax Purposes," in Valuing a Business: The Analysis and Appraisal of Closely Held Companies, 5th ed., by Shannon P. Pratt, Alina V. Nicolita, McGraw-Hill, 2008, pp. 633–637.

In the valuation of the stock of closely held corporations or corporate stock that lacks market quotations, all available financial data along with significant factors impacting the fair market value should be considered.

The value of financial assets, whether traded or not is generally based on the following:

- The level of expected distributable future cash flows
- The timing of these expected distributable cash flows
- The uncertainty in receiving expected future cash flows

Valuing your medical practice will require consideration of many other factors that influence value. A thorough valuation analysis will include a study of the economics of the health-care industry, reimbursement trends, competitive market conditions, historical earnings trends, as well as management experience. These factors, collectively considered, influence the future prospects of your medical practice and, ultimately, its estimate of value as a going concern.

The advisor, accountant, and appraiser need to understand the history of the practice, its operations, and local competition and payer-contracting issues. The business and management fundamentals studied are patient retention and potential for new patient growth, providing services efficiently and cost-effectively, timely collections for services, and maintaining competitive equipment and facilities.

After the need for an independent valuation is determined, here is what you can expect:

- Who pays the bill? An independent valuation appraiser may be engaged by the buyer or seller or, in some cases jointly by both the buyer and seller.
- Make sure the appraiser understands the health-care industry and most importantly, educates both the buyer and seller in the conduct of an appraisal. All too often, values are misunderstood and may result in deals unnecessarily falling apart.
- The appraiser will request financial information, operating statistics, and other information in advance of a site visit.
- The appraiser should visit your medical practice to conduct key interviews and review the physical condition of the facilities and medical equipment.
- The appraiser will review historical practice patterns, financial, and operating performance as a basis for forecasting future operations.
- The appraiser will adjust, or *normalize* historical financial data to eliminate one-time, non-recurring expenses, adjust for excessive or below-normal expenses, and eliminate expenses not expected to be a part of future practice costs. The rationale for adjusting practice costs is to estimate the fair market value price of the business that is transferable.
- The appraiser should work with you to assist with the development of key assumptions concerning future reimbursement trends, physician productivity, practice cost structure, and physician compensation for use in financial projections.
- The appraiser should review valuation assumptions and forecasts with you.

The choice of methodology primarily depends on the purpose of the valuation report, the specific characteristics of the medical practice, and the availability and reliability of data. Once the valuation consultant clearly understands the purpose of the appraisal assignment, has determined the standard of value and the premise of value, and has determined the availability and reliability of data, he or she must select one or more applicable methods. These methods can be classified by three major valuation approaches: income, cost, and market.

APPROACHES TO MEDICAL PRACTICE VALUE

In many cases, a significant amount of practice value may reside in the business operations as opposed to the physical assets. The value of a going-concern medical practice is directly linked to the value of the practice's ability to generate economic benefits to its owners, as measured by projected future cash flows. As a result, the development of a reasonable forecast of future operations is crucial to determining a meaningful practice value. Additionally, the three major valuation approaches are discussed below.

INCOME APPROACH

Since medical practice value directly correlates with the measurement of economic benefits to owners, earnings or cash-flow methods are the best tools for estimating practice value.

DISCOUNTED CASH FLOW (DCF) METHOD

The DCF method is accepted by the IRS and is considered relevant given the changing nature of the health care. The DCF is a sophisticated analysis requiring assumptions of forecasted practice operations regarding future reimbursements and physician productivity, practice efficiencies, and competitive market conditions. An estimate of practice value is developed by discounting future net cash flows to their present worth based on market rates of return required by an investor physician.

In other words, the discounting process converts future expected distributable cash flows to arrive at their present value, according to several core valuation principles.

- The discounting process is one of converting expected future practice cash flows into a present value.
- The value of an investment is based on the level of expected future practice cash flows, the timing of these cash flows, and the risk or uncertainty attached to these cash flows.
- The discount rate represents the purchaser's (investor's) required rate of return.
- The discount rate or required rate of return is based on a purchaser's (investor's) other opportunities to invest in alternative investments (AIs) whose cash flows have similar risk and duration.

Thus, the value of your medical practice is primarily dependent on future practice earnings that will provide an adequate return on an investment for the buyer. An informed buyer will not pay more than the present value of all anticipated future economic benefits of ownership. Supportable practice values are entirely dependent on realistic financial and operating assumptions about future practice operations.

KEY DCF ASSUMPTIONS

A DCF analysis includes a financial forecast projecting net cash flows for the business operations for usually a period of 3–5 years or until the practice achieves stable operations. In estimating practice value, key variables and assumptions used can have a significant impact to your value. The key DCF elements include

1. Reasonable supportable projections of future practice revenues based on historical practice patterns and with consideration of future physician productivity, reimbursement trends, and shifts in payer mix.
2. Reasonable supportable projections of future practice cost structure based on expected normal levels of practice expenses.
3. Projected physician compensation based on market rates for physicians with comparable age, experience, and productivity.
4. DCF model calculates after-tax cash flows regardless of the tax status of the buyer. The tax rate is based on a blend of federal and state rates.

5. Reinvestment in the business is necessary for funding working capital needs and capital expenditure requirements to replace and acquire new equipment or other medical assets.
6. Terminal value represents the going-concern value at the end of the projection period. Stated another way, it is a residual value for the expected remaining practice value at the end of the forecast period.
7. Discount rate is applied to the future net cash flows to arrive at the present (cash equivalent) value for the medical practice. The discount rate must be based on the industry's weighted average cost of capital that takes into consideration the specific risks for the practice.

The DCF analysis consistently produces higher values than other methods of estimating practice value because there may be supportable reasons to forecast improvements in future practice performance. Understanding the key DCF variables and assumptions used in the income method will assist in producing a meaningful estimate of practice value.

Determining the Required Rate of Return for DCFA

A physician's required rate of return takes into account that monies received sooner have a greater value than those received later, the greater the risk in receiving future cash flows, the lower their current value, and one must always keep in mind returns that can be earned on AIs.

The process of selecting an appropriate required rate of return begins with an assumption that all investors will require, at a minimum, the risk-less rate of return offered by government securities. Government securities with maturity similar to that of the duration of the investment in a private company are selected, and a normal duration of 10–20 years is used. Because of the minimal default risk associated with government securities, the rate is referred to as the risk-free rate.

Physician investors typically require returns greater than the risk-free rate. The additional return (in excess of the risk-free rate) is called the risk premium. Risk premiums are generally calculated through an analysis of historically realized rates of return segmented by varying levels of risk. This analysis illustrates that higher historical rates of return occur in situations of higher risk. For example, securities issued by the U.S. government have lower rates of return than securities issued by large corporations. Returns on the equity of large corporations are greater than those of debt securities issued by the same firms. Thus, historical rates of return are generally used as a proxy for future required rates of return.

When valuing a practice, one must compare the risk of the expected cash flows of the firm being valued to the risk of the cash flows of publicly traded securities, and to determine an appropriate required rate of return based on that assessment.

It is generally assumed that the expected cash flows from an investment in a closely held business are at least as risky as those of large publicly traded firms. The combination of the large firm equity risk premium and the riskless rate of return provide an indication of the required rate of return for an investor in a large public firm. Beyond that, additional risk premiums related to firm size, proportion of debt, and industry conditions and many other possible company-specific risk factors may be appropriate. When valuing a small medical practice, appraisers generally employ required rates of return 15–25% beyond the currently low long-term risk-free rate. However, this rate may vary greatly.

Capitalization of (Excess) Earnings Method

The *excess earnings method* estimates the present value of the medical practice by capitalizing a single representative (normalized) year of economic benefits to the owner, in contrast to a multiple-period discounting method.[*] The three variables on which a capitalization method depends are: (1) projected base level economic income flow; (2) cost of capital; and (3) expected long-term growth

---

[*] "ASA Business Valuation Standards," American Society of Appraisers, 2008, p. 26.

rate.[*] In cases where the anticipated future economic benefits are expected to be unstable, the discounted multiple-period DCF method is more appropriate. In contrast, the single-period capitalization method is useful for entities expecting a stable or relatively even growth in economic benefits.[†]

NET INCOME STATEMENT ADJUSTMENTS

When analyzing a set of financial statements, adjustments are generally needed to produce a clearer picture of likely future income and distributable cash flow. This normalization process usually consists of three types of adjustments to a medical practice's net income (profit and loss) statement.

Nonrecurring Items

Estimates of future distributable cash flow should exclude nonrecurring items. Proceeds from the settlement of litigation, one-time gains/losses from the selling of assets or equipment, and large write-offs that are not expected to reoccur, each of them represent potential nonrecurring items. The impact of nonrecurring events should be removed from the practice's financial statements to produce a clearer picture of likely future income and cash flow.

Perquisites

The buyer of a medical practice may plan to spend more or less than the current doctor–owner for physician executive compensation, travel and entertainment expenses, and other perquisites of the current management. When determining future distributable cash flow, income adjustments to the current level of expenditures should be made for these items.

Noncash Expenses

Depreciation expense, amortization expense, and bad-debt expense are all noncash items that impact reported profitability. When determining distributable cash flow, the link between noncash expenses and expected cash expenditures must be analyzed.

The annual depreciation expense is a proxy for likely capital expenditures over time. When capital expenditures and depreciation are not similar over time, an adjustment to the expected cash flow is necessary. For example, a practice may have radiographic equipment with a useful life of 14 years that are depreciated over 7 years for tax and financial reporting. Depreciation expense will likely overstate the funds needed to maintain the equipment as the useful life exceeds the depreciable life and distributable cash flow. In determining distributable cash flow, one must add back the annual noncash depreciation expense and subtract an estimate of funds needed to fund medical equipment replacement. In this way, the cash flow available for distribution to owners will be more properly stated.

Some practices reduce income through the use of bad-debt expense rather than direct write-offs. Bad-debt expense is a noncash expense that represents an estimate of the dollar volume of write-offs that are likely to occur during a year. If bad-debt expense is understated, practice profitability will be overstated. A close examination of accounts receivable to see if any past due accounts need to be written off is generally part of the due diligence a buyer of a practice will undertake. The calculation of distributable cash flow avoids this problem as the actual monies received from patients, and payers, rather than the revenue generated by patients is measured.

BALANCE SHEET ADJUSTMENTS

Adjustments can also be made to a practice's balance sheet to remove nonoperating assets and liabilities and to restate asset and liability value at market rates, rather than cost rates. Assets and

---

[*] "Valuing a Business," by Shannon P. Pratt and Alina V. Niculita, New York: McGraw-Hill, 2008, 5th ed., p. 256.

[†] "Valuing a Business," by Shannon P. Pratt and Alina V. Niculita, New York: McGraw-Hill, 2008, 5th ed., pp. 244–245.

liabilities that are unrelated to the core practice being valued should be added to or subtracted from the value depending on whether they are acquired by the buyer.

Examples include the asset value less outstanding debt of a vacant parcel of land and marketable securities that are not needed to operate the practice. Other nonoperating assets such as the cash surrender value of officer life insurance are generally liquidated by the seller and are not part of the business transaction.

Thus, the capitalization of earnings method can provide a reasonable estimate of practice value in situations where limited information is available, or when the practice is likely to maintain stable cash flows. The main advantage of this method is it does not require assumptions regarding future forecasted operations for the medical practice.

MARKET TRANSACTION APPROACH

The market transaction method is a useful gauge in setting a valuation bottom and top range for comparison with the income approach. Market multiples are ratios developed by correlating market sale prices of guideline practices to key practice performance measurements. Common physician practice market multiples include comparisons of sale price to revenues, sale price to earnings before interest and taxes (EBITs), sale price to earnings before interest, taxes, depreciation and amortization (EBITDA), and sale price to the number of physicians.

Market-transaction multiples are typically limited to serving as a benchmark for testing the reasonableness of the income approach. To apply the market approach, information on the guideline practices such as size of practice, specialty, number of physicians, growth potential, cost structure, payer mix, and profitability are necessary for determining comparability to the medical practice being valued. Often, information concerning transaction specifics and practice particulars is either insufficient or not available for direct comparison with the practice being valued.

ASSET/COST APPROACH

The asset/cost approach to estimating value calls for the identification and separate valuation of all the practice assets, including goodwill. Also referred to as "Accumulation of the Assets," this approach is more labor intensive and costly than using the business enterprise analysis to estimate practice value. Generally, this approach is not very useful for estimating going-concern value.

Although rarely used to estimate going-concern value, another cost approach method may be used to estimate the costs that would be incurred to start-up a medical practice and develop to the current level of practice operations. The costs of establishing a new medical practice typically include the expenses involved in the recruitment of physicians, acquisition of space, office furnishings, patient treatment equipment, computer software, and medical records; advertising for staff; and losses incurred during the start-up period.

This estimate of "replacement cost or cost avoidance" value represents an upper limit (or ceiling) of value. It has limited use as an accounting artifice, and no prudent buyer would pay for an existing medical practice a price equivalent to what it would cost to build and develop a new medical practice.

The most appropriate application of the cost approach involves the valuation of medical practice tangible assets. However, valuing only the tangible assets used in a profitable, medical practice is not representative of the business value of the company. Since the intangible assets typically represent a significant portion of practice value, the cost approach is generally not considered useful in estimating the value of a going-concern medical practice.

UNDERSTANDING CORPORATE DEALS STRUCTURE

Corporate deal structures often acquire substantially all of a medical practice's assets, excluding the working capital, and then enter into employment agreements with its physicians, which is becoming increasingly more common. In this scenario, the selling physician is left with the accounts receivable, cash, and the practice liabilities. Most of these asset purchases are cash deals. When the sale price is based on an enterprise value, this usually provides the physician with the ability to settle the practice debt.

STOCK PURCHASE VERSUS ASSET PURCHASE

There will be some variation in appraisal methods dependent on whether the transaction is structured as a stock purchase or an asset purchase. Owing to corporate practice of medicine laws in some states and desires of buyers not to assume practice liabilities, most practice acquisitions are structured as asset purchases. In an asset transaction, the buyer will receive a tax amortization benefit associated with the intangible value of the business. This tax amortization represents a noncash expense benefiting the buyer. In this case, the present value of those future tax benefits *is additive* to the business enterprise value.

RESTRICTIVE COVENANT VALUE IS GOODWILL

Restrictive covenants for physicians usually involve covenants-not-to-compete related to the sale of a medical practice or other assets. The value of covenant-not-to-compete lies in the protection it affords the buyer from potential loss of income due to competition from the selling physicians.

To estimate the value of a covenant-not-to-compete, the income approach is considered to be the most appropriate method. The cost to secure the agreement is irrelevant to the value of the protection afforded the buyer. The sales comparison approach requires sales of similar or like assets; because each medical practice is unique and public data are unavailable for transactions of the physician's noncompete agreements, the sales comparison approach is not useful. Generally, an income approach includes the value associated with a noncompete agreement as part of the intangible asset value. As such, the noncompete agreement value is not additive to your business enterprise practice value. Instead, it is a component of practice goodwill, which can be separately valued if desired.

BUYER MISTAKES ("CAVEAT EMPTOR")

Significant federal funding has been provided targeting physician transactions with penalties potentially imposed on both the physician and individuals in the acquiring organizations. Recently, there were several Federal investigations of for-profit hospital systems alleging those systems deliberately overpaid for physician practices as inducement to receive patient referrals (a violation of the anti-kickback statute). When selling your practice, beware of the following buyer blunders:

- *Overpaying physician practice value.* Some buyers obtain a business enterprise value, and will also obtain separate values for the medical equipment and noncompetition agreements. These values can be useful in allocating the overall purchase price. The business enterprise value, however, represents an estimate for a 100% ownership interest in the medical practice. The separate values for the assets are not added to the business enterprise value, but rather are components of the total value of the business. Some buyers have overpaid for physician practices by adding these separate asset values to the overall business enterprise value to determine the sale price. Not-understanding values can be misconstrued as overpaying in exchange for patient referrals.
- *Overpaying for physician compensation.* Industry surveys have reported that more than 75% of practices acquired fall short of projected productivity used in the valuation (Mergerstat Review Study). This fact coupled with exposure to IRS audit and intermediate

sanctions has increased the need to value practices based on reasonable appropriate projections of practice collections and market rates for physician compensation.

- *Not buying life insurance on the physician.* Much of the value to an investor rests with the physician's skill and talent to remain with the practice after acquisition. The buyer expects to achieve a return on the investment in the medical practice based on future cash flows and to eventually recoup the purchase price. Since most practice acquisitions are cash deals, the buyer is at significant financial risk due to a business interruption associated with an unexpected loss of life or permanent disability.

FINDING QUALIFIED VALUATION PROFESSIONALS

One landmark case in the business-valuation industry was *The Estate of Edgar A. Berg v Commissioner* (T. C. Memo, 1991–279). The court criticized its two CPAs for not being qualified and for failing to provide an analysis of the appropriate discount. The court observed that both CPAs made only general references to a prior court decision to justify their opinion of value. In rejecting the CPAs, the court accepted the IRS's expert because of his advanced education and demonstration of the discounting process.

This case marked the beginning of the tax court's tendency to lean toward the side with the most comprehensive appraisal. Previously, it had a tendency to split the difference. Some experts think that the Berg case launched the business-valuation profession. Since the Berg case, the corpus of knowledge for the valuation profession has grown exponentially. Valuation professionals include those with advanced degrees and designations by professional accrediting bodies.

Therefore, hire local or regional professionals with publishing, teaching, or academic experience—not commissioned agents. Medical specificity is paramount. Physician valuators with experience and deep subject-matter expertise are ideal. But finding a qualified medical practice appraiser is not always an easy task in a health-care environment with increasing levels of state and federal scrutiny regarding transactions and compensation related to medical practices. So, consider the following guidelines:

- Make sure appraisers use generally accepted IRS methods and have a proven track record with the government for medical appraisals.
- Make sure the valuation is written, substantiates medical practice value, provides detail to support conclusions, and is signed by the appraiser.
- Avoid conflict of interest or self-dealings. Seek an unbiased and independent viewpoint.
- Make sure the appraiser will qualify as an expert witness and is presentable on the witness stand, if needed.
- Request references and examples for previous medical practice appraisals.
- Inquire about experience in publishing, speaking, and teaching medical practice valuations techniques.

Organizations that accredit business appraisers (but not necessarily medical practice appraisers), include

- Health Capital Consultants, LLC. HCC specializes in health-care valuation, litigation support and expert testimony, financial analysis, and industry research services for hospitals and medical practices (www.HealthCapital.com) 1-800 FYI VALU.
- American Society of Appraisers (www.appraisers.org) offers their ASA designation for business appraisers.
- American Institute of Certified Public Accountants (www.aicpa.org) provides the accredited business valuation (ABV) only for CPAs.

- Institute of Business Appraisers (www.go-iba.org) awards the designations of certified business appraiser (CBA), Master-certified business appraiser (MCBA), and business valuators accredited in valuation (BVAL).
- National Association of Certified Valuation Analysts (CVAs) (www.nacva.com), awarding the designations of CVA, accredited valuation analyst (AVA), and certified forensic financial analyst (CFA).
- Fellow Royal Intuition of Chartered Surveyors (FRICS—Royal Institute of Chartered Surveyors); and certified merger and acquisition advisor (CM&AA—Alliance of merger and acquisition advisors).
- Institute of Medical Business Advisors, Inc; Atlanta, Georgia, 770-448-0769. Contact: Ann Miller RN MHA.

Since some appraisers feel that certain organizations set the bar for certification significantly higher than others, and the NACVA website at http://www.nacva.com offers a comparison of the accreditation criteria required by all four major organizations.

HOW MUCH MONEY IS A MEDICAL PRACTICE REALLY WORTH?

Now that you have a background of what factors influence value, the needs for valuation, a general understanding of appraisal theory and how industry regulations impact value, the valuation process, and methodologies employed, we get to the heart of the matter.

UNDERSTANDING VALUE

Understanding value is crucial to a successful negotiation. Both buyers and sellers too often misinterpret the value conclusions of appraisers straining buyer/seller relationships and unnecessarily jeopardizing deals.

HOW TO MAXIMIZE MEDICAL PRACTICE VALUE

There are a few critical areas you can review for opportunities to maximize your practice value. For example, use the DCF method to estimate practice value. This method consistently produces higher values than others, but recall the USPAP edicts.

Practice Revenue

- Can the practice and local market support adding additional providers such as physicians or mid-level providers? Providers usually take 2–3 years to ramp up their practice before they begin to significantly contribute to the bottom line. Generally, adding a mid-level provider will produce a greater impact to the value, as their compensation levels are lower than physicians.
- What future provider productivity is expected?
- Does the practice plan to offer new services?
- Is the current practice fee schedule at market rates? Is there an opportunity for fee increases?
- Is there an opportunity to improve payer mix?

Review Practice Costs

- Eliminate any unnecessary practice expenses. Identify any unusual, nonrecurring costs.
- Eliminate any physician-related costs not likely to be paid by a buyer.
- Eliminate any special perks of business ownership.
- Adjust for any overinflated salaries of relatives and eliminate any unnecessary salaries.

Physician Compensation Inverse Relationship to Value

- Although physician compensation must be based on market rates, fair market value is a range. Practice value directly correlates with the net cash flows available after all practice expenses including physician compensation. As a consequence, the higher the compensation, the lower the practice value, and conversely, the lower the compensation, the higher the practice value. As little as a $10,000 swing in salary can have a significant impact on value, and as physician compensation rises, practice value falls.

COMPLETING THE TRANSACTION

Depending on whether the likely buyer is a health system or a corporate partner, the deal structures will vary. From the physician's perspective, deal negotiations are based on consideration of personal and financial planning goals. Some of the key negotiations considered in the "art of the deal" include the following.

WORKING CAPITAL: IN OR OUT

Including working capital in the transaction will increase the sale price.

STOCK VERSUS ASSET TRANSACTION

Structuring the deal as an asset purchase will increase practice value due to the tax amortization benefits received by the buyer for intangible assets of the practice.

COMMON STOCK PREMIUM

The total sale price can be significantly higher than a cash-equivalent price for accepting the risk and relative illiquidity of the common stock as part of the payment.

PHYSICIAN COMPENSATION

If your personal financing planning goals are to maximize practice value, negotiating a lower salary within a range you feel comfortable with will increase the sale price.

UNDERSTANDING PRIVATE DEAL STRUCTURES

Now, assuming a practice sale is a private transaction, deal negotiations are based on the following discount and premium pricing methodologies, as presented below.

SELLER FINANCING

Many transactions involve an earn-out arrangement where the buyer puts money down and pays the balance under a formula based on future revenues, or gives the seller a promissory note under similar terms. Seller financing decreases a buyer's risks; the longer the terms, the lower the risk. Longer terms demand premiums, while shorter terms demand discounts. Premiums that buyers pay for a typical seller-financed practice are usually more than what you would expect from a simple time value of money calculation, as a result of buyer risk reduction from paying over time, rather than up front with a bank loan, or all cash.

DOWN PAYMENT

The greater the amount of the down payment for acquisition of a medical practice, the greater the risk is to the buyer. Consequently, sellers who will take less money up front can command a higher-than-average price for their practice, while sellers who want more down usually receive less in the end.

SELLER INVOLVEMENT

The key to practice purchase success boils down to how many of the selling doctor's patients and managed-care contracts can be transferred to the new doctor/owner. The most important factor in transitioning patients is the involvement of the selling doctor. The system of seller financing and earn-out arrangements can work well if the seller continues to be involved in the practice, and can create an incentive for the seller to make the transaction work. Sellers typically remain at least for 6 months, and usually for not more than a year, to ensure a seamless transaction. When a deal fails, it is usually due to lack of seller commitment.

LOCATION

Variations can be significant between the value of a practice in a major metropolitan city and one in a small town. Usually, practices in a small town have a larger, but less-affluent basis. Managed-care penetration is another factor to consider.

PROFIT MARGIN

Determining medical practice profitability is distinctly different from determining a practice's value. It is not unusual for selling doctors to run every expense imaginable through their practices, to reduce profit and hence, taxes. In many cases, however, a practice with high overhead can be sold for the same price as one with low overhead, because all expenses are not transferable.

TAXATION

Tax consequences can have a major impact on the price of a medical practice. For instance, a seller who obtains the majority of the sales price as capital gains can often afford to sell for a much lower price, and still pocket as much or more than if the sales price was paid as ordinary income. Value attributed to the seller's patient list, medical records, name brand, goodwill, and files qualify for capital gains treatment. Both the value paid for the selling doctor's continuing assistance after the sale and value attributed to a noncompete agreement are taxed at ordinary income. But, a buyer willing to allocate more for items with capital gains treatment, or a seller willing to take more in ordinary income, can frequently negotiate a better price.

AN ALTERNATE ASSET CLASS SURROGATE?

A medical practice is much like an AI, or alternate investment asset class in two respects. First, it provides the work environment that generates personal income that has been considered generous to date. Second, it has inherent appreciation and sales value that can be part of an exit (retirement) or succession-planning transfer strategy. So, unlike the emerging thought that offers Social Security payments as a surrogate for asset classes, or a federally insured AAA bond—a medical practice might also be considered by some as an asset class within a well-diversified modern investment portfolio.

ASSESSMENT

Do you think that considering Social Security or a medical practice as an asset class is too innovative for comfort? Well, some experts think that life insurance should also be considered as an asset class.

Why? The death benefits and steady growth of cash value over the years can improve an overall portfolio's risk-adjusted rate of return when combined with bond values. So, at the very least, when you design a portfolio by market capitalization and investment style, be sure to consider the cash value and death benefits of any existing life insurance policies.

CONCLUSION

This chapter described a modern model of medical practice valuation and mirrors how a typical practice would be inspected. Basically, with financial statements after mathematical spreadsheets, heuristics, industry market forces, and due diligence is performed. But, often, it is not easy; so, a price range with reasonable floor and ceiling is the usual result.

But, going forward in the era of patient centricity, valuation will be as much of an art as an economic science. Such information is becoming just one small piece of the puzzle and may not reflect the future definition of "value" at all. To be successful, a "new normal" based on value, outcomes, and patient satisfaction may be required, regardless of sales impetus or valuation methodology. And so, the next step in the process is just good old-fashioned negotiation.

Thereafter, it is left up to the informed new-era practitioner and/or his/her advisor to decide if a medical practice is considered an asset class or not. And then, how to invest the proceeds.

COLLABORATE

Discuss this chapter online with others at www.MedicalExecutivePost.com.

ACKNOWLEDGMENTS

To Bridget Bourgeois, CPA, CVA, partner at Ernst & Young Atlanta, Georgia, former medical practice valuation specialist from the American Appraisers Association, and member of the Global Pharma Congress; and to Robert James Cimasi, MHA, ASA, FRICS, MCBA, CVA, CM&AA, and CMP™ of Health Capital Consultants LLC, St. Louis, Missouri.

FURTHER READING

Bourgeois, B: Medical practice valuation and appraisal techniques. In, Marcinko DE [Editor]: *Business of Medical Practice*. Springer Publishing, New York, 2000.

Cimasi, RJ: *Healthcare Valuation—The Financial Appraisal of Enterprises, Assets, and Services*. Wiley, New York, 2014.

Cimasi, RJ: The role of the healthcare consultant. In, *ACOs [Value Metrics and Capital Formation]*. CRC and Productivity Press, New York, 2014.

Cimasi, RJ: Valuation of hospitals in a changing reimbursement and regulatory environment. In, Marcinko DE and Hetico, HR [Editors]: *Healthcare Organizations [Financial Management Strategies]*. iMBA Inc., Atlanta, GA, 2010.

Cimasi, RJ: Valuing specific assets in divorce. In, Robert D. Feder, Esq [Editors]: *Medical Practice Valuation in Divorce*. Aspen Law and Business, New York, 2000.

Lavine, A: *Life Insurance as an Asset Class*. Wealth Management, New York, April 15, 2014.

Marcinko, DE: Appraising a practice [The art of the deal for buyers and sellers—Parts I, II and III]. *Humana's Your Practice*. Louisville, KT, 2007.

Marcinko, DE: *Getting It Right: How Much Is a Plastic Surgery Practice Really Worth?* Plastic Surgery Practice, August 2006.

Marcinko, DE and Hetico, HR: *Dictionary of Health Economics and Finance*. Springer Publishing, New York, 2007.

Marcinko, DE and Hetico, HR: *Key Principles for Assessing Practice Value*. Podiatry Today, 2008.

Marcinko, DE and Hetico, HR: The science and art of medical practice valuation [Understanding fair market value]. In, *Business of Medical Practice*. Springer Publishing, New York, 2010.

Zack, GM: *Fair Value Accounting Fraud*. Wiley, New York, 2009.

18 Retirement Planning Practices
Transitioning to the End of Your Medical Career

Shikha Mittra and Alexander M. Kimura

CONTENTS

With the PP-ACA, increased compliance regulations, and higher tax rates, physicians are more concerned about their retirement and retirement planning than ever before, and with good reason. After payroll taxes, dividend taxes, limited itemized deductions, the new 3.8% surtax on net investment income, and an extra 0.9% Medicare tax, for every dollar earned by a high-earning physician, almost 50 cents can go to taxes!

Retirement planning is not about cherry-picking the best stocks or mutual funds or how to beat the short-term fluctuations in the market. It's disciplined long-term strategy based on scientific evidence and a prudent process. You increase the probability of success by following this process and monitoring on a regular basis to make sure you are on track.

INTRODUCTION

According to a survey by the Employee Benefit Research Institute (EBRI) and Greenwald & Associates, nearly half of workers without a retirement plan were not at all confident in their financial security, compared to 11% for those who participated in a plan, according to the 2014 Retirement Confidence Survey (RCS).

In addition, 35% of workers have not saved any money for retirement, while only 57% are actively saving for retirement. Thirty-six percent of workers said the total value of their savings and investments—not including the value of their home and defined benefit plan (DBP)—was less than $1000, up from 29% in the 2013 survey. But, when adjusted for those without a formal retirement plan, 73% have saved less than $1000.

Debt is also a concern, with 20% of workers saying they have a major problem with debt. Thirty-eight percent indicate they have a minor problem with debt. And, only 44% of workers said they or their spouse have tried to calculate how much money they'll need to save for retirement. But those who have done the calculation tend to save more.

The biggest shift in the last 24 years has been the number of workers who plan to work later in life. In 1991, 84% of workers indicated they plan to retire by age 65, versus only 9% who planned to work until at least age 70. In 2014, 50% plan on retiring by age 65; with 22% planning to work until they reach 70.

PHYSICIAN STATISTICS

Now, compare and contrast the above to these statistics according to a 2013 survey of physicians on financial preparedness by American Medical Association (AMA) Insurance. The statistics are still alarming:

- The top personal financial concern for all physicians is having enough money to retire.
- Only 6% of physicians consider themselves ahead of schedule in retirement preparedness.
- Nearly half feel they were behind.
- 41% of physicians average less than $500,000 in retirement savings.
- Nearly 70% of physicians don't have a long-term care plan.
- Only half of the U.S. physicians have a completed estate plan, including an updated will and medical directives.*

---

* www.AMAInsurance.com.

And so, this chapter will help make your golden years comfortable and worry free. It will discuss steps you can take to ensure the kind of retirement you look forward to and envision, not something to dread! The information is organized to provide answers to 10 important questions:

1. How much money do you need to retire?
2. What is your retirement cash flow?
3. What is your retirement vision?
4. How to stay on retirement track?
5. How to maximize retirement plan contributions such as 401(k) or 403(b)?
6. How to maximize retirement income from retirement plans?
7. What are some other retirement plan savings options?
8. What is your retirement plan and investing style?
9. What is the role of social security in retirement planning?
10. How to integrate retirement with estate planning?

HOW MUCH MONEY DO YOU NEED TO RETIRE?

One of the most critical steps for your future is to create a personal retirement cash flow plan to help you to know how much you need and how to get there. The cash flow planning process determines whether or not what you're currently doing will be adequate, helps you make informed decisions, points out areas that need improvement, and then tests those decisions to see if the plan is likely to work. While no one knows the future, a plan that's monitored and adjusted as time passes is the single most important step to take if you're in your mid- or late career.

PLANNING ISSUES: EARLY CAREER

Doing long-term projections early in your career will have the highest degree of inaccuracy, since there are many unknown factors to be considered. Projecting income increases, retirement expenses, savings, and other critical items would be very difficult without any history to base this on. The most important steps to be taken are

1. Live beneath your means. This is the primary reason "The Millionaire Next Door" has accumulated wealth, according to Tom Stanley's popular book. The real cost of an expensive lifestyle is the lost opportunity for your money to compound. For example, having a car payment of $250 per month instead of $500 per month means an extra $500,000 of retirement age savings over 30 years, assuming 10% annual returns.
2. Be an informed and prudent investor, since the compounding of your money over time accelerates the benefits of higher rates of return. In the example above, having a 7% return instead of a 10% return would cost you over $200,000!
3. Save as much as possible in your 401(k), 403(b) or other plan. Maximizing this benefit can literally create millions in retirement savings, and is critical for a comfortable retirement. For example, saving $2000 per year from age 22 to age 29 (8 years) and making no additional contributions, you'd have over $399,000 at age 60 (assuming 10% growth.) If you wait until age 30, then contribute $2000 every year until age 60 (30 years), you would have only $328,000! If you save $3000 per year from age 22 through age 60, you would have over $1,000,000!
4. Plan early for your children's college expenses, setting aside money in tax-efficient investments for their future. This prevents having to choose between retirement for you and college education for your children. Plans like 529 plans help save for educational expenses.

PLANNING ISSUES: MID-CAREER

1. This is the time to begin planning in earnest. Perform an in-depth retirement cash flow plan now, so you can make informed choices about your finances. **Note:** For a "snapshot" view of your retirement progress, consider doing a simple exercise. You might multiply all nonbusiness expenses per year times 20, which gives you an idea of the total investment assets you should have accumulated. Remember, this isn't a substitute for planning, since it ignores many other important factors.
2. Look at your savings and investments more critically since the development of an investment strategy becomes more important as you accumulate wealth. In particular, you need to have effective planning strategies for maximizing the after-tax returns on the investments outside of a retirement plan.
3. Implement your plan. Doing the analysis without taking action is like diagnosing cancer without treating it.

PLANNING ISSUES: LATE CAREER

1. If you haven't already done so, it's critically important to do your retirement cash flow planning now. Without planning, you're making decisions in a vacuum that may mean a severely restricted lifestyle later.
2. This is also the time to plan for the sale or succession of your medical practice. There are steps to be taken which can significantly enhance your benefits, but these often take a few years to provide meaningful results.
3. This may be the time to consider long-term care insurance (LTCI), depending on your financial situation. A good insurance agent or financial planner can help guide you on the appropriateness of this insurance since it may be questionable in many cases.
4. It's important to integrate both your estate and retirement planning, since the steps you take for one dramatically affect the other. For example, making gifts to your children may be prudent estate planning but terrible retirement advice, depending on your particular situation.
5. It's equally important to check beneficiary designations of your retirement plans as well and other investments, to make sure they are consistent with your estate planning objectives.

WHAT IS YOUR RETIREMENT CASH FLOW PLAN?

A retirement cash flow plan is a year-by-year analysis of how all your likely decisions will impact your finances. The result of planning is to learn if what you're doing will work, and how much money you should have accumulated at any time. You will need to know how your income stacks against your expenses; how your discretionary income is the starting point for saving for your retirement; how your time frame, risk tolerance, and amount of annual savings will determine if you will be able to achieve your retirement goal based on the assumptions made. Remember that time is your biggest friend.

WHAT NEEDS TO BE CONSIDERED IN A RETIREMENT CASH FLOW PLAN?

Income Sources

1. Your current balances in retirement accounts like individual retirement account's (IRA's) or 401(k) or 403(b) plans and the contributions you're making to your retirement and non-retirement accounts each year, with inflation increases as appropriate.
2. Savings and investments outside of your retirement plans, if this will be available for your retirement.

3. Income during retirement from part-time work or consulting, with any increases for inflation.
4. Other sources of retirement income, such as pensions or social security.
5. Installment payments from the sale of your practice, if any.
6. Rental property income, if you plan on keeping the property. Will there be annual increases?
7. Income from a reverse mortgage, if appropriate.
8. Any deferred compensation payments.

Other Sources of One-Time-Only Retirement Income
1. Expected proceeds from the sale of your home, less the cost of your new home and any taxes due. Will you pay cash or finance this home?
2. Any inheritances you expect.
3. After-tax cash from the sale of rental property.
4. After-tax cash from the sale of a medical practice.

Your Expenses

Fixed Expenses
1. Mortgage expenses, until the debt is paid off. If you've refinanced every few years in the past, thereby extending your mortgage term, will this continue?
2. Car payments, if any, including replacements as appropriate.
3. Insurance payments.
4. Loan payments.

Variable Expenses
1. Expected taxes when withdrawing money from your retirement accounts.
2. Likely cost of living, based on the retirement lifestyle you want, not on some "rule of thumb." If planning to move to another state, incorporate that as well.
3. The cost of supporting a parent or disabled child, or a boomerang child, if likely.

Significant One-Time Expenses
1. The payment of major debts, such as your mortgage.
2. The costs of educating your children or grandchildren, since this may occur at the same time as you begin retirement.
3. Other lump sum expenses, such as for weddings or buying a second home.
4. Major medical expenses such as dental work or out of pocket costs for a hospital stay or service that is not covered by insurance.

Planning Assumptions

1. *Retirement time period:* With medical advancement and healthy lifestyle, we may have a longer life span in retirement than in our working years. So, it is important to take longevity into consideration when designing a retirement portfolio. Your life expectancy and that of your spouse (if appropriate.) If your family has consistently lived to be 100, don't plan on dying at 78.
2. *Inflation rate:* The overall inflation rate you expect. The longer time you have before and during retirement, the more inflation will impact your buying power.
3. *Costs of living adjustments in retirement income*: Your pension and social security may have COLA (costs of living adjustments) to keep up with inflation. (Currently, the average social security rate is 2.8%). COLA will be based on where you live.
4. *Investment returns*: The expected long-term return on your retirement portfolio, and the after-tax return of your other accounts. Realistic projections have to be based on long-term

history, which shows stock market returns of about 9–10% and bonds at approximately 4–5%. The returns might be modified if academic research indicates lower or higher returns are likely.

5. *Withdrawal rates*: The rate of withdrawal from your portfolio in retirement.
6. *Medical expenses in retirement*: Unforeseen medical expenses.
7. Your other unexpected expenses that will start in retirement.
8. *Tax rates*: No one can predict the future tax rates.
9. Availability of social security and Medicare.

Estate Planning

As tax laws change, it is very important to review your estate planning needs. With increased exemption and gift limits, you need to make sure the current estate plan is meeting your objectives.

- How much you want to leave to your heirs or other beneficiaries can affect your required rate of return. Over many years, the compounding of even a 1% difference in return can make a huge difference.
- The cost of making gifts to your children and grandchildren.
- The cost of funding life insurance policies for your heirs.

DETERMINING RETIREMENT VISION

There's an aspect to retirement that many physicians do not plan for … the transition from work and practice to retirement. Your work has been an important part of your life. That's why the emotional adjustments of retirement may be some of the most difficult ones.

For example, what would you like to do in retirement? Your retirement vision will be unique to you. You are retiring to something, not from something that you envisioned. When you have more time, would you like to do more traveling, play golf, or visit family and friends more often? Would you relocate closer to your kids? Learn a new art or take a new class? Fund your grandchildren's education? Do you have philanthropic goals? Perhaps you would like to help your church, school, or favorite charity? If your net worth is above certain limits, it would be wise to take a serious look at these goals. With proper planning, there might be some tax benefits too. Then you have to figure how much each goal is going to cost you.

If you have a list of retirement goals, you need to prioritize which goal is most important. You can rate them on a scale of 1–10, 10 being the most important. Then, you can differentiate between wants and needs. Needs are things that are absolutely necessary for you to retire, while wants are things that still allow retirement but would just be nice to have.

Recent studies indicate there are three phases in retirement, each with a different spending pattern (Richard Greenberg, CFP®, Gardena, CA, personal communication). The three phases are

1. *The early retirement years.* There is a pent-up demand to take advantage of all the free time retirement affords. You can travel to exotic places, buy an RV and explore 49 states, or go on month-long sailing vacations. It's possible during these initial years that after-tax expenses increase, especially if the mortgage hasn't been paid off yet. Usually, the early years last about 10 years until most retirees are in their 70s.
2. *Middle years.* People decide to slow down on the exploration. This is when people start simplifying their life. They may sell their house and downsize to a condo or townhouse. They may relocate to an area they discovered during their travels, or to an area close to family and friends, to an area with a warm climate or to an area with low or no state taxes. People also do their most important estate planning during these years. They are concerned about leaving a legacy, taking care of their children and grandchildren, and

fulfilling charitable intent. This is a time when people spend more time in the local area. They may start taking extension or college classes. They spend more time volunteering at various nonprofits and helping out older and less healthy retirees. People often spend less during these years. This period starts when a retiree is in his or her mid to late 70s and can last up to 10 years, usually mid to late 80s.

3. *Late years.* This is when you may need assistance in your daily activities. You may receive care at home, in a nursing home, or an assisted-care facility. Most of the care options are very expensive. It's possible that these years might be more expensive than your preretirement expenses. This is especially true if both spouses need some sort of assisted care. This period usually starts when the retiree is in their 80s; however, they can sometimes start in the mid to late 70s.

Planning Issues: Early Career

Most retirement lifestyle issues do not have to be addressed at this point. Keeping a healthy, balanced lifestyle will help to ensure a more productive retirement. This is the time to focus on the financial aspects of retirement planning.

Planning Issues: Mid-Career

If early retirement is a major objective, start thinking about activities that will fill up your time during retirement. Maintaining your health is more critical, since your health habits at this time will often dictate how healthy you will be in retirement.

Planning Issues: Late Career

Three to five years before you retire, start making the transition from work to retirement:

- Try out different hobbies.
- Find activities that will give you a purpose in retirement.
- Establish friendships outside of the office or hospital.
- Discuss retirement plans with your spouse.
- If you plan to relocate to a new place, it is important to rent a place in that area and stay for few months and see if you like it. Making a drastic change like relocating and then finding you don't like the new town or state might be a very costly mistake. The key is to gradually make the transition.

STAYING ON TRACK

Developing a comprehensive plan that addresses different areas such as cash flow, insurance, investment, taxes, retirement, and estate with different retirement scenarios, such as best, worst, and moderate returns and how that impacts your retirement vision, will keep things in perspective. It gives a clear picture of your starting point, where you are in the retirement path at any given time, and how far you are from reaching your retirement vision. This is a blueprint that prevents you from getting lost or getting side tracked. To most physicians and medical professionals, needing millions of dollars in the future seems overwhelming, so breaking up your goals into small steps will make the task easier.

Planning Issues: Early Career

1. Use annual targets as a guide to your final objective at retirement.
2. Rebalance your portfolio whenever percentages drift significantly from your initial plan.
3. Revise and refine your analysis every few years as your objectives change.

Planning Issues: Mid-Career

1. Continue following the steps in early career.
2. Understand your assumptions more clearly.
3. Start to integrate your estate and charitable goals with your retirement plan.

Planning Issues: Late Career

1. You should be very comfortable with your retirement assumptions.
2. Understand how your estate and charitable intent influences your withdrawal rate.

Decide on a withdrawal rate that you are comfortable with and that incorporates your other sources of income.

Monitoring Your Progress

What If You're Behind Your Target for the Year?

If none of your assumptions have changed and you feel that you can make up the difference in the next year, you probably can use the same retirement cash flow plan. As a rule of thumb, if you're less than 10% off of your goal, you may not need to do anything. If you fall so far behind that each year's target seems unachievable, you will probably need to make some changes. However, before you change your planning, you need to see why you're behind.

If you haven't saved as much as you expected, take a look at your expenses and see where you can cut down. Remember, you need to pay yourself first before you spend on luxuries. Contribute as much as possible to your qualified retirement plan (QRP) at work.

Next, you need to look at your investment returns. Since the stock market has been in one of its inevitable "bull markets" for the past several years (since the 2008 crash), this can significantly impact your balances. Remember, your return assumptions are based on averages that should include the bad and good years. If you're close to retirement and have a large shortfall, you need to either postpone retirement by working few more years or save more to get back on track or cut down on your expenses in retirement. It is rarely a good idea to increase risk at this stage.

What If You're Ahead of Your Annual Goal?

Again, if the difference may be eliminated the next year, you probably don't want to make any changes.

If you're more than 20% ahead of your goal, you can either decrease the risk in your portfolio or change the planning. For example, you might decide to retire earlier, increase your retirement income, or fund another goal that was important to you such as paying for LTCI or pay off your debts.

Planning note: If you are working with a financial advisor, s/he may want to link your annual objective to the volatility of the portfolio developed for you using standard deviation as the measure of volatility. The advisor might suggest alternative actions if your results varied by more than two standard deviations, which indicates that you're probably outside of the expected range of results for your long-term plan.

How Should I Be Monitoring My Investments?

In addition to tracking whether you are close to your annual goal, you will want to make sure that your asset allocation percentages remain close to your plan. Whenever the percentages are significantly different than your plan, you will want to rebalance your portfolio (buy or sell your investments to bring them more in line).

Many times investors put more funds into sectors that are doing very well and take funds out of sectors that are doing poorly. This is the wrong thing to do because you might be making your portfolio more risky by exposing it to more variability or fluctuations. A properly diversified portfolio consists of negatively correlated assets with allocations based on risk tolerance, time frame, and investment objectives.

If your investments are in a taxable account, you can use new purchases to buy those areas that are underrepresented, rather than incurring taxes by selling the areas that represent too high a percentage of your portfolio.

The American Tax Relief Act of 2012 (ATRA) and the healthcare bill have raised the qualified dividend rates for high-income earners from 15% to 20%. A planning strategy would be for high-earning physicians to reduce their exposure to dividend paying stocks in their taxable accounts to capital appreciation.

What Is a Safe Withdrawal Rate from Retirement Assets?

An additional variable in staying on track after retirement is your withdrawal rate or the amount you take out of your accounts each year. Most people want to have a steady income, similar to the paycheck they received while they worked.

Most retirement analyses assume a certain inflation rate and assume your accounts go up a fixed percentage each year. Unfortunately, the stock market and inflation differs year to year. Therefore, high withdrawal rates can reduce your retirement assets and eat into your principal when the market is down, requiring you to decrease spending. You have several choices in selecting a safe withdrawal rate. You can choose the following:

1. Decide to minimize the amount of withdrawal while maintaining a high probability of not running out of money. You will invest for total return and may spend some of the principal.
2. Decide to live on only the income generated from the portfolio. The focus is on investment yield and not on total return.
3. Keep one to 2 year's worth of expenses in cash. This will prevent short-term market fluctuations having a severe effect on your portfolio and your withdrawal (Dr. David Edward Marcinko, MBA, CMP™, Atlanta, GA, personal communication).

The 4% Rule of Thumb

In 1994, William P. Bengen, CFP®, published an article on the optimal rate of withdrawal for retirees not to outlive their retirement portfolio. He suggested a 4% withdrawal rate, for a 30-year retirement, from a portfolio made of 50% bonds and 50% stocks. He used historical performance for his withdrawal strategy. Since then, however, this withdrawal rate has come under greater scrutiny with lower market returns and different inflation rates.

Why? The three-decade-long bull market in bonds and equities is over and if a "new-normal" prevails—meaning a 4.5% real annualized rate of return on equities and a 1.5% real rate on bonds—then standard wealth accumulation retirement planning rules like Bengen's 4.0 withdrawal rate for retirees and a 15% savings rate for working healthcare professionals won't be adequate.

Similarly, according to Wade Pfau, PhD, professor of retirement income and director of the Macroeconomic Policy Program at the American College in Bryn Mawr, Pennsylvania, the 4% withdrawal rate might not be considered safe when P/E ratios are high and dividend yields are low. So, Anthony Webb, PhD, senior research economist at the Center for Retirement Research at Boston University, suggests using IRS life expectancy tables for taking required minimum distributions (RMDs) by taking life expectancy into account.*

More recently, in 2006, John Guyton and Bill Klinger described a formula for how to adjust withdrawal rates for those who need to dip into a portfolio every year. It had two key rules:

---

* www.MedicalExecutivepost.com.

1. *Capital protection:* If over the course of a year the dollar amount of a withdrawal stays the same, but its percentage in relation to the entire account increases by 20% or more, the physician-client should reduce his or her withdrawal by 10% that year. Say, for example, a doctor makes a 5% withdrawal worth $50,000 in 2008, but in 2009, the same $50,000 is worth 6% of the entire account. He should reduce the year's withdrawal by $5000—10% of the $50,000 withdrawal—for a new withdrawal of $45,000.
2. *The prosperity rule:* The reverse of the first rule. If the dollar amount of a withdrawal stays the same but its percentage in relation to the entire account decreases by 20% or more, the doctor-client can increase his withdrawal by 10% for that year.

They then plugged this formula into a Monte Carlo (what-if scenario) simulation program. They ran a massive number of examples using different hypothetical portfolios to determine the effect of the capital protection and prosperity rules over the course of 30–40 years. They found that on average using their method, 99% of the original purchasing power of the portfolio was preserved.

However, striving for 99–100% Monte Carlo probability outcomes may be unduly harsh and constraining. In the real world, to assume as a "default" that investors will live well past age 100 (needed to ensure 100% success probabilities) are not appropriate as a baseline. It severely constrains spending when it will not be relevant in virtually all scenarios (by definition), and in practice one rarely see clients who want to plan this way anyway (there are a handful of "longevity-fearers" but they're certainly not the "default") (Mike Kitces, MSFS, CFP®, CLU, RHU, MTax, Reston, VA, personal communication).

Ask your advisor: To reduce your concern over yearly fluctuations, you may want to reserve 1–2 year's expenses in a money market and replenish the cash with the dividends from the retirement assets. Another way to reduce concern over portfolio fluctuations is to have enough bonds to cover your fixed expenses and rely on your stock portfolio to fund your variable expenses.

Another option is to look at fixed income sources such as pension and social security as the base for retirement income and, depending on the gap between your retirement income and expenses, use an immediate annuity to cover that gap.

MAXIMIZING QRP CONTRIBUTIONS

If you are an employee of a hospital or HMO health system, your employer selects the type of retirement plan that will be available for the employees.

The first step as an employee is to understand the type of plan that is available and understand all of its features. The best way to obtain a list of all the features is to look at the summary plan description that is provided by your company. The summary plan description should be updated annually. If the plan description has not been updated for a while and is not comprehensive enough to answer your questions, look at the plan document. Your human resource manager will be able to provide a copy of both the summary plan description and plan document.

Second, find out whether your employee can make salary deferrals into the plan or whether the plan is funded entirely by the employer.

Third, determine if investing decisions are made by the employer or the employee, depending on the kind of plan you have.

If the employer is responsible for all the funding and investment decisions, your responsibility is to understand how the benefits are determined, what is normal retirement age, and what happens if you leave your employer before normal retirement age.

Usually, if it is a defined benefit plan (DBP) the employer makes all the decisions. With a defined contribution plan (DCP), decisions as to where to invest lie solely with the employees. Sometimes, the sponsors may allow participants to choose their own brokerage account for their DCPs. It's a brokerage account option.

If you are responsible for either the investment or funding decisions, you have more influence over your retirement future and should do the following:

1. Perform a retirement analysis.
2. Include the employer contribution in the analysis and understand the impact of changing jobs or vesting.
3. Determine the savings rate and investment return needed to retire comfortably at the desired retirement age.
4. Develop an investment strategy to generate the desired investment return.
5. Understand the various investment options within the qualified plan and implement the investment strategy.
6. Monitor performance to make sure the plan is on target.

How Can I Benefit from an Employer-Sponsored Plan?

Often, your retirement plan is the single most important and effective savings method for retirement planning. If you participate in your employer's plan, or set one up, you receive the following benefits:

1. *Reduce your income taxes.* If you contribute to your employer's retirement plan, those contributions are deducted from your income, so you can reduce your income taxes.
2. *Employer gets a deduction.* If the employer contributes to the plan, the employer can deduct those contributions as an expense.
3. *Defer taxes on your investment earnings.* Usually, when you make money on your investments, you have to pay taxes that year. Within a retirement plan, you do not have to pay taxes on those earnings until you take the money out, which is usually after you turn 59½years old. This is true for your salary deferrals and the employer contributions.
4. *Employer gives you free money.* Often employers contribute to the retirement plans—either matching a portion of the employee's salary deferral or funding the entire employee benefit.
5. *Tax breaks on your retirement distribution.* If you decide to take a lump sum distribution (distribution of your entire balance), and you were born before January 1, 1936, you are allowed to pay taxes as if you received the money over 10 years.
6. *Your plan is portable—have plan will travel.* If you leave your employer, you are often allowed to leave your money in the QRP until retirement age. However, you can also roll-over your balance into an IRA or another QRP without paying taxes.
7. *Your spouse can continue tax deferral.* If you pass away, your spouse is allowed to rollover the account into his or her own IRA or allowed to keep the account in your name.
8. *Extra-strength creditor protection for QRPs.* In 1994, the U.S. Supreme Court held that a participant's interest in a QRP was exempt from the claims of creditors in a bankruptcy proceeding.

What Are the Most Important Features in My Employer's Retirement Plan?

Who Is Eligible to Participate?

When can you start participating in the employer's retirement plan? Generally, QRPs include all employees who are 21 years of age and who have been employed more than 1 year.

Does the Employer Match?

It's important to know if an employer matches your contribution and to what extent. Some employers may match dollar for dollar up to a certain percentage of your income and then a reduced amount such as 50 cents on the dollar up to certain percentage. These are free dollars that helps you save more for your retirement.

What Is Vesting and How Does It Affect Me?

Vesting defines how much you own of your employer's contribution. Employers have vesting schedules so that there is an incentive for an employee to stay at the company. If you're 100% vested, that means you own 100% of the employer contribution. Of course, you own 100% of the money you put into the plan.

There are two types of vesting schedules. First, if the plan has a gradual vesting schedule; you own an increasing portion of the employer's contribution every year you stay with the employer. The gradual vesting schedule cannot exceed 7 years (6 years if the plan has matching contributions). Second, if the plan has a cliff vesting schedule, you don't own any of the employer contribution until you stay with the employer for a certain period of time. The period of time cannot exceed 5 years (3 years if the plan has matching contributions).

Are Loans Available?

Many employers offer loans because employees often will not contribute without this feature. However, loans are not a requirement. The plan must specifically allow for loans. Loans are permitted for all qualified retirement or Section 403(b) plans. However, many DBPs do not allow for them because loans create difficult administrative issues for these types of plans.

Let's say you borrow money from your plan. In reality, you're borrowing money from yourself. The interest that you pay for the loan goes back into your account. However, you can't decide which interest rate you pay yourself. The plan administrator decides the interest rate, which is the current market rate or usually one or two percentage points above the prime rate, or what the banks are currently charging their best customers. The borrowed money is withdrawn from your balance and the return you receive on that borrowed money is based on the interest rate charged for the loan. Now, if the stock market has tremendous returns, you will lose out on those returns.

If your plan offers loans, you can take out a loan for the lesser of the following two amounts:

1. Up to $50,000
2. The greater of
   a. One-half the vested balance or
   b. $10,000

You must pay back the loan within 5 years unless you use the money to purchase your primary residence; in either case, the loan must provide for a fully amortized schedule of payments. You will usually repay the loan through payroll deductions.

If you leave your employment before paying off the loan, in most cases you have to pay it back immediately. If you don't, the loan is considered a premature withdrawal and you will have to pay income taxes on the outstanding balance and a 10% early withdrawal penalty if you are under age 59½.

Withdrawals While Still Working for the Same Employer

What happens if you have an emergency and you absolutely need to take money out of your retirement plan? This is known as an in-service distribution or withdrawal while you're still working for the hospital or healthcare employer who sponsored your retirement plan.

However, not all employer-sponsored retirement plans allow you to have in-service distributions. DBPs and DCPs that work like pensions (such as money purchase plans and target benefit plans) do not allow in-service distributions unless you've reached normal retirement age or early retirement age.

Profit-sharing plans (PSPs) usually allow in-service distributions but most require a hardship as defined by the plan. Most employers are liberal about defining a hardship. There are limits to the amount that can be withdrawn from PSPs. The amount cannot exceed the vested account balance and the vested balance must have been in the plan for at least 2 years.

401(k)s have very strict hardship withdrawal guidelines that must be satisfied before in-service distributions are allowed. According to the IRS, a qualifying hardship is a situation where the need is immediate and will incur a heavy burden and the participant doesn't have other resources easily accessible to satisfy the need. Some of the hardships allowed are

- Medical expenses
- Purchase of a principal residence
- Payment for education expenses for participant, spouse, or dependent
- Payment to prevent eviction or foreclosure on your home
- Funeral or burial expenses for owner, spouse, or dependents (since 2005)
- Expenses for repair or damage to the employee's principal residence that would qualify for casualty deductions under IRC Section 165

WHAT IF I'M THE OWNER? SHOULD I SPONSOR A RETIREMENT PLAN?

You should sponsor an employer-sponsored plan only if it is the best way to achieve your goals. So, we get back to your goals. Now, let's look at the new tax changes that might affect physicians:

- *Fewer deductions:* The deductions for people making more than the threshold are cut off. In 2014, physicians earning more than $305,050 for joint filers, the deductions are completely phased out.
- *Personal exemptions:* Personal exemptions are reduced if income is over a threshold.
- *Marginal tax rates:* Have slightly increased with the top bracket being 39.6%.
- *Capital gains:* The top tax bracket has increased from 15% to 20%.

New Tax Thresholds for Married Filing Jointly in 2014
- Taxable income is $457,600 and above are in 39.6% marginal tax bracket.
- Itemized deductions phased out over $305,050.
- If your adjusted gross income (AGI) is $250,000 or more, you will be subjected to 3.8% Medicare tax on investment income and 9% Medicare surtax, which is additional payroll tax. By contributing to your retirement plan on a pretax basis, it lowers your AGI, thus saving you on federal taxes and hopefully with the right advice on the new tax hikes as well.

Here are some of the major reasons why you may want to set up a retirement plan:

1. Tax savings as an employer: Your business gets a deduction for employer contributions within limits.
2. Employees don't pay taxes on contribution (except Roth) until distribution.
3. Accounts grow tax deferred (if pretax) and tax free (Roth).
4. Forced savings for your retirement.
5. Retain and reward key employees.
6. Attracts new employees as an employer benefit.

WHAT IS THE BEST PLAN FOR YOU? IF YOU ALREADY HAVE A PLAN, DO YOU NEED TO MAKE ANY CHANGES?

There are five major issues that need to be considered:

1. Objectives—The six questions addressed in the previous question of what motivated you to set up the retirement plan? Is it to shelter taxes or provide a benefit to the employees? What's your budget? Is it to maximize for the owners versus rank and file? Having a clear goal helps design a plan to meet that objective.
2. Census information—Who are all your employees, their ages, full- or part-time status, salaries, and length of service?
3. Employee funding capabilities—What will employees contribute?
4. How much you want to contribute—What does the owner want to contribute to the plan? Does the owner want to maximize savings for himself versus rank and file?
5. Monitor—It's very important to monitor the plan regularly to make sure it is meeting the objectives for setting up the retirement plan. Tax laws change, owner's funding capabilities change, employee census change, and monitoring it on a regular basis helps you to achieve your retirement goals faster than you thought possible.

So, what are the most common issues for an employer at each stage of his or her career? Each of the plan types is described in more detail in the next section.

Planning Issues: Early Career

1. Try to save early and let compound interest work in your favor. Save between 10% and 15% of your income at the minimum.
2. There will be additional cash needs at the start of your practice.
3. Start with a SIMPLE IRA or SEP IRA. If you are a practice owner without employees and would like to contribute a larger amount, you may want to consider an individual 401(k).

Planning Issues: Mid-Career

1. You may want to consider a 401(k) plan for employee contributions and for profit sharing.
2. With these additions, you may be able to save as much as $52,000 per year. If you are at least 50 years old, the limits increase to

Year	Limit	If 50 Years and Over
2009	$49,000	+$5500
2010	$49,000	+$5500
2011	$49,000	+$5500
2012	$50,000	+$5500
2013	$51,000	+$5500
2014	$52,000	+$5500

Planning Issues: Late Career

1. If you're just starting, you will need to save a large amount quickly.
2. If your practice has a steady cash flow and is well established, you may want to consider a DBP, where you may be able to save significantly above the levels shown above.
3. You might also consider some of the hybrid plans mentioned in the text.

Planning tip: If you are a physician-owner looking for a DCP that might benefit you more than your employees—and depending on your age—you might consider plans such as safe harbor 401(k) plan or age-weighted or cross-tested PSP.

If you have less time to accumulate retirement funds, and you have a steady cash flow from your practice with less employees, (e.g., less than 10 employees), a DBP will allow larger contributions, especially if you have less time to your retirement.

Some two-plan combinations might work to allow the sponsor to use two different plans with each designed for specific group of employees (physician-owners and key employees versus rank and file).

WHAT ARE INDIVIDUAL RETIREMENT PLANS?

IRA: It's a personal savings plan to which an eligible person can make pretax or posttax contributions and accounts grow tax deferred. In exchange for getting a tax deferral, the government wants you to keep that money saved until age 59½ otherwise, you pay a 10% penalty for early withdrawal.

- *Roth IRA:* Is also a personal savings plan to which an eligible person can contribute only after-tax dollars but the accounts grow tax free. Remember, eligible spouses can also contribute.

These types of plans are especially helpful in early career. If married, both spouses can contribute, if eligible.

WHAT ARE THE DIFFERENT TYPES OF EMPLOYER-SPONSORED IRA RETIREMENT PLANS FOR A SMALL MEDICAL PRACTICE?

a. *SIMPLE IRA (Savings Incentive Match Plan for Employees)* is for employers with 100 or fewer employees. The SIMPLE IRA is not a qualified plan. The maximum amount an employee can defer is $12,000 in 2014 ($12,000 in 2013, $11,500 in 2012, 2011, and 2010). If an employee is over the age of 50, an employee can defer $14,500 in 2014 and 2013 ($14,000 in 2012, $14,000 in 2011, $14,000 in 2010, $14,000 in 2009). The employer must provide contributions in the form of a match or as a contribution to all employees who qualify for the plan. In a SIMPLE IRA, the contributions are made to individual IRAs in the name of each participant. Employer contributions are always fully vested.

   SIMPLE IRAs must include all employees who made at least $5000 in the two preceding years and are expected to earn at least $5000 in the current year.

   Planning note: If creditor protection is important—consider a SIMPLE 401(k) plan! However, early distributions penalty from a SIMPLE IRA are subjected to 25% if made within 2 years of participation.

b. *Simplified Employee Pension Plans.* A SEP is not a qualified plan, so the qualified plan rules do not apply. It is especially attractive to small medical practices because of its simplicity. There is no plan document needed to set up the plan. There are no annual filings (unlike qualified plans) or any administration fees, since no administration is needed. Contributions are made by the employer and are made into individual IRA's for the benefit of the participant. All contributions are fully vested.

   An employer can deduct 25% of compensation paid to employees during a calendar year. In taking into account employee compensation for the year, there is a maximum compensation limit per employee, which was $260,000 in 2014.

   For plans beginning after 2013, the employer can contribute the lesser of 100% compensation or $52,000 in 2014 whichever is less. The rules for SEPs are in code section 408(k) and are as follows:

   1. Must contribute for each employee who is at least 21 years of age.
   2. Has performed services for the employer during the year in which contribution is made (including any such employee who because of death or termination, is no longer employed on the date distribution is made).

3. And at least three of the immediately preceding 5 years, has received $550 in compensation (2009–2014) from the employer.
4. Contributions do not need to be made to employees who make less than $550, in 2014 (indexed for inflation).
5. The plan cannot require 1 year of service and full-time employment, that is, 1000 h annually, requirement. Hence, it has to include both full- and part-time employees if they meet the criteria.
6. The plan can exclude employees who are covered under a collective bargaining agreement or are nonresident aliens.

This is a good plan for early-career medical professionals.

Example: Dr. Smith started his practice in February 2012 and adopted a SEP plan and contributed to his plan. If he hired a junior associate in 2012, and told her that she would not be eligible until 2016—4 years later—then this is not consistent with the plan. Why? If Dr. Smith had immediate vesting, so should his associate.

WHAT IS A QUALIFIED RETIREMENT PLAN?

There are two parts to the QRP. First, it is a retirement plan that the employer or the employee's organization (such as a union) sets up to provide retirement income for the employee. In addition, this retirement plan can allow the employees to defer income into the plan. Second, this retirement plan qualifies for special tax treatment from the IRS. In order to qualify for the special tax treatment, the retirement plan must meet all the Internal Revenue Code requirements, Employee Retirement Income Security Act of 1974 (ERISA), and Department of Labor (DOL) rulings.

What Are the Types of QRPs?

There are two major types of QRPs. DBPs provide a specified benefit to the participant. DCPs specify the contribution amount allowed by the employer and employee. These two major types of plans also differ in how the benefit is allocated to the participant. The participant in a DCP receives the accumulated account balance, whereas the participant in a DBP receives a monthly check or lump sum based on a formula established for the plan.

Defined Benefit Plans

The DBP is what most people consider a pension plan. The employer contributes all the money, which is pooled into one account, so there are no individual accounts for each participant. The employee has little or no choice in how the plan operates. The employer bears the risk. This plan promises to provide a monthly pension to the participant when he retires. Usually, this benefit depends on three factors:

1. The age of the participant at retirement
2. The number of years of service or how long the participant has worked at the practice or company
3. Salary at retirement, usually based on compensation over a number of years

The employee's benefits manual will provide more details regarding how the monthly pension is calculated. If you need additional information, ask your human resources manager for a summary plan description or a copy of the actual plan document.

Planning note: One caution concerning DBPs is to understand any "penalties" for retiring before normal retirement age! There can be a significant difference in payment amounts if you delay retiring for just 2–3 years.

Most DBPs require vesting before you are eligible to receive the benefit. Vesting can vary from immediate, to gradual, to full vesting in the future (known as "cliff" vesting). This kind of plan is appropriate only when your practice is well established and you have a surplus cash flow in the business that can be earmarked for retirement plans.

50/40 Test: A DBP must benefit the lesser of the following:

1. 50 employees
2. The greater of
   - 40% of all employees, or
   - 2 employees (if 1, that employee)

This is the 50/40 test.

Limits: According to Section 415 of IRC, the highest annual benefit payable in a DBP must not exceed the lesser of

- 100% of the participant's average compensation in his or her high 3 years or
- $210,000 in 2014

Example: John and Mary Jones, both 52 and physicians, are partners in their medical practice for 20 years with steady cash flow. They have two more employees who are 25 (receptionist) and 30 years old (administrator). John and Mary each make $400,000 per year. They want to defer taxes and start saving for retirement. They can benefit from a DBP.

Planning tip: These types of plans are good only if you have steady cash flow from the practice that enables you to fund the mandatory contributions regularly. If you have a large group of employees such as 10, or even more, or most of your employees are older than the practice owners, the plan may become very expensive and may not work.

Cash balance plans: One variation of the DBP is the cash balance pension plan. This plan is a cross between a DCP and a DBP. Like a DCP, the contribution rate is a percentage of salary; however, unlike a DCP, the actual contribution percentage is actuarially defined. The contribution rate is based on the expected benefit for the employee. There is an employer-guaranteed earnings rate that is predetermined. However, since the interest-crediting rate is never exactly the same as the investment return, the sum of all the account balances will not equal the total asset value of the plan. A DCP always has the sum of all the account balances equal to the total plan assets. Since the plan assets of cash balance account plan will have either a surplus or deficit, it cannot be a DCP. If the actual plan earnings are below the interest-crediting rate, the employer makes up the difference. After 2007, cash balance benefits must be 100% vested after 3 years of service.

Example: Dr. Murphy is married filing jointly, makes $510,000 from his medical practice and $100,000 from his investment portfolio, and does not have a retirement plan. He is 60 years old. He is in the highest tax bracket (39.6%). Contributing $210,000 to his cash balance plan reduces his AGI below the threshold ($450,000) saves him federal taxes and allows him to reduce the new tax increases (for illustrative purposes only).

412(i) plans: Another variation of the DBP is the Insured DBP or 412(i) Plan also known as fully insured DBP. After the Pension Protection Act of 2006, these plans are now controlled under Section 404(C) and Section 412(3) (4). This plan usually allows larger contributions and simpler administration because the assets are invested in either annuity or life insurance contracts, which guarantee the payments to plan participants. They are most commonly used in situations with very few employees and a desire to maximize the amount that can be contributed by the employer for their own benefit. Of course, since these are guaranteed investments, their rate of return may be lower than other more aggressive options.

Defined Contribution Plans

The DCP provides individual accounts for each of the participants. The participant's retirement benefit is dependent on the value of the participant's account at retirement. All allocations, including employer and employee contributions, investment returns, employee contributions forfeitures from participants who terminated before vesting, will contribute to each participant's account value. The 401(k) is an example of a DCP. Other common types of DCPs are

1. *PSPs.* The company makes discretionary contributions each year. The contribution limit is 25% of the total payroll of covered employees. These contributions are allocated among the participants based on a predetermined formula.

   Even though employer contributions are discretionary, there must be recurring and substantial contributions out of profits for the employees: (IRC401(K)(2),401(K)(3) (A)).

   Age-weighted PSPs: Allow discretionary contributions based on employees' age and compensation.

   New comparability PSPs (also known as cross-tested plans) allow the employer to make discretionary contributions of up to 25% of total payroll of covered employees based on employee's age, job group, or other business-related group.

   Safe harbor 401(k) plans: In order to meet its qualified status, 401(k) plans must meet certain nondiscrimination tests for deferrals, matching, and after-tax employee contributions to the plan. These are known as ADP, Actual Deferral Percentage (for deferrals) and ACP, Actual Contribution Percentage (for after-tax and matching contribution) tests. A plan is considered to have met those requirements, hence a "safe harbor" if it meets certain requirements such as

   - Fully vested employer contributions
   - One or more advance notices to participants
   - Certain restrictions on the level of discretionary matching contributions

   The safe harbor nonelective option: The safe harbor nonelective can be made by the employer by making a 3% of employee's compensation to all employees, including the non-highly compensated employees. Contributions should be fully vested. This meets the nondiscrimination tests.

   This plan will be good for mid- to late career medical providers.

   Planning note: If seeking to allocate a higher percentage to owners and highly paid physicians, safe harbor 401(k) plans will provide the benefit compared to a SIMPLE 401(k) for the same amount of employer contribution, even though the administration costs would be lower with a SIMPLE 401(k).

   Planning note: Often, a PSP can be considered when in mid-career, as PSPs allow you to save the full contribution while still maintaining flexibility.

2. *Money purchase plans.* The company makes the contribution and the contribution is fixed and determined ahead of time; for example, the company will contribute 5% of each employee's compensation each year. The company's contribution rate can vary from 0% to 25%. This contribution rate can only change if there is a formal amendment to the plan.

3. *Target benefit plans.* This is a money purchase plan that is age-weighted and based on compensation. It is subject to minimum funding requirements. It has features of a money purchase plan and DBP. The plan starts with a defined benefit formula that provides a target annual retirement benefit for each participant. The company's contribution percentages are determined actuarially so that each participant will receive the targeted benefit. The contribution percentage is determined for each employee as s/he enters the plan and does not change. Therefore, there are no periodic actuarial valuations. Individual accounts are maintained and the participant's benefit is dependent solely on the participant's account balance at retirement or termination. As with the money purchase plan, the employer deduction limit is 25% of total payroll of all covered employees.

Planning note: Target benefit plans may be appropriate for those of you in the late career stage. This plan provides a means to contribute a higher rate for the older employees than the younger employees.

4. *401(k) or cash or deferred arrangement plan.* This plan comes from a section of the IRS Tax Code, § 401, paragraph (k). A 401(k) is a type of PSP where the employees are allowed to contribute their own money on a pretax basis. The maximum amount the employee can contribute is $17,500 in 2014 and 2013 ($17,000 in 2012, $16,500 in 2011, and $16,500 in 2010). If you are over the age of 50, the limit in 2014 and 2013 was $23,000 ($22,500 in 2012, $22,000 in 2011, $22,000 in 2010). Usually, most 401(k) limit employee deductions to 15% of compensation. The employer has the option of s matching the employee's contribution. Instead of providing a match for every employee contribution, or in addition to a matching contribution, the employer has the option of providing a discretionary profit sharing based on the employee's salary.

401(k)s are popular because the employee is allowed to take more control of his retirement. Generally, if the employee leaves the healthcare organization before s/he retires, s/he can take his/her 401(k) with him/her. More employers are offering 401(k) plans because they want to attract and retain good employees.

Planning note: This plan is a good option for those medical professionals and doctors in mid-career.

Individual 401(k): Also known as the flexible 401(k) plan, this plan is applicable if there are no employees other than the owner. This type of 401(k) may enable you to contribute a larger amount. This type of plan can be used by the physician, his or her spouse (if working at the practice), and any partners in the practice and their spouses (if working at the practice). If any other employees are added, the plan becomes much more complicated and mandatory contributions to the new employees will likely come into play.

The Individual 401(k) is similar to a 401(k) plan, yet different: The physician acts as both employee and employer, thus creating an opportunity to make an elective deferral as an employee and a nonelective contribution or match as an employer.

If under 50, a physician is allowed to contribute up to a maximum 25% employer contribution, and as an employee, the physician can defer up to $17,500 maximum deferral in 2014. Total contribution is capped at $52,000 in 2014 and if over 50 years, its $57,500.

As an example, a sole physician owner of a C Corporation, who earned $75,000, may defer $17,500 in 2014. In addition, the owner can contribute 25% as an employer contribution or $18,750. The total contribution could be $36,250, even though the owner's income is $75,000. If the owner was 50 years old or older, the owner can contribute an additional $5500. One advantage over an IRA plan is the loan privileges, if allowed.

SIMPLE 401(k) plan: SIMPLE (Savings Incentive Match Plan for Employees) plan are for employers with 100 or fewer employees. The SIMPLE 401(k) is a qualified plan, whereas the SIMPLE IRA is not. In both plans, the maximum amount an employee can defer is $12,000 in 2014 ($12,000 in 2013, $11,500 in 2012, 2011, and 2010). If an employee is over the age of 50, an employee can defer $14,500 in 2014 and 2013 ($14,000 in 2012, $14,000 in 2011, $14,000 in 2010, $14,000 in 2009). The employer must provide contributions in the form of a match or as a contribution to all employees who qualify for the plan. In a SIMPLE 401(k), the contributions are made to a trust, whereas in a SIMPLE IRA, the contributions are made to individual IRA's in the name of each participant. Employer contributions are always fully vested in both plans.

Planning note: If creditor protection is important, then consider a SIMPLE 401(k). However, early distributions penalty from a SIMPLE IRA is subjected to 25% if made within 2 years of participation.

Roth 401(k)

Beginning January 1, 2006, Roth 401(k) contributions were allowed within a 401(k) plan. Roth 401(k) combines the benefits of both a Roth and a 401(k) plan style employee elective deferral plan. But unlike a 401(k) where the deferral is pretax, the Roth deferral is after tax, that is, it is included in employee's income. The deferrals will be considered wages, hence subjected to tax withholdings. It grows tax free if it meets certain requirements.

The maximum contribution is limited to elective deferrals for that year. For 2014 and 2013, it was $12,000. Catch up was an additional $2500 in 2013 and 2014. Roth contributions cannot be comingled with pre- or posttax contributions.

The major benefit of a Roth 401(k) is that there is no minimum required distribution at age 70½, but required distribution may apply at the death of owner.

As of January 1, 2013, provisions of the American Taxpayer Relief Act of 2012 allow 401(k) and other defined contribution (403(b)–(457) plans to be converted to a Roth account within the same plan, provided the sponsor offers that option. It's entirely at the discretion of the employer to decide if they want to offer this feature within their retirement plan.

Tax sheltered annuities (TSA): A tax-exempt organization, as described under IRC Section 501(C) (3) such as a hospital, clinic, university, and so on, or public school system may offer tax shelter annuities for their full- and part-time employees to save for their retirement. It is available only to employees, not contractors. A TSA is a tax-deferred arrangement approved by Congress under IRC Section 403(b). Contributions to TSA can be excluded from income.

Example: If a doctor works for a hospital as an employee, subject to social security and tax with holdings, s/he is eligible to participate in TSA.

Roth 403(b): According to IRC Sections 402 A (b) and 402(e), 403(b) plans are allowed to offer Roth accounts for employee deferrals. In these types of plans, employees can designate all or portion of their deferrals as Roth contributions. Roth contributions will be included in participant's income for the year and should be held in separate accounts.

Planning tip: Lowering 401(k) costs

Hospital and healthcare employer-sponsored retirement plans come with many investment choices. But employees often don't make sure they have access to the least expensive ones. The average index mutual fund carries an expense ratio of 0.76%—$7.60 in annual fees for every $1000 invested, according to *Morningstar.* For exchange-traded funds, it's 0.58%. However, for actively managed mutual funds, it's a heftier 1.27%. Over time, that can really add up.

For example, assuming a typical 401(k) size of $100,000 and annual contributions of $3000, with an expense ratio of 0.76%, a participating registered nurse (RN) would pay $43,759 over 25 years— while a registered physical therapist (RPT) with 1.27% would pay $68,189. With an expected return of 5% before costs, the final value for the fund with the 0.76% expense ratio is $412,317—versus $369,513 for the fund with the higher expense ratio; a difference of $42,804. So, always request a diversified group of low-cost index funds and exchange traded funds (ETFs) as investment choices, if possible.*

Long-Term Care Insurance

You might have done an excellent job of saving for retirement, but if a catastrophic illness or disease hits you and you have to go to a nursing home or need a home care aid, all your hard earned savings will evaporate very fast. There are limitations on how much Medicare covers. It's prudent to shift this risk to an insurance company by buying a long-term care policy, with a home care option and inflation option.

And, if you can afford it, it is better to apply early for both spouses (if married) than late, since premiums get very expensive at an advanced age. Depending on your age, the premiums can also be deducted from your income.

---

* Source: WageWorks.com.

Planning tip: If you are an employer, and you provide LTCI to your employees, the premiums can be deducted as a business expense; consult a tax advisor.

MAXIMIZING INCOME FROM RETIREMENT PLANS

So now you are successful with your retirement planning and you're ready to retire. A large portion of your retirement assets may be in a QRP your employer provided, or you sponsored yourself. What is the best way to handle the assets in the plan?

WHAT IF YOUR PLAN IS A TRADITIONAL PENSION OR DBP?

You will either receive a monthly check or have an option to receive a lump sum. If you select the monthly check, you have a short time after retirement to decide whether to take a check over your lifetime (known as the single life option) or a smaller check over your and your spouse's lifetime (known as the joint and survivor option). Often, you are provided several alternatives of joint and survivor options as follows:

1. Giving your spouse an equivalent monthly check if something should happen to you (known as 100% joint and survivor)
2. Giving your spouse a reduced monthly check if something should happen to you (e.g., 50% joint and survivor)

The single life option provides the largest check. If your spouse is much younger than you are, the check for both of your lives could be significantly less. Most people choose the 100% joint and survivor option because it's difficult to tell your spouse that everything will be fine while you're alive, but she or he will suffer if you die.

Another alternative instead of taking the 100% joint and survivor option is a technique called pension maximization. This technique may be used if the spouse is in poor health and would likely die before the participant. If you selected the 100% joint and survivor option and your spouse predeceased you, you will continue to receive the lower monthly check based on both lives. Therefore, to receive the higher income based on one life and still make sure your spouse receives a similar benefit if you should predecease him or her, you would use the pension maximization technique as follows:

1. Take the monthly benefit based just on your life.
2. Purchase life insurance on your life with a part of the increased monthly benefit. For this technique to work, the insurance death benefit should be large enough to provide your spouse the equivalent monthly income, assuming a reasonable investment return. Your spouse will probably not receive an equivalent income if he or she selects a risk-free investment, so this option will be more risky for him or her.
3. If your spouse predeceases you, cancel the insurance.

Before selecting the single life option, make sure you are insurable (have the policy in your hands before making the selection). The payout selection is irrevocable, so you want to be careful.

Planning note: You may want to consider pension maximization if your spouse is much younger than you. In this case, your 100% joint and survivor option may result in much lower monthly payments than a single life option.

WHAT IF YOUR PLAN IS LIKE A 401(K) OR ANOTHER TYPE OF DCP?

You have several alternatives as follows:

1. You can leave the money in your DCP. Each employer has rules for the qualified plan, dictating how long you can stay in the plan once you retire.

2. You can rollover the money to an IRA. A benefit of this option is that you will have more investment options than your current DCP.

3. You can take all the money out of the qualified plan, which is called a lump sum distribution. You may receive special tax treatment if you take this option (limited to very few). You will be taxed on the distribution and might put you in a higher tax bracket.

4. *SEP option*: If you're younger than age 55 and you are ready to retire, you can take money out of the plan in substantially equal payments over your life expectancy. You must continue to take these payments at least 5 years or to age 59½, whichever is longer. In addition, you must separate from service before starting the payments.

Planning note: You can also take substantially equal payments from an IRA if you are under age 59½. With an IRA, there is no requirement to separate from service.

Leave the Money in the Qualified Plan

The major benefit in staying in your employer's qualified plan is increased creditor protection. In addition, your spouse may have rights to an annuity income that he or she would give up if you move the money to an IRA. Your spouse also has these same rights to your pension or DBP. So, that's a consideration when taking the lump sum option instead of the monthly benefit.

If you are the employer, you may want to keep the money in the qualified plan. However, qualified plans must have a legitimate business entity to sponsor a plan. Usually, when doctors retire, that practice-business entity disappears. Therefore, you should see a pension attorney or Certified Public Accountant (CPA), if you want to keep your money in the qualified plan after retirement.

Rollover the Money to an IRA

Many people decide to move their funds from the QRP to an IRA and continue to defer taxes. Some of the benefits of the IRA are portability (you can move it to any custodian you want), control over the investment options, and possible tax advantages through greater control over beneficiary designations and minimum distribution elections.

If you decide to move money from a qualified plan to an IRA, you will want to elect a direct rollover. A direct rollover moves the funds directly from the qualified plan to the IRA custodian and is a trustee-to-trustee rollover. Money is never in your name (if the money is sent to you, it will be made out to the custodian for your benefit). If you don't select a direct rollover and decide to receive the money in your name, the qualified plan trustee will withhold 20% to make sure that taxes are covered. When you put the money in an IRA, you have to come up with the missing 20% or you'll be fined 10% if you're under age 59½ and taxed as if it were a distribution.

Planning note: You can roll over more after-tax money than you contributed! However, you will need to keep track of the accounting on your own. If you don't, you may have to pay tax on the money again because it will be considered pretax. If you elect to take out the after-tax money, you will receive a check for the after-tax amount, and the earning on that money will be rolled over.

Take a Lump Sum Distribution

Instead of moving money to an IRA, you can also decide to take a lump sum and pay taxes. If you qualify, you can elect to receive special tax treatment, called forward averaging.

Ten-year forward averaging is available only to people who were born on or before January 1, 1936, and allows you to pay taxes as if you received the money over 10 years. There's a catch, though. You must pay taxes at the 1986 tax rates, which were significantly higher than today. Also, you must pay all the taxes in the year you take the distribution.

You Are Retiring before You're Age 55 and Need the Money from the Qualified Plan

If you want to take the payments from your qualified plan, you need to make sure that your plan allows this option. If you decide to take the money from your qualified plan, you have to leave the company where you have the plan before you can start taking distributions.

If your plan doesn't allow substantially equal payments over your life, you can rollover the money to an IRA, then take the payments. Or, if you already have enough money in an IRA, you take the payments from the IRA and you're not required to leave the company.

If you are interested in this option, there are several ways to calculate how much you can take out each year. Once you select a method, you can't change it.

Planning Issues: Early Career

It's still early, so most of these issues don't apply to you. If you expect to retire at an early age, estimate how much of your money will be in qualified plans or IRAs at retirement. Then estimate how much you can withdraw each year. If that's not enough to support your lifestyle, you will want to save money outside of the retirement plans, so you can live comfortably before you're age 55.

Planning Issues: Mid-Career

Again, it's a little too early to worry about how you're going to take your money out of your retirement plans, unless you are planning to retire soon.

Planning Issues: Late Career

This is the time to start thinking about all your alternatives. Healthcare professionals need to integrate retirement plan distributions with tax planning. Depending on your age and on the type of plan that you have, you have some decisions to make before you retire. These decisions can get quite complicated, so it's wise to seek the advice of a CPA.

Required Minimum Distribution (RMD): You have to start taking money out of your retirement plans by age 70½; so you need to coordinate this with your tax planning.

RMDs are designed to ensure that owners of tax-deferred retirement accounts do not defer taxes on their retirement accounts indefinitely. You are allowed to begin taking penalty-free distributions from tax-deferred retirement accounts after age 59½, but you must begin taking them after reaching age 70½. If you delay your first distribution to April 1 following the year in which you turn 70½, you must take another distribution for that year. Annual RMDs must be taken each subsequent year no later than December 31.

The RMD amount depends on your age, the value of the account(s), and your life expectancy. You can use the IRS Uniform Lifetime Table (or the Joint and Last Survivor Table, in certain circumstances) to determine your life expectancy. To calculate your RMD, divide the value of your account balance at the end of the previous year by the number of years you're expected to live, based on the numbers in the IRS table. You must calculate RMDs for each account that you own. If you do not take RMDs, then you may be subject to a 50% federal income tax penalty on the amount that should have been withdrawn.

Remember that distributions from tax-deferred retirement plans are subject to ordinary income tax. Waiting until the April 1 deadline in the year after reaching age 70½ is a one-time option and requires that you take two RMDs in the same tax year. If these distributions are large, this method could push you into a higher tax bracket. It may be wise to plan ahead for RMDs to determine the best time to begin taking them.

OTHER RETIREMENT PLANS

Tax-qualified employer-based retirement plans may be the best way to save for retirement, but they are likely to fall short of providing enough income to support your lifestyle. While many Baby Boomer physicians expect to work in retirement, making work optional will most likely require additional investments, over and above contributing the maximum to your 401(k) or 403(b) plan.

Assuming you've set aside enough money for emergencies (remember, 3–6 month's expenses or more?), you should evaluate other personal plans. Let's cover these now.

Nonemployer Plans (Personal Plans)

The primary focus of these plans is for you to have complete control of your savings and investments. It's important to mentally segregate your investments based on their purpose, since near-term needs are best satisfied with more conservative approaches. You might think of this money as being in different "buckets," one for an emergency reserve, one for a home purchase, one for retirement, and so forth.

Tax Diversification

Since no one knows what our tax system will look like years from now, it's just as important to diversify the tax treatment of your investments as it is to diversify the types of investments you use! Using tax-deductible contributions, tax-free income, tax efficiency, and tax deferral can have a huge impact on your retirement security.

Retirement Assessment

You and your advisor will want to measure the effectiveness of the different tax strategies as they apply to your unique situations. For example, a strategy that appears best using 9% earning rates may not be best using 11% or 7% earning rates. Also, different time periods could result in different strategies appearing better.

Some tax strategies lend themselves to estate planning flexibility and others do not. It generally requires that the accumulated assets be taxable in your estate for federal estate tax purposes.

Most importantly, make your economic assumptions as consistent as possible when comparing different strategies.

How Can You Achieve Tax-Deferred or Even Tax-Free Growth?

IRA Accounts

First, and perhaps most complex, are various types of IRA accounts. There are five primary IRA types: traditional deductible and nondeductible IRAs, conduit (or rollover) IRAs, contributory Roth IRAs, and conversion Roth IRAs. Each of these provides tax deferral but has different tax treatments, advantages, and disadvantages.

There are many considerations in deciding on an IRA strategy; so here are some general rules to use, all subject to the particulars of your situation:

1. *Contributing to an IRA:* You should contribute to a Roth IRA if you can't qualify for a deductible traditional IRA. This provides tax-free income in retirement instead of taxable income. In addition, you are never forced to take distributions from the account until the death of the owner, so there may be estate planning and income tax benefits.

If your joint modified AGI is above $191,000 in 2014, you cannot contribute to a Roth IRA. Your only IRA option is the traditional nondeductible IRA, if you don't qualify for a deductible IRA.

2. *Roth Conversion:* "Qualified Rollover Contribution." You may convert your existing IRA or any eligible retirement plan to a Roth IRA. A rollover was not permitted prior to 2010 for individuals with certain AGI. You have other money to use in paying for the taxes due, and you have many years before retirement. Converting triggers current taxes on your account balance, but the tax-free income may more than offset the loss. Don't convert without calculating the likely results and talking to your advisors.

3. *Conduit IRA:* When you leave an employer, you should evaluate whether to leave the money in your old employer's plan or to rollover your money, either to your new employer's plan (if allowed) or to a conduit IRA. A 401(k) plan has certain advantages over an IRA, such as better creditor protection and, perhaps, the ability to borrow from the plan. In addition, there may be other distribution benefits from these plans. The disadvantage of these plans is your investments are limited to those offered by the plan, where with an IRA, the choice is virtually unlimited! You need to consider the investment options in the new plan to see if you're sacrificing performance.

What Other Tax-Deferred Choices Do You Have?

Planning tip: Use IRAs for a nonworking spouse.

Traditional IRAs allow investors to save in a retirement account and potentially get a deduction for their contribution, depending on their income and whether or not they or their spouse actively participate in an employer-sponsored retirement plan at work. But they may not be getting as big of a deduction as they could.

For example, if you have a nonworking spouse, spousal IRA contributions are often missed because they don't realize the spouse at home can make an IRA contribution and potentially get deductions on that as well. Though typical IRS rules require the IRA contributor to have earned income, working spouses may be able to make an additional deductible IRA contribution on behalf of a nonworking spouse. Deductions typically begin to phase out if a household's modified AGI exceeds $178,000 and the working spouse contributes to a retirement plan at work, like a 401(k). So, let's look at a couple where the working spouse makes the maximum contribution for a nonworking spouse— $6500. (For those under 50, it's $5500.) Now, assuming a federal income tax rate of 28%; that $6500 might bring a tax savings of $1000–$1800, depending on the couple's overall tax situation.[*]

Planning tip: Traditional IRA conversion as a workaround to Roth IRA income limits (so-called "back-door" Roth IRA).

Regardless of income, but subject to contribution limits, contributions can be made to a traditional IRA and then converted to a Roth IRA. This allows for "backdoor" contributions where individuals are able to avoid the income limitations of the Roth IRA. There is no limit to the frequency with which conversions can occur, so this process can be repeated indefinitely.

One major caveat to the entire "backdoor" Roth IRA contribution process, however, is that it only works for people who do not have any pretax contributed money in IRA accounts at the time of the "backdoor" conversion to Roth; conversions made when other IRA money exists are subject to pro-rata calculations and may lead to tax liabilities on the part of the converter.

For example, if a nurse has contributed $10,000 posttax and $30,000 pretax and wants to convert the posttax $10,000 into a Roth, the pro-rated amount (ratio of taxable contributions to total contributions) is taxable. In this example, $7500 of the posttax contribution is considered taxable

---

[*] Source: WageWorks.com.

when converting it to a Roth IRA. The pro-rata calculation is made based on all traditional IRA contributions across all the RNs traditional IRA accounts (even if they are in different institutions).

Variable Annuities

Variable annuities are described in the insurance chapter, but there is still a mighty controversy surrounding them.

The benefits of a variable annuity usually cost around 1.4% of your balance each year, plus money management averaging around 0.60%. If you invest in the average mutual fund at 1.4% per year, you would save 0.60% per year.* The issue you need to decide is if the 0.60% provides enough benefits to be worth the cost.

Most studies focus on an analysis comparing tax deferral versus mutual fund investing, not on the other features. This has become more of an issue with the reduction in capital gains rates to a maximum of 20% versus the ordinary income from the annuity. Unfortunately, this analysis is subject to the variability of mutual fund taxation from fund to fund, as well as how long you hold your fund without selling. One often ignored advantage of variable annuities is the ability to make changes in your investments without incurring any additional tax.

According to a Morningstar Study of January 2001, the average domestic equity mutual fund lost 21% of its return to taxes over the prior 15 years.

Using this example, $10,000 growing for 20 years in a taxable mutual fund at 10% (7.9% net) will be worth $45,754 while the annuity would be worth $60,304 (9.4% net). In 5 years, the taxable fund would be worth $14,625 versus the annuity at $15,670.

No matter how you analyze this, here are some general rules:

1. You might consider variable annuities with after-tax money after you've completely funded your qualified plan and IRA options.
2. Look for contracts with minimal surrender periods, meaning you can take your money out without penalty in a short time.
3. Consider the value to you of the additional features, such as riders, and only buy those you feel are worthwhile. Every additional feature adds cost to your annuity. As in all investments, watch your expenses.
4. Look for additional expenses: Contract charges as well as *mortality and expense* charges are added to your annuity.
5. Internal fund expenses need to be monitored.
6. Sometimes there are limitations how many times you can make interfund transfers.
7. Strength of the issuer and rating.

Modified Endowment Contract

The newest modified endowment contracts (MECs) are structured to use the joint lives of both you and your spouse, which can dramatically reduce your insurance costs. It's important to be clear on your goals and the costs inherent in the specific contract you're evaluating, to see if this is right for your situation.

Universal Life Insurance

Universal life insurance has also come under fire recently, mainly for lack of disclosure that people were actually buying life insurance. This type of life insurance should primarily be bought for the protection of your loved ones (or business) in the event of your death. There are two basic types of policies to be considered, as described in the chapter on insurance: (a) traditional universal life and (b) variable universal life.

---

* Morningstar Principia 12/31/2002.

Planning Hints

1. In general, this approach works best if you need life insurance, have reasonably stable income, have discretionary money to invest after funding your QRP, and can plan on keeping the contract for many years. If you're likely to need to stop making premium payments, or to cancel the contract prematurely, this isn't the right approach for you.
2. To maximize your benefits, plan on maximizing the funding of this contract while maintaining its' life insurance status.
3. Don't be a conservative investor here. To overcome the costs and grow your money over time, invest your money in the more aggressive options. If you're using this approach, you have many years to ride through the ups and downs of more aggressive investments.

Mutual Funds

Mutual funds are often used inside of IRAs and other retirement accounts and take on the tax characteristics of those accounts. What we're going to discuss now is the taxation of funds outside of these accounts, and how to use funds most effectively to supplement your QRP.

How should you manage your portfolio for maximum after-tax returns with whatever asset allocation mix you're using?

First, here's an explanation of how funds are taxed. Generally, you pay taxes on funds four ways: stock or bond dividends, tax-free dividends, capital gains from the sale of securities by the fund each year, and capital gains from the sale of your shares in the fund. Since mutual funds are jointly managed for many shareholders, the taxes generated by the fund are shared proportionately by the percentage of the fund assets you own.

Let's look at bonds for a moment. Most of your return in a bond fund is from the dividends paid by the bonds in the fund, although some funds have also generated capital gains through the active buying and selling of their holdings. The dividends paid on most bond funds is taxed as ordinary income, at a maximum tax rate today of 39.6%. Municipal bond funds invest in tax-free bonds, meaning the income is not subject to federal and sometimes state income tax (but may be a preference item for alternative minimum tax (AMT) calculations). This income is usually at a lower rate than similar quality taxable bonds.

Which is better? Your goal should be to get the highest after-tax return, not the lowest tax. The easiest way to decide whether tax-free or taxable bonds are better is to determine the "tax equivalent yield," which compares taxable and tax-free income. Just divide the tax-free rate by the inverse of your maximum tax bracket and you'll be able to compare. For example, if the tax-free rate is 4.5% and your bracket is 35%, here's the formula:

$$4.5\%/(1 - 0.35) = 4.5\%/0.65 = 6.92\% \text{ tax equivalent yield}$$

At this point, just choose the higher of the tax equivalent or taxable bond yield and you're (almost) home free. Be sure to consult your tax advisor before you act because the AMT calculation may change your results.

What about stock fund taxation? First, many companies pay out part of their profits to shareholders in the form of dividends, which are taxed as ordinary income. Since these are taxed at higher rates than capital gains, your goal might be to choose funds that minimize dividends, although over the last 70 years, about half of the return of the S&P 500 has been through dividends.[*]

Next is the issue of capital gains taxation, triggered by the selling of stocks within the fund at a profit. Since these are paid out by most funds on an annual basis, it's important to realize you may

---

[*] Ibbotson and Associates.

get a tax bill for gains that other people received. Be careful when investing in a fund near year end, since these distributions are usually paid in November or December. It's not unusual for an investor to be losing money and still have to pay taxes on gains.

Lastly, and easiest to control, are capital gains triggered by selling your shares in a fund. Any gains over your original investment, plus the value of all reinvested dividends and capital gains, are taxed at capital gains rates (if you've held the fund for at least 12 months; otherwise, this is a short-term gain taxed at the same rates as ordinary income.)

Planning hints: Here are ways to minimize taxes on a fund portfolio:

1. Don't reinvest dividends, so this money can be used when you rebalance your portfolio. This simplifies your record keeping and provides money to "buy low" without having to sell some of the better performing portions of your portfolio, which may trigger taxes. Don't forget to reinvest, though, since the loss of compounding on this money can be significant.
2. Use funds that have been tax efficient in the past, although past performance is not necessarily an indicator of future tax efficiency. Generally, lower turnover funds have been more tax efficient, as have those with lower dividend yields.
3. Another approach is to use index funds, which have been relatively tax efficient. One concern here may be the large capital gains already trapped inside some index funds, which might be paid out to you if the market drops and shareholders cash out.
4. If you can realize a loss, sell funds that have performed poorly each year before they pay out their capital gains distributions. This can be used to offset gains in other parts of portfolio for tax purposes. You might buy a similar fund to maintain your asset allocation mix, or buy the same fund back after waiting 31 days or more (wash rule). Remember, a fund with poor performance may not be a bad fund, it may be investing in part of the market that's not doing well. In a well-diversified portfolio, you almost always will have at least one asset class doing poorly, which is no reflection on the manager! Negatively correlated asset classes are the key to a diversified portfolio.

In the last decade, a category of mutual fund called "tax managed" funds has come out, with a certainty of more choices in the future. These funds are specifically managed to defer or minimize taxes on their investments, which can create significant advantages for you. First, they attempt to provide higher after-tax returns, and second, they provide a step-up in cost basis at your death. As opposed to IRAs and annuities, this eliminates any income taxes due at death (but not any estate taxes). It's important to recognize that money management issues have to come before taxes—if they do poorly at making you money, taxes are the least of your concerns.

Portfolios of Individual Stocks and Bonds

One of the primary choices you have is to either manage this portfolio yourself or to hire professional managers to take care of this for you. You may read more about this in the chapter on portfolio management and investments. One of the most important decisions you make is to determine your asset allocation, so don't forget to be properly diversified.

Planning Issues: Early Career

1. Maximize your retirement plan contributions now. This is the single most important step in having a comfortable retirement, since compounding on your money takes time to work. Remember, at 10%, your money doubles in value in around 7 years, and the difference between a fair retirement and a great one may be the last "doubling" of your account.

2. Consider your other life goals in developing a savings and investment plan. You may need to pay off student loans, save for your children's college education, buy a home, or have start-up expenses in your medical practice. Generally, the shorter the term for your goal, the more conservative you should be in your investments. In addition, obtaining tax deferral may not be consistent with your goals, since most of these approaches have penalties for withdrawal before retirement except hardship exceptions mentioned earlier.

3. Be sure to have 12–24 months expenses set aside for emergencies. This can protect you from having to borrow money and from large credit card interest payments (Dr. David Edward Marcinko, MBA, CMP™, Atlanta, GA, personal communication).

If you need life insurance and can make a long-term commitment, consider a properly structured variable universal life insurance policy as a method of saving for long-term goals.

PLANNING ISSUES: MID-CAREER

1. If you haven't done so yet, maximize your contributions to your retirement plan.

2. Assuming you've bought your home and you have a relatively stable situation, now is the time to be saving additional money outside of your plan. First, determine if you qualify to fund an IRA, since these provide the lowest cost tax deferral available. You should consider contributing to a Roth IRA, for each spouse and investing in growth-oriented securities. The tax-free income this provides in retirement can be a great complement to the taxable income from your qualified plan.

3. Remember to watch the tax efficiency of your personal investments. This can really add to your retirement security.

PLANNING ISSUES: LATE CAREER

1. One of the most critical issues is to determine which accounts your income will be taken from in retirement. As a general rule, you want to maximize tax deferral when you can, spending your after-tax money first. There are many planning issues surrounding this, so you might want to get professional advice.

2. The larger your nest egg, the more critical the need for a tax-efficient investment approach. This should be one of the criteria you use in selecting an investment advisor or financial planner. What process do they use to maximize your after-tax returns?

IRA PLANS AT A GLANCE

Contribution limits	2007	$4000
	2008–2012	$5000
	2013	$5500
	2014	$5500
Contribution limits if over 50	2007	$5000
	2008–2012	$6000
	2013	$6500
	2014	$6500

Type of Plan	Contributions and Withdrawals	Adjusted Gross Income Limits for Tax Deduction	Required Minimum Distributions
Deductible IRA	See above chart for maximum contribution limits Each spouse can contribute Withdrawals subject to ordinary income taxes when received Withdrawals before age 59½ subject to 10% tax penalty	If participating in a company retirement plan: Single: Full deduction at $60,000 or less, phased out at $70,000 MAGI (Y-2014) Married filing jointly: If both are active participants, full deduction limited to $96,000 MAGI and phased out at $116,000 MAGI (Y-2014) If your spouse is covered by a plan but you aren't, full deduction if your combined AGI is less than $181,000 and phased out at $191,000 MAGI.	Must begin by April 1 of the year following the year you turn 70½
Nondeductible IRA	See above chart for maximum contribution limits Each spouse can contribute Withdrawals are the same as above, except return of nondeductible contributions is tax free	None	Same as above
Conduit (rollover) IRA	No maximum, since this is moving the balance from your company retirement plan into your own IRA account Withdrawals are the same as in the deductible IRA above	None	Same as above
Contributory Roth IRA	See above chart for maximum contribution limits Each spouse can contribute Withdrawals are tax free if they meet certain qualifications	$181,000 MAGI limit for married filing jointly $191,000 MAGI limit for singles	None
Roth conversion IRA	Rollover qualified rollover from any retirement plan and IRA to Roth Withdrawals are the same as the contributory Roth except no "recharacterization" feature		None

Money Withdrawn from Tax-Deferred Accounts before Age 59½

Withdrawing funds from a tax-deferred retirement account before age 59½ generally triggers a 10% federal income tax penalty; all distributions are subject to ordinary income tax. However, there are certain situations in which you are allowed to make early withdrawals from a retirement account and avoid the tax penalty. IRAs and employer-sponsored retirement plans have different exceptions, although the regulations are similar.

IRA Exceptions

- *The death of the IRA owner:* Upon death, your designated beneficiaries may begin taking distributions from your account. Beneficiaries are subject to annual RMDs.
- *Disability:* Under certain conditions, you may begin to withdraw funds if you are disabled.
- *Unreimbursed medical expenses:* You can withdraw the amount you paid for unreimbursed medical expenses that exceed 10% of your AGI in a calendar year. Individuals older than 65 can claim expenses that surpass 7.5% of AGI through 2016.

- *Medical insurance:* If you lost your job or are receiving unemployment benefits, you may withdraw money to pay for health insurance.
- *Part of a substantially equal periodic payment (SEPP) plan:* If you receive a series of substantially equal payments over your life expectancy, or the combined life expectancies of you and your beneficiary, you may take payments over a period of 5 years or until you reach age 59½, whichever is longer, using one of three payment methods set by the government. Any change in the payment schedule after you begin distributions may subject you to paying the 10% tax penalty.
- *Qualified higher-education expenses:* For you and/or your dependents.
- *First home purchase:* up to $10,000 (lifetime limit).

Employer-Sponsored Plan Exceptions

- *The death of the plan owner:* Upon death, your designated beneficiaries may begin taking distributions from your account. Beneficiaries are subject to annual RMDs.
- *Disability:* Under certain conditions, you may begin to withdraw funds if you are disabled.
- *Part of a SEPP program (see above):* If you receive a series of substantially equal payments over your life expectancy, or the combined life expectancies of you and your beneficiary, you may take payments over a period of 5 years or until you reach age 59½, whichever is longer.
- *Separation of service from your employer:* Payments must be made annually over your life expectancy or the joint life expectancies of you and your beneficiary.
- *Attainment of age 55:* The payment is made to you upon separation of service from your employer and the separation occurred during or after the calendar year in which you reached the age of 55.
- *Qualified Domestic Relations Order (QDRO):* The payment is made to an alternate payee under a QDRO.
- *Medical care:* You can withdraw the amount allowable as a medical expense deduction.
- *To reduce excess contributions:* Withdrawals can be made if you or your employer made contributions over the allowable amount.
- *To reduce excess elective deferrals:* Withdrawals can be made if you elected to defer an amount over the allowable limit.

If you plan to withdraw funds from a tax-deferred account, make sure to carefully examine the rules on exemptions for early withdrawals. For more information on situations that are exempt from the early-withdrawal income tax penalty, visit the IRS website at www.irs.gov.

RETIREMENT PLANNING AND INVESTMENT STYLE

Contrary to popular belief, your investment policy should be driven by your retirement planning, not only by your tolerance for risk. This approach ensures you'll be comfortable in retirement, and gives you a context for decision making for both sides of the equation—you can balance your retirement planning with the likely returns your tolerance for risk will provide.

Planning Issues: Early Career

1. The focus at this point in your career might be on paying off student loans or buying a home, with retirement planning being secondary. These shorter-term goals might be best served with a more conservative approach, and your retirement needs with a more aggressive approach. You might view these as different "buckets" of money, each with their own investment policy.

2. For retirement investing, recognize that there's nothing inherently wrong with being a more conservative investor. The impact of lower returns, though, is a need to save more money each month.

3. Since you're likely to be saving money monthly and building up your nest egg, you need to realize the power of what's called *dollar cost averaging*, where you invest a fixed amount each month regardless of what the market is doing. This approach makes you appreciate the occasional market drops.

PLANNING ISSUES: MID-CAREER

1. You may well be faced with paying for your children's college tuition, weddings, or other shorter-term needs, while at the same time needing to prepare for retirement. You might want to consider having separate "buckets" of money, with more conservative investments for short-term needs and more aggressive ones for retirement.

2. The more money you accumulate for retirement, the less investment risk you may have to take in retirement. Many healthcare professionals find it comforting to take a conservative approach while they're retired, but this can only be achieved if you have adequate resources to provide for you and your family. Having an effective retirement plan can help you make this happen!

PLANNING ISSUES: LATE CAREER

1. While it's tempting to prefer a conservative investment approach, this might not be in your best interest. Remember, you're likely to live another 20–30 years or more in retirement, and your income will have to double or triple to keep up with inflation.

2. The most effective way to know how conservative you can be is to do a retirement cash flow plan, as shown elsewhere in this chapter. Your future spending needs savings to date and many other factors will determine how hard your money must work for you!

ROLE OF SOCIAL SECURITY IN RETIREMENT PLANNING

Social security maximization is a strategy and is part of retirement planning, where we look at ways to maximize income from social security.

Social security is like a DBP in the sense that you receive benefits as long as you live. The longer you live, the more you collect. And your benefits keep up with inflation.

Example: If you are receiving $2000 per month and if you lived 10 years you would get $304,256. If you lived 30 years, you would have received $1,160,479.

Many people wonder if social security will be there when they retire. The facts suggest that on December 2013, there was approximately $2.76 trillion dollars available, and if no reform occurs, then enough money exists to give full benefits until 2033. Thereafter, reduced benefits might occur (www.social security.gov). Congress is working to reform the system. So, it's important to coordinate your social security with your other retirement plan benefits such as pension, 401(k), 403(b) plans so that you can have a retirement income that you will not outlive.

MORE MONEY NEEDED?

So, if the above SS scenario is only partially true, more money may be needed for retirement than originally thought. For example, a 65-year-old RPT who wanted to pay for retirement with annuities tied to bonds needed 24% more wealth in 2013 than in 2005, National Bureau of Economic Research (NBER) President James Poterba opined in February 2014. The increase followed a drop in yields on top-rated corporate bonds to 3.8% from 5.4%.

INTEGRATING RETIREMENT PLANNING WITH ESTATE PLANNING

Just as every action has an opposite and equal reaction in physics, similarly, every action made for retirement has an effect on your estate. No action should be made in a vacuum. Planning for one and ignoring the other will cost your heirs in taxes! Thus, by ignoring estate planning and focusing only on retirement planning is a costly mistake. The money you worked so hard all your life might end up with Uncle Sam being your most favored heir!

It's important to realize that many of the decisions you make to provide a comfortable retirement may diminish your heirs' inheritances. It's particularly problematic when your estate-planning attorney tells you to make gifts to your kids, while your financial advisor is concerned that you may run out of money. Who should you listen to?

The most logical approach is to integrate both of these areas in your planning from the beginning, rather than piecemeal. The point here is to integrate and make decisions after evaluating them from both perspectives. All of these areas are intertwined in helping you make smarter decisions. Let's examine some of the issues you might consider.

The first step in effective estate planning is a quality retirement cash flow plan, which should help you have a secure retirement. It also projects the likely value of your assets at different times, which is invaluable in your estate planning.

Second, determine what part of your heirs' inheritance is likely to be from your QRP. It's common today to see healthcare professionals with very significant balances in their 401(k) and pension plans, and the technical issues in passing this money on are among the most complex parts of the law today. We'll be focusing on this for the balance of this section, since other estate planning issues are covered elsewhere.

Planning note: The beneficiary designation you've specified to your plan sponsor determines who gets your money when you die—not your will, your living trust, or anything else! Be sure to get legal advice.

Here's a quick review of the rules covering estate planning for qualified retirement benefits. Retirement plan money passes outside of probate directly to your beneficiary, who receives both the money and the income tax liability on the money. In addition, there may be estate taxes due, depending on the size of your total estate including these balances. So, with larger estates, it's not uncommon for income and estate taxes to take up to 75% of your retirement plan. Would you like to pass on only 25% of your money?

EMERGING THOUGHTS ON "AGE-BANDING"

Age banding is a model for retirement planning developed by Somnath Basu, PhD, MBA, CFP™ that may provide a new approach to retirement needs. The model reduces errors in estimating expenses, provides an algorithm to calculate replacement ratio, allows easier incorporation of LTCI benefits, and significantly reduces funding needs. For example, rather than doing a simple ratio of expected future expenses as compared to current living expenses and lumping 30–40 years of retirement into one big event, Dr. Basu breaks down retirement age into various groups or "bands." It is intuitive that the more active retirement years will be early on, and that more funds allocated to spending and enjoyment should be made for the beginning retirement years.

The current investment environment of low interest rates does not favor traditional retirement advice of moving more funds into bonds because they are "safe" money. So, coupled with Dr. Basu's age banding approach, physicians might consider more dividend-paying equities, in their portfolio, as an alternative (Somnath Basu, professor of finance at California Lutheran University and director of its California Institute of Finance, personal communication. Basu is involved in the National Endowment for Financial Education (NEFE), the CFP™ Board of Standards, International CFP™ Board of Standards, and the FPA). *Source*: http://healthcarefinancials.files.wordpress.com/2010/05/agebander.pdf.

How the 2015 Proposed Budget Impacts Retirement Accounts

President Barack Obama recently unveiled his proposed budget for 2015. Included in the proposal were the following potential changes to investor retirement accounts:

- *Apply required minimum distribution rule to Roth IRAs* As we have seen, there are currently two main reasons to invest in a Roth IRA—to pay taxes at your current rate in anticipation of being in a higher tax bracket in the future, and to invest in an account that does not require minimum distributions when the investor reaches age 70½. However, President Obama's 2015 budget called for Roth accounts to be subject to the same RMD requirements as other retirement accounts. This change would make Roth IRA accounts much less appealing for a good portion of the investment community. Additionally, if enacted, the rule would dramatically reduce the benefit for many individuals to convert their traditional retirement accounts to Roth accounts. Lastly, this rule would essentially betray all investors who already have converted their accounts to Roth IRAs by taking away a benefit they were counting on.
- *Eliminate stretch IRAs* Nonspouse beneficiaries of retirement accounts currently have the option of either withdrawing the funds from the inherited retirement account within 5 years of the original IRA owner's death or stretching IRA distributions over their expected lifetime. Stretching distributions is considered favorable because it allows the investor to spread the tax liability from the income over their lifetime and continue taking advantage of the tax-deferral provided by the retirement account. However, President Obama's proposal would eliminate non-spouse beneficiaries' ability to stretch distributions over a period of more than 5 years. If implemented, this change would have severe tax implications on people inheriting a retirement account and drastically reduce the value of tax-deferred accounts as estate planning tools.
- *Cap on tax benefit for retirement account contributions* Currently, investors obtain a full tax-deferral benefit on all contributions to retirement accounts. Under Obama's proposal, the maximum tax benefit that would be allowed on retirement contributions would be 28%. Consequently, an investor in the 39.6% tax bracket would only be able to deduct 28% and would still need to pay taxes at 11.6% (39.6%–28%) on all contributions made.
- *Eliminate RMDs for retirement accounts less than $100 k* Currently, investors over the age of 70½ must begin taking taxable distributions from their retirement accounts in the form of RMDs. Under Obama's proposal, individuals whose retirement accounts have a total value of less than $100 k would no longer be subject to RMD rules. This would enable retirees with less in their retirement accounts to take greater advantage of the tax-deferral benefit an IRA provides.
- *Retirement account value capping new contributions* Under the new proposal, once an individual's retirement account value grew to a certain cap, no further contributions would be allowed. This cap would be determined by calculating the lump sum payment that would be required to produce a joint and 100% survivor annuity of $210,000 starting when the investor turns 62. Currently, this formula would indicate a cap of $3.2 million. This cap would be adjusted for inflation.

Proposals, Not Law...

Keep in mind that these potential changes are currently just proposals and are not certain to be implemented into law. In fact, with the exception of RMDs for Roth accounts, all of these suggested adjustments were proposed last year and none were approved by congress. Consequently, history suggests that the President may have a hard time getting these changes implemented. Still, examining the proposals provides some insight into the direction President Obama would like to proceed.

"BREAKING NEWS": IRA ROLLOVER RULING STUNS FINANCIAL ADVISORS, DOCTORS, AND ALL SAVERS

In April 2014, the U.S. Tax Court ruled that the one-rollover-per-year rule applies to all of a taxpayer's IRAs rather than to each IRA separately. And, the ruling is in direct conflict with IRS Publication 590.

To recap, there are two ways to move money between IRAs:

1. *Transfers*: Not reported to the IRS and not reported on a tax return. The IRA owner never touches the money. You can do this as often as you like, whenever you like.
2. *Rollovers:* With this method, the IRA owner takes the money as a distribution and they have 60 days to rollover (put back) the amount in an IRA. And this, you can do only once per 12-month period.

So, the IRS has said for at least 20 years that the rollover method applies on a "per-IRA" basis. In other words, if you have 10 IRAs, you can do 10 rollovers for the year (12-month period), as long as an IRA does it only once (or the year).

Generally, if you make a tax-free rollover of any part of a distribution from a traditional IRA, you cannot, within a 1-year period, make a tax-free rollover of any later distribution from that same IRA. You also cannot make a tax-free rollover of any amount distributed, within the same 1-year period, from the IRA into which you made the tax-free rollover. The 1-year period begins on the date you receive the IRA distribution, not on the date you roll it over into an IRA.

Example: You have two traditional IRAs, IRA-1 and IRA-2. You make a tax-free rollover of a distribution from IRA-1 into a new traditional IRA (IRA-3). You cannot, within 1 year of the distribution from IRA-1, make a tax-free rollover of any distribution from either IRA-1 or IRA-3 into another traditional IRA.

However, the rollover from IRA-1 into IRA-3 does not prevent you from making a tax-free rollover from IRA-2 into any other traditional IRA. This is because you have not, within the past year, rolled over, tax free, any distribution from IRA-2 or made a tax-free rollover into IRA-2. *Source*: http://www.ustaxcourt.gov/InOpHistoric/BobrowMemo.Nega.TCM.WPD.pdf

So what now? You should plan ahead so that you avoid making more than one IRA rollover in 2015, and in years beyond.

ASSESSMENT

Far too many physicians incorrectly believe that by having a few brokerage accounts, or insurance products, their retirement planning needs are being met. Retirement planning however involves an in-depth analysis of needs, wants, resources, and alternative what-if scenarios to develop a long-term strategy. It also takes into account other areas of financial planning such as cash flow analysis, insurance and asset protection, investments, tax, and estate planning. It is based on risk tolerance, time frame, annual savings, and prioritized goals. The probability of success is increased by following this process and monitoring the plan on a regular basis. All assumptions are strictly unique and there is no one-size-fits-all strategy! More planning time decreases risk and enhances the chance to make any retirement vision a reality.

CONCLUSION

Proper retirement planning allows doctors, nurses, therapists, and medical professionals to live comfortably beyond their practice and work years, where work is optional. You work because you want to, not because you have to. This strategy can add millions of dollars to the benefits you receive, and may even allow retirement plan balances to pass on to heirs, or help your favorite religious charity, medical school, or cause of choice.

COLLABORATE

Discuss this chapter online with others at www.MedicalExecutivePost.com.

ACKNOWLEDGMENTS

To Richard J. Greenberg, CFP® and Richard P. Moran, CFP® of the Financial Network Investment Corporation, in Gardena, California; David K. Luke, MIM, CMP™ and Lon Jefferies, MBA, CFP® of the Net Worth Advisory Group, Sandy, Utah; and J. Christopher JD of www.North FultonWills.com.

FURTHER READING

Basu, S: Current retirement investing options for physicians. *Medical Executive Post.com*. Atlanta, GA, June 10, 2010.

Basu, S: Doctors: Are you ready to retire? *Medical Executive Post.com*. Atlanta, GA, March 4, 2010.

Bengen, WP: Asset allocation for a lifetime. *Journal of Financial Planning*, August, 58–67, 1996.

Bengen, WP. Conserving client portfolios during retirement, Part III. *Journal of Financial Planning*, December, 84–97, 1997.

Bengen, WP: Determining withdrawal rates using historical data. *Journal of Financial Planning*, October, 14–24, 1994.

Britton, D: The retirement illusion. *Wealth Management*, April, 13, 2014.

Edelman, R: *The Truth about Retirement Plans*. Simon & Schuster, New York, 2014.

Glover, R: *Preparing for Retirement: A Comprehensive Guide to Financial Planning*. Tarheel Advisors LLC, Cary, NC, 2013.

Guyton, J and Klinger, B: Decision rules and maximum initial withdrawal rates. *Journal of Financial Planning*, March, 50–58, 2006.

Guyton, JT: Decision rules and portfolio management for retirees: Is the "Safe" initial withdrawal rate too safe? *Journal of Financial Planning*, October, 54–62, 2004.

Hirt, GA, Block, SB and Basu, S: *Investment Planning*. McGraw-Hill, New York, 2006.

Kapadia, R: Revisiting the 4% rule. *Barron's*, November 11, 2013.

Kimura, A, Greenberg, R and Moran, R: Retirement planning. In: Marcinko, DE (editor). *Financial Planner's Library on CD-ROM*. Aspen Publishing, New York, 2001, 2002, and 2003.

Kimura, A and Moran, R: Retirement planning. In: Marcinko, DE (editor). *Financial Planner's Library on CD-ROM*. Aspen Publishing, New York, 2000.

Mittra, S: Starting early: Retirement planning. In: Mittra, S (editor). *Finance for Non-Finance Majors*. McGraw-Hill, New York, 2012.

Pfau, WD: Can we predict the sustainable withdrawal rate for new retirees. *Journal of Financial Planning*, August, 24(8), 40–47, 2011.

Stout, RG: Stochastic optimization in retirement portfolio management and withdrawal planning. *Financial Analysts Journal*, 61(6), 89–100, 2005.

Vincent, M: *Retirement Planning: A Guide to All Important Financial Decisions [How to Manage Your Money, Get Out of Debt and Plan Investments?]*. Amazon Kindle edition, New York, 2014.

Webb, A and Anspach, D: *Control Your Retirement Destiny: Achieving Financial Security before the Big Transition [Paperback]*. Apress Publishing, New York, 2013.

Williams, AJ: *Retirement: The Ultimate Retirement Planning Guide!* Amazon Kindle edition, New York, 2014.

WEBSITE

www.401k.org

Section IV

For Mature Practitioners

Several years ago, a group of highly trusted and deeply experienced financial service professionals and estate planners noted that far too many of their mature retiring physician clients, using traditional stock brokers, management consultants, and financial advisors, seemed to be less successful than those who went it alone. These do-it-yourselfers (DIYs) had setbacks and made mistakes, for sure. But, the ME Inc. doctors seemed to learn from their mistakes and did not incur the high management and service fees demanded from general or retail one-size-fits-all "advisors."

In fact, an informal inverse-related relationship was noted, and dubbed the "doctor effect." In others words, the more consultants an individual doctor retained, the less well they did in all disciplines of the financial planning and medical practice management, continuum.

Of course, the reason for this discrepancy eluded many of them as Wall Street brokerages and wire-houses flooded the media with messages, infomercials, print, radio, TV, texts, tweets, and Internet ads to the contrary. Rather than self-learn the basics, the prevailing sentiment seemed to pursue the holy grail of finding the "perfect financial advisor." This realization, topically noted in Section IV, was a confirmation of the industry culture, which seemed to be: *Bread for the advisor—Crumbs for the client*!

And so, the Institute of Medical Business Advisors Inc. (iMBA) formed a cadre of technology-focused and highly educated doctors, nurses, financial advisors, attorneys, accountants, psychologists, and educational visionaries who decided there must be a better way for their healthcare colleagues to receive financial planning advice, products, and related management services within a culture of fiduciary responsibility.

We trust you agree with this ME Inc., and Certified Medical Planner™ consulting philosophy, as illustrated in Section IV, and the entirety of this text book.

19 Professional Portfolio Construction
Investing Assets and Their Management

Timothy J. McIntosh, Jeffrey S. Coons,
and David Edward Marcinko

CONTENTS

In 1952, *The Journal of Finance* published an article titled "Portfolio Selection" authored by Dr. Harry Markowitz. The thoughts introduced in this editorial have come to form the underpinning of what is now widely referred to as modern portfolio theory (MPT). Initially, MPT generated relatively little interest, but with time, the financial community has ultimately adopted this thesis. Fifty years later, a multitude of financial models are based on the theory. In the paper, he argued in favor of portfolio diversification. Markowitz shared the Nobel Prize in Economics in 1990 with two other scholars "for their pioneering work in the theory of financial economics."

MODERN PORTFOLIO THEORY

MPT approaches investing by examining the complete market and the full economy. MPT places a great emphasis on the correlation between investments. Correlation is a measure of how frequently one event tends to happen when another event happens. High positive correlation means two events usually happen together—high SAT scores and getting through college for instance. High negative correlation means two events tend not to happen together—high SATs and a poor grade record. No correlation means the two events are independent of one another. In statistical terms, two events that are perfectly correlated have a "correlation coefficient" of 1; two events that are perfectly negatively correlated have a correlation coefficient of −1; and two events that have zero correlation have a coefficient of 0.

Correlation has been used over the past 20 years by institutions and financial advisors to assemble portfolios of moderate risk. In calculating correlation, a statistician would examine the possibility of two events happening together, namely,

- If the probability of A happening is $1/X$
- And the probability of B happening is $1/Y$; then
- The probability of A and B happening together is $(1/X)$ times $(1/Y)$, or $1/(X$ times $Y)$

There are several laws of correlation, including

1. Combining assets with a perfect positive correlation offers no reduction in portfolio risk. These two assets will simply move in tandem with each other.
2. Combining assets with zero correlation (statistically independent) reduces the risk of the portfolio. If more assets with uncorrelated returns are added to the portfolio, significant risk reduction can be achieved.
3. Combing assets with a perfect negative correlation could eliminate risk entirely. This is the principle with "hedging strategies." These strategies are discussed later in the book.

In the real world, negative correlations are very rare. Most assets maintain a positive correlation with each other. The goal of a prudent investor is to assemble a portfolio that contains uncorrelated assets. When a portfolio contains assets that possess low correlations, the upward movement of one asset class will help offset the downward movement of another. This is especially important when

TABLE 19.1
Historical Correlation of Asset Classes

Benchmark	1	2	3	4	5	6
1 U.S. Treasury Bill	1.00					
2 U.S. Bonds	0.73	1.00				
3 S&P 500	0.03	0.34	1.00			
4 Commodities	0.15	0.04	0.08	1.00		
5 International stocks	−0.13	−0.31	0.77	0.14	1.00	
6 Real estate	0.11	0.43	0.81	−0.02	0.66	1.00

Source: Ibbotson (1980–2012), Chicago, IL.

economic and market conditions change. As a result, including assets in your portfolio that are not highly correlated will reduce the overall volatility (as measured by standard deviation) and may also increase long-term investment returns. This is the primary argument for including dissimilar asset classes in your portfolio. Keep in mind that this type of diversification does not guarantee that you will avoid a loss. It simply minimizes the chance of loss. In Table 19.1, provided by Ibbotson, the average correlation between the five major asset classes is displayed. The lowest correlation is between the U.S. Treasury Bonds and the EAFE (international stocks). The highest correlation is between the S&P 500 and the EAFE; 0.77 or 77%. This signifies a prominent level of correlation that has grown even larger during this decade. Low correlations within the table appear most with the U.S. Treasury Bills.

RISK

One of the major concepts that most investors should be aware of is the relationship between the risk and the return of a financial asset. It is common knowledge that there is a positive relationship between the risk and the expected return of a financial asset. In other words, when the risk of an asset increases, so does its expected return. What this means is that if an investor is taking on more risk, he/she is expected to be compensated for doing so with a higher return. Similarly, if the investor wants to boost the expected return of the investment, he/she needs to be prepared to take on more risk.

One important thing to understand about MPT is that Markowitz's calculations treat *volatility* and *risk* as the same thing. In layman's terms, Markowitz uses *risk* as a measurement of the likelihood that an investment will go up and down in value—and how often and by how much. The theory assumes that investors prefer to minimize risk. The theory assumes that given the choice of two portfolios with equal returns, investors will choose the one with the least risk. If investors take on additional risk, they will expect to be compensated with additional return.

According to MPT, risk comes in two major categories:

- *Systematic risk*—The possibility that the entire market and economy will show losses, negatively affecting nearly every investment; also called *market risk*.
- *Unsystematic risk*—The possibility that an investment or a category of investments will decline in value without having a major impact upon the entire market.

Diversification generally does not protect against systematic risk because a drop in the entire market and economy typically affects all investments. However, diversification is designed to decrease unsystematic risk. Since unsystematic risk is the possibility that one single thing will decline in value, having a portfolio invested in a variety of stocks, a variety of asset classes and a variety of sectors will lower the risk of losing much money when one investment type declines in value. Thus, putting together assets with low correlations can reduce unsystematic risks.

Understanding the Risk

Although broad risks can be quickly summarized as "the failure to achieve spending and inflation-adjusted growth goals," individual assets may face any number of other subsidiary risks:

- *Call risk*—The risk faced by a holder of a callable bond that a bond issuer will take advantage of the callable bond feature and redeem the issue prior to maturity. This means the bondholder will receive payment on the value of the bond and, in most cases, will be reinvesting in a less favorable environment (one with a lower interest rate).
- *Capital risk*—The risk an investor faces that he or she may lose all or part of the principal amount invested.
- *Commodity risk*—The threat that a change in the price of a production input will adversely impact a producer who uses that input.
- *Company risk*—The risk that certain factors affecting a specific company may cause its stock to change in price in a different way from stocks as a whole.
- *Concentration risk*—Probability of loss arising from heavily lopsided exposure to a particular group of counterparties.
- *Counterparty risk*—The risk that the other party to an agreement will default.
- *Credit risk*—The risk of loss of principal or loss of a financial reward stemming from a borrower's failure to repay a loan or otherwise meet a contractual obligation.
- *Currency risk*—A form of risk that arises from the change in price of one currency against another.
- *Deflation risk*—A general decline in prices, often caused by a reduction in the supply of money or credit.
- *Economic risk*—The likelihood that an investment will be affected by macroeconomic conditions such as government regulation, exchange rates, or political stability.
- *Hedging risk*—Making an investment to reduce the risk of adverse price movements in an asset.
- *Inflation risk*—The uncertainty over the future real value (after inflation) of your investment.
- *Interest rate risk*—Risk to the earnings or market value of a portfolio due to uncertain future interest rates.
- *Legal risk*—Risk from uncertainty due to legal actions or uncertainty in the applicability or interpretation of contracts, laws, or regulations.
- *Liquidity risk*—The risks stemming from the lack of marketability of an investment that cannot be bought or sold quickly enough to prevent or minimize a loss.

VALUE AT RISK

Value at Risk (VAR) is another risk measure that has been gaining in popularity for several reasons. First, financial advisors (FAs) and doctors should intuitively evaluate risk in monetary terms rather than standard deviation. Second, in marketable portfolios, deviations of a given amount below the mean are less common than deviations above the mean for that same amount. Unfortunately, measures such as standard deviation assume symmetrical risk. VAR measures the risk of loss at some probability level over a given period of time.

For example, a physician-investor or FA may desire to know the portfolio's risk over a 1-day time period. The VAR can be reported as being within a desired quantile of a single day's loss. In other words, assume a portfolio possesses a one-day 90% VAR of $5 million. This means that in any one of 10 days the portfolio's value could be expected to decline by more than $5 million. Note that VAR is only useful for the liquid portions of an endowment's portfolio and cannot be used to assess risks in classes such as private equity or real assets.

Thus, it would seem self-evident that a risk that is not fully understood cannot be consciously managed or mitigated.

THE EFFICIENT FRONTIER

In order to compare investment options, Markowitz developed a system to describe each investment or each asset class with math, using unsystematic risk statistics. Then he further applied that to the portfolios that contain the investment options. He looked at the expected rate of return and the expected volatility for each investment. He named his risk–reward equation *the Efficient Frontier*. The graph in Figure 19.1 is an example of what the Efficient Frontier equation looks like when plotted. The purpose of the Efficient Frontier is to maximize returns while minimizing volatility. The outgrowth of Markowitz's work on MPT was the development of a plotted graph identifying portfolios that have the maximum expected return for any given level of risk, or the minimum level of risk for an infinite number of asset class combinations. By plotting each portfolio or combination of asset classes on one axis, and the volatility measures—or standard deviations—on another, a line graph representing the optimal combination of asset classes for various levels of risk is produced. This graph is known as the Efficient Frontier.

Points on or under the curve (in dots) represent the achievable combinations of investments. Points higher than the curve are unobtainable combinations given the particular set of accessible asset class categories. The portfolios that are positioned directly on the curve are viewed as efficient, which is why the curve itself is called the Efficient Frontier. Portfolios that lie underneath the curve are considered inefficient, as interchangeable portfolios exist with higher returns, lower volatility, or both.

Utilizing Efficient Frontier analysis, a medical professional can select which asset classes to include in a given portfolio and then view all possible combinations of those asset classes to help establish the most appropriate mix of assets. Until recently, the remuneration for the revolutionary

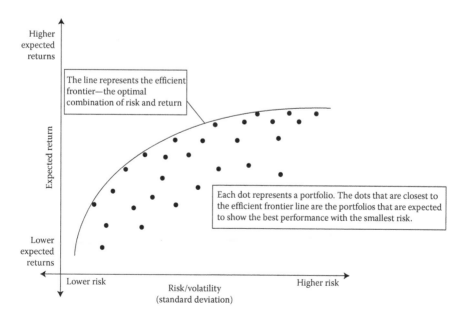

FIGURE 19.1   Efficient frontier. (From Ibbotson, Chicago, IL.)

efforts of Markowitz and others in the financial arena have been largely reserved for institutional and high-net-worth investors who were able to utilize the high-level mathematicians and computer systems needed to capture, calculate, and report risk and return data on a multitude of asset class categories. Now, with advances in computer technology and additional studies done to measure the accurate value of the asset allocation decision, sophisticated software has proliferated at a reasonable cost (Figure 19.2).

Utilizing MPT in the simplest form is about finding equilibrium between *maximizing your return* and *minimizing your portfolio risk*. The purpose is to select your investments in such a way as to diversify your risks while not impacting your expected return. Understanding how portfolio theory works will allow a medical professional to make informed decisions regarding which investment categories to include in their personal retirement accounts. Asset allocation is the process of dividing your investment dollars among an assortment of complementary asset classes, such as stocks, bonds, and real estate, so that your portfolio is well diversified. The decisive objective of an asset allocation program is to develop an investment portfolio that is properly aligned with your investment objectives and risk tolerance. A well-diversified investment portfolio will rarely outperform the top investment in any certain year, but over time it has frequently been one of the most resourceful methods to meet a person's long-term financial goals. Asset allocation gained national prominence after a landmark study conducted in 1986 by Brinson, Hood, and Beebower [1]. These gentlemen found that 93.6% of the total variation in portfolio results were attributable to asset allocation. A follow-up study by Brinson, Beebower, and Singer [2] confirmed this result, indicating that asset allocation explained 91.5% of variation in returns. These results underscored the importance of a well-thought-out asset allocation strategy. The process of determining which asset classes to include and the appropriate weights to assign to each is, in part, defined by your time horizon, risk tolerance, and familiarity or comfort level with the financial markets and various investment products.

Key benefits of a sound asset allocation strategy include

1. *Reduced risk:* An appropriately allocated portfolio produces lower volatility, or a lower fluctuation in yearly return, by simultaneously spreading market risk across numerous asset class categories (i.e., stocks and bonds).
2. *Steady returns:* By investing in a mixture of asset classes, you can advance your chances of participating in market gains and lessen the blow of poor-performing asset class categories on overall yearly results.
3. *Meeting long-term goals:* A diversified portfolio is designed to assuage the need to constantly adjust investment holdings to chase market trends.

Believers of the asset allocation philosophy concur that rather than investing in a single asset, investors should consider allocating a segment of their investment portfolios to numerous asset class

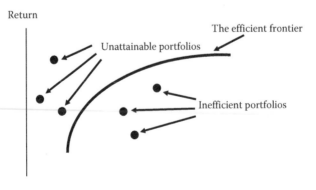

FIGURE 19.2 Efficient frontier portfolios.

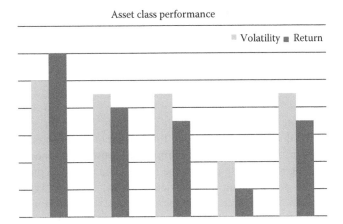

FIGURE 19.3   Asset allocation example—1983–2013. Stocks measured by S&P 500, bonds by the Barclays Aggregate Bond Index Real Estate by the NAREIT Index, and cash by IBC Money Market Fund Average. Diversified portfolio = 35% stocks, 45% bonds, 10% real estate, 10% cash. (From Factset, Norwalk, CT.)

categories in an effort to achieve higher risk-adjusted returns over time. The true power of asset allocation is illustrated by the chart in Figure 19.3 with examines performance of a diversified portfolio over a 30-year period. The diversified assortment of assets, which held 35% in stocks, 45% in bonds, 10% in real estate, and 10% in cash, performed nearly as well as the all-stock portfolio. It secured 80% of the return of the all-stock portfolio, with a 55% reduction of volatility.

CAPITAL ASSET PRICING MODEL

While Dr. Markowitz is credited with developing the framework for constructing investment portfolios based on the risk–return trade-off, William Sharpe, John Lintner, and Jan Mossin are credited with developing the capital asset pricing model (CAPM). CAPM is an economic model based upon the idea that there is a single portfolio representing all investments (i.e., the market portfolio) at the point of the optimal portfolio on the capital market line (CML) and a single source of systematic risk, beta, to that market portfolio. The resulting conclusion is that there should be a "fair" return investors should expect to receive given the level of risk (beta) they are willing to assume. Thus, the excess return or return above the risk-free rate that may be expected from an asset is equal to the risk-free return, plus the excess return of the market portfolio, times the sensitivity of the asset's excess return to the market portfolio excess return. Beta, then, is a measure of the sensitivity of an asset's returns to the market as a whole. A particular security's beta depends on the volatility of the individual security's returns relative to the volatility of the market's returns, as well as the correlation between the security's returns and the markets returns. Thus, while a stock may have significantly greater volatility than the market, if that stock's returns are not highly correlated with the returns of the overall market (i.e., the stock's returns are independent of the overall market's returns), then the stock's beta would be relatively low. A beta in excess of 1.0 implies that the security is more exposed to systematic risk than the overall market portfolio, and likewise, a beta of less 1.0 means that the security has less exposure to systematic risk than the overall market.

MPT has helped focus investors on two extremely critical elements of investing that are central to successful investment strategies. First, MPT offers the first framework for investors to build a diversified portfolio. Furthermore, an important conclusion that can be drawn from MPT is that diversification does in fact help reduce portfolio risk. Thus, MPT approaches are generally consistent with the first investment rule of thumb, "understand and diversify risk to the extent possible." Additionally, the risk/return trade-off (i.e., higher returns are generally consistent with higher risk) central to MPT-based strategies has helped investors recognize that if it looks too good to be true, it probably is.

PASSIVE INVESTING

Passive investing is a monetary plan in which an investor invests in accordance with a predetermined strategy that doesn't necessitate any forecasting of the economy or an individual company's prospects. The primary premise is to minimize investing fees and to avoid the unpleasant consequences of failing to correctly predict the future. The most accepted method to invest passively is to mimic the performance of a particular index. Investors typically do this today by purchasing one or more "index funds." By tracking an index, an investor will achieve solid diversification with low expenses. Thus, an investor could potentially earn a higher rate of return than an investor paying higher management fees. Passive management is most widespread in the stock markets. But with the explosion of exchange-traded funds on the major exchanges, index investing has become more popular in other categories of investing. There are now literally hundreds of different index funds.

Passive management is based upon the efficient market hypothesis (EMH) theory. The EMH states that securities are fairly priced based on information regarding their underlying cash flows and that investors should not anticipate to consistently outperform the market over the long term. The EMH evolved in the 1960s from the PhD dissertation of Eugene Fama. Fama persuasively made the case that in an active market that includes many well-informed and intelligent investors, securities will be appropriately priced and reflect all available information. If a market is efficient, no information or analysis can be expected to result in outperformance of an appropriate benchmark. There are three distinct forms of EMH that vary by the type of information that is reflected in a security's price:

- *Weak form*: This form holds that investors will not be able to use historical data to earn superior returns on a consistent basis. In other words, the financial markets price securities in a manner that fully reflects all information contained in past prices.
- *Semistrong form*: This form asserts that security prices fully reflect all publicly available information. Therefore, investors cannot consistently earn above-normal returns based solely on publicly available information, such as earnings, dividend, and sales data.
- *Strong form*: This form states that the financial markets price securities such that all information (public and nonpublic) is fully reflected in the securities price; investors should not expect to earn superior returns on a consistent basis, no matter what insight or research they may bring to the table.

While a rich literature has been established regarding whether EMH actually applies in any of its three forms in real-world markets, probably the most difficult evidence to overcome for backers of EMH is the existence of a vibrant money management and mutual fund industry charging value-added fees for their services.

The notion of passive management is counterintuitive to many investors. Passive investing proponents follow the strong market theory of EMH. These proponents argue several points, including

1. In the long term, the average investor will have a typical before-costs performance equal to the market average. Therefore, the standard investor will gain more from reducing investment costs than from attempting to beat the market over time.
2. The efficient-market hypothesis argues that equilibrium market prices fully reflect all existing market information. Even in the case where some of the market information is not

currently reflected in the price level, EMH indicates that an individual investor still cannot make use of that information. It is widely interpreted by many academics that to try and systematically "beat the market" through active management is a fool's game.

Not everyone believes in the efficient market. Numerous researchers over the previous decades have found stock market anomalies that indicate a contradiction with the hypothesis. The search for anomalies is effectively the hunt for market patterns that can be utilized to outperform passive strategies. Such stock market anomalies that have been proven to go against the findings of the EMH theory include

1. Low price to book effect
2. January effect
3. Size effect
4. Insider transaction effect
5. Value line effect

All the above anomalies have been proven over time to outperform the market. For example, the first anomaly listed above is the low price to book effect. The first and most discussed study on the performance of low price to book value stocks was by Dr. Eugene Fama and Dr. Kenneth R. French. The study covered the time period from 1963 to 1990 and included nearly all the stocks on the NYSE, AMEX, and NASDAQ. The stocks were divided into 10 subgroups by book/market and were reranked annually. In the study, Fama and French found that the lowest book/market stocks outperformed the highest book/market stocks by a substantial margin (21.4% vs. 8%). Remarkably, as they examined each upward decile, performance for that decile was below that of the higher book value decile. Fama and French also ordered the deciles by beta (measure of systematic risk) and found that the stocks with the lowest book value also had the lowest risk.

Today, most researchers now deem that "value" represents a hazard feature that investors are compensated for over time. The theory being that value stocks trading at very low price book ratios are inherently risky, thus investors are simply compensated with higher returns in exchange for taking the risk of investing in these value stocks. The Fama and French research has been confirmed through several additional studies. In a *Forbes* magazine 5/6/96 column titled "Ben Graham was right— again," author David Dreman published his data from the largest 1500 stocks on Compustat for the 25 years ending 1994. He found that the lowest 20% of price/book stocks appreciably outperformed the market.

One item a medical professional should be aware of is the strong paradox of the efficient market theory. If each investor believes the stock market were efficient, then all investors would give up analyzing and forecasting. All investors would then accept passive management and invest in index funds. But if this were to happen, the market would no longer be efficient because no one would be scrutinizing the markets. In actuality, the EMH actually depends on active investors attempting to outperform the market through diligent research.

The case for passive investing and in favor of the EMH is that a preponderance of active managers do actually underperform the markets over time. The latest study by Standard and Poor's (S&P) confirms this fact. S&P recently compared the performance of actively managed mutual funds to passive market indexes twice per year. The 2012 S&P study indicated that indexes were once again outperforming actively managed funds in nearly every asset class, style, and fund category. The lone exception in the 2012 report was international equity, where active outperformed the index that S&P chose. The study examined 1-year, 3-year, and 5-year time periods. Within the U.S. equity space, active equity managers in all the categories failed to outperform the corresponding benchmarks in the past 5-year period. More than 65% of the large-cap active managers lagged behind the S&P 500 stock index. More than 81% of mid-cap mutual funds were outperformed by the S&P MidCap 400 index. Lastly, 77% of the small-cap mutual funds were outperformed by the S&P SmallCap 600 index. The U.S. bond active managers fared no better than equity managers over a 5-year period. More than 83% of general municipal mutual funds underperformed the S&P National AMT-Free Municipal Bond index, 93% of government long-term funds underperformed the Barclays Long Government index, and nearly 95% of high-yield corporate bond funds underperformed the Barclays High Yield index. Although the performance measurements for index investing are very strong, many analysts find three negative elements of passive investing:

1. Downside protection: When the stock market collapses as it did in 2008, an index investor will assume the same loss as the market. In the case of 2008, the S&P 500 stock index fell by more than 50%, offering index investors no downside protection.
2. Portfolio control: An index investor has no control over the holdings in the fund. In the event that a certain sector becomes overowned (i.e., technology stocks in 2000), an index investor maintains the same weight as the index.
3. Average returns: An index investor will never have the opportunity to outperform the market, but will always follow. Although the markets are very efficient, an investor can perhaps take advantage of market anomalies and invest with those managers who have maintained a long-term performance edge over the respective index.

ACTIVE ASSET ALLOCATION

Proponents of active and passive investment management styles have made extensive and legitimate arguments for and against both approaches. For medical professionals who believe from time to time the financial markets misprice securities and want to take advantage of anomalies, an active investment selection policy can make sense. Investors who feel that the markets either overreact or underreact to a given piece of news related to a specific security are generally willing to commit their time and resources, or to hire an investment manager, to find mispriced securities. For example, a medical professional with a long time horizon may feel that financial markets are too focused on the near term following a decline in a pharmaceutical company's stock from a disappointing FDA report. While the short-term disappointment associated with an unsuccessful research and development effort may be significant, long-term investors may believe that the company's product pipeline as a whole is strong, and that the company's long-term future is still very bright. Thus, the healthcare provider may feel that the markets have overreacted to a short-term variable, and lost sight of the long-term prospects for the particular investment. The investor may conclude that the financial markets have mispriced the security relative to his/her time horizon and expectations regarding the company's future. An actively managed individual portfolio also allows tax considerations to be taken into account. For example, an active manager can harvest capital losses to offset any capital gains realized by its owner, or time a sale to minimize any capital gains. An actively managed mutual fund can do the same on behalf of its communal shareholders.

If active asset allocation makes sense based upon the limitations of passive asset allocation in managing risk over even long periods of time, how do investors and their advisors make active asset allocation decisions? There are two distinct active asset allocation approaches used by financial professionals to build an investment portfolio. They are the top-down method and the bottom-up method, and they differ based on how important economic and industry variables are to the decision-making process relative to individual security variables. The top-down approach establishes and adjusts asset allocation based primarily upon an overview of the overall economy and/or the industry in which the particular security operates. In contrast, bottom-up portfolio management approaches are geared toward identifying attractive investments on a security-by-security basis.

Top-Down Approach

Advocates of the top-down approach generally begin their investment process by formulating an outlook for the domestic economy, and in certain circumstances, the outlook is constructed for the global economy. This may be a direct result of a quantitative model using various market and economic data as input to reach a conclusion regarding the best asset mix on a tactical basis, or it may be a more subjective process resulting from a qualitative assessment of the market and economic outlook. In developing an economic overview for qualitative top-down asset allocation decisions, the medical professional and/or his advisors typically consider factors such as monetary policy, fiscal policy, trade relations, and inflation. Clearly, macroeconomic factors such as those listed above are likely to have a significant impact on the performance of a wide range of investment alternatives. After a thorough analysis of the overall economy has been completed, top-down investors will either buy broad baskets of stocks representing an asset class or perform an analysis of industries that they believe will benefit from the economic overview that has been developed. Factors that may influence the attractiveness of particular industries include regulatory environment, supply and demand of resources, taxes, and import/export quotas. The top-down approach generally views the best company in a weak industry as being unlikely to provide satisfactory returns. The final step in the top-down process involves analyzing individual companies in industries that are expected to benefit from the forecasted economic environment.

Bottom-Up Approach

In contrast, investors employing a bottom-up approach will focus their attention on identifying securities that are priced below the investor's estimate of their value. Investors using the bottom-up approach to asset allocation and portfolio construction will only purchase securities deemed attractive according to their basic pricing and security selection criteria, thus adjusting the overall mix of investments by the limit of securities considered attractive at current valuations. A truly bottom-up approach will consider economic and industry factors as clearly secondary in identifying investment opportunities. Investors using this approach will focus solely on company analysis. However, they must recognize that investment decisions cannot be made in a vacuum. Macroeconomic factors, as well as industry characteristics and traits are likely to be key elements in identifying attractive investment opportunities even on a security-by-security basis.

The key to bottom-up asset allocation and portfolio management is to realize that the decision variables driving the basic mix of assets in the portfolio are more related to the availability of attractive individual investments than to a general top-down market or economic overview.

Technical Analysis

There are two distinct forms of analysis often used by investors who desire to pursue an active investment strategy. The first strategy is referred to as technical analysis. Technical analysts, sometimes referred to as chartists, use historical price and transaction volume data to identify mispriced securities. A key belief shared by technical analysts is that stock prices follow recurring patterns, and that once these historical patterns are identified, they can be used to identify future security prices. The heart of technical analysis is identifying significant shifts in the supply and demand factors for a particular investment. Skeptics of technical analysis generally subscribe to the notion that the markets efficiently and accurately price securities. In fact, the weak form of the EMH is based on the view that investors cannot consistently earn superior returns using historical data alone.

Fundamental Analysis

In contrast to technical analysis, which relies on historical market return/transactions data, fundamental analysis focuses on the underlying company's earnings, risk, dividends, and economic factors to identify mispriced securities. The central theme behind fundamental analysis is the determination of a security's intrinsic value, or the value that is justified by the security's earnings, assets, dividends, or other economic measures. While technical analysis focuses on market prices, a security's intrinsic value is determined independently of the security's market value. A medical professional utilizing fundamental analysis is attempting to find securities that are trading at market prices below their intrinsic value.

How do healthcare providers or their advisors determine a security's intrinsic value? The methods used to place a value on a stock are too numerous to list. The methods range from very simple methods (e.g., price-to-earnings multiplier) to more complex (e.g., the dividend discount model (DDM)).

The price-to-earnings multiplier method of determining a stock's fundamental value is appealing to certain investors because of its simplicity. Under the price-to-earnings multiplier method, a stock's intrinsic value is determined by multiplying the stock's expected earnings per share by the stock's expected price-to-earnings ratio. For example, if a physician feels that Stock Y will earn $2.00 per share and that a reasonable estimate for Stock Y's price-to-earnings ratio is 15, then Stock Y's intrinsic value as determined under the price-to-earnings multiplier method is $30. While the price-to-earnings multiplier method appears simple on the surface, an investor's success using this method lies not only in his/her ability to estimate a stock's earnings per share, but also the stock's price-to-earnings ratio. Unfortunately, it is often a difficult task to estimate the multiple to its earnings that a stock should trade. While an analysis of multiples of other stocks in the same industry may provide insight as to what kind of earnings multiples could be reasonable, it is important for medical professionals to recognize that a stock's price-to-earnings ratio is determined by such factors as interest rates, stock market bullishness, and investor expectations regarding the company. Each of these variables can change dramatically in a short period of time.

The DDM is one of the most widely used valuation methods for estimating a stock's intrinsic value. As mentioned previously, a stock can be thought of as the right to receive future dividends. A stock's intrinsic value is defined as the present value of its dividends under the DDM. In its simplest form (i.e., zero growth), the DDM determines a stock's value by dividing the stock's dividend by the investor's required rate of return. The investor's required rate of return should reflect current interest rates plus the risk associated with investing in the stock.

The rate of return determined under the CAPM is frequently used in the DDM. For example, assuming that ABC Corporation pays a $2.00 dividend per share and that an investor requires a 10% return for holding ABC stock, the stock's intrinsic value is $20 ($2/0.10).

Shortcomings of the zero-growth DDM include the following:

- The model assumes that the stock's dividends will remain constant over time.
- The model assumes that dividends are the only source of return available to stock investors, ignoring the effect of reinvested earnings.
- The model can only be used to value stocks that pay dividends.
- The model assumes that the company and the dividends last forever.

Despite its shortcomings, the DDM highlights the point that the stock market is a discounting mechanism and that financial investments should be assessed in light of the future cash flows that they are expected to provide investors.

One variation on the DDM that may be appealing to healthcare professionals involves determining the present value of a stock's earnings rather than simply its dividends. Theoretically, owning a stock entitles investors to a claim on the earnings that are left after accounting for the company's costs (including interest costs). A model accounting for a stock's earnings rather than just dividends may help account for the capital appreciation element of owning stocks because a corporation can either invest its earnings back into the company to pursue growth opportunities or distribute the earnings to shareholders in the form of dividends.

COMBINING ASSET CLASSES

Combining disparate information into a workable asset allocation is as much art as it is science, perhaps more so. Most portfolios will use a combination of quantitative and qualitative analyses to develop their allocations. The quantitative portion of the analyses generally uses a variety of statistical techniques to develop a top-down approach to the general allocation. After developing a general sense of their desired range of returns, many endowments will use one of several "optimizer" techniques to assist in constructing an allocation. Commonly used optimization techniques include mean variance optimization (MVO) and Monte Carlo simulation (MCS).

MEAN VARIANCE OPTIMIZATION

MVO has at its core MPT, which seeks to find the "efficient frontier" that defines the minimum risk for any given level of return. In order to find this frontier, MVO will consider the expected returns, standard deviations (i.e., volatility), and correlation coefficients of individual asset classes. All things being equal, the endowment manager would generally choose the investments with the highest expected long-term return. However, the current funding needs placed upon endowments require that they be sensitive to the volatility of asset classes.

Expected volatility is often defined as "risk" and measured by the standard deviation of investment returns around an expected average return for that same investment. In other words, an asset class with an expected return of 10% and standard deviation of 5% would have its returns range from 5% to 15% approximately two-thirds of the time. This assumes that returns are normally distributed around a mean although a fair amount of evidence suggests that they are not. The below table summarizes periodic returns and standard deviations for selected classes of assets.

Average Annual Returns and Standard Deviations: 2006 through 2012 (Presented for Illustrative Purposes Only)

	Return	Standard Deviation
Wilshire 5000	1.15%	19.24%
MSCI EAFE	−5.37%	22.69%
MSCI EAFE emerging markets	−1.7%	29.01%
Hedge fund	2.95%	9.20%
Timber	6.39%	25.67%
Real estate	6.77%	6.41%
Long-term U.S. government	11.21%	1.01%
Intermediate U.S. government	6.34%	1.40%
Short-term U.S. government	2.69%	1.50%
Medical inflation	4.20%	1.14%

Cross-asset correlation is measured by the correlation coefficients between two categories of investments. Correlation coefficients range from −1.0 to +1.0. A correlation coefficient of −1.0 means two investment classes move exactly inverse to one another. On the other hand, a +1.0 correlation coefficient means that two asset classes have totally positive correlation. A 0.0 correlation coefficient means that movement in one asset class cannot be used to predict the level of return in another asset class. By holding asset classes with imperfect correlation, volatility in the portfolio can be reduced as classes with higher returns balance those with low or negative returns. The below table summarizes correlation coefficients for the same asset classes described in the above table.

Selected Asset Class Correlations Annual Return Historical: (Presented for Illustrative Purposes Only)

	Wilshire 5000	MSCI EAFE	MSCI EAFE Emerging Markets	Hedge Fund	Timber	Real Estate	Long-Term U.S. Government	Intermediate U.S. Government	Short-Term U.S. Government	Medical Inflation
Wilshire 5000	1.00									
MSCI EAFE	0.71	1.00								
MSCI EAFE Emerging Markets	0.41	0.67	1.00							
Hedge Fund	0.70	0.60	0.82	1.00						
Timber	0.38	0.18	0.32	0.58	1.00					
Real Estate	0.07	0.16	-0.42	-0.38	-0.59	1.00				
Long-Term U.S. Government	0.08	-0.26	0.01	0.25	0.63	-0.65	1.00			
Intermediate U.S. Government	0.07	-0.32	-0.20	0.13	0.42	-0.34	0.91	1.00		
Short-Term U.S. Government	0.10	-0.30	-0.36	0.01	0.09	0.04	0.64	0.89	1.00	
Medical Inflation	-0.30	-0.40	0.12	0.02	0.30	-0.80	0.73	0.55	0.30	1.00

The MVO optimizer will then mathematically plot a series of portfolio options that represent the maximum level of return for a given level of risk. By definition, there can be only one such efficient frontier of portfolios. Also, explicit in MPT is the idea that a portfolio below the efficient frontier is inefficient while a portfolio above the efficient frontier is impossible to sustain on a long-term basis. The efficient frontiers provide a graphical representation of the efficient frontier and portfolios that would be considered either inefficient or impossible to attain.

MONTE CARLO SIMULATION

Named after Monte Carlo, Monaco, which is famous for its games of chance, MCS is a technique that randomly changes a variable over numerous iterations in order to simulate an outcome and develop a probability forecast of successfully achieving an outcome. In endowment management, MCS is used to demonstrate the probability of "success" as defined by achieving the endowment's asset growth and payout goals. In other words, MCS can provide the endowment manager with a comfort level that a given payout policy and asset allocation success will not deplete the real value of the endowment.

The problem with many quantitative tools is the divorce of judgment from their use. Although useful, both MVO and MCS have limitations that make it so they should not supplant the endowment manager's experience. As noted, MVO generates an efficient frontier by relying upon several inputs: expected return, expected volatility, and correlation coefficients. These variables are commonly input using historical measures as proxies for estimated future performance. This poses a variety of problems.

First, the MVO will generally assume that returns are normally distributed and that this distribution is stationary. As such, asset classes with high historical returns are assumed to have high future returns. Second, an MVO optimizer is not generally time sensitive. In other words, the optimizer may ignore current environmental conditions that would cause a secular shift in a given asset class returns. Finally, an MVO optimizer may be subject to selection bias for certain asset classes. For example, private equity firms that fail will no longer report results and will be eliminated from the index used to provide the optimizer's historical data.

Twenty-Year Risk and Return Small Cap versus Large Cap (Ibbotson Data)

	1979			2010		
	Risk (%)	Return (%)	Correlation (%)	Risk (%)	Return (%)	Correlation (%)
Small-Cap Stocks	30.8	17.4	78.0	18.1	26.85	59.0
Large-Cap Stocks	16.5	8.1		13.1	15.06	

Source: Reproduced with permission from Loeper, DB, CIMA, CIMC: Asset Allocation Math, Methods and Mistakes. Wealthcare Capital Management White Paper, June 2, 2001.

David Nawrocki identified a number of problems with typical MCS as being that most optimizers assume "normal distributions and correlation coefficients of zero, neither of which are typical in the world of financial markets." Dr. Nawrocki subsequently describes a number of other issues with MCS, including nonstationary distributions and nonlinear correlations. Finally, Dr. Nawrocki quotes Harold Evensky, MS, CFP®, who eloquently notes that "[t]he problem is the confusion of risk with uncertainty. Risk assumes knowledge of the distribution of future outcomes (i.e., the input to the MCS). Uncertainty or ambiguity describes a world (our world) in which the shape and location of the distribution is open to question. Contrary to academic orthodoxy, the distribution of the U.S. stock market returns is far from normal." Other critics have noted that many MCS simulators do not run enough iterations to provide a meaningful probability analysis.

Some of these criticisms have been addressed by using MCS simulators with more robust correlation assumptions and with a greater number of iterative trials. In addition, some simulators now combine MVO and MCS to determine probabilities along the efficient frontier.

IMPACT OF TAXES

The general goal of a medical professional's investment program should be to provide capital growth and control investment risk in line with his/her overall investment objectives. However, an important issue for medical professionals to keep in mind when evaluating their investment program is the tax implications of their investment decisions. Certain types of accounts, such as qualified retirement plans, individual retirement accounts (IRAs), and variable annuities, provide growth on a tax-deferred basis, which means that income or capital gains earned within the account are not taxed until funds are withdrawn. As a result, investment decisions within these accounts may be made without concern for the interim tax implications of those decisions. In contrast, investors with nonqualified or taxable investment portfolios may incur taxes as the result of their investment decisions and should understand the basic income tax implications of buying and selling securities.

CAPITAL GAINS

The sale of a security typically results in either a capital gain, which results from shares being sold at a higher price than their original cost (after adjusting for splits, etc.), or a capital loss, which results from shares sold at a price below their original cost. Capital gains and losses are categorized as either short-term or long-term depending on how long the security was held. In order for a capital gain or loss to qualify as long-term, the underlying security being sold must have been held more than 12 months based upon the tax laws as of this writing.

The Internal Revenue Code provides an incentive for investors to take a long-term view when making their investment decisions by taxing long-term capital gains at 20%, while short-term capital gains are taxed at the investor's marginal federal income tax rate, which can run as high as 39.6%. Thus, investors (especially those in high income tax rates) prefer long-term gains to short-term gains due to the tax rate differential (i.e. 20% vs. 39.6%).

Investors are generally allowed to reduce their capital gains by their capital losses, but long-term losses must be used to offset long-term gains before they can be used to offset short-term losses and vice versa. For example, an investor with $1000 in long-term losses, $500 in long-term gains, $500 in short-term losses, and $2000 in short-term gains must first net his/her long-term gains and losses (resulting in a $500 net long-term loss), then his/her short-term gains and losses (resulting in a net $1500 short-term gain), and finally the $500 net long-term loss can be used to reduce the $1500 net short-term gain resulting in a $1000 overall short-term gain.

COST BASIS

A key element in calculating capital gains is the concept of cost basis. In order to calculate the gain or loss on the sale of a particular security, the investor's cost basis, or the amount they originally paid to acquire the security adjusted for share splits, spin-offs, and so on, is subtracted from the proceeds of the sale. Thus, a higher cost basis results in a lower capital gain, which in turn results in a lower capital gains tax liability.

The determination of cost basis is relatively straightforward in the case of a security that is purchased in one single transaction with no subsequent splits, with the security's cost basis equaling the total purchase price (including commissions and sales charges). However, there are several methods for determining the cost basis of a security that was acquired via multiple transactions, such as reinvested mutual fund dividends, systematic purchases (i.e., dollar cost averaging), or simply the purchase of multiple lots of the same stock at different points in time. The simplest method is referred to as the average cost method, where the security's cost basis is determined by calculating the weighted average purchase price. The last-in-first-out (LIFO) method assumes that the shares that were acquired most recently are the first shares sold, while the first-in-first-out (FIFO) method assumes that the shares that have been held the longest are the first shares sold. Finally, the specific shares method allows an investor to identify the specific shares that he/she sold. The following example illustrates these various methods of determining a security's cost basis:

Shares	Acquisition Date	Purchase Price
200	1/1/2006	$25.00
100	7/1/2013	$35.00

If the healthcare professional subsequently sells 150 shares of the security on 12/31/2013 what is his/her cost basis under the various methods?

Average cost method:	$28.33 [(200 × $25.00) + (100 × $35.00)]/300
LIFO method:	$31.67 [(100 × $35.00) + (50 × $25.00)]/150
FIFO method:	$25.00 (150 × $25.00)/150
Specific shares method:	$31.67 [(100 × $35.00) + (50 × $25.00)]/150

The specific shares calculation above assumes that the investor's goal is to minimize his/her capital gain by using the highest possible cost basis.

While medical professionals and their advisors should be aware of the tax implications of buying and selling securities in taxable investment portfolios, they must also not fall into the trap of letting the tax tail wag the investment management dog. While paying taxes is not an enjoyable experience for any investor, there is a clear trade-off between tax avoidance and risk management. Tax avoidance requires that the medical professional buy and hold securities in their taxable portfolio. Managing risk generally requires adjusting investments as market conditions and an investor's time horizon change. A buy-and-hold approach in the face of variable returns across the portfolio's securities is likely to lead to overweighted investments, usually at the time when those overweighted investments have the greatest price risk. Failing to properly diversify a portfolio as a result of avoiding capital gains increases the risk of the portfolio experiencing dramatic declines if the large, concentrated positions fall on hard times.

Thus, like risk, taxes are not necessarily something that should be avoided, but rather something that should be managed. One step that a medical professional can take with his/her taxable assets is to consider tax-exempt (i.e., municipal) bonds in the place of the taxable government or corporate bond investments of the portfolio. While tax-exempt bonds generally have lower yields than taxable bonds of similar credit quality, investors with a high income tax bracket are often able to achieve a higher after-tax yield from tax-exempt bonds. Another step is to evaluate the investments in the taxable portfolio for potential tax loss candidates that may be sold to offset capital gains realized in the portfolio. While it is important to consider the opportunity cost of selling a security at a loss, a security below original cost with deteriorating fundamentals may provide a benefit of reducing a tax liability already incurred. Finally, mutual fund investors can take steps to limit their tax liability by avoiding the purchase of funds that already have significant unrealized capital gains in their portfolio (i.e., buying someone else's capital gains), since all shareholders generally pay taxes on a fund's capital gains irrespective of when the gain was achieved.

PERFORMANCE MEASUREMENT

If securities are the pharmaceuticals and medical devices, and if portfolio management and investment strategies are the treatments, then performance measurement is the check-up and physical examination that ensures the patient's health is on the right track. While there has been a host of performance measurement statistics developed to assist in the evaluation of an investment program, the risk of misdiagnosis remains significant. In fact, the increase in computing power available to analyze investment performance has resulted in a proliferation of new statistical tools, but this improved capability to slice and dice performance has not necessarily coincided with improved understanding of the health of the investment program. Thus, it is important to grasp the various performance measurement calculations, but also to be able to evaluate the results in the context of the market and economic environment.

Calculating Returns

The first step in analyzing the results of an investment program is the calculation of total returns for the program. Total return represents the accumulated percentage increase in wealth from an investment, and is measured by the sum of capital appreciation (i.e., realized and unrealized capital gains and losses) and income over the time period divided by the amount invested. For example, assume a portfolio starts the period with a market value of $100,000, earns $5000 in income over the period, and securities appreciate in value another $3000 to achieve an ending value of $108,000. The total return is $8000/$100,000 or 8% over the period.

In most situations, however, the total return calculation must be adjusted to deal with cash flow that may come in and out of a portfolio. The standard total return calculation for a portfolio in the investment industry to take into account cash flow is the time-weighted return. The time-weighted return is the compounded periodic return with each period's return calculated as follows:

$$R_t = \frac{EV - BV - CF}{BV + WCF} \text{ for period } t$$

where EV = ending market value
BV = beginning market value
CF = cash flow = contributions – withdrawals

$$WCF = \frac{\left[(\text{day of } CF) - (\text{total days in period})\right] \times CF}{\text{total days in period}}$$

The time-weighted return, R, over T periods is calculated as

$$R = (1 + R_1)*(1 + R_2)* \cdots *(1 + R_T) - 1 \text{ for } t = 1, 2, \ldots, T$$

- *Example:* Dr. Hansen starts with $100,000 in a mutual fund on 12/31 and buys $10,000 per month at the mid-month point for 1 year, with one $50,000 withdrawal at the end of June and no fund dividends.

  Dr. Hansen started with $100,000 and added net cash flow over the full period of $70,000. The market value was $176,073 at the end of the year. The total investment gain was $6073. The return reported in the newspaper for the mutual fund would be 10.0% (i.e., $1.00/$10.00), which is also the time-weighted return achieved by Dr. Hansen.

Month Ending	NAV	Total Market Value	Contributions	Withdrawals	WCF	Monthly Time-Weighted Returns	Compound Time-Weighted Returns
December	$10.00	$100,000	–	–	$5000	–	–
January	$11.00	$120,500	$10,000	–	$5000	10.0%	10.0%
February	$11.50	$136,205	$10,000	–	$5000	4.5%	15.0%
March	$12.00	$152,344	$10,000	–	$5000	4.3%	20.0%
April	$11.50	$155,788	$10,000	–	$5000	–4.2%	15.0%
May	$11.75	$169,283	$10,000	–	$5000	2.2%	12.5%
June	$10.50	$110,742	$10,000	$50,000	$5000	–10.6%	5.0%
July	$11.00	$126,254	$10,000	–	$5000	4.8%	10.0%
August	$10.50	$130,288	$10,000	–	$5000	–4.5%	5.0%
September	$11.00	$146,730	$10,000	–	$5000	4.8%	10.0%
October	$11.25	$160,179	$10,000	–	$5000	2.3%	12.5%
November	$11.50	$173,849	$10,000	–	$5000	2.2%	15.0%
December	$11.00	$176,073	$10,000	–	$5000	–4.3%	10.0%

As is evident from the example, the time-weighted return calculation is intended to minimize the impact of cash flows and offers a performance number that can be used against other portfolios or investment vehicles. However, given a gain of only $6073 on a total net investment of $170,000, the time-weighted does not necessarily capture the rate of return achieved on each invested dollar. The calculation needed to measure the return on investment is called the internal rate of return or dollar-weighted return, which is defined as the percentage return needed to equate the initial market value plus a series of cash flows to the ending market value. The internal rate of return in our example is 4.5%.

The return calculations discussed so far measure the periodic return for an investment, which is then compounded to calculate the cumulative return. If the cumulative return covers a period of more than 1 year, the return is often annualized to reflect the rate of return on a yearly basis reflected in the cumulative return. To annualize a cumulative return R:

$$R_{ann.} = (1 + R)^{(P/TP)} - 1$$

where
P = # of periods in a year
TP = total # of periods in the cumulative return

As an example, a cumulative return of 18.9% over a 2¼ year period is

$$R_{ann.} = (1 + 0.159)^{(4/9)} - 1 = 8.0\%$$

While it is reasonable to annualize cumulative returns for periods greater than a year, it is generally inappropriate to annualize returns of less than a year. Why shouldn't an investor annualize a partial year return? An annualized number is intended to bring a return achieved by a portfolio down to a rate experienced over a standardized time period, in this case, 1 year. However, when an investor or his/her advisor increases the period covered by the performance measurement to calculate an annualized return for a partial year period, the implication is that this rate would be achievable over a full year. Just as the stock market's +21.3% rise in the first quarter of 1987 should not be annualized to +116%, the –22.6% fourth quarter should not be annualized to –64%. Neither of these annualized numbers shed any light on the actual 1987 calendar year return of +5.2% for the stock market.

Performance Benchmarks

Performance measurement has an important role in monitoring progress toward the portfolio's goals. The portfolio's objective may be to preserve the purchasing power of the assets by achieving returns above inflation or to have total returns adequate to satisfy an annual spending need without eroding original capital, and so on. Whatever the absolute goal, performance numbers need to be evaluated based on an understanding of the market environment over the period being measured.

One way to put a portfolio's a time-weighted return in the context of the overall market environment is to compare the performance to relevant alternative investment vehicles. This can be done through comparisons to either market indices, which are board baskets of investable securities, or peer groups, which are collections of returns from managers or funds investing in a similar universe of securities with similar objectives as the portfolio. By evaluating the performance of alternatives that were available over the period, the investor and his/her advisor are able to gain insight to the general investment environment over the time period.

Market indices are frequently used to gain perspective on the market environment and to evaluate how well the portfolio performed relative to that environment. Market indices are typically segmented into different asset classes.

Common stock market indices include the following:

- Dow Jones Industrial Average—a price-weighted index of 30 large U.S. corporations
- Standard & Poor's (S&P) 500 Index—a capitalization-weighted index of 500 large U.S. corporations
- Value Line Index—an equally weighted index of 1700 large U.S. corporations
- Russell 2000—a capitalization-weighted index of smaller capitalization U.S. companies
- Wilshire 5000—a cap-weighted index of the 5000 largest U.S. corporations
- Morgan Stanley Europe Australia, Far East (EAFE) Index—a capitalization-weighted index of the stocks traded in developed economies

Common bond market indices include the following:

- Barclays Aggregate Bond Index—a broad index of bonds
- Merrill Lynch High Yield Index—an index of below investment grade bonds
- JP Morgan Global Government Bond—an index of domestic and foreign government-issued fixed-income securities

The selection of an appropriate market index depends on the goals of the portfolio and the universe of securities from which the portfolio was selected. Just as a portfolio with a short-time horizon and a primary goal of capital preservation should not be expected to perform in line with the S&P 500, a portfolio with a long-term horizon and a primary goal of capital growth should not be evaluated versus Treasury Bills.

While the Dow Jones Industrial Average and S&P 500 are often quoted in the newspapers, there are clearly broader market indices available to describe the overall performance of the U.S. stock market. Likewise, indices like the S&P 500 and Wilshire 5000 are capitalization-weighted, so their returns are generally dominated by the largest 50 of their 500–5000 stocks. While this capitalization bias does not typically affect long-term performance comparisons, there may be periods of time in which large cap stocks out- or underperform mid-to-small cap stocks, thus creating a bias when cap-weighted indices are used versus what is usually non-cap-weighted strategies of managers or mutual funds. Finally, the fixed income indices tend to have a bias toward intermediate-term securities versus longer-term bonds. Thus, an investor with a long-term time horizon, and therefore potentially a higher allocation to long bonds, should keep this bias in mind when evaluating performance.

Peer group comparisons tend to avoid the capitalization bias of many market indices, although identifying an appropriate peer group is as difficult as identifying an appropriate market index. Further, peer group universes will tend to have an additional problem of survivorship bias, which is the loss of (generally weaker) performance track records from the database. This is the greatest concern with databases used for marketing purposes by managers, since investment products in these generally self-disclosure databases will be added when a track record looks good and dropped when the product's returns falter. Whether mutual funds or managers, the potential for survivorship bias and inappropriate manager universes make it important to evaluate the details of how a database is constructed before using it for relative performance comparisons.

Time Periods for Comparison

What is the appropriate time period for comparison? Performance measurements over trailing calendar periods, such as the last one, 3 and 5 years, are often used in the mutual fund and investment industry. While 3–5 years may seem like a long enough time for an investment strategy to show its value added, these time periods will often be dominated by either a bull or bear market environment, a large-cap- or small-cap-dominated environment.

One way to lessen the possibility of the market environment biasing a performance comparison is to focus on a time period that captures the full range of market environments: a market cycle. The market cycle is defined as a market peak, with high investor confidence and speculation, through a market trough, in which investor bullishness and speculation subsides, to the next market peak. A bull market is a market environment of generally rising prices and investor optimism. While there have been several definitions of a bear market based upon market returns (e.g., a decline of –15% or more, and two consecutive negative quarters), the idea implied by its name is a period of high pessimism and sustained losses. Thus, one returns-based rule-of-thumb that can be used to identify a bear market is a negative return in the market that takes at least four quarters to overcome. By examining performance over a full market cycle, there is a greater likelihood that short-term market dislocations will not bias the performance comparison.

Risk-Adjusted Performance

Performance measurement, like an annual physical, is an important feedback loop to monitor progress toward the goals of the medical professional's investment program. Performance comparisons to market indices and/or peer groups are a useful part of this feedback loop, as long as they are considered in the context of the market environment and with the limitations of market index and manager database construction. Inherent to performance comparisons is the reality that portfolios taking greater risk will tend to outperform less risky investments during bullish phases of a market cycle, but are also more likely to underperform during the bearish phase. The reason for focusing on performance comparisons over a full market cycle is that the phases biasing results in favor of higher-risk approaches can be balanced with less favorable environments for aggressive approaches to lessen/eliminate those biases.

Can we eliminate the biases of the market environment by adjusting performance for the risk assumed by the portfolio? While several interesting calculations have been developed to measure risk-adjusted performance, the unfortunate answer is that the biases of the market environment still tend to have an impact even after adjusting returns for various measures of risk. However, medical professionals and their advisors will have many different risk-adjusted return statistics presented to them, so understanding, for example, the Sharpe ratio, Treynor ratio, Jensen's measure or alpha, *Morningstar* star ratings, and their limitations should help to improve the decisions made from the performance measurement feedback loop.

Treynor Ratio

The Treynor ratio measures the excess return achieved over the risk-free return per unit of systematic risk as identified by beta to the market portfolio. In practice, the Treynor ratio is often calculated using the T-Bill return for the risk-free return and the S&P 500 for the market portfolio.

Sharpe Ratio

The Sharpe ratio, named after CAPM pioneer William F. Sharpe, was originally formulated by substituting the standard deviation of portfolio returns (i.e., systematic plus unsystematic risk) in the place of beta of the Treynor ratio. Thus, a fully diversified portfolio with no unsystematic risk will have a Sharpe ratio equal to its Treynor ratio, while a less diversified portfolio may have significantly different Sharpe and Treynor ratios.

Jensen Alpha Measure

The Jensen measure, named after CAPM research Michael C. Jensen, takes advantage of the CAPM equation discussed in the Portfolio Management section to identify a statistically significant excess return or alpha of a portfolio [3]. The essential idea is that to investigate the performance of an investment manager, you must look not only at the overall return of a portfolio, but also at the risk of that portfolio. For instance, if there are two mutual funds that both have a 12% return, a lucid investor will want the fund that is less risky. Jensen's gauge is one of the ways to help decide if a portfolio is earning the appropriate return for its level of risk. If the value is positive, then the portfolio is earning excess returns. In other words, a positive value for Jensen's alpha means a fund manager has "beat the market" with his or her stock picking skills compared with the risk the manager has taken.

Database Ratings

The ratings given to mutual funds by databases, such as *Morningstar,* and various financial magazines are another attempt to develop risk-adjusted return measures. These ratings are generally based on a ranking system for funds calculated from return and risk statistics. A popular example is *Morningstar's* star ratings, representing a weighting of 3, 5, and 10 year risk/return ratings. This measure uses a return score from cumulative excess monthly fund returns above T-Bills and a risk score derived from the cumulative monthly return below T-Bills, both of which are normalized by the average for the fund's asset class. These scores are then subtracted from each other and funds in the asset class are ranked on the difference. The top 10% receive five stars, the next 22.5% get four stars, the subsequent 35% receive three stars, the next 22.5% receive two stars, and the remaining 10% get one star.

Unfortunately, these ratings systems tend to have the same problems of consistency and environmental bias seen in both non-risk-adjusted comparisons over 3 and 5 year time periods and the other risk-adjusted return measures discussed above. The bottom line on performance measurement is that the medical professional should not take the easy way out and accept independent comparisons, no matter how sophisticated, at face value. Returning to our original rules-of-thumb, understanding the limitations of performance statistics is the key to using those statistics to monitor progress toward one's goals. This requires an understanding of performance numbers and comparisons in the context of the market environment and the composition/construction of the indices and peer group universes used as benchmarks. Another important rule-of-thumb is to avoid projecting forward historical average returns, especially when it comes to strong performance in a bull market environment. Much of an investment or manager's performance may be environment-driven, and environments can change dramatically.

SETTING OBJECTIVES

The portfolio management process begins with the medical professional's investment objectives for a given portfolio. In general, establishing reasonable investment objectives requires prioritization of various risk management goals, since there is often a trade-off between coverage of one investment risk and exposure to another. While most investors would like to have a portfolio that beats the stock market every year and never loses money over any single year, such investments simply do not exist (irrespective of any manager or fund's marketing material to the contrary). Therefore, when the medical professional sets the goals for a given portfolio, it is important to identify the basic need he/she has for these assets and the time horizon over which the need will be realized.

OVERHEARD IN THE DOCTOR'S LOUNGE: ON INVESTING PSYCHOLOGY

Of course you don't need a human financial advisor . . . until you do. Today, we've had unfettered Internet access to a wide range of investments, opinions and models for at least two decades. So, why the bravado to go it alone; five straight positive years for equities, since 2009!

The financial advisor's role is to remove the human element and emotion from investing decisions for something as personal as your wealth. Emotion drives the retail investor to sell low (fear) and buy high (greed). This is the reason why the average equity returns for retail investors is less than half of the S&Ps returns.

No, of course you don't need a human financial advisor . . . until you do. And when you do, it may be too late.

Dan Ariely, PhD
(The Irrational Economist)

COMMON INVESTING MISTAKES

There are many investment mistakes that medical professionals and their advisors need to be aware of and avoid. Here are some of the most common problems, along with suggested solutions.

FAILING TO DIVERSIFY

A single investment may become a large portion of a medical professional's portfolio as a result of market growth, a desire to avoid capital gains taxes, as a result of solid returns lulling an investor into a false sense of security, or some other reason.

Guideline: Understand and diversify risk to the greatest extent possible. Diversification is the only free lunch in investing. One key contribution of MPT is an understanding that diversification can in fact reduce portfolio risk, and the specific risk of a single stock may well overwhelm taxes or any other justification for failing to diversify.

CHASING PERFORMANCE

A medical professional can easily fall into the trap of chasing securities or mutual funds showing or promising the highest return, without understanding the risk involved in the investment. It's an article of assurance among many investors that they should only purchase mutual funds sporting the best recent performance. But in fact, it actually pays to shun mutual funds with strong recent performance. The latest report from S&P demonstrates that choosing a mutual fund purely based on performance is statistically a losing game as very few funds can consistently stay on top. Out of 703 funds that were top performers in their respective category as of March 2011, only 4.69% managed to stay on top over three consecutive 12-month periods. Looking longer term, only 2.41% of large-cap stock, 4.65% mid-cap stock, and 4.65% of small-cap stock funds were able to stay in the top half of their peers over five consecutive years. Unfortunately, many investors struggle to appreciate the benefits of their investment strategy because in jaunty markets, people tend to run after strong performance and purchase last year's winners.

In a market downturn, investors tend to move to lower-risk investment options, which can lead to missed opportunities during subsequent market recoveries. The extent of underperformance by individual investors has often been the most awful during bear markets. Academic studies have consistently shown that the returns achieved by the typical stock or bond fund investors have lagged substantially.

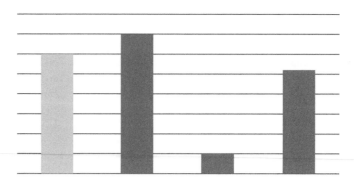

FIGURE 19.4   Investors have averaged lower returns than some market indexes due to chasing performance. January 1, 2002, to December 31, 2013. (From DALBAR, Boston, MA.)

The data in Figure 19.4 from independent research company DALBAR demonstrates that fund investors almost always follow behind the market. This means the choices made by investors of when to get into or out of the market, as well as enter into certain fund categories, have catastrophic results. Investors thus generate far lower returns than the overall market.

Guideline: Understand chasing performance does not work. Continually monitor your investments and don't feel the need to invest in the hottest fund or asset category. In fact, it is much better to increase investments in poor-performing categories (i.e., buy low). Also keep in remind rebalancing of assets each year is key. If stocks perform poorly and bonds do exceptionally well, then rebalance at the end of the year. In following this strategy, this will force a medical professional into buying low and selling high each year.

ASSUMING ANNUAL RETURNS WILL FOLLOW HISTORICAL AVERAGES

Many medical professionals and even some investment professionals make their investment decisions under the belief that stocks will consistently give them solid double-digit returns and bonds mid-digits. But both the stock and bond markets go through extended long-term cycles. In examining stock market history, there have been six secular bull markets (market goes up for an extended period) and five secular bear markets (market goes down) since 1900. There have been five distinct secular bull markets in the past 100+ years. Each bull market lasted for an extended period and rewarded investors. As with analysis of primary market cycles, secular cycles are analyzed from one top to the next. In Tables 19.2 and 19.3 are listed the major bull and bear stock market cycles since 1900.

If an investor had started investing in stocks either at the top of the markets in 1966 or 2000, future stock market returns would have been exceptionally below average for the proceeding decade. On the other hand, those investors fortunate enough to start building wealth in 1982 would have enjoyed a near two-decade period of well above-average stock market returns. The key element to remember for a medical professional is that future historical returns in stocks are not guaranteed. If stock market returns are poor, a medical professional must consider that he or she will have to accept lower projected returns and ultimately save more money to make up for the shortfall.

Stocks are not the only investment category to suffer through extended period of underperformance. Bond type investments can also do poorly and give below-average returns, especially if interest rates are historically low and interest rates are expected to rise. As of December 2013, the yield on the Barclays U.S. Aggregate Bond Index stood at 2.8%, with a weighted average duration of 5.5 years. To use a simplistic example, a 1-percentage-point rise in yields during a 12-month period would lead to a new yield of 3.8% and a capital loss of –5.5%. Following the 1-percentage-point rise in rates, the initial expected return for year two would be 3.1%, instead of 2.1%. Over a 2-year holding period, an investor would approximately breakeven in this case.

TABLE 19.2
Top Six Secular Bull Markets

Secular Event	Date	High	Low	Secular Bull Market Duration (Years)	Percent Change (%)	Annualized Compound Return (%)
Top 1	1/19/1906	103				
Bottom 1	12/24/1914		53.17	14.75	617	14
Top 2	9/3/1929	381.17				
Bottom 2	7/8/1932		41.22	4.67	371	39
Top 3	3/6/1937	194.15				
Bottom 3	4/28/1942		92.92	23.75	971	10
Top 4	2/9/1966	995.15				
Bottom 4	5/26/1970		631.16	2.58	67	22
Top 5	1/11/1973	1051.7				
Bottom 5	12/6/1974		577.6	32.75	2352	10
Top 6	03/1/2000	14,164.53				
				15.7	876	18
Average standard deviation				12.7	890	10

TABLE 19.3
Top Six Secular Bear Markets

Secular Event	Date	High	Low	Secular Bear Market Duration (Years)	Percent Change (%)	Annualized Compound Return (%)
Top 1	1/19/1906	103				
Bottom 1	12/24/1914		53.17	8.93	−48	−7
Top 2	9/3/1929	381.17				
Bottom 2	7/8/1932		41.22	2.85	−89	−54
Top 3	3/6/1937	194.15				
Bottom 3	4/28/1942		92.92	5.14	−52	−13
Top 4	2/9/1966	995.15				
Bottom 4	5/26/1970		631.16	4.3	−37	−10
Top 5	1/11/1973	1051.7				
Bottom 5	12/6/1974		577.6	1.9	−45	−27
Top 6	10/9/2007	14,164.53				
				4.6	−54	−22
Average standard deviation				2.7	20	19

Hypothetical Example of Impact of 3-Percentage-Point Increase in Interest Rates

	+1 year	+2 years	+3 years	+4 years	+5 years
Yield	5.8%	5.8%	5.8%	5.8%	5.8%
Price change	−16.5	0.0	0.0	0.0	0.0
Total return	−12.9	5.1	5.1	5.1	5.1
Cumulative total return	−12.9	−8.5	−3.8	1.1	6.3
Annualized total return	−12.9	−4.3	−1.3	0.3	1.2

Source: Vanguard—This hypothetical example does not represent the return on any particular investment. "Today's" yields are as of May 31, 2013, based on Barclays U.S. Aggregate Bond Index. For simplicity, duration was assumed to remain at 5.5 years, but in practice, as yields change, duration also changes. Such a dramatic change in yields as this example assumes would likely constitute a rather significant adjustment to a fund's weighted average duration. For purposes of illustration, we assumed no changes to yields in subsequent years.

If interest rates jumped from 2.8% to 5.8%, that rise would represent a 143% alteration in rates. The theoretical impact of an actual 3% increase in interest rates on an investment linked to the broad U.S. bond market is demonstrated in the above table. As expected, in year one, the price decline would be considerable, potentially leading to the second-worst 12-month return ever for the U.S. bond investors of −12.9%. If rates stayed at that level for the next 3 years, a bond investor would maintain a loss of 3.8% for the entire period.

Guideline: Beware of projecting forward historical returns. Medical professionals should realize that the stock and bond markets are inherently volatile and that, while it is easy to rely on past historical averages, there are long periods of time where returns and risk deviate meaningfully from historical averages.

ATTEMPTING TO TIME THE MARKET

Some medical professionals or their advisors believe they are "smarter than the market" and can time when to jump in and buy stocks or sell everything and go to cash. Wouldn't it be nice to have the clairvoyance to be out of stocks on the market's worst days and in on the best days? Using the S&P 500 Index, our agile imaginary investor managed to steer clear of the worst market day each year from January 1, 1992, to March 31, 2012. The outcome: he compiled a 12.42% annualized return (*including reinvestment of dividends and capital gains*) during the 20+ years, sufficient to compound a $10,000 investment into $107,100.

But what about another unfortunate investor that has the wonderful mistiming to be out of the market on the best day of each year? This ill-fated investor's portfolio returned only 4.31% annualized from January 1992 to March 2012, increasing the $10,000 portfolio value to just $23,500 during the 20 years. The design of timing markets may sound easy, but for most investors, it is a losing strategy.

Guideline: If it looks too good to be true, it probably is. While jumping into the market at its low and selling right at the high is appealing in theory, medical professionals should recognize the difficulties and potential opportunity and trading costs associated with trying to time the stock market in practice. In general, healthcare providers will be best served by matching their investment with their time horizon and looking past the peaks and valleys along the way.

FAILING TO RECOGNIZE THE IMPACT OF FEES AND EXPENSES

An attractive investment and a polished sales pitch can often hide the underlying costs of the investment, leading some medical professionals to give up a significant portion of the long-term growth of their assets to fees. Fees absolutely matter. In a good market investors have a propensity to ignore them and in challenging markets they are scrutinized, but in the end no matter what type of market we are in, fees do make a substantial difference in your long-term investment returns.

The first step in assessing the worth of the investment under consideration is figuring out what the fees actually are. If a medical professional is investing in a mutual fund, these costs are found in mutual fund company's now obligatory "Fund Facts." This manuscript clearly outlines all the fees paid—including upfront fees (or commissions/loads), deferred sales charges (DSCs), and any switching fees. Fund management expense ratios are also part of the overall cost of ownership. Trading costs within the mutual fund can also impact performance.

Here is a list of the traditional fees from investing in a mutual fund:

- Front-end load: It is the commission charged to purchase the fund through a broker or financial advisor. The commission reduces the amount you have available to invest. Thus, if you start with $100,000 to invest and the advisor charges a 5% front-end load, you end up actually investing $95,000.
- DSC or back-end load: Charge imposed if you sell your position in the mutual fund within a prespecified period of time (normally 5 years). It is initiated at a higher start percentage (i.e., as high as 10%) and declines over a specific period of time.
- Operating fees: These are costs charged by the mutual fund, including the management fee rewarded to the manager for investment services. It also includes legal, custodial, auditing, and marketing.
- Annual administration fee: Many mutual fund companies also charge an additional fee just for administering the account—usually under $150 per year.

A 1% disparity in fees for a medical professional may not seem like a lot, but fees do make a considerable impact over a longer time period. For example, a $100,000 portfolio that earns 8% before fees grows to $320,714 after 20 years if the client pays a 2% operating fee. In comparison, if the investor opted for a fund that charges a more reasonable 1% fee, after 20 years, the portfolio grows to be $386,968—a divergence of over $66,000! For many investors, this is the value of passive or index investing. In the case of an index fund, fees are generally under 0.5%, thus offering even more fee savings over an elongated period of time.

Guideline: Keep fees and commissions to a minimum. Fees and expenses can have significant impact on the performance of your investments. Always monitor the costs of an investment program to ensure that fees and expenses are reasonable for the services provided and are not consuming a disproportionate amount of the investment returns.

ASSESSMENT

Health economist and colleague Austin Frakt, PhD, of the *Incidental Economist*, alerted us to the publication: "Achieving Cost Control, Care Coordination, and Quality Improvement through Incremental Payment System Reform," by R.F. Averill et al., *JACM*, 2010. In it, the following prescient query is presented: "Is there an 'Efficient-Frontier' for Medicare Reform?" The paper, released prior to the PP-ACA, described various Medicare payment reform methods (personal communication).

Paper Abstract

The healthcare reform goal of increasing eligibility and coverage cannot be realized without simultaneously achieving control over healthcare costs. The reform of existing payment systems can provide the financial incentive for providers to deliver care in a more coordinated and efficient manner with minimal changes to existing payer and provider infrastructure. Pay for performance,

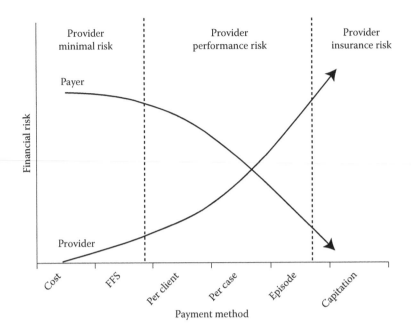

FIGURE 19.5   Modern portfolio theory.

best practice pricing, price discounting, alignment of incentives, the medical home, payment by episodes, and provider performance reports are a set of payment reforms that can result in lower costs, better coordination of care, improved quality of care, and increased consumer involvement. These reforms can produce immediate Medicare annual savings of $10 billion and create the framework for future savings by establishing financial incentives for long-term provider behavior changes that can lead to lower costs.[*]

MODERN PORTFOLIO THEORY IN MEDICARE

Of course, the third dimension of risk (beyond traditional doctor/hospital provider and Medicare insurer) would be the risk borne by the patient insured (degree of cost-sharing or "consumer responsibility"). This relationship is represented diagrammatically in Figure 19.5.

CONCLUSION

MPT attempts to maximize investment portfolio expected returns for a given level of risk by carefully choosing the proportions of various asset classes. As a mathematical formulation, the concept of diversification aims to select a collection of assets that collectively lowers risk (measured by standard deviation) more than any individual asset class. This is the "efficient frontier." And, it can be seen intuitively because different types of assets often change in value in opposite ways.

Health insurance (Medicare payment reform) econometric considerations may now be extended in this analogy to suggest that medical providers and CMS payers are the surrogates for two dimensions in the MPT. The third might be the risks borne by the insured patient (degree of cost-sharing or "consumer responsibility"), as above. Then, patients could self-select where they wish to fall on the health insurance "efficient frontier," balancing all three dimensions as in MPT, along with lifestyle and moral hazard considerations, and so on.

---

[*] *Source:* http://www.ncbi.nlm.nih.gov/pubmed/20026992.

COLLABORATE

Discuss this chapter online with others at www.MedicalExecutivePost.com.

ACKNOWLEDGMENT

To Christopher Cummings, CFA, CFP® of Manning-Napier Investment Advisors, New York.

REFERENCES

1. Brinson, GP, Hood, R, and Beebower, GL: Determinants of portfolio preference. *Financial Analysts Journal* 1986; 42(4):39–44.
2. Brinson, GP, Singer, BD, and Beebower, GL: Determinants of portfolio performance II: An update. *Financial Analysts Journal* May/June 1991.
3. Jensen, MC: The performance of mutual funds in the period 1945–1964. *Journal of Finance* 1967; 23(2):389–416.

FURTHER READING

2007 Annual US Corporate Pension Plan Best and Worst Investment Performance Report. FutureMetrics, April 20, 2007.

Avrill, RF, Goldfield, NI, Vertrees, JC, McCullough, EC, Fuller, RL, and Eisenhandler, J: Achieving cost control, care coordination, and quality improvement through incremental payment system reform. *The Journal of Ambulatory Care Management* January–March 2010; 33(1):2–23, doi: 10.1097/JAC.0b013e3181c9f437.

Boogle, J: *The Little Book of Common Sense Investing*. Wiley, New York, 2007.

Brinson, GP, Hood, R, and Beebower, GL: Determinants of portfolio performance. *Financial Analysts Journal* 1986; July/August, 39–44.

Clark, SE and Yates, TT, Jr.: How Efficient Is Your Frontier? Commonfund Institute White Paper, November 2003.

Coons, J and Cumming, C: In: Marcinko DE (editor): *Financial Planning for Physicians*. Jones and Bartlett, Sudbury, MA, 2004.

Dimensional Fund Advisors. Basic 60/40 Balanced Strategy vs. Company Pension Plans Results of 192 Corporate Pension Plans. Annual: 1988–2006 PowerPoint Slides.

Doody, D: Measuring Up Investment Policies and Practices in Not-for-Profit Healthcare: Investment Management Is an Area That Lends Itself to Quantitative Analysis to Produce Information That Can Inform and Guide Your Decision Making. Healthcare Financial Management Association and Gale Group, 2007.

Ibbotson, RG and Patel, AK: *Do Winners Repeat with Style? Summary of Findings*. Ibbotson & Associates, Chicago, February 2002.

Kacperczyk, MT, Sialm, C, and Lu Z: *On Industry Concentration of Actively Managed Equity Mutual Funds*. University of Michigan Business School, Ann Arbor, MI, November 2002.

Loeper, DB, CIMA, CIMC: Asset Allocation Math, Methods and Mistakes. Wealthcare Capital Management White Paper, June 2001.

Malkalkiel, BG: *A Random Walk Down Wall Street: The Time-Tested Strategy for Successful Investing* (10th edition). Norton, New York, 2012.

Nawrocki, D, PhD: The problems with Monte Carlo simulation. *FPA Journal* November 2001.

Sedlacek, V: Currents & commentary enter the matrix. *CFQ, Commonfund*, Fall, 2004.

Swensen, DF: *Pioneering Portfolio Management*. The Free Press, a division of Simon and Schuster, Inc., New York, 2000.

WEBSITES OF INTEREST

Investment Theory and Research Sites
  www.stanford.edu/~wfsharpe/
  www.efficientfrontier.com
  http://advisorperspectives.com/dshort/
  http://www.bespokeinvest.com/

Investor Research Sites
      www.sec.gov
      www.morningstar.com
      www.marketguide.com
      www.yardeni.com
      www.aima.org
Investment News Sites
      www.bloomberg.com
      www.thestreet.com
      www.finance.yahoo.com
      www.wsj.com
      http://www.marketwatch.com/
      http://online.barrons.com/home-page
Investment Blog Sites
      http://www.ritholtz.com/blog/
      http://www.zerohedge.com/
      http://abnormalreturns.com/
      http://www.businessinsider.com/
      http://www.peridotcapitalist.com/

20 Investment Policy Statement Construction

The Essential Document for Physician Investors and Healthcare Organizations

David Edward Marcinko

CONTENTS

To create and monitor an investment portfolio for personal or institutional use, the physician executive, financial advisor, wealth manager, or healthcare institutional endowment fund manager should ask three questions:

1. How much have we invested?
2. How much did we make on our investments?
3. How much risk did we take to get that rate of return?

INTRODUCTION

Most doctors, and hospital endowment fund executives, know how much money they have invested. If they don't, they can add a few statements together to obtain a total. But, few actually know the rate of return achieved last year; or so far this year. Everyone can get this number by simply subtracting the ending balance from the beginning balance and dividing the difference. But, few take the time to do it. Why? A typical response to the question is, "We're doing fine."

Now, ask how much risk is in the portfolio and if help is needed. In fact, Nobel laureate Harry Markowitz, PhD said, "If you take more risk, you deserve more return." Using standard deviation, he referred to the "variability of returns"; in other words, how much the portfolio goes up and down—its volatility (Markowitz, H: Portfolio selection. *Journal of Finance*, March, 1952).

PART I: THE IPS FOR INDIVIDUAL PHYSICIAN INVESTORS

How to manage risk and create your own portfolio (ME Inc.) is what the first part of this chapter is about. First, you must determine what to do with your investments. How much risk can be taken and what is the time frame? You must understand the concept of risk versus reward and write an Investment Policy Statement (IPS). Next, the assets that will be used for investment must be selected. This involves asset allocation and mixing different styles of investing to achieve the desired results, and is the point where you go it alone, or hire a financial advisor. Be sure to review expenses, service fees, commissions, and compare mutual funds with private money management. Once the initial portfolio is in place, performance must be monitored to assure compliance with the IPS. Now after all of this, if you still want to do it yourself, the entire process will be reviewed.

THE BASICS

You would not think of building a house without a set of construction drawings and detailed written specifications. An IPS sets forth plans and specifications for the portfolio, just like construction drawings and detailed written specifications tell the contractor how to build a house. The physician investor who writes the IPS is like the architect who draws up plans for a building. Both must ask many questions to determine the wishes of the owner. The same is true with a portfolio.

In a personal communication, Fred Rice, a senior vice president of Carolinas Physicians Network in Charlotte, North Carolina, who writes medical institutional and foundation IPS documents explains:

> To me, the Investment Policy Statement is the most important investment document. It must be a clear statement of precisely what you want your money to do for you. Everyone involved; physicians, board

members, money managers, administrators, investment consultants and beneficiaries of the trust must have a single clear statement of investment parameters. There should be no misunderstanding of who is to do what and how they are suppose to do it with a properly written Investment Policy Statement.

A personal Investment Policy Statement (IPS) has six parts:

1. Statement of purpose
2. Statement of responsibilities
3. Objectives and goals
4. Asset mix guidelines
5. Performance review
6. Communication

First, consider why you are writing the document and what you are trying to accomplish. This is the *Statement of Purpose*. The *Statement of Responsibilities* identifies the parties associated with the portfolio and the functions, responsibilities, and activities of each with respect to management of the assets (ME, Inc.). Then, establish some *Objectives and Goals* for risk tolerance and expected returns. Which assets (stocks, bonds, cash or international equities, etc.) will you use? What net return do you desire after inflation? Net after taxes? Net after fees and commissions? Now, consider the direction you must give to the selection of securities. In the *Asset Mix Guidelines* section, you need to identify specific securities or types of securities that you want to use in the portfolio and which are to be excluded. Consider benchmarks, the use of margin, foreign stocks, short selling, futures trading, and so on. The *Performance Review* section involves how to measure performance, what benchmark you will use and how to evaluate your progress. Finally, you want to consider the procedures for employee or self-reporting in your *Communications* policy. Quarterly reports are usually required. You need to make a complete performance measurement and analysis.

In reality, the solo doctor's written IPS can be as simple as a single page. For a healthcare organization, it can be an elaborate, detailed, and multi-page tome. So, let us review all six parts.

Statement of Purpose

The purpose of this document is to guide the investment of (usually) retirement plan accounts. You want details about goals and objectives, as well as the performance measurement techniques that you will employ in evaluating the plan. Realizing that your overall objective is best accomplished by employing a variety of styles, and that you will adjust your asset tolerances and volatility to incorporate specific styles.

Statement of Responsibilities

The physician-executive is responsible for the daily investment management of plan assets, including specific security selection and timing of purchases and sales.

The custodian is responsible for safekeeping the securities, collections and disbursements and periodic accounting statements. The prompt credit of all dividends and interest to accounts on the payment date is required. The custodian shall provide monthly account statements and reconcile all statements. A financial advisor, if used, is responsible for assisting in developing the IPS and monitoring the overall performance of the Plan.

Investment Goals and Objectives

The asset value of the funds, exclusive of contributions or withdrawals, should grow in the long-run and earn through a combination of investment income and capital appreciation a rate-of-return in excess of a specified market index for each investment style, while incurring less risk than such index. It is recognized that short-term fluctuations in the capital markets may result in a loss of capital on occasion, commonly expressed as negative rates of return. The amount of volatility and specific frequency of negative returns shall be detailed for each investment style.

The IPS is based on the assumption that the volatility of the portfolio will be similar to that of the market. A specific index or combination of indexes will be assigned to each class of securities and style of selection to be employed. The physician investor will determine an overall index for volatility and asset allocation within the Plan as a whole. It will be the duty of the physician to monitor this section closely and make changes to comply with the overall policy. Expect that the accounts in total will meet or exceed the rate of return of a balanced market index comprised of the S&P 500 stock index, Government/Corporate Bond Index and the U.S. treasury bills in similar proportion to the asset allocation policy. Recognizing that short-term market fluctuations may cause variations in the account performance, expect the combined accounts to achieve the following objectives over a three-year moving time frame. For example,

1. The account's total expected return will exceed the increase in the Consumer Price Index by 7.0 percentage points annually. Actual returns should exceed the expected returns about half the time. Expected returns should exceed actual returns about half the time (i.e., if the CPI increases from 5.0% to 7.0%, then expected return should exceed 9%).
2. The total annual return of the account is expected to exceed the average CPI for the year by an absolute of 3.0 percentage points (i.e., if the average CPI is 5.0%, then the expected annual return should exceed 8.0%).
3. The average total expected return will exceed 8–10% annually.

Index for Performance Comparisons

Style	Index
Small cap growth	Russell 2000 Growth
Medium cap value	Russell Medium Cap Value
Small cap value	Russell 2000 Value
Growth	Russell 1000 Growth
Value	Russell 1000 Value
Tax-free bonds	Federal/State
Taxable bonds	Federal/State
Blended account	S&P 500/Govt/Corp

Trading and Execution Guidelines

Trading shall be done through a discount-brokerage firm. Instruction to execute transactions assumes that their service is equal to, and the rates are competitive with, other nationally recognized investment firms. Additionally, it is understood that block transactions or participation in certain initial public offerings might not be available through a primary broker. In this case the doctor should execute those trades through a broker offering the product and service necessary to best serve the account.

Social Responsibility

No (some) assets shall be invested in securities of any organization that does not meet the standard for socially and morally responsible as determined by the physician investor.

Asset Mix Guidelines

The Plan shall have the assets invested in accordance with the maximum and minimum range for each asset category: selected and illustrated below. Separate asset category guidelines will be provided according to specified style and standard deviation tolerances.

Asset Class	Minimum Weight	Target Weight	Maximum Weight	REP Index
Equities	50	60	70	S&P 500/FRC 2000 Index
Fixed income	25	40	55	LB Muni/LBGC Inter
Cash & Equiv	0	0	30	90 Day Treasury

Portfolio Limitation

The following are general requirements, as these limitations would be adjusted for a different physician-executive whose performance expectation might make it necessary to expand definitions.

Equities: Equity securities shall mean common stock or equivalents (American Depository Receipts plus issues convertible into common stocks). Preferred stocks with the exception of convertible preferreds are considered part of the fixed income section. The equity portfolio shall be well diversified to avoid undo exposure to any single economic sector, industry group, or individual security. No more than 5% of the equity portfolio based on the market value shall be invested in securities of any one issue or corporation at the time of purchase. No more than 10% of the equity portfolio based on the market value shall be invested in any one industry at the time of purchase. Capitalization/stocks must be of those corporations with a market capitalization exceeding $250,000,000. Common and convertible preferred stocks should be of good quality and listed on either the New York or American Stock Exchange or in the NASDAQ System with requirements that such stocks have adequate market liquidity relative to the size of the investment.

Fixed Income Investments: Types of securities of funds not invested in cash equivalents (securities maturing in one year or less) shall be invested entirely in marketable debt securities issued either by the U.S. Government or agency of the Government, domestic corporations, including industrial and utilities, domestic banks, and other United States financial institutions. In terms of quality, only fixed income securities that are rated BBB or better by Standard and Poor's or Baa by Moody's shall be purchased. The maturity of individual fixed income securities purchased in the portfolio shall not exceed 30 years. No more than 30% of the fixed income portion of the portfolio may be placed in these lower rated issues. The average quality rating of the fixed income section shall be A, or better.

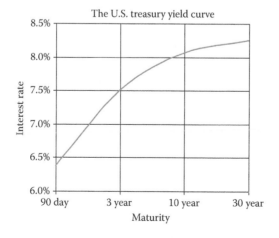

Restricted Investments: Categories of securities that are not eligible might include

1. Short Sales
2. Margin Purchases
3. Private Placements
4. Commodities
5. Foreign Securities
6. Unregistered/Restricted Stock
7. Options
8. Futures

Administration

The custodian will be responsible for settling trades executed by the physician in his/her accounts. From time to time, they will request disbursements from the accounts. Checks covering must be mailed on the date of the request providing notification is received before 2:00 pm; EST.

Investment Performance Review and Evaluation

Performance is measured on a quarterly basis against a balanced index posed of commonly accepted benchmarks weighted to match the long-term asset allocation policy of the Plan. Additionally, performance will be measured against commonly accepted benchmarks applicable to that particular investment style and strategy. The custodian shall report performance results in compliance with standards formerly established by AIMR (Association for Investment Management and Research); now the CFA Institute (https://www.cfainstitute.org). Reports shall be generated on a quarterly basis and delivered within four weeks of the end of the quarter.

Communications

Copies of all transactions will be maintained on a daily basis and will conform to the IPS. Monthly statements will detail each transaction and summarize the account, identifying unrealized and realized gains and losses as needed. A review will be prepared quarterly and delivered within six weeks from the end of the quarter. The doctor and custodian of the report will review past performance and evaluate the current investment outlook. These reports will compare the performance with the respective market benchmarks measuring return and volatility and compare it with their respective peer groups. If a financial advisor is used, s/he will be required to forward SEC Form ADV Parts 1 and 2 annually, or if the ADV is substantially revised.

Now that we have written a personal IPS, let's select the assets.

Asset Allocation

Asset allocation is the most important decision made in effecting your total return in keeping with your risk tolerance. It has been said that over 90% of the variability of returns come from asset allocation. This is a hard concept to grasp. Most doctors believe that picking the right stocks (those that go up fast) is all that is necessary to be successful. That certainly would make you successful, but it just isn't that simple. Over an extended period of time, if stocks go up and you own a diversified portfolio of stocks, your portfolio will most likely be worth more. If on the other hand, bonds go up (and stocks go down) your portfolio will most likely be worth less. A combination of asset classes is the better way to go. This is why professional money managers spend so much time and money on the subject of asset allocation.

Periodically, the "C" section in the *Wall Street Journal,* or from other online resources, illustrates various asset allocation models proposed by major brokerage firms. These firms are attempting to forecast the best asset mix going forward. The following is an illustration printed in the *Wall Street Journal* on Wednesday, August 1, 1999. Now, self-compare and contrast this with findings at the time as you read this chapter 15 years or so later.

Who Has the Best Blend?

Brokerage Houses	Performance			Recommended Blend		
	Three-Month	One Year	Five Year	Stocks	Bonds	Cash
Prudential Securities[a]	5.00%	19.81%	151.14%	75%	10%	10%
Lehman Brothers	4.77%	17.87%	162.51%	80%	20%	0%
A.G. Edwards & Sons	3.03%	17.01%	140.08%	55%	40%	5%
Goldman Sachs[b]	4.07%	16.72%	154.63%	70%	27%	0%
PaineWebber	3.12%	16.44%	144.81%	53%	35%	12%
Edward D. Jones[c]	3.99%	15.19%	139.87%	71%	24%	5%
J.P. Morgan	2.94%	15.12%	NA	50%	25%	25%
Morgan Stanley D.W.[d]	4.30%	14.93%	152.01%	65%	15%	20%
Bear Stearns	2.96%	14.55%	NA	55%	35%	10%
Credit Suisse F.B.	3.06%	13.87%	140.23%	55%	30%	15%
Salomon Smith Barney	2.83%	12.16%	128.62%	60%	35%	5%
Raymond James[e]	5.10%	11.46%	110.71%	55%	20%	10%
Merrill Lynch[f]	1.10%	7.59%	101.89%	40%	55%	5%
AVERAGE	3.56%	14.82%	138.77%	60%	29%	9%
By Comparison						
Robot Blend[g]	2.83%	12.97%	137.69%			
100% Stock	6.64%	22.62%	244.52%			
100% Cash	1.14%	4.90%	30.26%			
100% Bond	−2.60%	−0.56%	51.75%			

Sources: Wilshire Associates, Carpenter Analytical Services company documents

Note: Performance of asset-allocation blends recommended by 13 major brokerage houses in periods ended June 30, 1999. Figures do not include transaction costs. Houses are ranked by 12-month performance. Also shown is the mix each house now recommends.

[a] 5% in Real Estate
[b] 3% in Commodities
[c] 12% in International Stocks
[d] 10% in International Stocks
[e] 15% in Real Estate; 6% in Intl Stocks
[f] 14% in International Stocks
[g] Always 55% Stocks, 35% Bonds, 10% cash
NA = not available

Most asset allocation studies illustrate historical data giving various combinations of asset classes that can best satisfy your investment risk and return objectives. Basic asset allocation assigns a percentage weighting to stocks, bonds, cash, and international stocks. A more elaborate proposal would include various classes of these four main categories.

Stocks can be broken down into small, mid, and large capitalization. Value and growth styles are also used to diversify the mix. Bonds can be of varying quality and maturity as well as corporate, government, and municipal.

The first thing to realize about asset allocation is that it can reduce risk; adding "international" stocks, for example, to a portfolio made up of exclusively US investments reduces standard deviation over a long period of time. There is a feeling among doctors that international stocks are risky. By themselves they are a more volatile asset class, but historically they have had a very low correlation to domestic stocks and, therefore, over time will reduce overall volatility.

Correlation is used in reference to assets selected for use in the portfolio. Low "correlation" means that when one asset class goes up 50%, the other asset class goes up by a lesser amount; let us say 10% for purposes of this illustration. Inverse "correlation" means two asset classes go in different directions (when one goes up, the other goes down). You want to have a group of assets that have low, or in some cases, even inverse "correlation" to reduce the volatility of the account.

Asset Class	Correlation Matrix					
	1	2	3	4	5	6
1. Domestic Equity	1.00	0.32	0.51	−0.03	0.12	0.32
2. Domestic Bonds	0.32	1.00	0.14	0.35	0.32	0.99
3. Non-U.S. Equity	0.51	0.14	1.00	0.27	−0.02	0.14
4. Non-U.S. Bonds	−0.03	0.35	0.27	1.00	0.11	0.35
5. Cash	0.12	0.32	−0.02	0.11	1.00	0.32
6. Municipal Bonds	0.32	0.99	0.14	0.35	0.32	1.00

Here is an asset allocation proposal that offers several combinations, which obviously produce varying degrees of risk and return.

First, note that various assets have different return and risk expectations. Cash (90-day Treasury Bills) have very low risk and commensurate return. Non-U.S. equity, on the other hand, had experienced high return and high risk (standard deviation). The time frame used is 1926–1928 experimentally weighted in favor of more recent years.

QUALIFIED RETIREMENT PLANS

For healthcare employees, 401(k) and 403(b) plans offer great opportunities to change asset allocations. For example, Karen Markland, a Certified Registered Nurse Anesthetist (CRNA) at Carolina's Medical Center, found it was relatively easy to shift from bonds to stocks. No taxes or commissions were involved. A simple phone call moved her allocation from 40% bonds, 50% stocks and 10% international to 20% bonds, 70% stocks and 10% international after a recent stock market decline (personal communication).

One point of caution when using 401(k) or 403(b) plans for asset allocation is required. Quite often the trustees of the plans will decide on a single group of mutual or index funds for the participants. Not all funds in the group are worthy of your money. Jean Surber, another Certified Registered Nurse Anesthetist (CRNA) at Presbyterian Hospital, did not have a good international option and so had to limit her allocation in that 403 bk plan to stocks, bonds and cash. So, she used her Individual Retirement Account (IRA) at a brokerage firm for international investing (personal communication).

The status of 401(k) and 403(b) plans is normally sent to participants' quarterly. This is an excellent time to do some asset allocation and review performance. Since most 401(k)s use mutual funds and offer daily valuations by telephone or online, you don't have to wait for the quarterly report, which is often received 60 days after the end of the quarter. When changes are made in the allocation of existing positions, the percentage allocation of future contributions should be made as well. When Karen repositioned her 401(k) portfolio, she also changed her future contribution percentages.

Morningstar, a Chicago-based company that analyzes and computes statistics on most of the mutual funds produces a monthly report that you can review at the library; or online. Most banks and brokerage firms subscribe to this service. They can send you an up-to-date single page analysis of each of your funds. This is good material, well researched, but it is historical data. "Past performance is no assurance of future results." The Morningstar system rates funds from 1 star (worst) to 5 stars (best). This is sometimes referred to as the *Sesame Street* method of selecting mutual funds. If you can count to 5, you can pick the best fund. Using this report alone is like driving on an Interstate highway at 80 miles per hour using only the rear view mirror (that can be fatal). Fund portfolio managers' change; good managers are hired away by their competitors and bad managers are fired. Managers themselves are not always consistent in maintaining their style or in their performance.

Morningstar is a good place to start however, because you can review much information on a single page. You can see historical returns, sector weightings, manager tenure, investment style, costs (except trading commission expense) and statistics concerning risk. Here you may have a suggestion of the performance you can reasonably expect. Few physicians, but many financial advisors, are well versed in a variety of mutual funds. Representatives of the funds call on them frequently. Many brokerage firms perform independent due diligence research. Mutual funds and ETFs are a large part of the financial services industry and you can expect the availability of extensive information.

Most 401(k) plans should be invested for growth of capital. You are generally talking about long-term investment objectives. You should be very reluctant to withdraw funds from this tax-sheltered environment. Unfortunately far too often, the participant becomes discouraged (usually in a down market cycle) and moves the money out of stocks and into a money market fund at the wrong time. It is not unusual to see doctor participants assume a very defensive posture a year or so before retirement. This is shortsighted. The investments are meant to provide income and growth of capital for many years, not just until retirement. Upon retirement, the funds will be rolled out directly into an IRA and invested with almost the same asset allocation.

Although you need to adjust portfolios to provide more income in retirement, the basic risk tolerance of individuals does not change just because the person retired. If you were comfortable with moderate volatility before retirement, you will be comfortable with moderate volatility during retirement.

MANAGING YOUR OWN PORTFOLIO

Most individual portfolios are simply a list of stocks. Doctors with such lists usually know the cost of each position and when they acquired it. It is not unusual to find inherited low-cost stocks in the account that have been held for many years.

When you inherit securities, a new cost basis is established (the price of the stock on the date of death or six months later—the executor of the estate makes this determination). Even though there would be no capital gain liability if the stock were sold immediately after date of death, most people simply don't do anything, just hold the stock. Of course, taxes should be considered when selling securities, but the investment merit should be the overriding factor.

In a personal communication, Mr L. Eddie Dutton, CPA said, "First make an investment decision and if it fits into the tax plan, so much the better. Doctors often wonder where they will get the money to pay the taxes. I say to get it from the sale of the appreciated stock and cry all the way to the bank with your profit."

Dr. Ernest Duty, a very successful private investor advises, "Ask yourself this question: If you had the money instead of the stock, would you buy the stock? If your answer is 'Yes' then, hold on to the stock but if you say 'No, I wouldn't buy that stock today' then, sell it" (personal communication).

Why Average Investors Fail to Keep Up with the Markets

This chart was recently released by our colleague Bob Doll at *Nuveen Investments,* Boston, Massachusetts (now TIAA-CREF).

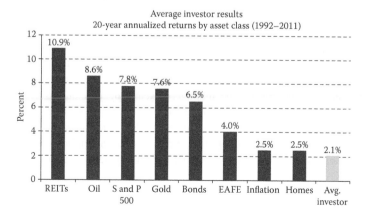

Average investor results
20-year annualized returns by asset class (1992–2011)

Doll attributes the failure of the average investor to keep up with investment markets (or even inflation, for that matter); to market timing and emotionally driven decisions to move into and out of the markets. How long has it supposedly been common knowledge that we are better off choosing an investment strategy that represents risk tolerance and sticking to it both in the good times and bad?

Still, these data illustrate that investors are terrible at sticking to their strategy when markets stall, and still have an overwhelming urge to buy after the market has already done well, and then sell shortly after a market drop (i.e., buy high and sell low). This is where having a written IPS can be invaluable.

Additionally, working with a financial advisor with a history of executing a steady buy-and-hold approach can provide important support in avoiding detrimental behaviors during the rough times (personal communication, with permission, Lon Jefferies; MBA, CFP®).

Whither ME, Inc., and Self-Portfolio Management

So, if you elect to manage your own portfolio, you are going to be competing with some of the best investment talent in the world; others not so much. Some have studied and practiced for years to attain the level of competence they enjoy, others are salesmen. Some have been educated in some of the finest schools in the world and initially practiced under the tutelage of the most successful in the profession, others may labor in virtual, or real, boiler rooms (THINK: Jordan Belfort, and The Wolf of Wall Street). So, always remember, it is your portfolio.

PART II: THE IPS FOR HEALTHCARE ORGANIZATIONS

Hospital endowment fund management aims for accountability on the part of each financial advisor or major player sharing responsibility for the endowment, and for a management model likely to make most of their resources while protecting against major risks. In a period of extreme uncertainty like today, endowments should give heightened attention to the composition of their investment committees and to the skills and time priorities of members.

Just as the field of medicine continuously changes—so too does endowment fund management. Endowment managers continue to increase their knowledge of the science and expand their skill in the art. However, successful endowment managers will continue to focus on the areas that they can control in order to minimize the risk of the areas they cannot.

Sample Hospital Endowment Fund IPS

Goals and Objectives

Objective of the Policy Statement

In recognition of the inter-generational character of the fund, the Plan has as its objective the attainment of real growth on the total asset value after current spending. The principle purpose of the IPS is to protect the portfolio from ad hoc revisions of sound long-term policy. The written policy will serve to guide and direct various investment managers in the investment of funds when short-term market outlooks are troubling. The Board wants to detail, to the extent reasonably possible, the goals and objectives as well as the performance measurement techniques that will be employed in evaluating the service rendered by the managers. Realizing that our overall objective is best accomplished by employing a variety of management styles, we will adjust our asset tolerances and permissible volatility to incorporate specific manager styles. The Board hopes that the net result of the process used to develop investment policy and formalize that policy into a written statement will increase the likelihood that the Plan can meet the inter-generational needs of the sponsoring organization.

Performance Objectives and Goals

The Plan's target performance, on an annualized basis net of fees, will be expected to

- Equal or exceed the spending rate plus inflation over the market cycle
- Equal or exceed the average return of the appropriate capital market index as weight by the asset allocation target percentages

Interim fluctuations in the value of the fund will be viewed in perspective since the Plan is considered to have a long-term horizon. However, within an individual asset class, the fund's short-term performance and volatility should not be materially worse than those of the appropriate benchmark for that class.

Investment Philosophy

The Plan will allocate its investments in accordance with the belief that it has a long-term investment horizon. We believe that long-term investment success requires discipline and consistency of approach. The Plan will be managed on a total return basis recognizing the importance of capital preservation while remaining cognizant that real returns require the assumption of some level of investment risk. The Plan shall seek appropriate compensation for the risks that must inevitably be assumed while using prudent investment practices to mitigate or eliminate those risks that can be diversified without sacrificing return. The basic tenets of the Plan's management include the following:

- The portfolio as a whole is more important that any individual asset class or investment
- At any given level of risk, there is an optimal combination of asset classes that will maximize returns
- Equities and similar investments generally offer higher long-term returns than fixed income investments while also generally having higher short-term volatility
- Overall portfolio risk can be decreased by combining asset classes with low correlations of market behavior

INVESTMENT POLICIES AND PROCEDURES

Investment Program Policy

The investment program is intended to result in a policy that allows the greatest probability that the goals set forth in the Objective of the Policy Statement can be met. This process includes the following broad actions:

- Projecting the organization's spending needs
- Maintaining sufficient liquidity for near-term spending commitments
- Assessing expected market returns and risks for the individual asset classes

The policy recognizes that diversification among and across asset classes can result in lower portfolio risk while simultaneously providing higher portfolio returns. Modeling and simulation are used to identify the asset classes the Plan will use as well as the approximate percentage of the Plan that each class will represent. It is recognized that fluctuation in market values will occur, or that tactical movements can be made to recognize temporary market inefficiencies. As such, the asset allocation provides ranges around each asset class target. It is generally anticipated that the investment program which gives rise to the asset allocation will be periodically repeated and that asset class target ranges will be modified or affirmed.

Asset Allocation Targets and Ranges

As a result of the above investment process, the Board has adopted the following asset allocation policy with the indicated targets and ranges.

Asset Class	Minimum Weight	Target Weight	Maximum Weight
Domestic equities	xoxox%	xoxox%	xoxox%
Fixed income	xoxox%	xoxox%	xoxox%
International equities	xoxox%	xoxox%	xoxox%
Absolute return	xoxox%	xoxox%	xoxox%
Private equity	xoxox%	xoxox%	xoxox%
Real assets	xoxox%	xoxox%	xoxox%

It is expected that the fund's daily management team will utilize external managers to implement areas within individual asset classes for which those managers have the requisite expertise, resources, and sustainable investment selection process. These external managers will have discretion over matters related to security selection and timing within their area of mandate.

Spending Policy

It is the organization's intent to distribute ___ percent annually based on the ___ payout methodology. This intent is subject to the understanding that the spending rate plus the organization's rate of inflation will not normally exceed the rate of return. It is understood that the total return basis for calculating spending, as sanctioned by the Uniform Management of Investment Funds Act (UMIFA), allows the organization to spend an amount in excess of the current yield (interest and dividends earned) including realized and unrealized appreciation. However, it is also understood that from time-to-time the inevitable volatility in the portfolio may require that payouts be reduced to preserve the purchasing power of the fund.

Rebalancing Policy

The organization recognizes that a disciplined approach to investing is the best way to secure consistent performance. As such, the fund should be rebalanced within target ranges on no less than an annual basis in a manner consistent with not incurring inappropriately excessive costs.

INVESTMENT MANAGEMENT POLICIES AND PROCEDURES

Equity Securities

Both domestic and international securities are intended to provide capital appreciation and current income to the Plan. It is generally recognized that the higher return potential of equities entails higher market volatility and potential for loss. This asset class shall mean domestic and international common stocks or equivalents (American Depository Receipts plus issues convertible into common stocks). The equity portfolio shall be well diversified to avoid undue exposure to any single economic sector, industry group, or individual security. No more than 5% of the equity portfolio based on the market value shall be invested in securities of any one issue or corporation at the time of purchase. No more than 10% of the equity portfolio based on the market value shall be invested in any one industry at the time of purchase. Capitalization/stocks must be of those corporations with a market capitalization exceeding $50,000,000. Common and convertible preferred stocks should be of good quality and traded on a major exchange, including NASDAQ, with requirements that such stocks have adequate market liquidity relative to the size of the investment.

Fixed Income Securities

Fixed income securities are intended to provide additional diversification to the Plan and to provide dependable sources of income to the Plan. It is anticipated that the Plan will include fixed income investments of various maturities and durations. Allowable types of such securities include marketable debt securities issued by the United States Government or an agency of the United States Government, foreign governments, domestic corporations, mortgages and asset-backed securities, and high yield debt. These investments should be managed actively to take advantage of opportunities presented by such factors as interest rate fluctuations and credit ratings. These investments are subject to the following limitations:

- No issues may be purchased with more than 30 years until maturity
- Investments of single issuers other than direct obligations of the United States government or its agencies may not represent more than 5% of the Plan's assets
- No more than 25% of the fixed income securities portion of the Plan's assets may be allocated to below investment grade debt issues

Cash and Equivalents

All cash equivalent investments should be a pooled investment vehicle, such as money market funds, where the fund's share price is intended to remain constant and the yield is comparable to the then current risk-free rate of return. The Plan is also permitted to purchase United States agency guaranteed certificates of deposit or short-term U.S. government securities. Cash and equivalents are not generally considered to be appropriate vehicles for purposes of investment return. As such, these investments should typically be limited to serving as temporary placements for funds awaiting distribution to the sponsoring organization or investment into an approved asset class.

Other Securities

- *Private Capital Partnerships:* Investments may be made into venture capital, leveraged buy-out, or other private equity managed pools. Such investments should only be made through managers having the requisite experience, resources, and track record of superior performance with the given type of private equity.
- *Real Estate:* Investments in real estate should be in the form of professionally managed, income producing commercial or residential properties. Such investments should be made only through pooled investment real estate funds as managed by professionals with track records of superior long-term performance.
- *Natural Resources:* Investments may include timber, oil, or gas interests held in the form of professionally managed pooled limited partnership interests. Such investments should only be made through managers having the requisite experience, resources, and track record of superior performance with the given type of natural resource.
- *Absolute Return Investments:* Investments may include equity-oriented or market-neutral hedge funds (i.e., long/short, event driven, arbitrage, etc.).
- *Derivatives and Derivative Securities:* Derivatives are securities whose value depends upon the value of some other security or index. Examples of such investments include futures, options, options on futures, interest-only or principal-only strips, and so forth. Certain managers may be permitted to use derivatives. However, no derivative positions can be utilized if such positions would cause the portfolio to fall outside of portfolio guidelines. In addition, such derivative positions must be fully collateralized. Examples of appropriate derivative strategies include hedging a position, maintaining exposure to an asset class while making changes to the allocation where maintaining the derivative position is more cost-effective than holding a cash position, or changing the duration of a fixed income position. Such investments should only be made through managers having the requisite experience, resources, and track record of superior performance with the given type of derivative. The manager must also be able to demonstrate that such derivatives are integral to their mandate and that the counterparty to the derivative strategy can fulfill their obligations.

Restrictions

The Board is authorized to waive or modify any of the restrictions in these guidelines after thorough investigation of the manager and the rationale for the deviation.

Roles and Responsibilities

To achieve our overall goals and objectives, we want to identify the parties associated with our accounts and the functions, responsibilities, and activities of each with respect to the management of fund assets. Our investment managers are responsible for the day-to-day investment management of the Plan assets, including specific security selection and timing of purchases and sales. The custodian is responsible for safekeeping the securities, collections, and disbursements and periodic accounting statements. The prompt credit of all dividends and interest to our accounts on payment date is required. The custodian shall provide monthly account statements and reconcile account statements with manager summary account statements. The investment consultant is responsible for assisting the client in developing the IPS and for monitoring the overall performance of the Plan and the specific investment managers.

Duties of the Board

The Board's primary duties shall include, but not be limited to, the following items:

- Hiring and evaluating the members of the management team
- Approving the investment policy as prepared by the management team
- Reviewing, no less than annually, the Plan's allocation and performance

Duties of the Management and Staff

Management and staff will be primarily responsible for the day-to-day administration of the Plan. It is anticipated that their primary duties shall include, but not be limited to, the following items:

- Selecting, retaining, and terminating investment managers as necessary to implement the investment policy
- Selecting, retaining, and terminating consultants as necessary to prepare the asset allocation, hire and evaluate managers, perform topical research, and review performance
- Developing investment policy for the Board's review and approval
- Implementing investment policy within the target ranges set forth by the Board
- Reviewing no less than quarterly the Plan's investment performance
- Administering the Plan's investments in a cost-effective manner
- Developing a contingency Plan for the protection of the Plan's assets and ensuring appropriate communication with the public in the face of a catastrophic event
- Selecting an appropriate custodian to hold and safeguard the Plan's securities investments
- Maintaining sufficient records to allow for the necessary oversight and management of the Plan's investments

Duties of External Investment Managers

Management and staff will be primarily responsible for the day-to-day administration of the Plan. It is anticipated that their primary duties shall include, but not be limited to, the following items:

- Complying with the provisions of this policy statement
- Staying within the style and risk parameters of their respective mandates
- Providing proof of liability and fiduciary insurance coverages
- Maintaining necessary risk controls

- Using best possible execution for trades made on the Plan's behalf in order to ensure the most timely, cost-effective execution
- Reconciling transaction data no less than monthly with the custodian
- Disclosing material changes in personnel, processes, investment outlook, financial condition, or other matters that could be reasonably deemed to be of interest to the Plan

OTHER CONSIDERATIONS

Trading Guidelines

All trading in accounts shall be done through a recognized national or regional brokerage firm. Additionally, it is understood that block transactions or participation in certain initial public offerings might not be available through a primary broker. In this case, the manager should execute those trades through the broker offering the product and service necessary to best serve the account. It should be the responsibility of the manager to see that duplicate trade confirmations and duplicate monthly statements are mailed to your consultant.

Proxy Voting

The investment manager shall have the sole and exclusive right to vote any and all policies solicited in connection with securities held by the client.

Performance Review and Evaluation

Performance results for the investment managers will be measured on a quarterly basis. Total fund performance will be measured against a balanced index posed of commonly accepted benchmarks weighted to match the long-term asset allocation policy of the Plan. Additionally, the investment performances specific for individual portfolios will be measured against commonly accepted benchmarks applicable to that particular investment style and strategy. The consultant will be responsible for complying with this section of our policy statement. The managers shall report performance results in compliance with the standards established by the Association for Investment Management and Research (AIMR). Reports shall be generated on a quarterly basis and delivered to the client with a copy to the consultant within four weeks of the end of the quarter.

CONCLUSION

Investing and managing your own portfolio or pension plan, or the endowment funds of a healthcare organization, is serious business. It should not be a hobby. You need the best advice you can obtain, because mistakes may not be discovered until it is too late. Remember, when considering money management, be sure to understand the ultimate fiscal consequences and your own personal liability?

COLLABORATE

Discuss this chapter online with others at www.MedicalExecutivePost.com.

ACKNOWLEDGMENTS

To Clifton N. McIntire, CFP®, CIMA and Lisa McIntire Shaw, CFP®, CIMA® of Cygnus Asset Management, LLC, Charlotte, North Carolina; and to J. Wayne Firebaugh, CPA, CLU, CFP®, CMP™, Roanoke, Virginia.

FURTHER READING

Cimasi, RJ, Zigrang, TA and Sharamitaro, AP: Research and financial benchmarking in the healthcare industry. In: Marcinko, DE and Hetico HR (editors): *Financial Management Strategies for Hospitals and Healthcare Organizations*. CRC and Productivity Press, New York, 2014.

Commonfund Institute: *see* www.commonfund.org

Craig, JE, Jr.: Rethinking the management of foundation endowments. The Commonwealth Fund 2009 Annual Report.

D'Alessio, P and Marcinko, DE: Investment policy statement construction for hospital endowment fund management. In: Marcinko, DE and Hetico HR (editors): *Financial Management Strategies for Hospitals and Healthcare Organizations*. CRC and Productivity Press, New York, 2014.

Firebaugh, W: Hospital endowment fund management. In: Marcinko DE (editor): *Hospitals and Healthcare Organizations*. ST Publications, Vancouver, BC, 2006.

Foundation for Fiduciary Studies: *see* www.fiduciary360.com

McIntire, C: Wither self-portfolio management? In: Marcinko, DE (editor): *Financial Planning for Physicians and Healthcare Professionals*. Aspen Publishers, New York, 2003.

Schachter, B: *An Irreverent Guide to Value at Risk*. 1997. *See* www.gloriamundi.org.

Swensen, DF: *CIO. Pioneering Portfolio Management: An Unconventional Approach to Institutional Management*. The Free Press, Yale University, 2003.

21 Special Situations Planning
Nontraditional Financial Planning Topics

Anju D. Jessani and David Edward Marcinko

CONTENTS

Although one can hardly plan for an event like divorce, or the other special situation topics covered in this chapter, there are certain steps to take that may lessen the financial impact of them all.

PART I: DIVORCE PLANNING AND CONSCIOUS UNCOUPLING

Married couples strive to stay together for richer or poorer, and in sickness and health. But the reality is that more than 2 million people get divorced each year in the United States. Divorce is a $50 billion annual industry. Divorce rates for first marriages are 52% and 60% (75–90% if there's a special needs child) with the second. So, it pays for all medical professionals to be aware of this reality.

DIVORCE-PRONE MEDICAL SPECIALTIES*

A Johns Hopkins University study, by Michael J. Klag, MD, in 1997, found that physicians in some specialties—chiefly psychiatry and surgery—are at higher risk for divorce than their medical brethren in other fields. But the results did not support the common view that job-related anxiety and depression are linked to marital breakup. Alerting medical students to the risks of divorce in some specialties may influence their career choices and strengthen their marriages whatever field they choose. The study, supported by the National Institutes of Health (NIH), was published in the

---

* Coauthors of the study, which was part of the Johns Hopkins Precursors Study, an ongoing, prospective study of physicians from the Hopkins medical school graduating classes of 1948 through 1964, were lead author Bruce L. Rollman, MD, Lucy A. Mead, ScM, and Nae-Yuh Wang, MS.

March 13 issue of *The New England Journal of Medicine*. Results also strongly suggested that the high divorce risk in some specialties may result from the inherent demands of the job as well as the emotional experiences of physicians who enter those fields.

For example, the Hopkins team assessed the specialty choices, marriage histories, psychological characteristics, and other career and personal factors of 1118 physicians who graduated from The Johns Hopkins University School of Medicine from 1948 through 1964. Over 30 years of follow-up, the divorce rate was 51% for psychiatrists, 33% for surgeons, 24% for internists, 22% for pediatricians and pathologists, and 31% for other specialties. The overall divorce rate was 29% after three decades of follow-up and 32% after nearly four decades of follow-up.

Physicians who married before medical school graduation had a higher divorce rate than those who waited until after graduation (33% vs. 23%). The year of first marriage was linked with divorce rates: 11% for marriages before 1953, 17% for those from 1953 to 1957, 24% for those from 1958 to 1962, and 21% for those after 1962. Those who had a parent die before medical school graduation had a lower divorce rate.

Female physicians had a higher divorce rate (37%) than their male colleagues (28%). Physicians who were members of an academic honor society in medical school had a lower divorce rate, although there was no difference in divorce rates according to class rank. Religious affiliation, being an only child, having a parent who was a physician, and having a divorced parent were not associated with divorce rates. Physicians who reported themselves to be less emotionally close to their parents and who expressed more anger under stress also had a significantly higher divorce rate, but anxiety and depression levels were not associated with divorce rate.

DIVORCE-PRONE CITIES

The divorce laws in all 50 states were evaluated relative to the waiting period required before a divorce is finalized, residency requirements, whether mandatory counseling exists, or whether a separation period is required for a no-fault divorce.

The 10 worst cities for marriage are[*]

- Toledo, Ohio
- Boise City, Idaho
- Las Vegas, Nevada
- Tulsa, Oklahoma
- Jacksonville, Florida
- Little Rock, Arkansas
- Cheyenne, Wyoming
- Norfolk, Virginia
- Albuquerque, New Mexico
- Charleston, West Virginia

"The Commitment Conversation" brochure is a resource that can be downloaded at www.equalityinmarriage.org/cc.pdf. It's an excellent tool that allows couples to sit together and review some important issues they need to discuss prior to taking their vows, regardless of state residence.

PRENUPTIAL AGREEMENTS

A *prenuptial agreement* is a contract between prospective spouses. Most prenuptial agreements contain provisions limiting the distribution of marital property and alimony in the event of divorce and limiting the distribution of property to a spouse in the event of death. It is important to note that most states specifically prohibit provisions regarding child support.

---

[*] *Source*: Covert, J: MensHealth.com, March 31, 2014.

Because of past uncertainty whether courts could enforce prenuptial agreements, a uniform treatment of prenuptial agreements was sought through the Uniform Premarital Agreement Act (UPAA). The UPAA was approved by the National Conference on Uniform State Laws in 1983, and has been adopted in whole or in part by approximately half the states. While the standards for enforcing prenuptial agreements vary from state to state, in almost all states, four conditions are imposed:

- Each party must make complete disclosure to the other of his or her assets, liabilities, sources of income, and any other facts likely to affect his or her financial position.
- Each party must be represented by separate and independent legal counsel (or must make a voluntary and well-considered decision to waive such independent legal counsel).
- The terms of the agreement must be fair at the time the agreement is entered into, a standard with respect to which even reasonable people may differ.
- Finally, the agreement may be set aside by the courts if enforcement of the agreement would impoverish either party and thereby create a risk that either party (or any minor children of either party) would require public assistance.

Life Insurance and Prenuptial Agreements

Medical professionals and other high-net-worth clients getting married might also consider a life insurance policy along with their prenuptial agreements. Why? Death benefit proceeds can provide future money to a spouse who gets alimony due to a divorce. The policy can also make a breakup more palatable for clients who have children from a first marriage.

The book *Pre-Nups for Lovers* by Arlene Dubin, a New York City matrimonial lawyer who specializes in prenuptial agreements, may be helpful in this regard.

DIVORCE MEDIATION

Mediation is a court-approved process, in which a trained neutral person, called a mediator, encourages and facilitates the resolution of a dispute between two or more parties. The mediator does not replace the services of attorneys, but supplements their role to an advisory position. Mediators include attorneys, mental health practitioners, accountants, doctors, and other professionals with special training. Some benefits of mediation include the following:

- *Mediation is not adversarial.* The nature of the legal system requires the participants to be adversarial. Many people in disputes are not adversaries. Rather, they may want to problem solve because they understand the importance of maintaining their ongoing relationship.
- *Mediation is private.* In many states, divorce records and divorce proceedings are open to outsiders. Resolving the conflict in the confines of the mediator's office limits the information available to what the parties agree will be included in their divorce judgment.
- *Mediation is faster.* Since all discussions are held face-to-face, resolving the dispute takes less time in mediation than resolving it through intermediaries.

The mediator usually meets with the client for three to eight sessions. At the end of the process the mediator will draft a memorandum of understanding (MOU), which summarizes in plain English what the clients agreed to and where appropriate, why they made the agreement. The spouses take the MOU to their respective separate attorney for review, advice, and incorporation into their formal legal agreement, which is ultimately filed with the court as part of the divorce decree.

CHOOSING A DIVORCE ATTORNEY

Whether you choose to mediate or litigate, you will still require the services of an attorney. As a medical professional or the spouse of a medical professional, you will probably have more at stake in your divorce than the average person getting divorced.

The following tips on how to choose a divorce lawyer are from the late Elaine Majewski, an advocate for divorce reform (personal communication):

1. *Qualifications*—Ask the attorney to describe their legal training, how long they have practiced family law, how many family law cases they have handled, and what proportion of their time is spent on family and divorce matters. If the answer is less than 30%, this attorney may not spend sufficient time in this practice area to stay abreast of new developments and current case law.
2. *Attorney's philosophy*—Ask the attorney about his/her view on child custody, visitation/parenting time, support, and so on. What are his/her feelings about shared custody? Inquire about his/her outside activities and professional associations, as they will tell you a lot about his views. Will the lawyer first seek to resolve the matter amicably in lieu of the traditional adversarial approach? Seek to work with any attorney who is receptive to your ideas and desires.
3. *Fees*—Inquire how much do they charge, in what increment of billable time, who will actually do the work, and whether a flat or mixed fee arrangement can be worked out. Be aware that novices often charge less for an hour, but may require more time to handle a problem. What are the specifics of the retainer arrangement as well as costs for travel, meals, administrative assistance, and so on? Is the attorney willing to submit an itemized bill each month?
4. *Point of view*—Once you have presented the facts, the attorney should be able to point out the strengths and weaknesses of your case, assess your probability of achieving your goals, and be able to give you an estimate of how long your matter will take to resolve and make an estimate of the approximate legal fees they would anticipate. Some lawyers neglect to give honest appraisals, and clients are then misled and spend large sums of money on losing causes. Ask the lawyer to also estimate what the minimum and maximum of the fee might be.
5. *Work style*—Will the attorney return phone calls within 24 h? In his/her absence, how will your inquiries be answered? How are you charged for these inquiries? Does the attorney utilize e-mail or text messaging? Will the attorney agree to keep you apprised of all developments in your case and make no offers or agreements without first consulting you? Make sure that the attorney will be available to you, and that you are comfortable with his/her work style and manner.

OVERVIEW OF FAMILY AND DIVORCE LAW

Which state you live will determine grounds for filing, child custody and parenting time options, how property is divided, and guidelines for child and spousal support. As a result, a New York divorce decided by the courts may look very different from a California divorce, even though the circumstances of the parties may be quite similar. We will take a look at each of these major components you need to decide as you face a divorce:

- Custody options and parenting time issues
- Child support and other financial issues related to the children
- Distribution of marital assets and liabilities
- Spousal support/alimony and tax issues related to alimony

Custody Options and Parenting Time Issues

James Cooke, president of *The Joint Custody Association*, Los Angeles, California, offers the following custody definitions (personal communication):

- *Sole custody*: An award of custody to one parent with parenting/visitation rights to the noncustodial parent. The custodial parent retains exclusive authority and control regarding the education, medical care, religion, discipline, and financial support of the child or children.

- *Joint legal custody*: Both parents retain and share responsibility and authority for the care and control of the child or children. The sharing of that responsibility can traverse an entire spectrum, from casual cooperation to delineated time and functions. In its broadest interpretation, joint legal custody has encompassed nearly all major responsibilities and opportunities that are relegated to custodians (e.g., medical, schooling, and religion), except for day-to-day residence.
- *Joint physical and legal custody*: This is joint legal custody plus the allocation of significant periods of time for the child or children with each parent. Variations for sharing physical custody can include freedom of movement between two homes, school year versus summer vacation with exchange weekends and nights, workday versus weekends, special vacation periods, and so on.
- *Split custody*: This awards one or more of the children to one parent and the other child or remaining children to the alternate parent. Parents and courts considering the split custody alternative will wish to weigh carefully the wisdom and necessity of assuring that the children do, or do not, have significant time together with their siblings.

CHILD SUPPORT AND OTHER FINANCIAL ISSUES RELATED TO THE CHILDREN

Parents have a legal and moral obligation to provide their children with the necessities of life. Child support is mandated by law. Most states have a variation of the following formula—17% of net income for one child, 25% of net income for two children, 29% of net income for three children, 31% of net income for four children and 35% of net income for five or more children. If physical custody is shared for long or frequent periods of time, depending on the financial circumstances of the parents, the needs of the children, and the time spent with each parent, child support payments may or may not be required and may be subject to state guidelines.

In most instances, child support is paid to the custodial parent and not the children. Child support covers food, clothing, and shelter for the child. Additional expenses usually not included in the basic child support obligation include medical insurance, child care needs, and private school tuition if appropriate. Such states provide for these expenses to be shared, while other states suggest that the parents pay for these expenses based on their percentage of income. As opposed to alimony, child support is not taxed as income to the recipient and is not deductible to the payer.

DISTRIBUTION OF MARITAL ASSETS AND DEBTS

In the United States, a few states, influenced by their French or Spanish heritage, have the continental system of community property (50–50), which essentially means that property or assets acquired by either husband or wife during the marriage, except for gifts from third parties, belong equally to the husband or wife. Community property does not mean that each asset is divided 50–50. Rather that the net value of the assets received by each spouse must be equal. Thus, it is not uncommon for one spouse to be awarded the family residence, with the other spouse receiving the family business and investment real estate. Community property states include Arizona, California, Idaho, Louisiana, Nevada, New Mexico, Texas, and Washington.

The majority of states base marital law on British common law and provide for equitable rather than equal distribution. In equitable distribution states, the court determines a fair and reasonable distribution that may be more than or less than 50% of any asset to either party. The equitable distribution laws vary from state to state. Each state has their own factors in determining equitable, fair, and just division of assets. State factors may include

- The duration of the marriage
- The age and physical and emotional health of the parties
- The income or property brought to the marriage by each party

- The standard of living established during the marriage
- Any written agreement made by the parties before or during the marriage
- The economic circumstances of each party at the time property division is effective
- The income and earning capacity of each party including education and training
- The contribution by each party to the education, training or earnings of the other
- The contribution amount or value of property, as well as contribution as homemaker
- The tax consequences of the proposed distribution to each party
- The present value of the property
- The need of a parent with physical child custody to own/occupy the marital residence
- The debts and liabilities of the parties
- Loss of inheritance rights upon dissolution as of date of dissolution
- Loss of pension rights upon dissolution as of date of dissolution
- Any award of maintenance
- The amount of each person's separate property
- The need for creation, now or in the future, of a trust fund to secure reasonably foreseeable medical or educational costs for a spouse or children
- Any other factors that the court may deem relevant

BUSINESSES AND PROFESSIONAL PRACTICES

Business appraisers are hired to determine the value of a business or professional medical practice. The appraiser who is hired reviews the books and records of the practice and prepares a written report. Usually, judges will look to provide the other spouse with an offset for the value of the practice.

PENSION PLANS (DEFINED BENEFIT PLANS)

Pension plans usually specify the monthly benefit the retiree will receive upon retirement at a specified age. If there are no other assets to offset the present value of a pension plan as determined by an actuary, the other spouse may receive a percentage of each future pension check, or at some other designated time as allowed by the pension plan, based on the numbers of years the spouses lived together as husband and wife and the total number of years the employed spouse has been participating in the pension plan.

The laws governing pensions are different for private corporate physicians than they are for government and military healthcare workers. Private corporate employees are usually covered under the Federal Retirement Equity Act of 1984, which created what is known as the "Qualified Domestic Relations Order," or "QDRO" (pronounced "quadro"). The QDRO is a court order to designate how a specific retirement plan will be divided, to whom it will be paid, and whom, and requires the employer to comply with the terms of the order. If you or your spouse is a government, VA, or military employee, you and your attorney should seek to understand the nuances of the specific plan.

401(k) PLANS, OTHER QUALIFIED PLANS (DEFINED CONTRIBUTION PLANS), AND INDIVIDUAL RETIREMENT ACCOUNTS

If there are no other assets to offset the net value of a 401(k) plan, a Qualified Plan, or individual retirement account (IRA), the other spouse may receive a percentage of these accounts. This distribution usually occurs concurrent with the divorce. He or she will be able to defer taxes on the distribution by placing the funds in a rollover IRA account. Be aware that while there is usually an additional 10% penalty for early liquidation of these accounts, the early distribution tax does not apply for receipts from 401(k) plans and other qualified plans paid to an alternate payee through a QDRO.

REAL ESTATE/MARITAL RESIDENCE

There are some financial pitfalls that must be considered in dealing with the marital residence. For physicians, ignoring these could be a financial disaster since it is not unusual for a doctor to have a significant part of his or her net worth tied up in home ownership; or as a disaster after the 2008 debacle.

The Taxpayer Relief Act of 1997 provided new rules for home sales. The Act provides for a couple to exclude $500,000 in capital gains and for an individual to exclude $250,000 in capital gains, every 2 years. Additionally, the Act states that to qualify for these exclusion, this home must have been your primary residence for 2 of the past 5 years. (As a medical professional, if you have an office at home, any portion that qualified for the home office tax deduction, does not qualify for this tax free profit).

There are special rules in the Taxpayer Relief Act for divorcing couples regarding home sales. Divorcing couples should be entitled to a partial exclusion of taxes, even if they don't meet the 2 year time test. For example, if a divorcing couple had a $375,000 gain during their 18 months of home ownership (i.e., $500,000 × 75%), they could exclude the whole gain. Additionally, a taxpayer is treated as using his home as his principal residence during any period that the taxpayer's spouse or former spouse is granted use of the residence under a divorce or separation agreement.

Where minor children are involved, it is common for the custodial parent to be allowed to live in the residence with the children for a specified period of time after the Dissolution of Marriage is finalized. During that period of time, the spouse who lives in the home is usually required to make all mortgage, property tax and homeowner insurance payments when due. The house may be sold when there are no children living at the property, the youngest child attains the age of majority, or any date as otherwise agreed by the parties or specified by the court, with the proceeds to be divided based on the agreement in the divorce settlement. In this situation, the parties will still be entitled to take the $500,000 joint exclusion after the divorce.

If there is a large gain on the house at the time of the divorce, a pitfall to avoid is transferring the entire house to one of the parties in the divorce settlement. If that spouse subsequently were to sell the house and have to report the entire gain on his/her separate return, only $250,000 of the gain (from the time of the original purchase of the house), would escape taxation.

SPOUSAL SUPPORT/ALIMONY AND TAX ISSUES RELATED TO ALIMONY

During the divorce process, no one word seems to incite riot as easily as "alimony" (also known as spousal support or maintenance). Issues such as closure, dependency, and deservedness come into play. However, once you separate the emotions and stereotypes from the actual mechanics, alimony can offer some couples financial advantages. Publication 504 issued by the Department of the Treasury provides information for divorced or separated individuals, including the Federal rules regarding alimony. "Alimony is a payment to or for a spouse of former spouse under a divorce or separation instrument. Alimony is deductible by the payer and must be included in the spouse's or former spouse's income." To be alimony, a payment must meet certain requirements:

- The payment is made pursuant to divorce or separation—not a verbal agreement.
- The instrument does not designate the payment as not alimony.
- Alimony doesn't include child support or payments pursuant to equitable distribution.
- The parties should live in separate households (there are some exceptions).
- The parties must file separate tax returns and also live in separate households.
- The payment must be in cash (check); transfer of services or property is not permitted.
- There is no liability to make payment after the death of the recipient spouse.
- Alimony cannot terminate or drop by more than $15,000 from the prior year in the first three calendar years of payment. There is the potential to have to recapture if this does occur, unless the drop is due to death, or the remarriage of the person receiving payments.

- There must be no contingency related to payment of alimony based on an event impacting your child or children such as leaving school or the children becoming employed.

There is always some risk involved with actually getting payments over a period of time versus getting a lump sum payment upfront. To avoid some of these risks, another way to receive alimony is through a so-called *alimony substitution trust*. In this vehicle, liquid investments such as stocks and bonds are placed in trust with a custodian with generated interest and dividends sufficient to pay each month's agreed alimony stipend. Stipulations are made in the trust provisions to sell portions of the portfolio if sufficient cash is not generated by the portfolio's investments. Some professionals feel this arrangement is a better vehicle for periodic alimony payments than the goodwill of the payer spouse, as the "check is in the mail" syndrome is avoided.

While many people believe alimony is assumed, it is not as common as one may think. Nearly one of six divorce cases even considers it as an option. Temporary spousal support is more common and occurs at the time of separation, mostly to help the receiving spouse get on his or her feet again. It is either agreed upon or an order is issued. However, if your marriage is a long-term marriage in the eyes of the court (this usually means over 20 years), and your spouse has income that is less than one-third of your income, you may be expected to pay alimony. While few states have alimony guidelines as they do for child support, most have statutory criteria for an award of alimony. Some of the factors that may be part of your state's criteria may include

- Parental responsibility
- Income available to either party through investments or any assets held by that party
- Tax treatment of alimony includes a designation of all or a portion of the award
- The actual need and ability of the parties to pay
- The duration of the marriage
- The age and physical and emotional health of the parties
- The marriage standard of living and the likelihood that it be maintained
- The earning capacities, educational levels, skills, and employability of the parties
- The absence from the job market and custodial responsibilities for children of the party seeking maintenance
- The time and expense necessary to acquire sufficient education or training to enable the party seeking maintenance to find appropriate employment, the availability of the training and employment, and the opportunity for future acquisitions of capital assets and income
- The history of the financial or nonfinancial contributions to the marriage by each party, including contributions to the care and education of the children and interruption of personal careers or educational opportunities
- The equitable distribution of property ordered and any payout on equitable distribution directly or indirectly, out of current income, to the extent this consideration is reasonable, just, and fair
- Any other factors that the court may deem relevant

OTHER TAX CONSIDERATIONS OF SEPARATION AND DIVORCE

Filing Status

As mentioned, child support is not taxed as income to the recipient and is not deductible to the payer, while alimony is usually taxed as income to the recipient and is deductible to the payer.

Exemptions for Dependents

Only one parent can claim a child on their tax return. The parent who had custody of the child for the greater part of the year is generally treated as the parent who provided more than half the child's support is usually allowed to claim the exemption for a child. Noncustodial parents can still claim the child exemption if the custodial parent signs a statement (using Form 8332), agreeing not to claim the child's exemption, and the noncustodial parent attaches this statement to his or her return, or attaches a copy of certain pages of his/her divorce decree or separation agreement addressing exemptions. There are separate rules for divorce agreements made prior to 1985.

Child Tax Credit

The Child Tax Credit is an important tax credit that may be worth as much as $1000 per qualifying child, depending upon income.

- *Amount*—With the Child Tax Credit, you may be able to reduce your federal income tax by up to $1000 for each qualifying child under the age of 17.
- *Qualification*—A qualifying child for this credit is someone who meets the qualifying criteria of six tests: age, relationship, support, dependent, citizenship, and residence.
- *Age test*—To qualify, a child must have been under age 17—age 16 or younger—at the end of the year.
- *Relationship test*—To claim a child for purposes of the Child Tax Credit, they must be your son, daughter, stepchild, foster child, brother, sister, stepbrother, stepsister, or a descendant of any of these individuals, which includes your grandchild, niece, or nephew. An adopted child is always treated as your own child. An adopted child includes a child lawfully placed with you for legal adoption.
- *Support test*—In order to claim a child for this credit, the child must not have provided more than half of their own support.
- *Dependent test*—You must claim the child as a dependent on your federal tax return.
- *Citizenship test*—To meet the citizenship test, the child must be a U.S. citizen, U.S. national, or U.S. resident alien.
- *Residence test*—The child must have lived with you for more than half of 2015. There are some exceptions to the residence test, which can be found in IRS Publication 972, Child Tax Credit.
- *Limitations*—The credit is limited if your modified adjusted gross income is above a certain amount. The amount at which this phase-out begins varies depending on your filing status. For married taxpayers filing a joint return, the phase-out begins at $110,000. For married taxpayers filing a separate return, it begins at $55,000. For all other taxpayers, the phase-out begins at $75,000. In addition, the Child Tax Credit is generally limited by the amount of the income tax you owe as well as any alternative minimum tax you owe.
- *Additional Child Tax Credit*—If the amount of your Child Tax Credit is greater than the amount of income tax you owe, you may be able to claim the Additional Child Tax Credit.

Child Care Tax Credit

If you paid someone to care for your child under age 13, or other qualifying person, so you could work or look for work *and you have physical custody of a child*, you may be able to take the credit for child and dependent care. If you are divorced or separated and you have physical custody of the child, you can treat your child as a qualifying person, even if you cannot claim the child's exemption. If you are the noncustodial parent, you cannot treat your child as a qualifying person even if you can claim the child's exemption.

Education Credits

This credit allows for the first $1200 in "qualified tuition and related expenses," as well as half of qualifying expenses between $1200 and $2400, to be fully creditable against the taxpayer's total tax liability. The maximum amount of the credit is $1800 per eligible student. Students in a qualified Midwestern disaster area may receive up to $3600. And in 2015 the Hope Scholarship Credit cannot exceed $2500. The amount you can claim is equal to 100% of qualified tuition and related expenses not in excess of $2000 plus 25% of those expenses in excess of $2000 but not to exceed $4000.

Earned Income Credit

The earned income credit (EIC) is a tax credit for certain people who work have earned income under a specified threshold. There are different thresholds for people without children, people with one child, and people with two or more children. As with the child care tax credit, you must have custody of a child for s/he to be considered a qualified child.

Child's Investment Income

If your dependent child has unearned income of more than $1000 in 2015, s/he will have a tax liability on these earnings. The custodial parent or parents may choose to include this income on their return rather than file a return for the child. The Internal Revenue Service (IRS) specifically states not to use the return of the noncustodial parent. Note that if your child's interests, dividends, and other investment income exceed thresholds, part of that income may be taxed at the parent's tax rate instead of the child's tax rate.

Adoption Credit

For taxable years beginning in 2014, the credit allowed for the adoption of a child with special needs is $13,190; the maximum credit allowed for other adoptions is the amount of qualified adoption expenses up to $13,190. Phase-outs do apply beginning with modified adjusted gross income (MAGI) in excess of $197,880.

Marital Review

To reduce the chance of divorce, or at least mitigate potential financial consequences, some financial advisors (FAs) suggest married couples perform an annual "State of the Marital Financial Union" address to sit down with a spouse and review the following:

- Financial statements and accounts
- Tax returns with CPA
- Investment performance of separate and maritally created accounts
- Spending deficits or a surplus for the year?
- Miscellaneous

Surprises aren't uncommon, so couples should discuss financials to remove ambiguity. Unfortunately, many busy medical professionals skip this review.

OVERHEARD IN THE DOCTOR'S LOUNGE

I recently accepted the dinner invitation of a financial planner even though I told him I already had a lawyer, CPA, securities analyst and insurance counselor. So, at the end of the meal I asked him what he could do for me … that the others could not.

His reply: I want to be the "quarterback for your consulting team."

My reply: I already have a secretary!

Anonymous, MD
(Atlanta, GA)

PART II: FINANCIAL PLANNING FOR OTHER SPECIAL SITUATIONS

Like divorce, although one can hardly plan for these situations, there are certain specials cases that medical professionals might encounter.

WORKING ABROAD

If you are a U.S. citizen and medical professional working abroad, you may be able to minimize what you owe in the U.S. income tax if you qualify for the foreign income exclusion. If you qualify, you may exclude up to $97,600 in foreign income from the U.S. income tax liability in 2013. If you are married, your spouse is allowed an additional $97,600 exclusion. To qualify, you and your spouse must satisfy the following requirements:

- You must reside in a foreign country for an entire tax year or for at least 330 days during a 12-month period.
- Your salary must be paid by a company or agency in your country of residence or by a U.S. company operating in that country.

Also, only earned income—salaries, wages, and fringe benefits, plus allowances and expenses for housing—qualifies for the exclusion. Dividends, interest, capital gains, pension or retirement distributions, and alimony do not qualify. If you are a member of the U.S. military or other government service and are living abroad, your income is not considered foreign income. You'll have to pay taxes as if you were a taxpayer living in the United States.

Even if you avoid the U.S. income tax, you will likely pay some form of income tax to the country in which you reside and earn a salary. Should you fail to meet its residency requirements, or if you receive income above the allowable exclusion, you'll probably end up paying both foreign and the U.S. income tax. If you do pay foreign income tax, you can apply for a separate U.S. tax credit (using Form 1116) in the amount of foreign income tax you are required to pay.

You'll also owe the U.S. Social Security taxes if your country of residence has no treaty to coordinate its social service coverage with the United States. However, if such a treaty is in force, you'll pay foreign social service taxes to your host nation and will not be required to pay the U.S. Social Security taxes. In addition, you may be subject to estate and gift taxes if you transfer property, no matter where that property is located. If you maintain a house in the United States, you may owe state income tax and local property tax. For more information, consult a tax advisor or contact the IRS at (800) 829-3676 or http://www.irs.gov and request Publication 54, "Tax Guide for U.S. Citizens and Resident Aliens Abroad."

NONCITIZEN SPOUSE

Currently, the IRS offers an unlimited estate tax deduction (unlimited marital deduction) by which a spouse can receive an estate tax free, regardless of amount. The IRS Code has a much different view of the noncitizen spouse, limiting the marital deduction for a legal resident alien to only $$136,000 gift tax exemption since 2011. Fortunately, this spouse is offered a safe harbor in the Qualified Domestic Trust. The QDOT has the effect of narrowing the gap between a citizen and noncitizen spouse and is a valuable tool when draw up according to the IRS Code. Sans a proper QDOT, the noncitizen spouse is subject to the same treatment as a nonspouse beneficiary. The rules are somewhat less favorable for a noncitizen spouse who is not a resident alien.

A noncitizen spouse cannot use the applicable exclusion amount to shelter assets in a QDOT from estate taxes upon his or her death. However, the surviving noncitizen spouse may use the applicable exclusion amount ($5,340,000) in 2014 to shelter his or her own assets from federal estate taxes.

DUAL CITIZENSHIP

There may be a number of reasons why a foreign medical professional, especially a physician, may choose to remain a nonresident alien. But few realize that the U.S. income tax applies worldwide, and when a doctor becomes a U.S. dual citizen, the IRS is with them forever. Also, there is the $136,000 annual limitation on gifts to a noncitizen spouse. At his death, a doctor can't leave his possessions to a noncitizen spouse since the U.S. government is concerned that the foreign survivor will take her inheritance to her home country. Accordingly, the estate is tax immediately due after the first death. Separate savings accounts may mitigate this so that the dual-citizen spouse can acquire assets personally and have something to pass on to children. Otherwise, any assets that can't be proven, at least a one half contribution, even if jointly owned, will be taxed as if they solely belong to the American-citizen spouse.

EXPATRIATES

Here are three reasons for the recent increase in the number of the U.S. expatriations:

1. *Increased awareness of new tax filing laws.* Many people with the U.S. passports who live permanently overseas have been unaware of the rules requiring all citizens to file tax returns. The Swiss Bank UBS tax scandal and crackdown on Americans with overseas assets has made more people aware of the requirement. And they have simply given up their citizenship rather than comply.
2. *Growing compliance burden.* A new law, known as the Foreign Account Tax Compliance Act, was enacted in 2010 and may soon require foreign financial institutions to report to the Internal Revenue Service accounts held by the U.S. taxpayers. Some banks are simply closing the accounts of the U.S. clients as a result.
3. *Big penalties.* The standard penalty for unintentionally failing to file a tax return is $10,000. But the penalty for intentionally failing to file is far more. For example, a physician retired overseas with savings of $1 million in a foreign bank account. If s/he intentionally failed to file for 4 years, the penalty could be $2 million.

SPOUSE DEBT

The general rule is that spouses are not responsible for each other's debts, but there are exceptions. Many states will hold both spouses responsible for a debt incurred by one spouse if the debt constituted a family expense (e.g., child care or groceries). In addition, community property states will hold one spouse responsible for the other's debts because both spouses have equal rights to each other's income. Also, you are both responsible for any debt that you have in both names (e.g., mortgage, home equity loan, and credit card).

MEDICAL OFFICE CRISIS MANAGEMENT

The medical professional who remains in practice long enough is sure to undergo some adverse situation that may negatively affect the practice. A patient may die, your hospital may close, or a patient may go ballistic and injure your staff or yourself. When, not *if*, this scenario occurs, you must have a crisis management business plan in place to deal swiftly and successfully with the matter. Some management experts suggest the following course of actions when tragedy strikes:

- Stay calm and relaxed; act immediately.
- Release detrimental, but accurate, information as soon as possible. Try to stay neutral.
- Educate your staff about the crisis, then your local community, if relevant.

- Fix the problem, or find an alternate solution to minimize recurrence and disruption.
- Continually release information about the crisis if it is ongoing.
- Monitor and report the results of your strategy to all affected parties.
- Thank everyone and turn a negative story into a positive one through good public relations.

Remember, speed and productivity are the keys to adverse public relations fallout. Recall Johnson & Johnson, which recovered beautifully from the Tylenol-R tragedy three decades ago, and not only recovered lost profits but trust in the marketplace as well.

EMPLOYMENT CRISIS MANAGEMENT

Sooner or later, the employed medical professional or hospitalist will be terminated or reduced in force due to the current managed-care crisis. In the future, it will not be unusual to have a career with several different companies throughout a lifetime. This form of employment crisis management encompasses two different perspectives. If you become aware that you may lose your job, the following proactive steps will be helpful to your financial condition:

- Decrease retirement contributions to the minimum required to get the company match. Place the difference in your after-tax emergency fund.
- Eliminate unnecessary payroll deductions and deposit the difference to cash.
- Replace group term life insurance with personal term, or universal life insurance. Take your old group term policy with you, if possible.
- Establish a home equity line of credit to verify employment.
- Borrow against your pension plan only as a last resort.

After you have lost your job, negotiate your departure and get an attorney if you believe you lost your position through breach of contract or discrimination. Then, the following retroactive steps will be helpful to your financial condition:

- Prioritize fixed monthly bills in the following order: rent/mortgage; utility bills; minimum credit card payments; and restructured long-term debt.
- Consider liquidating assets to pay off debts, in this order: emergency fund, checking accounts, investment accounts, or asset held in your children's names.
- Review insurance coverage. Increase deductibles on homeowner's and automobile insurance for needed cash.
- Then, sell stocks or mutual funds; personal valuables, such as furnishings, jewelry, and real estate; and finally assets not in pension or annuities, if needed.
- Keep or rollover any lump sum pension or savings plan distribution directly to your new company, if possible, when you get rehired. Pay taxes and penalties, and use the money only as a last resort.
- Apply for unemployment insurance.
- Review your medical insurance, COBRA coverage, and the PP-ACA.
- Eliminate unnecessary variable, charitable, and/or discretionary expenses.
- Become very frugal.

NONTRADITIONAL RELATIONSHIPS

Medical practitioners who cohabitate in less than traditional relationships may find their personal financial assets at risk. Gay and lesbian couples frequently keep property and bank accounts separate and might not be aware that a joint account is possible, or that documentation is possible that can protect their finances within the context of their relationship. So if one dies, the other knows what to expect. Other potential problems include estate planning, wills, advanced directives, living trusts, guardianship for children, Do Not Resuscitate (DNR) orders, a power of attorney, or a healthcare power of attorney.

There are other problems as well. For example, if one member of a married couple dies, the surviving spouse receives an inheritance based on state law, but state laws do not have similar provisions for unmarried, or gay couples, and there are no QDROs available.

Even in today's environment, where an increasing number of employers are providing unmarried couples the same benefits as the traditional family, many state and federal laws are not so openminded. Familial interference notwithstanding, disability, Medicare, Social Security, and estate tax laws do not recognize cohabitation, whether a same-sex couple or a woman–man relationship. As an example, the Defense of Marriage Act, 1996, passed by Congress, provides that same-sex marriages will not be recognized for any federal purposes. This includes Social Security benefits, income tax, and pension distribution laws. The result is that the benefits available to husband and wife may simply still not be available to unmarried couples, regardless of their sexual orientation. But currently, federal statue are changing dramatically.

Understanding What Is at Risk

A function of Social Security is to be an old-age pension plan supplement. However, it also offers survivor benefits for a spouse and children. This benefit is not paid to a live-in companion. Social Security also offers a disability payment for those unable to work. This benefit will be available to those who qualify, but calculated at a single individual's rate for those unmarried. One area where a bonus may be earned is the old-age pension program. This will be paid to every qualifying individual. In other words, if both you and your significant other qualify for maximum benefits, these will be received for your lifetime. You will not be subject to a reduced survivor benefit.

Medicare pays health insurance benefits based upon the individual. These benefits will be affected by a nontraditional relationship. The family pieces of this puzzle are missing under current Medicaid guidelines. Estate law is also unforgiving and its penalties are truly gender and relationship blind. As an example, the powerful first tool in a well-written estate plan, the unlimited marital deduction, is not possible. This is a fact that must be recognized and dealt with in a proactive manner. Do not be misled by your local or state law that may recognize a relationship involving a significant other. The federal estate tax code simply does not exist for such a relationship, but this is changing going forward.

ABCs of Marriage Benefits

The federal and state government—as well as corporate America—confers many benefits, protections, and obligations to married couples. Among them are

- Assumption of spouse's pension
- Automatic housing lease transfer
- Automatic inheritance
- Bereavement leave
- Burial determination
- Child custody
- Confidentiality of conversations
- Crime victim's recovery benefits
- Divorce protections
- Domestic violence protection
- Exemption on property tax upon partner's death
- Family leave to care for sick partner
- Immunity from testimony against spouse

- Insurance benefits and breaks
- Joint adoption, foster care, and custody
- Joint bankruptcy
- Joint parenting to care for partner
- Medical decisions on behalf of partner
- Property rights
- Reduced rate membership
- Social security benefits
- Tax advantages
- Visitation of partner's children
- Visitation of partner in hospital or prison
- Wrongful death benefits

Minimizing the Impact of Nontraditional Relationships

The year 2014 will be the first time any married gay couple has ever filed Federal taxes together in the United States. It's been a decade since Massachusetts became the first state to start granting marriage licenses, and some states have previously accepted joint returns for state taxes. But until the Supreme Court struck down the Federal prohibition against gay marriage in *The United States v. Windsor* last summer, the Internal Revenue Service didn't recognize joint returns for married same-sex couples. So, filing will be on a state-by-state basis.

On the other hand, Social Security regulations are more set in stone. To combat reduced disability payments, for example, it is advised that both partners in these relationships purchase additional disability insurance, above and beyond what may be offered with your medical office group plan.

To combat the lack of death benefit from Social Security and some restrictive employer plans, it is recommended that sufficient life insurance be purchased on both parties. View this as a business buy–sell arrangement, so that one either partner will be left with sufficient financial means if an untimely death should take place.

And a charitable remainder trust, for estate planning, may be an appropriate document that allows a medical professional with an alternative lifestyle to insure an income stream for the rest of both partner's lives. It may result in reduced estate taxes, relief from capital gains, and the opportunity to diversify your investments. In this way, the legacy that is left to a significant other comes without familial meddling.

Same-Sex Divorce

Here are the residency requirements to get divorced in the 17 states (plus D.C.) that recognize same-sex marriages:

- California—6 months
- Connecticut—12 months (unless "the cause for the dissolution of the marriage arose after either party moved into this state")
- Delaware—6 months
- Hawaii—6 months
- Illinois—90 days
- Iowa—12 months
- Maine—6 months
- Maryland—12 months
- Massachusetts—12 months
- Minnesota—180 days
- New Hampshire—1 year
- New Jersey—12 months
- New Mexico—6 months

- New York—12 months
- Rhode Island—12 months
- Vermont—You can file after 6 months, but no divorce can be granted before 1 year
- Washington—90 days
- Washington, D.C.—6 months

Conservative LGBT Investors

An emerging body of evidence suggests that wealthy lesbian, gay, bisexual, and transgender (LGBT) investors take a more conservative approach to investing and may be less diversified than non-LGBT investors. In fact, according to the Spectrem Group, LGBT investors had 15% of their assets in stocks and bonds and 13% in mutual funds, versus 19% and 16% for non-LGBT investors, respectively. The difference may be attributed to the fact that such investors have less confidence in investment knowledge. Only 20% of ultra-high-net-worth LGBTs were knowledgeable about financial products and investments, compared to 40% of those in the non-LGBT community. The study also found that LGBT investors had fewer investable assets (47% vs. 60% for non-LGBT respondents). A principal residence accounted for 17% of overall assets, while non-LGBT households accounted for 14% of assets.

The types of FAs used by both groups are very similar. However, LGBT investors were more satisfied with their advisors at 82%, compared to 73% of non-LGBT respondents who were satisfied with their advisors. At the same time, LGBT investors felt their legal and advising needs were not well understood. Only about a third believed their FA understood the unique situations of the LGBT community, and only 21% felt financial advisory and services firms were doing a good job of meeting needs. The extent to which the LGBT medical community mirrors this study has yet to be determined.[*]

HEALTHCARE WORKFORCE COMMUTERS

Employees can use pretax dollars from their paychecks to pay for qualified commuting expenses, including mass-transit passes and parking. You reduce your taxable income—and potentially get a lower tax bill—while getting something you were going to pay for anyway. But while roughly 11.7 million workers have access to a commuter-benefit plan, fewer than three million sign up for it. For example, commuters can set aside up to $250 a month for qualified parking expenses, up from $245 last year. Assuming a total tax rate—federal, state, local, and FICA taxes—of about 40%, lowering your pretax income by $250 a month could end up saving you about $1200 a year in taxes. If a commuter invested that $1200 every year and got a 5% return, he would have more than $41,000 after two decades. While the monthly contribution limit for mass-transit riders has dropped to $130 from $245, there could be about $624 in tax-bill savings, using the same tax assumptions.[†]

OLDER PARENTS

Since more medical professionals are delaying marriage and child rearing until their own careers are well underway, it may be especially difficult in the cost-constrained future to fund college expenses. Older parents can therefore improve their chances for aid with the following strategies:

- Shift income, such as bonuses, withholds, and capitation disbursements, since more or less income in any given year can affect the potential for aid significantly. Keep in mind that financial eligibility for the current year is based on tax information from the prior year.
- Shift assets away from student and toward the professional parents, since the student contribution percentage is expected to be larger.

---

[*] *Source*: Diana Britton, Rep Magazine, North Hollywood, CA, page 11, February 2014.
[†] *Source*: www.WageWorks.com.

- Death, loss of job earnings, divorce, medical expenses, and the like will affect eligibility for aid and the amount offered.
- Use cash assets to reduce nonhousing debt and pay for major purchases to increase your loan potential. You will also get a tax break with a home equity loan.
- Apply each and every year, even if rejected the previous year.
- Do not ever offer information on a college aid application that is not requested.

SECOND AND SENIOR MARRIAGES

Financial and estate planning for a second marriage can be complicated, especially when children from a prior marriage are involved. Finding the right planning technique for your situation can not only ease family tensions but also help you pass more assets to the children at a lower tax cost. For example, a qualified terminal interest property (QTIP) trust marital trust can maximize estate tax deferral while benefiting the surviving spouse for his or her lifetime and the children after the spouse's death. Combining a QTIP with life insurance benefiting the children or creatively using joint gifts or generation skipping transfer (GST) tax exemptions can further leverage your gifting ability. A prenuptial agreement can also help you achieve your estate planning goals. But any of these strategies must be tailored to your particular situation, and the help of qualified advisors is suggested.

Healthcare professionals who marry as older folks also encounter special concerns that must be considered in order to maintain optimal financial health. For example,

- A surviving spouse will not lose survivor's pension benefits upon remarriage. However, this may occur if the deceased spouse retired from the military or federal government, and get remarried before the age of 55.
- A widow or widower, age 60 or older, may remarry and still collect benefits on a dead spouse's record. If you remarry prior to age 60, you lose your deceased spouse's benefit. If this occurs with a second spouse, you may keep either deceased spouse's full benefit, or your own, whichever is greater.
- It is not illegal for an employer, even an HMO, to deny healthcare coverage to a surviving spouse who remarries. The PP-ACA may be helpful in this case.

Today, the above situations even cause some senior medical professionals to live together, without the "benefit" of marriage.

THE UNMARRIEDS: THE CASE AGAINST MARRIAGE

For couples that decide not to marry, the potential tax planning is ripe with opportunity. Such couples can do anything that the tax code or state statutes prohibit married or related parties from doing. This provides some great tax savings and asset protection opportunities. For example, spouses cannot be the trustees of each other's irrevocable or asset protection trusts, but unmarried partners absolutely can. Choosing not to marry is becoming especially popular with older couples. This is because many older people with previous marriages have accumulated two things: assets and children. They find marriage less compelling when they and their new partner won't have children together.

Insurance and Tax Examples

Laws relating to Worker's Compensation (WC) insurance are one example of this. Someone whose spouse has died in a work-related accident may be eligible to receive a monthly benefit, paid for the rest of his or her life. However, most state laws provide that the benefits end if the recipient remarries. This puts a real cost to remarrying.

Example

Consider an RN who at age 50 loses her husband to a work-related accident and receives a settlement of $2000 a month for life. Assuming she will live another 35 years and could invest the proceeds in a 3% bond, the present value of that income stream is $520,000. That means a person would need $520,000, invested at 3%, to give a monthly income of $2000 for 35 years. Therefore, if this nurse fell in love and wanted to remarry 2 years into receiving the payments, the remaining 33 years of monthly payments she would forfeit has a value of $502,000. This puts a rather quantifiable cost on one's social, emotional, and religious values.

Tax Code

The tax code also encourages couples to remain unmarried.

Example

Now, consider a physician couple who both earn high incomes. Suppose each has a taxable income of $400,000, which is the breakpoint where the 39.6% tax bracket begins. As two singles, as long as their taxable income is $400,000 or less, they both remain in the 35% tax bracket. However, if they marry, their joint income goes to $800,000 while the 35% tax bracket only expands to $450,000 for couples. That means they now pay an additional 4.6% in federal income taxes on the excess of $350,000, or $12,600. Some may be quick to dismiss that amount as trivial, given their income level, but the point is still that marriage for them brings a tangible cost in higher taxes.

Of course, younger couples who do plan to have children still recognize that marriage is important. For many reasons, marriage isn't going out of style any time soon. Few of those reasons, however, are financial ones.

FINANCIAL WINDFALLS

If you are fortunate enough to win the lottery, or receive a large inheritance, the following simple rules will help maintain your emotional stability, as well as financial health. And, answering these questions may help you evaluate your short- and long-term needs and goals:

- Do you have outstanding debt that you'd like to pay off?
- Do you need more current income?
- Do you plan to pay for your children's education?
- Do you need to bolster your retirement savings?
- Are you planning to buy a first or second home?
- Are you considering giving to loved ones or a favorite charity?
- Are there ways to minimize any upcoming income and estate taxes?
- Do you have enough money to pay your bills and your taxes?
- How might investing increase or decrease your taxes?
- Do you have assets that you could quickly sell if you needed cash in an emergency?
- Are your investments growing quickly enough to keep up with or beat inflation?
- Will you have enough money to meet your retirement needs and other long-term goals?
- How much risk can you tolerate when investing?
- How diversified are your investments?

Now, consider the following:

- Deposit cash into a money market account in your name, or into a joint account with your spouse, and limit access. If a doctor is the executor of an estate, be aware that significant tax benefits may result by freezing the estate for 6 months and using the alternate valuation method of size determination. Similarly, if a windfall is in the form of securities, make sure they are titled correctly. Limit those to whom you tell about your luck.

- Hire a team of financial advisors, accountants, lawyers, and insurance agents. Get tax advice immediately.
- Do not quit your job, sell your practice, or initially disrupt your life materially.
- Maintain your routine and limit new expenditures. Consider your lifestyle options.
- Redefine your financial plans, and continue to save and invest. Pay down your debt.
- Nondeductible debt costs the stated APR, while deductible debt costs less if you itemize.
- Review your insurance policies, will, estate plan, or trusts.
- Avoid friends or relatives who petition you for money. Consider charitable interests and gifting strategies carefully.
- Exercise, stay healthy, and enjoy your windfall.

Receiving a settlement from a lawsuit may also bring added financial concerns. If the lawsuit is injury related, for example, one should address the issues of budgeting and health care, projecting the effects of inflation on the settlement to help make the money last long enough to take care of your needs.

Financial Aid for College

Feel at ease medical professionals of all sorts; you don't have to be "poor" to qualify for financial aid for your children. In some circumstances, families with incomes of $100,000 or more can qualify.

Federal Government Grants

The federal government provides student aid through a variety of programs. The most prominent of these are Pell Grants and Federal Supplemental Educational Opportunity Grants (FSEOGs). Pell Grants are administered by the U.S. government. They are awarded on the basis of college costs and a financial aid eligibility index. The eligibility index takes into account factors such as family income and assets, family size, and the number of college students in the family. By law, Pell Grants can provide up to $5645 per student for the 2013–2014 year. However, only about 28% of recipients currently qualify for the maximum. The average grant was $3650 in 2012–2013. Students must reapply every year to receive aid. Most colleges will not process applications for Stafford loans until needy students have applied for Pell Grants. Students with Pell Grants also receive priority consideration for FSEOGs. Students who can demonstrate severe financial need may also receive an FSEOG. FSEOGs award up to $4000 per year per student.

State Grants

Many states offer grant programs as well. Each state's grant program is different, but they do tend to award grants exclusively to state residents who are planning to attend an in-state school. Many give special preference to students planning to attend a state school.

College Grants

Some colleges and universities offer specialized grant programs. This is particularly true of older schools with many alumni and large endowments. These grants are usually based on need or scholastic ability. Consult the college or university's financial aid office for full details.

Independent College 500–Indexed Certificates of Deposit

The I.C. 500 is the College Board's index of college inflation based on a survey of the costs at 500 independent colleges and universities. I.C. 500-indexed Certificates of Deposit are a relatively new funding vehicle offered by a few savings institutions. Their rate of return is linked to the I.C. 500 index.

Section 529 Plans

Section 529 Plans are also known as Qualified Tuition Plans (QTPs). These state-sponsored and college-sponsored plans offer higher contributions than Coverdell IRAs along with tax-deferred accumulation. Once withdrawals begin, they are tax exempt as long as the funds are used to pay for qualified higher education expenses. As with other investments, there are generally fees and expenses associated with participation in a Section 529 savings plan. In addition, there are no guarantees regarding the performance of the underlying investments in Section 529 plans. The tax implications of a Section 529 savings plan should be discussed with a CPA because they can vary significantly from state to state. Most states offer their own Section 529 plans, which may provide advantages and benefits exclusively for their residents and taxpayers. The 529 plan is also a way for grandparents to shelter inheritance money from estate taxes and contribute substantial amounts to a student's college fund. At the same time, they also control the assets and can retain the power to control withdrawals from the account. By accelerating use of the annual gift tax exclusion, a grandparent—as well as anyone, for that matter—could elect to use 5 years' worth of annual exclusions by making a single contribution of as much as $70,000 per beneficiary in 2013 (or a couple could contribute $140,000 in 2013), as long as no other contributions are made for that beneficiary for 5 years. If the account owner dies, the 529 plan balance is not considered part of his or her estate for tax purposes.

Tip: Many states offer an income tax deduction for residents that make contributions to 529 college-savings plans. For example, consider a single CRNA, or married physician, in Ohio with $150,000 in taxable income, a 28% marginal federal tax bracket, and a 5.45% state marginal tax bracket. Investing $4000 in the Ohio State 529 plan accounts for two children would save roughly $218 come tax time.

PHYSICAL DISABILITIES

Studies of the physician community estimate the need for treatment of physical disabilities to number about 8–10% of the total community. Early intervention is the key to successful treatment. The original Physical Healing Foundation of the American Medical Association (AMA) has been replaced by the new Federation of State Physician Health Programs. Disability re-education remains on the agenda and is usually included in the annual International Conference on Physicians Health. The Disabled Physicians Association, headquartered in Louisiana, as well state medical associations is the intervention starting point for disabled physicians.

CHEMISTRY DEPENDENCY

Chemical or mental disorders may be effectively hidden, with admirable coping mechanisms developed to deny its existence. Chemical dependency includes alcoholism, substance abuse, gambling, sex addiction, and similar diseases. Often, these are coupled with other mental health problems, such as depression. The rank of healthcare providers needing treatment is growing as a lack of self-recognition and denial is a powerful force precluding success. Unfortunately, recidivism rates are higher than desired from many traditional treatment programs, and centers that have higher rates of success are sometimes the last stop on the road to recovery.

THE ELDERLY FAMILY

Care and concern for elderly family members bring questions about Medicare supplement insurance planning, trusts and wills, long-term care planning, assisted living search and selection, home health or nursing home selection, living wills, inflation protection planning, and others. Caring for an Alzheimer's disease patient or similar patient takes both an emotional and financial commitment on the part of the family member(s) or other caregiver who is responsible. When faced with this unfortunate situation, advice may be needed for establishing powers of attorney, living trusts, addressing long-term care issues, and working with an elder-law attorney to prepare appropriate legal documents.

ENGAGE WITH GRACE

According to the website, *Engage with Grace*, we all make choices throughout our lives—where we want to live, what types of activities will fill our days, and with whom we spend our time, and so on. These choices are often a balance between our desires and our means, but at the end of the day, they are decisions made with intent. Somehow when we get close to death, however, we stop making decisions. We get frozen in our tracks and can't talk about our preferences for end-of-life care (Mathew Holt, personal communication).

Can you and your loved ones answer these questions?

1. On a scale of 1 to 5, where do you fall on this continuum?

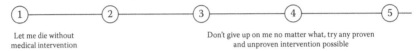

Let me die without medical intervention   Don't give up on me no matter what, try any proven and unproven intervention possible

2. If there were a choice, would you prefer to die at home, or in a hospital?

3. Could a loved one correctly describe how you'd like to be treated in the case of a terminal illness?

4. Is there someone you trust whom you've appointed to advocate on your behalf when the time in near?

5. Have you completed any of the following: written a living will, appointed a healthcare power of attorney, or completed an advance directive?

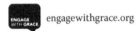 engagewithgrace.org   The one slide project

So, the *One Slide Project* was designed with one simple goal: to help MDs/DOs and FAs get the conversation about the end-of-life experience started. The idea is simple: Create a tool to help get people talking. One Slide, with just five questions on it. Five questions designed to help get us talking with each other, with our loved ones, about our preferences. And, we're asking readers to share this One Slide—wherever and whenever they can.

Download the One Slide—http://engagewithgrace.org/Download.aspx

Share it any time you can—in the doctor's lounge, at the end of a client-prospect presentation, or at a pharmaceutical company-sponsored dinner. Think of the slide as currency and donate just 2 minutes whenever you can. Commit to being able to answer these five questions about end-of-life experience for yourself and family, and your patients and clients. Then, commit to helping other colleagues do the same. Get the conversation started.

Just *One Slide*, just one goal. Think of the enormous difference that all doctors, medical professionals, and financial advisors can make together.

CHARITABLE GIFT SECURITIES

By gifting stock that has increased in value instead of selling it and donating the cash, a donor can avoid paying capital-gains tax, which has the potential to save thousands come tax time.

For example, if Dr. Markus bought 500 shares of a stock at $10 each and it's now worth $50, he wouldn't have to pay the capital-gains taxes on the $20,000 profit. That's a potential tax savings of $3000 if that stock was held for more than a year and taxed at the 15% long-term capital-gains rate. That savings increases to $4760 for joint filers with taxable income of $450,000 or more in 2013, who are subject to a 20% long-term capital-gains rate and a 3.8% Medicare surtax on net investment income.

Terminal Illness and Anatomic Gifts

If you are diagnosed with a terminal illness, the following may not be helpful to you, but might be of help to your survivors:

- Increase liquidity to cover the costs of pre- and postdeath expenses.
- Contact your local social security office to determine eligibility for disability and death benefits.
- Determine the contents, and those you wish to have access to, of your safety deposit box(es).
- Since some states do not have death taxes, consider changing your domicile.
- Preserve your testimony to any outstanding claims or litigation regarding personal or professional affairs, through a formal legal deposition or other means.

As a medical professional, consider organ donation since the supply of donated organs is dwarfed by the demand for them. The Coalition on Donation is a campaign to raise awareness of this need. The decision to be an organ donor is personal and some healthcare professionals have philosophical or religious beliefs that prohibit this option. However, if you decide to be an organ donor, documentation and communication are the critical steps to insuring your wishes are carried out. First, contact your local motor vehicle department and inform your family and loved ones. You should also inform your own personal physician, in writing, and wear a donor identification bracelet, or something similar, that fits in your wallet or purse, so your wishes are known.

Funeral Finances

When one considers the cost of a funeral, with casket, embalming, burial, and other itemized costs and service-related expenses, the average price tag is about $8500 and, of course, purchasing the burial plot is extra. The cost of the average cremation is about $750. Further information relating to burial finances can be obtained from Consumer Caskets USA at 800-611-8778, the Choice in Dying at 202-338-9790, and the Funeral and Memorial Society of America at 802-482-3437. Remember, life is a perilous journey. The above information will help turn potential financial disasters into manageable pitfalls.

CONCLUSION

Standard financial planning strategies don't fit every situation. Single people, unmarried couples, noncitizen spouses, individuals planning a second marriage, and grandparents are among those who might benefit from less common techniques.

In this chapter, we looked at several special situations that may apply to physicians and some medical professionals.

COLLABORATE

Discuss this chapter online with others at www.MedicalExecutivePost.com.

ACKNOWLEDGMENTS

To Brian S. Orol, CFP®, president, Strategic Wealth Management, Raleigh, North Carolina, Rick Kahler, MS, CFP®, ChFC, CCIM of the Kahler Financial Group, in Rapid City, South Dakota, and Perry D'Alessio, CPA, New York, NY.

FURTHER READING

Braver, S with O'Connell, D: *Divorced Dads—Shattering the Myths*. Penguin Putnam, New York, 1998.

Jessani, AD: Divorce planning for doctors. In Marcinko, DE [editor]: *Insurance and Risk Management Strategies for Physicians and Advisors*. Jones and Bartlett, Sudbury, MA, 2007.

Jessani, AD: Ten common parenting-related mistakes in drafting divorce agreements. *American Journal of Family Law*, 14, pages 102–107, Summer 2000.

Lavine, A: Life insurance and pre-nuptial agreements. *Wealth Management*, page 36, March 2014.

Muldowney, TM, Marcinko, DE and Hetico, HR: In Margolis, HS [editor]: *The Elder Law Portfolio Series*. Aspen Publishers, New York, 2008.

Pavia, A: Finding hidden assets: Digging deep in HNW divorce. *Financial Planning*, pages 1–2, March 24, 2014.

Seiffer, A: Suddenly single. *Wealth Management*, page 17, April 2, 2014.

Wilson, CA: Five errors financial planners commonly make when working with divorcing clients. *JFP*, October 2000.

22 Sales Contracting for Medical Practice Succession Planning

Reviewing Terms, Conditions, and Selling Agreements

Charles F. Fenton III

CONTENTS

Dealing with many issues concerning the actual contract that affects the purchase or sale of a medical practice can be daunting. For example, this chapter will not deal with the issue of determining whether or not a physician should retire. Nor will it determine the proper fair market value (FMV) of the practice. However, physicians may be assisted in both instances by a medically focused financial advisor (FA), or valuation specialist, AVA, CPA-CVA, Certified Medical Planner™, etc. who will work in conjunction with an experienced health-care contract attorney to act as an advocate and determine certain contingencies that might occur, and protect him/her from them.

THE PARTIES

The first determination is whether the party at interest is an individual, group of individuals, or an entity (such as a partnership, limited liability partnership, limited partnership, limited liability company, or corporation—whether an S corporation, C corporation, or a professional corporation). In many instances, even if the party at interest is an individual or an entity, the individual(s) behind the entity should be made parties to the agreement.

From the buyer's perspective, the purchase of a medical practice is a highly person-oriented business. The practice value depends much upon the personality of the current-treating physicians. If the current-treating physicians are also the owners of the entity, then binding these individuals (especially as applies to the restrictive covenant) is of primary importance.

If the current-treating physicians are not owners of the entity, but rather employees, then a determination of whether they will continue in their same positions or whether the buyer will be taking over the treatment of patients becomes the prime focus. If the current-treating physicians will be continuing in their same positions, then their current employment contract must be reviewed to determine whether the rights of the seller will accrue to the buyer.

If the rights of the seller will not accrue to the buyer, then the purchase and sale agreement must have a provision that makes the continued employment of those current-treating physicians a condition to consummation of the sale. In such instances, the new employment agreement might be an exhibit to the main agreement and executed contemporaneously with the main agreement.

If the current-treating physicians will not be continuing in their same position and if the purchaser will be assuming treatment of the patients, then the main agreement must provide for the dissolution of the employment agreement and provision must be made for restricting the ability of those physicians from competing with the buyer. If the employment contract with the seller contains a restrictive covenant, then the buyer must ensure that such covenants will accrue to the buyers' benefit. Otherwise, the buyer should insist that those physicians sign restrictive covenants. In such an instance, a portion of the purchase price may need to be allocated toward the consideration for those restrictive covenants and paid directly to those physicians.

DATE OF AGREEMENT AND CLOSING DATE

In general, it usually does not matter when the agreement is dated. It should usually be dated once all the terms are agreed to and the parties desire to bind each other and to be bound. In a certain instance, the parties may have reached an agreement, but certain issues (such as the obtaining of a state license to practice medicine) may be outstanding. In such a case, then an option can be given by either the seller or the buyer to bind the other to sell or buy the practice upon exercise of the option. Giving an option can also push the agreement date into the future. The option will usually be given with token consideration (e.g., $100) and will have a fixed expiration date (e.g., 30–90 days).

The determination of the closing date is more important than the date that the agreement is dated. Just as in the purchase of a house where certain issues (such as obtaining a mortgage and home inspection) must occur before closing, in the purchase of a practice, there may be certain issues that require time to undertake before the actual transfer can be consummated. For example, the buyer may still need to obtain financing or the landlord may need to approve the assignment of the lease.

RECITALS

The recitals—or "whereas" clauses—traditionally enunciate the reasons the parties are entering into the agreement. In the sale of the practice, the recitals may simply state that the buyer wishes to buy the practice and the seller wishes to sell the practice. Yet, there is a modern growing tendency among contract attorneys to eliminate the "whereas" clauses as some attorneys feel that such language is antiquated. In such instances, the agreement will simply have a paragraph or two delineations of the "Purpose" of the agreement.

ARTICLES, SECTIONS, AND PARAGRAPHS

The agreement will often be divided and numbered in some logical manner, into articles, sections, paragraphs, or a combination of these. The reason for doing so is twofold. First, it allows ready reference to the numbered paragraph, and second, it allows the agreement to be divided and grouped in logical associations.

BINDING THE PARTIES

The first paragraph of the first article will often bind the seller to sell and the buyer to buy the practice under the terms of the agreement. The rest of the agreement simply spells out those terms.

WHAT IS PURCHASED?

The agreement must disclose the items that are being transferred and the items that are not considered part of the agreement. This section should be crystal clear, so that anybody reading the contract (and hence a court which may be called upon to enforce the contract) and not privy to the preliminary negotiations will know what is part of the agreement and what is not part of the agreement.

SALE OF STOCK VERSUS SALE OF ASSETS

In most cases, well-informed FAs will recommend that the buyer solely purchases the assets of the practice and not the stock of the practice. By purchasing selected assets, the buyer is ensured that he will not become responsible for the known or unknown liabilities of the corporation. In prior days, avoiding purchasing the stock of the corporation was a wise recommendation.

However, with the advent of managed care, the purchase of the stock of the corporation can provide the new practitioner with certain competitive advantages. It may take a new practitioner 3–9 months to get onto enough managed care panels to make the practice profitable. Purchase of the stock of the corporation ensures the new practitioner of acquiring the federal tax identification number (TIN), personal identification number (PIN), Drug Enforcement Agency (DEA), Centers for Medicare and Medicaid (CMS), global location number (GLN), national provider identifier (NPI), HIE-Form 834 transmission number, durable medical equipment number (DME), and so on, of the corporate entity. Since most managed care corporations identify providers by the federal TIN, purchase of the stock of the corporation should allow the new practitioner to be enrolled on managed care panels in a shorter period of time.

Items Purchased

Items purchased often list the tangible and intangible property of the seller that will be transferred to the buyer. Such items often include

1. A detailed inventory of the tangible assets to be purchased
2. A detailed listing of the inventory of the practice
3. The names and addresses of all the patients of record treated by the seller
4. The patient medical records maintained by the seller
5. The computer records maintained by the seller
6. All licenses, permits, accreditation, and franchises issued by any federal, state, municipal, or quasi-government authority relating to the use, maintenance, or operation of the practice, running to or in favor of the seller, but only to the extent that they are accepted by the buyer
7. All of the sellers' right, title, and interest in and to all real estate and equipment leases, if any, services agreements, employment, and professional service contracts relate to the practice but only to the extent that the foregoing contracts are accepted by the buyer
8. Assignment of lease should be attached and be incorporated to the agreement
9. All existing telephone numbers are used in connection with the operation of the practice and all yellow-page advertising of the practice
10. The goodwill of the practice, which includes the seller's assistance and cooperation in transfer of all sellers' rights and interests in the practice to the buyer and any other intangible assets of the practice are not listed in any other category

Certain items purchased, such as (paper or electronic) medical records, governmental licenses, fax, e-mail, website, and telephone numbers have special considerations as discussed below.

Medical Records

The seller should protect its future need to use the transferred patient medical records. In the current managed care environment, providers are subject to strict scrutiny. Even after leaving practice, the provider may find himself subject to a government or third-party audit or subject to a medical malpractice lawsuit. Therefore, the provider should ensure that the contract allows for him to take future possession of the specific medical record(s) of the practice to mount an appropriate defense.

Governmental Licenses

Certain government licenses and permits may be nontransferable. These would include items such as the federal and state employer identification numbers, as these are unique to the seller as a corporate entity. Likewise, other items unique to the seller include Medicare identification numbers, Medicaid identification numbers, NPIs, and unique provider identification numbers (UPINs). The buyer would have to purchase the stock of the corporation order to acquire such items, which is another advantage of a stock transaction versus an asset transaction. Likewise, some local business licenses may or may not be transferable.

Telephone and Fax Numbers, Website URLs, Twitter Accounts, and So On

Transference of the telephone numbers often requires that a special local telephone company performs the authorizing transfer of the telephone numbers to the buyer. Often, the new owner of the telephone number will also become liable for any current yellow-page advertisement monthly fees. It is the same with a uniform resource locator (URL) or website address or office Twitter account, and so on.

ITEMS NOT PURCHASED

Items not purchased or "excluded items" often list the personal items of the parties or of the employees of the parties. Such items would often include

1. All cash on hand or on deposit
2. All accounts receivable generated prior to the closing date
3. All prepaid expenses, utility deposits, tax rebates, insurance claims, credits due from suppliers, and other allowances after the closing date
4. The personal effects, including but not limited to photographs, diplomas, uniforms, books, mementos, memorabilia, personally owned art, and any personal property owned by them
5. Life insurance, disability insurance, and disability buy-out insurance on the seller
6. Motor vehicles used in connection with the practice
7. Any or all tangible–intangible assets used in conjunction with another practice of the seller
8. All other assets owned by the seller other than those specifically described as items purchased

The exact items transferred will often depend on the prior negotiations of the parties. For example, the parties may have agreed that the accounts receivable will be transferred with the practice. In such an instance, the accounts receivable will be listed as an item to be purchased.

PURCHASE PRICE AND TERMS

The price of the transaction (or the value of the practice) is often one item that is aggressively negotiated between the parties. That is because both the buyer and the seller are overly concerned with "how much?" As this chapter demonstrates, there are a lot more details that go into the negotiation and final contract than just the price. The buyer or seller would be doing him/herself a disservice to consider the other factors simply "lawyer details." Many additional terms of the agreement should be considered by one side or the other as "walk-way" conditions. The party that fully adheres to their additional terms is likely to find the other party capitulating to them. This is because the other party will most likely be fixated on the price.

The purchase price should be delineated in the agreement. Furthermore, the method of payment of the purchase price should be delineated. Although the usual method of payment would be cash, there are other methods available as well.

Cash payment can be made by an official bank cashier's check, by a certified check, by deposit of funds into an escrow account, or by other methods agreed upon by the parties.

Non-cash-type transactions include loan agreements and exchanges. Exchanges can provide certain tax benefits if the exchange is a "like kind" exchange. A like kind exchange would occur when parties swap practices. For example, a group practice might have several offices. As part of the breakup of the group, the parties might exchange their stock of one office for all of the stock of another office. Like kind exchanges have strict guidelines that must be adhered to or the tax advantages will disappear. The reader is cautioned to get the current legal and financial advice prior to the time of exchange.

It is in the seller's best interest to get all cash at the time of closing. Then the seller can walk away and not worry about the success or failure of his predecessor. The seller will not have to worry about collecting periodic payments. The seller will not have to worry about placing the buyer in default or about eventually having to repossess the practice and begin to practice medicine at that office again. If a seller repossesses a practice, the buyer may have driven the patients away or lost the managed care contracts (why else would the buyer not be able to honor the loan agreement?). So, the repossessed practice will have a significantly lower market value—if it is even marketable at that time.

On the opposite end of the spectrum, it is in the buyer's best interest to get long and lean loan terms. First, by getting loan terms, the buyer will often have to come up with much less initial capital. Second, because of the discussion in the preceding paragraph, the seller has a vested interest in ensuring that the buyer succeeds once the practice changes hands.

If the transaction involves a seller-financed loan, then the agreement should specify the terms. Additionally, a separate loan agreement and security agreement should be attached as exhibits to the agreement. Finally, to perfect the security agreement, the lien should be recorded at the local courthouse in accordance to local rules and customs.

ALLOCATION OF PURCHASE PRICE

The final purchase price will actually be the amalgamation of various assets of the practice. These assets include the tangible and intangible assets. The tangible assets include the hard assets (such as computers, treatment tables, chairs and furniture, DME and x-ray machines, etc.) and the soft assets (such as Q-tips, paper, and cotton balls). The intangible assets will include the going-concern value, goodwill, and the value of any restrictive covenant.

The parties should delineate the allocation of the purchase price among those various categories to reach a mutual best fit with the potential tax obligations. The buyer is the one who should strive to make the allocation fit his needs as best as possible.

Generally, the sale of the assets will be ordinary income to the seller and taxed at the seller's usual rate. The buyer will be able to depreciate the purchased items. However, the characterization of those assets and the allocated portion of the purchase price will determine how much can be depreciated and over what time period the items can be depreciated.

As a general rule, soft assets can be depreciated fully in the year of purchase. Generally, hard assets can be depreciated over a 3–7-year time period, depending on the class of the asset. Also, under Section §179, a certain dollar amount can be "expensed" or deducted in the year of purchase. The sooner and faster that the assets can be deducted, the less current taxes the buyer will be required to pay. However, intangible assets generally must be deducted over a 15-year period. This prolongs the tax benefits of any payments characterized as such.

Nonetheless, purchase of the assets results in better tax consequences than purchase of the stock of the practice. When the stock is purchased, there is no depreciation allowance allocated in the current or subsequent years. Instead, the cost of the stock becomes the "basis" of the buyer in the practice. Any gain or loss from that basis will only have tax benefits or tax consequences in the year that the stock is sold or becomes worthless.

Because of the tax consequences of the characterization of the allocations of the purchase price, it is important that the agreement delineates the portion of the practice price that is allocated to each category. Each party should further agree never to claim a different allocation in any future tax filings. Generally, the soft and hard assets will be valued at their current actual cash value. In no event should the purchase price allocated to the soft and hard assets exceed the actual initial cost that the seller paid for the item. The only exception to the foregoing would be if the sale involved the transfer of an appreciable asset.

LEASE ASSIGNMENT

The agreement should provide that upon closing that the seller will assign the lease to the buyer. The buyer then acquires possession of the premises and assumes responsibility for the lease payments.

Sellers often do not understand that even though they do not practice at the leased premises and even though the buyer is making the lease payments, that the seller still remains liable to the landlord under the original lease. Usually, this does not present a problem for the seller. But if the buyer abandons the premises or stops making the lease payments, then the landlord will look to the seller for the lease payments through the expiration of the lease.

If the seller has signed a restrictive covenant, then the seller may find himself in the unenviable position of making lease payments for the premises and prohibited from practicing at the premises. The seller should protect himself from this possibility. Therefore, the seller should ensure that the original agreement contains a provision that if the seller becomes liable under the lease, the seller can enter onto the premises, take possession of the practice and the practice assets, and can practice medicine at the location until the seller's liabilities are extinguished.

INDEMNIFICATION AND EXCLUSION/INCLUSION OF LIABILITIES

During the sale of a medical practice, each party will have certain liabilities that the other party should not assume and should not be required to assume. A mutual indemnification clause will act to ensure that each party remains liable for its own liabilities.

In a medical practice, the most common liability is a claim of medical malpractice against the provider. The seller has an interest in insuring that he is not liable for any claim brought by a patient that resulted after he leaves the practice, and the buyer has an interest in insuring that she is not liable for any claim brought by a patient that resulted before she acquired the practice.

There are other areas of liability in the sale of a medical practice that may not be readily apparent. These include premise liability (e.g., slip and fall claims), employment claims (e.g., unemployment liability, sexual harassment, discrimination, and wrongful termination claims), tax claims (e.g., unpaid employment taxes and income or sales tax liabilities), and third-party payer claims (e.g., Medicare recoupment claims). Consult your insurance agent to determine whether you can obtain insurance coverage to limit your liability under these clauses.

Medical practitioners should understand the full risk of signing an indemnification or a hold harmless clause. If a claim is brought against the other party, then the party giving indemnification can be forced to pay any judgment or settlement incurred by that other party. The party giving indemnification can even be required to pay the other party's attorney bills. This is an important point that the reader should consider carefully: *Even if the other party successfully defends a claim, the indemnifying party can be held liable for the other party's attorney's fees.* Since attorney fees can mount up rapidly, the indemnifying party can find itself responsible for thousands or even tens of thousands of dollars of attorneys' fees.

If at all possible, one should never sign an indemnification agreement, whether in the sale of a medical practice, a managed-care contract, or even a home security-monitoring contract. Sometimes, one has no choice but to assume the risk and sign the contract. If at all possible, one should strive to sign such clauses in a corporate capacity and not in an individual capacity. If that is not possible, then seek insurance to minimize the risk. Indemnification clauses and the potential unlimited risk that they pose is one reason why the professional should undertake a carefully planned asset protection program.

OTHER FACTORS AND CLAUSES

INTEGRATION

As a general rule, once parties have seen fit to put their agreement in writing, then no prior oral agreement regarding the same subject is binding. A paragraph stating that the written agreement contains the entire understanding of the parties simply reflects this rule of contract construction. Such a paragraph also places the parties on notice that any oral representation of the other party that has not been placed in the contract will be worthless.

CONSTRUCTION

At times, a court may hold any ambiguities in a contract against the party that prepared the agreement or that had the agreement prepared for them. If the party on the other side of the contract is an individual who was not represented by the counsel and especially if that party has had very little business experience (such as a physician or medical provider recently in practice), courts are much more likely to hold ambiguities against the drafter of the agreement.

A paragraph regarding the construction of the agreement and stating that the agreement was formed from negotiation (as opposed to a "take-it-or-leave-it" proposition) can identify for any court constructing the contract that the court should not hold any ambiguities against the drafter. After all, even with negotiated contracts, one party or the other draws up the agreement.

CHOICE OF LAW

In the United States today, it is common for parties in different states to have business dealings with each other. Likewise, in the sale of a medical practice, the buyer may begin negotiations in one state and then move to the practice state after consummation of the sale. In a similar vein, following the sale, the buyer may move to another state.

In most cases, the various state laws should be similar on the contractual issues involved in the sale of a medical practice. However, a statement in the contract identifying the state whose laws will govern the contract will eliminate one possible source of dispute involving a side issue to the contract. In the vast majority of contracts, the laws of the state where the practice is physically located should be chosen by the parties to govern the contract.

CHOICE OF VENUE

Just like providing for choice of law, a side issue to the contract can be eliminated by choosing ahead of time the venue to resolve any conflicts that may arise. The venue is simply the place where the conflict will be decided. In most cases, the parties should choose the trial court of the county in which the practice is located.

SURVIVAL OF OBLIGATIONS

An agreement to purchase a medical practice contains two aspects. First is the transference of the practice assets in exchange for the purchase price. Second are the various other terms, such as preservation of the medical records. By providing that these obligations survive the closing, each party is assured that the other party will not claim that the actual closing of the agreement extinguished the rights of the parties under the agreement.

NO-WAIVER CLAUSE

A provision providing that a party does not waive its rights unless such a waiver is committed to writing allows a party to be a "nice guy" without risking its future rights. In some instances, if a party does not insist upon full compliance by the other party, then the first party may be considered to have waived its rights and may have no recourse against the other party.

There may be instances when the forbearance to exercise a right under the contract will benefit both parties. For example, if the buyer cannot pay the seller an installment on time, the seller may agree to extend the time for payment of that installment. The no-waiver clause allows the seller to refuse to extend the time for payment of a future installment. Without the clause, the buyer might be able to argue that the seller had waived its future rights to timely payments.

NOTICES

There may be various reasons under the contract why one party may need to give a notice to the other party. Most often, such notice will be that a party is claiming that the other is in breach of some provision of the agreement.

By specifying the address and method of any delivery notice, the sending party can be assured that a court will rule that the receiver had actual or constructive notice.

Such a provision should also provide that one type of notice would be a change of address. Such a change of address notification would then supersede the address delineated in the agreement.

In most cases, the agreement should provide that the counsel to the party would receive a copy of any notice. This accomplishes two goals. First, there is a greater likelihood that the receiving party would receive actual notice. If the receiving party had moved and had failed to provide notice of the change of address, then the party's counsel would have received the notice. Second, the party's counsel would have received the notice in a timely manner and could take any immediate action that may be necessary.

SEVERABILITY CLAUSE

A severability clause helps to ensure that if one provision is held by a court to be illegal or unenforceable, then the offending clause will be stricken from the agreement and the parties will be held to the agreement without the clause.

Without a severability clause, if a court finds that one provision of the agreement is illegal or unenforceable, then the court has the power to strike down the entire agreement. Although, even with a severability clause a court could strike down the entire agreement, the severability clause tells the court that the intent of the parties was that only the offending clause could be stricken and essentially asks the court to honor the parties' intent.

FURTHER ASSURANCES CLAUSE

After execution of the agreement, the parties may discover that certain other documents are necessary to complete the transaction. Unless such documents materially change the meaning and purpose of the agreement, a further assurance clause requires the party or parties to execute and deliver the document.

CLOSING: SETTLEMENT

The closing or settlement date should be chosen for a mutual time and place. Generally, the date will be between 30 and 90 days from the execution of the agreement. This will allow the buyer and the seller adequate time to complete any conditions precedent to closing. At closing, the buyer will tender to the seller the agreed-upon funds and will execute any loan and security agreements required under the purchase and sale agreement. If the restrictive covenant also contains a buyer's covenant, then the buyer will execute that document. The seller will deliver to the buyer a bill of sale for the assets of the practice, will execute the restrictive covenant, will deliver the keys to the practice, and will surrender the assets and the premises to the buyer. Both the buyer and the seller will execute the lease assignment.

Many of the provisions of the agreement will survive the closing. This includes any agreement to prorate expenses not allocated in at the closing, the restrictive covenant agreement, the indemnifications, and any seller's right maintained in the medical records.

TRANSITION

Both the seller and the buyer have certain interests to protect after the closing that would require the seller to stay with the practice for a period of time following the closing. The seller may have ongoing treatment plans with certain patients (such as postoperative follow-up treatment). The agreement should specify that the seller must be allowed to continue at the practice location for the purpose of finishing such treatment plans. Although the buyer may be fully capable of completing such treatment plans, both the buyer and seller should be cognizant that the patient may claim abandonment. Allowing the seller to complete treatment plans in progress will mitigate against any perceived or actual claims of abandonment.

The buyer will want to require the seller to stay with the practice for a certain period of time, usually between 3 and 6 months. During that time, the seller will act to introduce the buyer to the current patients and the buyer will begin treatment of any new patients to the practice. In this way, the transition will appear smooth and natural to the current patients.

Of course, during the transition period, the seller will have the right to be paid by the buyer. To avoid misunderstanding, the method of payment should be reduced to writing. Usually, the rate of compensation will be the profit margin percentage of the practice allocated to all income collected from the seller's efforts during the time period in question. An astute negotiator might be able to require the seller to function during the transition period as an implicit condition for the payment of the practice price.

RESTRICTIVE COVENANTS

As part of the purchase price, the buyer is paying for intangible assets of the practice. A medical practice is a highly individual-based business. The practice depends in large part on the reputation of the selling physician. For that reason, the buyer must ensure that the seller cannot use that highly individualized asset to compete against the practice for which she has just paid a high sum. The restrictive covenant protects this interest of the buyer.

A restrictive covenant actually contains several covenants to protect the buyer's interests. These include not only the obvious covenant not to compete, but also a covenant regarding financial interests, a covenant regarding solicitations, and a covenant regarding proprietary information.

The first is the covenant not to compete. In this covenant, the seller agrees not to compete with the practice in the geographic area during the time term of the agreement. This covenant prohibits the seller from actually practicing or from practicing indirectly. For example, the seller could not set up a clinic within the geographic area during the time period and employ a nurse practitioner to treat patients under his medical license.

The next covenant would be the covenant regarding financial interests. In this, the seller is prohibited from investing in a competing business (i.e., medical practice), within the geographic area during the time period. This provision prevents the seller from investing in such a medical practice, even if he does not directly treat patients at that location.

The third would be the covenant regarding solicitation. In this covenant, the seller agrees not only to refrain from contacting patients of the practice during the time period, but also to refrain from contacting employees of the practice. If the seller maintains another office location that will not be sold, then the seller should ensure that the agreement provides that the seller is allowed to treat patients who find themselves to that practice location. Otherwise, the seller may be liable for patient abandonment and may also violate managed-care contracts.

A final covenant would be a covenant regarding proprietary information. Simply by the fact of operating the practice, the seller has obtained certain proprietary information about the practice. This includes patient lists, accounting information, managed care contracts, and forms and handbooks. The seller should be prohibited from using such knowledge to the detriment of the practice.

TIME AND DISTANCE

The time and distance covered by the restrictive covenants must be reasonable. If either the time or distance is unreasonable, then a court might strike down the entire restrictive covenant.

A reasonable time is usually between 2 and 5 years. A 2-year time period should be the minimum that the buyer should insist upon. The purpose of the time period is to allow sufficient time for the practice patients to consider the buyer as their "doctor" and to lose confidence in the selling doctor. For that reason, any time period over 5 years is likely to be considered as an unreasonable restraint.

On the other hand, a reasonable distance depends on many individual factors. A reasonable distance in an urban area such as New York City would most likely be completely unreasonable in rural areas, such as rural Iowa. In most metropolitan areas, a 5–10-mile radius from the practice location is likely to be considered reasonable. In rural areas, an entire county or even several contiguous counties may be considered reasonable. The main determination of the reasonableness of the distance factor is the total area from which the practice draws its patients.

Most practice management software programs allow for delineation of the practice patient base determined by zip code. That will provide the parties a starting point from which to negotiate the distance factor of the restrictive covenant.

BUYER'S COVENANTS

The restrictive covenant should also contain buyer's covenants, although it may seem counterintuitive that the buyer, having paid the seller tens of thousands of dollars for the practice, should be required to sign the buyer's covenants. However, a buyer's covenant is an important part of the restrictive covenant. Under the purchase agreement, the seller might retain the right to repossess the practice, the practice assets, and the premises. This is most likely to happen when the seller finances the purchase price and the buyer defaults on the payments. It can also happen when the seller assigns the lease to the buyer and the buyer either abandons the premises or otherwise causes a default under the lease. The seller then remains liable as a principle under the lease.

For these reasons, the restrictive covenant should provide that if the seller is required to enter onto the premises and take possession of the practice, then the seller is relieved of his obligations under the restrictive covenants and the buyer now becomes bound by those same obligations. Such buyer's covenants will prevent the buyer from abandoning the practice and then setting up a nearby competing practice.

CORPORATE RESOLUTION

Most of the medical practices being sold are corporate entities. If the transaction is a sale for stock, then the transaction is between private parties—the buyer paying cash and the seller transferring the stock.

However, in these cases where the buyer is purchasing the assets of the corporate practice, then the corporation must take certain prerequisite steps. Generally, a corporation, through its officers and directors, is prohibited from selling significant assets without permission of the shareholders.

For that reason, a shareholder meeting must be held and the shareholders at that meeting must approve a resolution allowing the officers and directors to sell significant assets of the corporation.

ASSESSMENT

The contract regarding the sale of a medical practice is the final agreement of the parties. Such a contract should only be executed after sufficient investigation into the practice and upon consultation with proficient professionals, including attorneys, accountants, FAs, and practice management consultants. Understanding the basic terms and conditions of a contract regarding the sale of a medical practice is the first step in successfully negotiating the best agreement possible. Before one can negotiate for a certain provision, one must first be aware of the possibility of such a provision and its possible ramifications.

So, what else can FAs and consultants do to help plan properly for the sale of a medical practice, physician succession planning, and this major life liquidity event? Some experienced FAs suggest constructing a "dry run template analysis" so that the doctor can envision what life will be like after the sale, and what their corresponding financial needs might be. When the practice is sold, life is very different because many expenses that the practice paid become expenses the doctor now must pay. And so, the use of an astute FA, practice valuation specialist, and health-care contract attorney is highly advised.

CONCLUSION

As we have seen, the purchase price of a medical practice, although an important part of any sale, should only be considered as one element of the negotiations. There are many clauses and provisions of a contract regarding the sale of the medical practice, which if not negotiated favorably, should be considered as factors to initiate the party to walk away from the sale.

COLLABORATE

Discuss this chapter online with others at www.MedicalExecutivePost.com.

FURTHER READING

Boundy, C: *Business Contracts Handbook*. Gower Publication, New York, 2010.

Fenton, CF: *Contracts regarding the Sales of a Medical Practice. Financial Planning for Physicians and Healthcare Professionals*. Aspen Publishers, New York, 2003.

Hekman, K: *Buying, Selling and Merging a Medical Practice*. Keneth Hekman, New York, 2008.

Katz, D: Psychic income, Financial Advisor, p. 36, 2014.

Schatzki, M: *Negotiation Speak: Winning Words and Phrases for Sales, Purchasing, Contract and Other Business Negotiations—All the Dialogue and Skills You Need to Come Out Ahead*. Dynamic Negotiations, Chicago, IL, 2009.

UCC, Commercial Contracts and Business Law Blog: LexisNexis, 2010.

Walker, L: The ultimate transition. *Financial Advisor*, p. 33, 2014.

23 Techniques of Estate Planning
Avoiding End-of-Life Government Confiscation

Lawrence E. Howes and Stephen P. Weatherby

CONTENTS

Estate planning is an ongoing process and it should be considered a vital part of every medical professional's overall financial plan. Your estate is the total value of everything you own: your home and everything in it, the car, minivan, diamond brooch, wine collection, portfolio of mutual funds, other investments, retirement plans, medical practice, ownership in a family business, vacation homes, furniture, and clothing. It all adds up very quickly, especially when you consider any positive effect that the stock market may have had on your investments and the escalation in the price of homes in many parts of the United States.

All too often, estate planning decisions are routinely made for you, without your knowledge. For example,

1. When you buy a house, the title agent or closing attorney may assume that you want the house titled as joint tenants with your spouse.
2. Your investment account is opened and it is titled in joint tenancy.
3. Your life insurance agent names your spouse as primary beneficiary and your minor children as contingent beneficiary.
4. You don't take the time to draft a will, so by default the state you live in has prepared one for you.
5. Your medical practice agreement doesn't address death or disability.
6. Your ex-spouse is still the beneficiary of your IRA and 401(k) plan.
7. Your parents are still the beneficiaries of your life insurance.

Regardless of your current planning, let someone know the whereabouts of your existing estate planning documents and the names of your advisors. Some medical professionals keep these critically important wishes a secret, which adds a frustrating search process to an already sad and disruptive time in the lives of loved ones.

Estate planning is probably the last bastion for the sincere procrastinator. As a medical professional, you are likely so busy pursuing your career that you think that you do not have time to plan. Perhaps the current state of flux in health care keeps you too unsettled to think about long-term planning. Maybe a fear of family conflicts, unresolved issues, or believing it will be too expensive to develop a proper estate plan keeps you from acting.

There are three common impediments to estate planning:

1. Having to contemplate the consequences of one's own death
2. A lack of understanding of the terms that advisors often use
3. Having to think through the allocation of money between providing a family legacy or funding a charitable cause

This chapter will educate you on how to avoid common estate planning errors and guide you through key elements that should be part of your thinking and ultimately included in your estate plan.

No one can predict what future laws will look like. The best we can do is plan based upon current law. If there is pending legislation, then it behooves you to evaluate the potential impact of any changes. In 2010, Congress passed a new estate tax bill that imposes a federal estate tax only on estates valued at more than $5 million, indexed for inflation. At the beginning of 2013, Congress removed the expiration date from this estate tax starting point, but it could always change the rules, so you have to stay flexible. A more detailed explanation of the federal estate tax and several examples are found later in this chapter.

ESTATE PLANNING OVERVIEW

Planning for the disposition of worldly possessions begins with the wishes of the individual. Although estate planning is a team process, the individual must have a clear objective or the final result will be confusion.

The four primary goals to consider are

1. To maintain financial independence during your lifetime
2. To reduce costs and not delay settling the estate
3. To minimize estate taxes
4. To maximize the inheritance to chosen beneficiaries

The entire estate planning team can consist of a lawyer, accountant, life insurance agent, trust officer, and financial planner. Each of the team members has a specific focus that is usually predicated on how they are compensated. The lawyer wants to draft your documents, the accountant wants to run the numbers, the life insurance agent wants to sell insurance, and the trust officer wants the money from your estate to fund the trusts. The financial planner should make sure that your estate planning goals and objectives are achieved by coordinating the efforts of the other team members.

The first step is to pull together all the information about yourself and your family. Create a balance sheet or a net worth statement. Make copies of all your existing wills, trusts, powers of attorney, durable power of attorney for health care (DPOAHC), and business agreements. When were they last reviewed? Do they still name the correct people in the correct jobs? Is the guardian for your children still your first choice? Does the guardian know of his or her responsibilities and your wishes for the future of your children? Have your children grown up making guardians unnecessary?

What about your life insurance? Has your agent checked the ownership or beneficiaries recently? Is the amount of insurance still correct? Are you able to keep any financial promises that you have made?

At this point, thoroughly review your current estate plan and see if it still adequately represents your goals and objectives. Remember that a good estate plan is an ongoing process with stages of implementation, and careful review at least every 5 years.

Meeting with Advisors

Make an appointment with a financial advisor to help you organize all your financial information and work through your goals and objectives. Once you have a plan in mind, then meet with an attorney to get documents drafted, talk with your life insurance agent, and if needed, meet with a trust officer if you are drafting a trust with a corporate trustee. Meet with all other relevant advisors.

Finalizing the Estate Plan

Make sure all your assets are retitled appropriately, and that your retirement plan and life insurance beneficiaries are coordinated with your new estate plan. The next step is to sign the documents.

CHOOSING A PERSONAL REPRESENTATIVE

Your executor or personal representative is named in your will and is responsible for management of assets subject to probate. A basic checklist of the duties of the personal representative looks like this:

1. Gather all estate assets
2. Collect all amounts owed to the decedent
3. Notify creditors and pay all valid debts
4. Sell assets as needed to pay expenses or as directed by the will
5. Distribute assets to beneficiaries
6. File decedents final federal income tax return
7. File an estate tax return if the estate is large enough
8. File inventories and annual returns with the probate court, if required

The position requires a lot of responsibility and involves many duties and a considerable commitment of time. The personal representative must petition the probate court for formal appointment.

Selection of your personal representative should not be made lightly, or as a favor to a friend. It requires a lot of work and very often for little or no pay. Friends and family typically will not charge the estate for their time and work. Outside advisors like attorneys and accountants will not hesitate to bill for their work effort. A few items for your selection criteria should be

1. Longevity—the person should have a likelihood of being able to serve after your death
2. Skill in managing legal and financial affairs
3. Familiarity with your estate and wishes
4. Integrity and loyalty
5. Impartiality and absence of conflicts of interest

Alternatives to family or friends might be a corporate executor, such as a bank, an attorney, or other advisor. Similar criteria should be used in the selection of a trustee.

PROBATE

The motivating issue and primary purpose of estate planning is to assure the proper transfer of property to desired heirs with a minimum of expenses and taxation. The process of transferring property owned by an individual who has died is called probate. Probate, meaning "to prove," is the legal process of a court-supervised property transfer whose disposition is guided by either your will, or if you do not have a will, by the state laws of intestacy. Other property or nonprobate assets include property held in trust, in joint tenancy, most life insurance policies (because they have a named beneficiary), and most retirement plan assets again because of a named beneficiary. All property is subject to estate taxation— whether or not it goes through probate. Avoiding probate does not mean you can also avoid estate taxes.

Probate avoidance is the subject of numerous seminars across the country. These programs rely mainly on people's fears of the unknown. In actuality, many states have adopted all, or part, of the Uniform Probate Code (UPC). The UPC provides for a streamlined probate process and in most situations, residents of these states have little to fear when it comes to probate. However, the probate process is a public process. Anyone can go to the court and look up the will of a decedent and delve into their personal life and bequests.

An estate is usually probated, distributed, and taxed under the laws of the state in which you are domiciled. A majority of states, mostly those in the Southern and Western halves of the nation, have no additional death taxes beyond what the federal estate tax would be. Changing your residence to one of these states may avoid significant death taxes at the state level.

You can do several things to establish domicile in a particular state. Examples involve voter registration, automobile registration, driver's license, safe-deposit boxes, and having a principal residence there. Owning property in more than one state may cause multiple taxation by multiple states claiming jurisdiction, if you are not careful. Determine the requirements for each state and take a definitive position on where you wish your property to be taxed and probated. This needs to be included specifically in your estate planning documents.

NONPROBATE ASSETS

There are situations where avoiding probate is desirable especially for those who want a lot of privacy for their finances after their death. There are relatively simple ways to avoid probate, but they all have consequences.

JOINT TENANCY

Joint tenancy is the most common way that property between spouses is titled. Each spouse maintains a 50% undivided interest in the property. For bank accounts, it is simple, usually requiring only the check of a box on an application or loan form. For real estate, however, joint tenancy often needs to be written into the deed. Upon death, joint tenancy property automatically, by operation of law, passes to the surviving spouse and avoids probate.

The automatic aspect of joint tenancy means that a will does not control the disposition of the asset. Before you title anything, think about the consequences. There may be situations where you have an asset, for example a brokerage account that you would like to leave to a charity. If you have titled the account as joint tenants with your spouse, the brokerage account will go automatically to your spouse, and not to the charity as was intended. If a joint bank account is created between spouses, then each spouse owns one half of the account. If the account is established with a non-spouse, different rules apply. Be careful when establishing the ownership of all property.

COMMUNITY PROPERTY

Community property is another form of coownership limited to the interests held between husband and wife. Community property does not automatically pass to your spouse. When one spouse dies, the survivor continues to own only his or her half of the assets. The decedent's will determines the transfer of the other half. Only eight of the 50 states are community property states, but it is estimated that 25% of the population resides in these states. The eight states are Arizona, California, Idaho, Louisiana, Nevada, New Mexico, Texas, and Washington. Wisconsin has a form of community property called marital partnership property. It is similar but as in all states, the specifics vary. While not a community property state, Alaska does allow couples to opt into a community property arrangement; property is separate property unless both parties agree to make it community property through a community property agreement or a community property trust. The territory of Puerto Rico allows property to be owned as community property as do several Native American jurisdictions. In the case of Puerto Rico, the island had been under community property law since its inception to the Spanish Crown upon its discovery in 1493. The laws of the particular state must be examined to determine the effect on the married couple's property.

LIFE INSURANCE

Life insurance is also property. The two aspects of the property are the face amount and unless it is a term life insurance policy, the cash value. The critical item to remember is: if you own the policy, then the face amount or death benefit is included in your estate and probably subject to estate taxes. The death benefit passes through the operation of a beneficiary designation. At the time of death, most cash value policies include the existing cash value in the death benefit. This is known as a type A policy. Type B excludes the cash value from the death benefit so it would be added to the face amount.

RETIREMENT PLANS

Your retirement plans and IRAs are transferred by beneficiary designation. It is common to see a client who is divorced still have an ex-spouse as the named beneficiary on a retirement plan or life insurance policy. Making sure that all beneficiary designations are consistent with your current estate plan will avoid these unintended consequences.

REVOCABLE LIVING TRUST

A revocable living trust is another legal arrangement that gets a lot of attention. Here, your assets are voluntarily placed in a trust, thereby making you a *trustor*. The control of the assets in the trust is then transferred to a *trustee*. You can make yourself the trustee as well. The key word here is revocable, which means the terms of the trust can be changed, altered, amended, or terminated. Legal title to the property however is retained by the trust.

The trust document specifies what happens to the property upon death of the trustor and hence property transfer occurs by operation of law. An interesting aspect of this trust is its ability to handle property upon disability or incompetence. Many single medical professionals who do not have relatives to manage their financial affairs or prefer not to use relatives could benefit from their assets being placed in a revocable living trust. The trust can provide continuity of investment management, bill paying, collection of accounts receivable, and general financial stability until the medical professional is able to resume control of his or her financial affairs. In addition, if property is owned in more than one state, ownership of that property by a revocable living trust would eliminate the necessity of dealing with probate in several states.

BUY–SELL AGREEMENTS

All of your business agreements, which dictate what happens to property, should be addressed in what is called a buy–sell agreement. This agreement stipulates what would happen to your practice should you die, become disabled, leave, or wish to retire. The agreement states that your partner or partners will buy your interest upon your death and stipulates that your estate will sell your interest. It is a binding agreement to both parties. The agreement will have a valuation method, which might be a stated fixed price, or a formula. If a fixed price is selected, then a procedure should be in place to assure at least an annual revaluation of the practice. Formulas provide a better ongoing representation of the value of the practice. However, the dynamic healthcare environment might warrant a review of the validity of your existing formula. If the practice is valued highly, having sufficient cash to buy out a deceased partner might be difficult and possibly an overwhelming financial burden. Life insurance is commonly considered the best vehicle to provide the cash when it is needed the most.

DOCUMENTS OF PROPERTY TRANSFER

WILLS

The will is a legally enforceable document that expresses directions for disposing of your probate property at death. In most states, any individual 18 or older who is of sound mind may draw up a will.

One of the most important aspects of a will, for those of you who have minor children, is the nomination of a guardian for your children and a trustee for your money in the event of death. For a married couple the surviving parent would become the guardian; however, in the case of a common accident, a guardian and trust would be beneficial. A divorced parent must consider that their ex-spouse would be the natural guardian. Special concerns should be addressed if there are reasons the ex-spouse would not be a suitable guardian. If you are a widowed parent, special considerations should be made when addressing the nomination of a guardian. The word "nomination" is important, as the selection of a guardian is only a recommendation to the court. Selection of a guardian is extremely important, as it is your intention that this person would be responsible for raising your children. The guardian is generally used when both parents are deceased. Prior to including this person or persons in your will, you should discuss your expectations and desires and make sure the person is willing to take on what could be a tremendous responsibility.

Divorced couples still retain their natural rights as parents independent of who was the custodial parent. If a divorced spouse is, in the other parent's estimation, not suitable to being a parent, then these issues must be addressed in the guardian section of the will.

Wills are regularly contested if someone is unhappy. Normally, a will contest occurs when an expectant heir believes they were not treated properly under the terms of the will. Many lawyers now draft a "no contest clause," which simply states, "I have only provided for the persons set forth in this will."

TRUSTS

A very commonly used planning tool is a trust. They come in numerous types with countless different purposes. There are three parties to a trust:

1. The trustor (the person putting the property into the trust)
2. The trustee (the person in charge of managing the trust according to its terms)
3. The beneficiary (the person(s) entitled to the enjoyment or ultimate disposition of the trust property)

The beneficiary or beneficiaries might be entitled to receive money now or upon certain events like the attainment of a specific age. A trust usually contains two different legal types of property: *principal* and *income*. The principal of a trust is its invested wealth, and its size will fluctuate based upon the performance of the investments and any withdrawals made from it. Income, on the other hand, is money derived from the use of the principal, for example, dividends, rents, and interest.

Many trust documents are written to provide the beneficiary with income only during their lifetime. Hence, only income from the trust investments may be distributed to the beneficiary with the intent that the principal will remain intact and be available to the remainderman or ultimate beneficiary when the income beneficiary dies.

Modern investment theory takes a different approach. Instead of the trust investing for the separate components of principal and income, many trusts are invested to seek total return. This is portfolio appreciation without regard for the difference between principal and income. For example, a stock that appreciates 10% (additional principal) yet pays no dividend (no income) still provides a successful investment result to the trust in the form of additional capital. In this case, the trustee can sell some of the shares of the appreciated stock to provide income to the beneficiary. Here, a trust might provide a stated payout percentage like the greater of trust income or 4% of trust principal. Many lawyers have recognized that states are enacting this concept and have adjusted the drafting of their trusts.

Testamentary Trust

A testamentary trust can be established as part of your estate planning but does not become effective until you or your spouse dies. This vehicle is not subject to court supervision, but its terms become part of the public record because it is described in your will. It offers great flexibility and the terms can be tailored to meet your individual needs.

EXAMPLE 23.1

Dr. Cheung is married and has a child who is a minor. He has established a testamentary trust to receive assets upon his or his spouse's death. The asset that is funding this trust is simply a beneficiary designation on a life insurance policy, which names the "Testamentary Trust created under the last will and testament of Dr. Cheung." The trust provisions allow the trustee to spend money on behalf of the child for health, education, maintenance, and support (HEMS). Additional money will be spent on certain birthdays, such as 13, 18, and 21, and upon marriage. Ultimately, the balance in the trust funds will be distributed, when the child reaches age 25.

Marital Trust

You may leave property outright to your spouse or in a marital trust. A marital trust is established to receive all property and assets that you intend to go to your surviving spouse and puts some boundaries on who your spouse can leave the money to at his or her subsequent death. If the portion of the estate that will go to the surviving spouse is large, it is best left in trust. The trust provides a container for all assets and simplifies the management of those assets for the surviving spouse. If also named as trustee, the spouse has total control over the assets and may remove the assets from the trust, at any time. A variation on the marital trust, a qualified terminal interest property (QTIP) trust, allows assets to pass to a spouse only for the spouse's lifetime.

Incentive Trusts

These provisions in testamentary trusts are a way to transfer assets while trying to influence the behavior of the beneficiary(ies). They offer incentives to the beneficiary to achieve some predetermined goal, usually to seek achievements important to the decedent or other family members. For example, each heir shall receive $100,000 upon graduation from medical, business, law, or dental school or each heir shall receive an income distribution equal to three times the charitable contribution they make each year. The possibilities are endless and these provisions can be a very powerful incentive to maintain and fulfill cherished family behavior and values.

Irrevocable Life Insurance Trust

Life insurance has extreme leverage. By that we mean that a relatively small premium can produce a large asset at death. Avoiding inclusion of this large asset in your estate can be achieved by using an irrevocable life insurance trust (ILIT). This trust uses life insurance as its primary asset. Upon death, the insurance proceeds are paid into the trust and the money is then available to pay estate expenses, taxes, and ultimately distributed to the beneficiaries of the trust. If a cash value life insurance policy is used, the build-up of equity may be accessible by the trust beneficiaries for limited uses before death.

The important issue is to ensure that ownership of the trust never reverts to the insured because this would defeat the whole purpose of an ILIT. Life insurance policies also require ongoing premium payments. Hence, the ILIT needs cash, assets, or periodic contributions to enable it (through the trustee) to pay the premiums. Because this is an irrevocable trust, any contribution is removed from the donors' estate, and the contribution cannot be taken back. The contribution does not qualify for the $14,000 annual gift tax exclusion, because the intent of the $14,000 exclusion is for a current gift, called a gift of a *present interest*, that is, money or property that can be used immediately by the recipient. Any gift that is deemed to be a gift of a *future interest* or one that is accessible sometime in the future falls outside of the $14,000 annual exclusion ($28,000 per married couple). Therefore, when money is contributed to an ILIT the beneficiaries would have to wait until death before they could receive the money. That defines a gift of a future interest. Hence, a gift tax return would have to be filed with each contribution and a portion of your unified credit would be utilized.

About Clifford Crummey, DDS

Fortunately, this administrative nightmare was addressed by Dr. D. Clifford Crummey, DDS, who went to court to solve this problem. Under what is now termed the *Crummey trust* or *Crummey provision* each time money is contributed to the trust, the trustee writes a letter to the beneficiaries stating that money has been placed in the ILIT and they have 30–45 days to request, in writing, their money. As the beneficiaries at that time have access to the money, the contribution is deemed to be a gift of a current interest and qualifies for the $14,000 exclusion [*Crummey v. Commissioner* No. 21, 607 (9th Cir. 25 June 1968)].

Another way to remove a life insurance policy from your estate is to have another person own it. A life insurance policy is a piece of property, with an owner, a beneficiary, and a premium payer. Ownership means inclusion in your estate. Hence, it is preferable to have the owner be the ILIT as described above or, at least another individual. Naming a spouse as the owner at first glance seems simple and effective and avoids the expenses of setting up a trust. However, if your spouse is the owner and beneficiary of your policy, when you die, the policy is not included in your estate, but the proceeds are included in your spouse's estate. So naming the spouse accomplishes only one half of the goal of removing a life insurance policy from your combined estates. In this situation, if your spouse predeceases you, then any cash value of your life insurance policy will be included in his or her estate. Naming adult children as owners solves the inclusion of the proceeds in the combined estate, but if they are the beneficiaries, they do not have an obligation to use the proceeds for estate settlement costs. The use of an ILIT is normally the best solution to removing life insurance proceeds from your estate even though there is a cost to establish and maintain them.

You may have an existing life insurance policy that you would like to remove from your estate by transferring the ownership to your children or to an ILIT. If you die within 3 years of transferring ownership of a life insurance policy, the policy proceeds are brought back into your estate. It is normally best to apply for a new insurance policy when you are doing estate planning. This eliminates the concern over the 3-year rule. If you have a health condition that makes you uninsurable or life insurance underwriting establishes a premium that is not acceptable, then using a current policy may be the only alternative.

Note: President Obama's recently released budget proposal for 2015 requested a Crummey crackdown. The IRS is concerned that taxpayers could inappropriately exclude from gift tax a large total amount of contributions to the trusts. Under the proposed change, the present interest requirement would be replaced by a $50,000 annual cap on gift tax exclusions for transfers to trusts. Such a change might never be passed, or might be scaled back, but Crummey appears to be in the IRS crosshairs. For now, though, the Crummey rules remain in effect.

DISCLAIMERS

In some situations, an inheritance might complicate an estate and add to the estate tax burden. If there are sufficient assets and income to accomplish financial goals, more assets are not needed. A disclaimer may be useful. This is an unqualified refusal to accept a gift or inheritance, that is, when you "just say no." You have decided not to accept a sizable gift made under a will, trust, or other document. When you disclaim the property, certain requirements must be met:

- The disclaimer must be irrevocable
- The refusal must be in writing
- The refusal must be received within nine months
- You must not have accepted any interest in the property
- As a result of the refusal, the property will pass to someone else

The property passes under the terms of the decedents will, as if you had predeceased the decedent. If the filer of the disclaimer has control, the property will be included in the disclaimant's estate and can only be passed to another as a gift for as an inheritance. The intent of the disclaimer is to renounce and never take control of the property.

UNIFIED ESTATE AND GIFT TAXES

Over the years, the lifetime exemption from federal gift taxes has significantly increased while the gift tax rate has significantly decreased. Below is a chart that shows the changes in the lifetime gift tax exemption and top gift tax rate from 1997 through 2014.

Tax years 2010 through 2012 are based on the Tax Relief, Unemployment Insurance Reauthorization, and Job Creation Act ("TRUIRJCA" for short) that was signed into law by President Obama on December 17, 2010. While this law was only supposed to be in effect for 3 years, on January 2, 2013, President Obama signed the American Taxpayer Relief Act ("ATRA" for short) into law, which has made the rules governing federal estate taxes, gift taxes, and generation-skipping transfer taxes as enacted by TRUIRJCA permanent for 2013 and later years with one notable exception—the top estate tax, gift tax, and generation-skipping transfer tax rate is increased from 35% under TRUIRJCA to 40% under ATRA.

HISTORICAL AND FUTURE FEDERAL GIFT TAX EXEMPTIONS AND RATES

Year	Gift Tax Exemption	Top Gift Tax Rate
1997	$600,000	55%
1998	$625,000	55%
1999	$650,000	55%
2000	$675,000	55%
2001	$675,000	55%
2002	$1,000,000	50%
2003	$1,000,000	49%

Year	Gift Tax Exemption	Top Gift Tax Rate
2004	$1,000,000	48%
2005	$1,000,000	47%
2006	$1,000,000	46%
2007	$1,000,000	45%
2008	$1,000,000	45%
2009	$1,000,000	45%
2010	$1,000,000	35%
2011	$5,000,000	35%
2012	$5,120,000	35%
2013	$5,250,000	40%
2014	$5,340,000	40%

Calculation

Estate tax calculations are similar to income tax calculations in the methods used. First, we add up all of your estate assets to determine your total gross estate. Items included in assets are cash, CDs, money market funds, life insurance proceeds, stocks, bonds, mutual funds, retirement benefits and IRAs, personal property, real estate, vacation homes, jewelry, art, coins, stamp collections, business interests, and all receivables.

Deductions are taken for estate administration, funeral expenses, debts, mortgages, and credit cards. The assets minus the deductions yield the adjusted gross estate.

Another set of deductions is taken for charitable gifts and transfers to your spouse. The resulting figure is the *taxable estate* from which the final deduction is made for the unified credit.

EXAMPLE 23.2

Dr. Cheung decided to calculate the amount of his taxable estate in 2014, assuming he and his wife die in the same accident. He has a $1,000,000 life insurance policy on himself and a $750,000 life insurance policy on his spouse. Here is the chart he came up with:

Dr. Cheung made the following observations:

Federal Estate Tax Calculation

GROSS ESTATE	$13,930,000
FUNERAL AND ADM*	$ 20,000
DEBTS AND TAXES*	$ 155,000
LOSSES	$____$0____
TOTAL DEDUCTIONS	$ 175,000
ADJUSTED GROSS ESTATE	$ 13,755,000
MARITAL DEDUCTION AT FIRST DEATH	$ 8,415,000[a]
EXEMPTION AMOUNT PLACED IN SPECIAL TRUST	$ 5,340,000
(PRESERVED EXEMPTION FOR SURVIVOR)	
CHARITABLE DEDUCTION	$0
TOTAL DEDUCTIONS AT FIRST DEATH	$ 13,755,000
REMAINING ADJUSTED GROSS ESTATE AT SECOND DEATH	$8,415,000[a]
EXEMPTION AMOUNT AT SECOND DEATH	$5,340,000
TAXABLE ESTATE	$3,075,000
ADJUSTED TAXABLE GIFTS	$ 0
TENTATIVE TAX BASE	$3,075,000
TENTATIVE TAX	$1,230,000
GIFT TAXES PAYABLE	$ 0
TAX PAYABLE BEFORE CREDITS	$1,230,000
NET FEDERAL ESTATE TAX	$1,230,000

* Property claimed under the marital deduction at the first death is counted toward the taxable estate at the second death.

1. Because the estate is taxed in the 40% bracket, each additional dollar added to the estate would lose 40 cents to taxes. Or alternatively, a dollar reduction in the estate saves 40 cents.
2. Any gifts to charity can save significant estate taxes.
3. The addition of the $1,750,000 in total life insurance proceeds included in the estate generated $630,000 in taxes. The heirs enjoyed only $1,120,000 of the policy proceeds.
4. Without the inclusion of the life insurance proceeds, the estate tax would have been reduced to $600,000.

Although the unified estate and gift tax rates are high, they only apply after the unified credit is deducted. Everyone is entitled to the unified credit. A tax credit is a dollar for dollar offset, which in the year 2014 is set at $2,081,800, which is the tax that is calculated on an estate worth $5,340,000, sometimes called the "exclusion amount." The credit applies only to property that is owned by the decedent at death. Hence, great attention must be paid to the correct titling and ownership of assets, especially within marriages.

Exclusion Amount

The exclusion amount is the amount of property that can be passed without taxation. In the year 2014, this amount is $5,340,000. Now that the estate tax exclusion is portable, a married couple can pass $10,680,000 free of estate taxes. This does require some effort as described later in the chapter because the surviving spouse must either claim the unused exclusion amount or use a Unified Credit Shelter Trust.

ESTATE LIQUIDITY PLANNING

It has been said that you need credit to live but cash to die. Unfortunately, in many cases this is so because cash may be needed quickly following a death to pay a variety of obligations that can be subdivided into three general categories:

- Last expenses. These include federal estate and income taxes along with state inheritance taxes, lawyers, accountants, appraisers, last illness, and funeral expenses. Federal estate taxes are due 9 months after the death of the taxpayer.
- Funds to allow the family to readjust their lives. The amount is determined by the nature of the family.
- Money for family needs. The money could be needed for upcoming college expenses or basic annual income requirements.

Determining the amount of cash needed for your estate requirements can be accomplished by a Certified Financial Planner (CFP)®, CPA, or life insurance agent.

The three major sources of cash for your estate are as follows:

1. Cash in checking or money market accounts, assets in brokerage accounts, certificates of deposit, and mutual funds
2. Life insurance proceeds not designated to individual beneficiaries
3. Loans

You may not want your heirs to have to sell real estate or other assets, perhaps at reduced prices because of the need to raise cash quickly. The sale of existing assets can provide some liquidity but frequently there are insufficient saleable assets to satisfy the total cash requirements of your estate. When there are cash shortages, the least expensive way to provide for the shortage may be with a life insurance policy.

Life insurance premiums are relatively small when compared to the potential benefits. A properly structured life insurance policy will never have you paying more in premiums than the death benefit. Hence, life insurance provides tremendous leverage and that is a small price to pay for a potentially large benefit when it is needed the most. With the increased exclusion amount, the need for life insurance on a long-term basis appears to be reduced. Estates that are subject to taxes should consider the purchase of term life insurance for liquidity purposes. With proper planning, the spouse with the lowest premium should be the one insured. If the law is amended and a more permanent need for life insurance arises, the term insurance may be converted.

Some medical professionals have been told that the beneficiary of a life insurance policy receives the proceeds tax-free. That means *income* tax-free, not *estate* tax-free. Without proper planning, your estate is automatically increased by the amount of insurance proceeds.

If you do not want to buy life insurance, then loans to pay the taxes may be an alternative. However, securing a loan for an estate may be difficult. Banks want to be repaid and because estate liquidity is the issue, the banking community is frequently an unwilling partner. Estate loans may come from potential beneficiaries and other family members. This is a technique of last resort.

Section 6161

The IRS has discretion under IRC § 6161 to grant an extension to any estate for up to 10 years to pay estate tax upon a showing of "reasonable cause." The IRS charges interest, but if the estate does not have the money to pay all the estate taxes when initially due, then § 6161 is a potential opportunity to reduce the immediate payment burden on the estate. Unfortunately, this extension does keep the estate open for the duration of the payment plan and will incur additional accounting and administrative costs.

Section 303 Redemption

A family business or medical practice may make up the majority of your estate. The business has a value, but very little cash. In recognition of the closely held business owner, the IRS allows stock in the company to be redeemed to pay federal and state death taxes, generation-skipping transfer taxes, and funeral and administration expenses. There are few tax deductible ways of getting money out of a corporation and salaries and business expenses head the list. The IRS maintains that if a business is at least 35% of your adjusted gross estate, the business owner can redeem stock to pay for approved expenses. Since you get a step-up in basis at death, the shares redeemed should not generate a capital gain. The transaction is deemed a sale of a capital asset, and not a dividend. (A dividend is not deductible so it is taxable to the corporation as well as taxed to you personally upon receipt.)

The strategy of a § 303 redemption is prudent. However, there must be cash available to redeem the stock. Typically, a life insurance policy is purchased to provide the cash for the redemption.

Section 6166

Another benefit the IRS allows on the death of a qualifying small business owner is estate tax deferral under Section 6166 of the tax code. This provides for the extension of the payment of estate taxes over a period of 14 years, but there are three levels of qualification. The first is the same as for § 303. The second adds a strict definition of a closely held business. The third requires that the business must have been actually engaged in carrying on a trade or business *at the time of death*. The first four annual payments are interest only and then the next 10 annual payments are principal and interest. One of the best attributes of Section 6166 is that the interest rate on the first $580,000 of deferred tax is set by statute at a fixed 2%. Calculating the tax that qualifies for the extension requires applying the percentage of the adjusted gross estate attributed to the small business, multiplied by the total federal estate tax.

Section 2032A Special Use Valuation

Suppose you own a farm that for many years was located well outside the city limits of a growing community and now the farm is in the path of this growth. The dynamics of determining the fair market value of your farm have changed. You might be inclined to value it as a farm and your estate would make the argument that it is a farm. The IRS would argue the property should be valued at its highest and best use. Unfortunately, for your estate, the "highest and best use" might be as a mega mall, apartment buildings, or a high-rise office building. All worth considerably more than the farm might be.

Valuation of a property at the highest and best use might force the survivors to sell the land to pay a large estate tax. On the other hand, valuation at its present use might enable the survivors to carry on the farm business. Section 2032A permits qualifying estates to value at least a portion of the real property at its "qualified use." This section applies to farms or other trades or businesses.

Five major requirements and conditions must be satisfied. Ultimately, the maximum amount by which the value of the special use real estate can be reduced is $1,090,000. While this is not an insignificant amount, if there is a large disparity between "highest and best use" and present use value, then planning to avoid the potential liquidity deficit is imperative.

FAMILY GIFTING AND LOANS

The annual gift tax exclusion allows you to give any individual $14,000 per year without paying or filing a gift tax return in 2014. There is no limit on the number of individuals who might benefit from your generosity. If you are married, then you and your spouse together may gift $28,000 to any number of individuals. The recipients do not owe any tax on the money either. Gifts in excess of $14,000 reduce your lifetime gift tax exemption of $5,340,000 (tied to the estate tax exclusion). You only have to send a check in with the gift tax return if your lifetime gifts are more than this amount, but the gift tax return must be filed by April 15 of the year following the gift. Gifts to qualified charities are subject to a different set of income tax rules discussed later.

Gifting assets to family members or others during your lifetime can be an effective estate planning technique. A gift of money or stock to your children automatically reduces your estate. If the combined *taxable estate* of you and your spouse exceeds $10,680,000, then your estate is in the 40% estate tax bracket. This means that each dollar you can remove from your estate, and allow to appreciate in your children's estate can help reduce a significant potential estate tax liability so long as your exemption is not used up while doing so. We must remember that tax laws are always subject to change. Gifting strategies may still be appropriate depending on your expectation of law changes and where the estate is large and life expectancy is limited. There are gifting traps in these situations, so consult proper counsel.

When you gift stock, you also give the recipient your cost basis. If you have low basis stock that you are thinking about selling but are concerned about paying up to 28% in capital gains tax, you could gift portions of the stock to your children (or anyone in the 15% income tax bracket) and sell just enough to qualify for 0% capital gains tax in their bracket. The gift value is the market price of the stock on date of gift. We are talking about an outright gift, so before you really do it make sure you can afford to give up the cash or the asset forever.

EXAMPLE 23.3

Dr. Jay Miller recently gave his son $4,340,000. He had an exemption equivalent amount of $5,340,000 in 2014. His gift reduced this by $4,340,000, leaving $1,000,000. (If you can't remember, your gift tax returns will be a formal reminder.)

EXAMPLE 23.4

Dr. Eva Gray has already given gifts in 2014 of $5,340,000, the maximum allowed under the exemption equivalent. She now wants to give an additional $100,000.

The tax table shows that the tax on this extra gift is $40,000 (40% tax rate). Conventional tax wisdom has always been to delay paying taxes whenever possible. However, Dr. Gray has taken a closer look at what will happen if she gives $100,000 of property that is likely to rapidly appreciate to her adult daughter.

Dr. Gray is in good health and believes her life expectancy to be at least 15 years. If the property were to appreciate at 9% per year for the next 15 years until 2029, $100,000 would grow to approximately $360,000. All of this appreciation is outside of Dr. Gray's estate if she makes the gift now.

If Dr. Gray kept the property then the $360,000 would be included in the estate and taxed at 40%.

This example shows the leverage available with a gifting strategy. If appropriate in your estate planning, paying taxes now could benefit your estate later. However, as mentioned above, this technique has limited applicability.

Uniform Transfer to Minors Act

The Uniform Transfer to Minors Act (UTMA) or Uniform Gift to Minors Act (UGMA) provides for an account established by a checkmark on most mutual fund applications and/or brokerage accounts. No trust documents have to be prepared. A uniform trust has been adopted by each state. A custodian, normally a parent or grandparent, is named as the party responsible for making investment decisions and distributing assets for the benefit of the child. The account is primarily used as a tool for accumulating assets to pay for a child's college education; however, money may be used for most any purpose that benefits the child, for example, reading classes, computer camp, ballet classes, and so on. Money gifted to an UTMA account qualifies under the annual gift tax exclusion.

This money is a gift to the child and depending upon state law, the child has control of it at age 18 or 21. The assets are removed from the donor's estate, unless the giver dies while still the custodian of the account. In that case, the assets are taxed at the giver's bracket until the child reaches age 14, at which time they are taxed directly to the child. Investments can be selected to minimize or eliminate taxation. For example, individual stocks with no dividend might provide the appreciation without generating a taxable event until the stock is sold after the child reaches age 14. Alternatively, low turnover, growth-oriented mutual funds, or tax-efficient mutual funds, offer account growth with little or no taxable distributions.

Section 529 Plans

Section 529 Plans are for college education funding. These plans allow assets to grow tax-free if the money is used to pay for qualified higher education expenses. These costs include tuition, room and board, books, and some miscellaneous expenses. There are penalties if the money is not used for qualified higher education expenses. Some states have what they call prepaid tuition plans and they vary dramatically from state to state. Contributions qualify for the $14,000 annual exclusion and the annual gift of $14,000 may be aggregated into one payment of $70,000. However, the right to use the $14,000 gift is eliminated for the subsequent 4 years. The maximum amount per beneficiary varies by state. The account may be structured so that the proceeds will be part of the child's estate versus the UTMA where the account is included in the custodian's estate. Some states permit contributions to be income tax deductible.

Medical Care and Tuition Payments

Medical care and tuition payments are either direct payments to a healthcare provider for the medical care of another person or direct payments of tuition to an educational institution for another person and are not transfers for gift tax purposes. For instance, your parents may pay all the college tuition for their grandchildren free of gift tax. This is limited to tuition, so room and board and other personal expenses are not included.

Intrafamily Loans

You may consider loaning money to your children or other family member. These are referred to as intrafamily loans. These must respect the formality of any business arrangement, with a signed promissory note, a market interest rate, and term and amortization schedule. Without documentation, the loan will more than likely turn out to be a gift. If a gift is your intention, make it a gift. The advantage of a loan is the ability to provide a favorable interest rate and repayment schedule. However, if you set the interest rate at zero or below the applicable federal rate, then you will be deemed to have made a gift. The forgone interest will be taxed to you as ordinary income. This consequence does not apply to loans of up to $10,000 for non-income-producing property or loans of up to $100,000 if the borrower's net investment income is less than $1000.

Sometimes parents or grandparents will invest only in bank savings accounts or CDs. Some of these investments are yielding 1–3%. Loaning this money to a family member, who would be willing to pay 4–6%, would benefit everyone involved. In addition, if the lender is wealthy and does not necessarily need the interest income, this can be a good strategy. If a loan is placed for $50,000 at 6% interest, the interest cost is $3000 per year. The family member/lender may elect to waive the interest each year, which constitutes a gift. Since the gift amount is less than the $14,000 annual exclusion, no gift tax return needs to be filed.

COMMON ESTATE PLANNING TECHNIQUES

By-Pass Trust

A By-Pass Trust is commonly referred to as a Unified Credit Shelter Trust, a Family Trust, or an A-B Marital Trust. All references are commonly used terminology in the estate planning profession, much like the medical profession has its own terminology.

A By-Pass Trust is established to receive property at death equal to the exclusion amount. Thus, the amount in the trust is carved out of your estate and does not go directly to your spouse but is still subject to estate taxes. However, the amount subject to taxes is offset by the unified credit and hence no tax is due. Under the new estate tax rules, the increased exclusion amount, currently $5,340,000, presents another planning issue. Smaller estates need to be careful, so that the majority of the estate doesn't end up in the credit shelter trust.

For example, a medical practitioner with a $6 million estate, dying in 2014 would have $5,340,000 allocated to the credit shelter trust, leaving only $660,000 outright to the surviving spouse. The surviving spouse may be surprised to find out that the majority of the estate is in trust and will be subject to withdrawal limitations. These trusts need to contain provisions to allow the spouse access to the money under what is called an "ascertainable standard." This standard permits money to be paid out for health, education, support, or maintenance.

This language has been approved by the IRS and should never be tampered with. If the trust document provides the spouse broader withdrawal power, the risk is that the assets in this trust could be included in the spouse's estate, which defeats the purpose of carving out the trust assets in the first place. Upon your spouse's death, the assets in the trust are paid to your beneficiaries, commonly the children. If the beneficiaries are minors, provisions are included for their well-being until ultimate distribution, similar to the terms indicated previously under the testamentary trust.

A powerful effect of the trust is the potential for appreciation in trust value. If, for example, the trust starts out at $5,340,000 and then 7 years later the spouse dies, the trust might have appreciated to $7 million or more and the appreciation is not subject to estate taxation. Drafting of trust language to allow for changing amounts and to accommodate different wording by Congress is important to avoid having to create new documents every time Congress decides to make changes. However, owing to the far-reaching effects of recent changes in the tax code, all estate plans and documents should be reviewed by estate planning lawyers.

Unlimited Marital Deduction

Under the unlimited marital deduction, virtually all transfers to a spouse, whether made during lifetime or at death, are tax-free. However, there may be a tax consequence for leaving your entire estate to your spouse. Leaving everything to your spouse does not utilize your exclusion amount, which is $5,340,000 in 2014. If your spouse is reasonably likely to die with a greater net worth than his or her own exclusion amount, then he or she will need to claim the unused exclusion by filing an estate tax return within 9 months after your death. Failing to claim the exclusion after the first death still means there is zero tax at that point, but when your spouse dies, the estate of the spouse may pay higher taxes.

EXAMPLE 23.5

Dr. Welch died in 2014 and left to his wife the entire estate, which amounted to $5,925,000. This approach qualifies for the unlimited marital deduction, so there is no estate tax due at his death.

However, if Mrs. Welch subsequently dies without claiming Dr. Welch's unused exclusion, her estate tax in the year 2014 would amount to $234,000. The simplified calculations are as follows:

Gross taxable estate	$5,925,000
Exclusion amount	(5,340,000)
Taxable estate	$585,000

From the tax tables, the tax on an estate of $585,000 is $234,000.

If Dr. Welch had created a credit shelter trust, his estate plan calculations would look like this:

Gross taxable estate	$5,925,000
By-Pass Trust	($5,340,000)
Unlimited marital deduction	($585,000)
Taxable estate	$0

At Mrs. Welch's subsequent death, calculations would be as follows:

Gross taxable estate	$585,000
Exclusion amount	($585,000)
Taxable estate	$0

Mrs. Welch would include in her estate the amount she received by the unlimited marital deduction. While alive, she would have reasonable access to the 5,340,000 that was allocated to this trust in the husband's estate, but it will not be included in her estate.

At an estate amount of $585,000, the new estate tax due is $0 with the net savings of this approach calculated as follows:

First tax calculated	$234,000
New tax calculated	$0
Savings with planning	$234,000

Subsequently, Congress passed the American Tax Relief Act of 2012 ("ATRA"), which President Obama signed on January 2, 2013.

One of the key provisions of ATRA is to make permanent the so-called portability of the applicable exclusion amount between spouses, which was enacted by TRUIRJCA of 2010.

Portability allows the first spouse to die to transfer his/her unused estate tax applicable exclusion amount to the surviving spouse, who can then use it for his/her gift or estate tax purposes.

More specifically, if the estate of the first spouse to die makes the appropriate portability election, the surviving spouse's applicable exclusion amount may be calculated as follows:

EXAMPLE 23.6

Dr. Welch dies in 2011 and his estate makes the portability election. Assume the "deceased spousal unused exclusion amount" or DSUE amount from Dr. Welch's estate is $4 million. In 2014, when the basic applicable exclusion amount equals $5.34 million, Mrs. Welch dies. Here, the applicable exclusion amount available to Mrs. Welch's estate equals $9.34 million, which is calculated as follows:

Mrs. Welch's basic applicable exclusion amount	$5,340,000
Aggregate deceased spousal unused exclusion amount	$4,000,000
Updated applicable exclusion amount	$9,340,000

Any applicable exclusion amount of the first spouse to die that is used to reduce the estate tax liability of that spouse's estate tax reduces the amount of the excess applicable exclusion amount that carries over to the surviving spouse in the form of DSUE amount.

Qualified Terminal Interest Property Trust

A QTIP trust was designed for those who have children from a prior marriage. The QTIP rules are complicated and deal with legal rights to assets and in whose estate the assets are titled. Suffice it to say that Congress has allowed a qualification to be put on the normal terminal interest rules to provide for this situation. The result provides assets that qualify for the unlimited marital deduction, but your spouse does not control where the assets go upon the spouse's death. The spouse is entitled to the income generated from the trust for life and is also entitled to the use of tangible property, such as the home and contents. In addition, these trusts provide the surviving spouse a limited power to access principal for health, education, maintenance, or support.

ADVANCED ESTATE PLANNING CONCEPTS

All of the following concepts provide family benefits in addition to potential estate tax savings. Structuring gifts to charity, transferring businesses to family members, and gifting large sums to children or grandchildren may still be part of a person's financial planning desires even if estate tax is no longer a concern.

Charitable Giving

Charitable giving or transfers to charity, whether lifetime or at death, are supported by several provisions of the Internal Revenue Code that usually allows generous deductions on a contributor's income tax, gift tax, and estate tax returns. Compelling as the tax benefits are, they do not offset the loss of wealth to the family. Considering charitable giving must be in conjunction with a sincere desire to support and provide for one or more charities with a true gift of the heart. Without this charitable intent, the best of strategies most likely will not have any appeal.

Selecting an asset to give to a charity may provide additional value for you. Most of you are familiar with the gift of cash. You write a check, the charity receives the money and you receive an income tax deduction. The money gifted to the charity is out of your estate and therefore will not grow and enhance the value of your estate. More importantly, the charity gets the current use of the cash.

In addition to cash, you may want to gift mutual fund shares or other assets that you deem appropriate. You could sell the stock or other assets, pay the capital gains, and give the charity the net cash. A better alternative is to gift the stock or other asset directly to the charity. You may actually deliver the stock certificate, or in today's electronic age, have the brokerage firm that holds the stock or fund deliver the shares directly to the charity's investment account. The value of your deduction is based upon the price of the stock the day it is delivered. There is no capital gains tax for the giver or the charity. Subsequently, the charity can sell the stock and receives the full value of the deductible gift.

Occasionally, we make investments that go down in value. In that case, it is best to sell the stock, realize the tax loss personally, and deliver cash to the charity.

Charitable Remainder Trust

You may have a greatly appreciated asset with a low cost basis. If you sold the asset, you would have to pay capital gains on the difference between your cost basis and the selling price. Under current law, this amounts to a 20% tax liability in the 39.6% tax bracket, with a few exceptions that could result in a 25% or 28% tax liability. You may want to be free of the asset anyway for various reasons: the medical company stock is paying low dividends, and the real estate is requiring extensive management and maintenance.

One common solution to this problem is a charitable remainder trust (CRT). Gifting low basis assets into a CRT accomplishes several goals.

- Capital gains are avoided on any subsequent sale.
- An income of 5–8% of the value of the asset can be generated. This percentage may be as high as 50%, but requires special planning.
- A current income tax deduction is received for the gift. Because you are also receiving income back from the trust until you die, a complicated calculation is necessary to determine the value of the tax deduction. In general, depending on your age or the term of the CRT, the deduction will be worth 25–50% of the value of the asset.
- After you and your spouse both die, you leave the value of the trust to your named charity or charities.

Net Income Charitable Trust

A net income charitable trust is a variation of the CRT. Upon establishing the trust, you determine a percentage of the asset value that will be paid out each year, just as you would do with a CRT. The trust may state that only income earned by the trust will be paid out. Trust expenses are deducted from the income before it is paid out. This technique allows you to contribute to a charitable trust and then have the trust invested in growth stocks (non-dividend-paying stocks). If there is no income, there will be no payout. The contribution, which can be a one-time payment or a series of payments over several years, will be partially tax-deductible. This creates a vehicle that can accumulate investments on a tax-deferred basis. Trading stock in the trust generates capital gains that pass through to you in the form of a K-1.

When you are ready to receive income, you change the investments to start generating an income. Every year that the trust did not pay out the percentage you originally chose, it owes it to you. Based upon trust accounting rules, part of the payout to you will be taxed at capital gains rates. Upon your retirement, the trust would likely owe a large payout, and if the trust earns the income, it can pay it to you.

If you are looking for a way to set aside additional money for retirement and have maximized your qualified plans, this approach has merit. The downside is when you die the assets go to your favorite charity rather than your family. If you begin making contributions and never get to the point of taking an income from the trust, the entire value of the charitable trust goes to the charitable beneficiary when you die.

Charitable Lead Trust

A charitable lead trust is a technique that allows you to provide a charity or charities current income (the lead), and at the end of a designated period, the money in the trust passes to designated family members. This is an excellent family wealth transfer technique, while providing an immediate benefit to designated charities. Any appreciation in trust assets passes to the family free of gift or estate taxes. As a result of the current low interest rate environment, this trust can be especially attractive because lower interest rates cause the gift or estate tax deduction to increase and cause the transfer tax value of the gift of the family interest to decrease.

INTRAFAMILY SALES

Family limited partnerships (FLPs) have become a popular planning tool for almost any business that is family owned and operated. This structure provides numerous advantages, including the following:

1. Parents can give away wealth and still retain control.
2. Transfers can be made at substantial discounts as compared to the value of underlying assets, thus saving unified credit and gift taxes.
3. Restrictions can be placed on transfers by children.
4. There is some protection from creditors.

To establish an FLP, you must follow the requirements of your state's limited partnership act. The Uniform Limited Partnership Act requires that there be at least one general partner and one limited partner. The general partner retains all management control over the business or property, while the limited partner retains only an ownership interest. The limited partner has no voting power or authority over decision making. In addition, the limited partner cannot take assets from the partnership or otherwise force liquidation of the partnership before the term is up.

EXAMPLE 23.7

Dr. Savely and his spouse have a medical office building valued at $30,000,000. He establishes an FLP with the limited partnership representing 95% of the total value of the building and the other 5% being allocated to the general partnership interest. The limited partnership portion will be divided into 95 limited partnership units. Dr. Savely and his wife plan to transfer 20 units to each of their three children. Each unit represents 1% of the total building. At full value, 20% of $30,000,000 equals $6,000,000. Without the FLP, Dr. Savely would be giving a $6,000,000 gift to each child and paying the associated gift taxes.

However, owing to the structure of the FLP, your children are limited partners. They would not control the assets they own. In addition, each child will have only a minority interest in the building. The IRS allows a valuation discount due to the minority ownership. That is, the children have an undivided interest in real property, which is neither easily partitioned nor readily marketable. In addition, their interest is noncontrolling.

Giving up control over property is normally the biggest roadblock to an aggressive and substantial gifting strategy but this is less of an issue with an FLP. The FLP is also advantageous in getting children involved in the business entity. Once they have a beneficial interest in the business, they should take a greater interest and role in how it works. Annual partnership meetings with all family members should be established on a formal basis. Financial reports and a discussion about why the business performed well or poorly should be included. This can be a good opportunity for a family retreat.

Income generated by the FLP must be distributed equally by partnership ownership. This can be a unique opportunity to shift income from the enterprise to your children's lower tax bracket. The adult might be in the 39.6% bracket while your children might be in the 15% bracket. Children under 19, or 24 if full-time student, will be subject to the "kiddie tax" for annual unearned income over $1000 (the 2014 amount), which is taxed at the adult rate.

Additional concerns arise in today's society where divorce is commonplace. Language should be included in the FLP to identify a child's limited partnership interest as separate property and not subject to divorce. It would seem unlikely that the family would want to stay in business with a child's former spouse.

Gifts of partnership interests retain the cost basis. This is one of the disadvantages of gifting assets to your children. If the children were to sell an asset, then a potentially large capital gains tax would be incurred. Alternatively, if your children received the property at the parent's death, they would receive a step-up in basis. That means their cost basis would be the value of the property on the date they received it. Of course, if the children have no intention of ever selling the property, the low cost basis is a small price to pay to avoid a large estate tax payment.

FLPs also provide limited asset protection as long as the transfer was not a fraudulent transfer. By definition, that means you did not transfer assets to an FLP to avoid a malpractice suit. It is also true that limited partnership units given several years before any financial difficulty should not be subject to attachment by creditors.

Costs to set up an FLP consist mainly of attorney's fees to draft documents that establish the partnership. These range between $4000 and $15,000 depending on the nature of the business assets. The appraisal fees to establish the asset value and appropriate discounts may range from $5000 to $20,000. In addition, there will be annual accounting fees for preparation of the partnership returns and K-1s that must be distributed to all partners. In most cases, a large gift is made when the FLP is established. Future gifting of limited partnership shares will require an updated appraisal to establish property value and applicable valuation discounts.

DONOR-ADVISED FUNDS

There are a variety of charitable organizations, mutual funds, and custodians such as Charles Schwab and Fidelity that offer donor-advised funds. A gift to a donor-advised fund is a gift for estate planning purposes that offers special opportunities for the donor to retain control over the money. The control is exercised by choosing which charity the funds are distributed to over time without any permanent commitments.

EXAMPLE 23.8

Dr. Shela Brinker donates $50,000 to a donor-advised fund. She takes a current year charitable income-tax deduction based upon the $50,000 gift in the year the gift is made. The donor-advised fund invests the money aggressively to grow for the future and Dr. Brinker selects a $5000 gift every year to a different charity. Her one-time gift is spread to many worthy causes and gives her the opportunity to reevaluate her bequeath every year. With good investment results, the original gift will ultimately supply much more money and be spread much further than the initial lump sum. For example, if $50,000 were invested and Dr. Brinker waited 5 years prior to beginning her charitable giving, the amount that could be gifted, with a 6% annualized return, would be approximately $67,442.

LIMITED LIABILITY COMPANY

This device is more flexible than the S Corporation, which it is designed to replace. A limited liability company (LLC) offers business owners the limited liability of a corporation with the pass-through tax advantages of a partnership. Each owner-investor is called a member and an ownership share is called a member interest. Creating an LLC requires compliance with state statute and avoidance of certain characteristics that the federal government looks for to try to tax the entity as a corporation. Proper legal advice will ensure pass-through taxation. LLCs also do not have the restrictions on stock ownership that S corporations have. S corporations are limited to one class of stock, whereas LLCs can have membership interests with different rights such as income, capital preferences, or voting. Trusts, foreign individuals, and other corporations can be members. Usually, LLCs are closely held. However, there is no restriction on the number of owners. Federal law limits the number of S Corporation shareholders to 75.

GENERATION-SKIPPING TRANSFER TAX

When strategies are put in place that are deemed as tax avoidance, Congress acts to close the loopholes. One of these loopholes existed for more than 50 years. Prior to 1986 (laws were enacted in 1976, but repealed retroactively), it was possible to pass property to any generation with only one layer of gift or estate tax. If you wanted to leave or give property to your grandchildren or great-grandchildren, that was fine. Members of Congress finally were bothered by this because with property passing down several generations, it could take 80 or even 100 years before that property would again be subject to estate taxes. So, in 1986 the Generation-Skipping Transfer Tax (GSTT) was enacted to make up for the lost tax revenue when wealth is transferred and skips a generation.

The GSTT is assessed on amounts in excess of $5,340,000. The tax is in addition to normal taxes and is equal to the maximum federal estate tax rate in effect at the time of the gift. Currently, the maximum tax rate is 40%. The example below is a simplistic representation of how the GSTT tax is calculated. This is a very complicated area and the fact situation may greatly affect the actual calculation.

EXAMPLE 23.9

In 2003, Dr. Skye gave $5,600,000 to her grandchildren in a generation-skipping trust. The taxes were calculated as follows:

Gift	$5,600,000
Exclusion	5,340,000
Taxable gift	260,000

Taxes on 260,000 = $104,000 (40% tax bracket)

Generation-skipping transfers do not always need to be along bloodlines. Congress created a methodology for those who may wish to gift or bequest money to a younger person, but not necessarily related person. If the person or persons receiving the gift are more than 37.5 years younger than the giver, the GSTT applies.

PRIVATE ANNUITIES

Private annuities are an interesting version of the more familiar commercial annuities purchased from an insurance company. The difference is that in private annuities, the parties involved are usually family members. An asset is sold to a family member in exchange for an unsecured promise to provide a life annuity (income) to the seller. A life annuity is a predetermined annual income, which is paid for the lifetime of the recipient. Under a private annuity arrangement the tax code has tables that determine the annual payment. This could be paid monthly. The giver's age and the current interest rate environment determine the payment. The federal government publishes various interest rates that are used for calculations and planning purposes.

EXAMPLE 23.10

Dr. McCourt has shares in IBM worth $100,000 with a cost basis of $20,000. He plans to transfer the shares to his son, which will achieve an estate freeze on this asset. The payout is determined by the date he enters into the private annuity arrangement. All future appreciation occurs in the son's estate. Dr. McCourt is 65 years old. Assuming that annuity interest rates are 6%, he will receive $10,600 for life from his son. There is no gift taxation as long as, when the private annuity is established, Dr. McCourt has greater than 50% probability of living more than 1 year.

The use of a private annuity can be effective in transferring property when the seller is in poor health. There is no immediate income taxation upon creation of the annuity. However, as each payment is received, there is recognition of the gain. Taxation is under §72, which deals with annuity payments.

At Dr. McCourt's age, 65, life expectancy using the tables is 20 years. The annual taxation would break out this way:

$1000 is return of principal and income tax-free
$4000 is capital gain
$5600 is ordinary income
$10,600 total annual income

If Dr. McCourt lives longer than 20 years, then all payments are treated as ordinary income.

The annuity is for life-only, so, upon the death of Dr. McCourt no value of the IBM stock will be included in his estate. If he dies after 2 years, his estate would have received two $10,600 payments and his son would receive the balance tax-free.

Dr. McCourt's plan has three disadvantages:

1. There is no security and this lack of security might increase the risk that the son will not pay the required amount.
2. No part of the annuity payment is tax deductible for the son.
3. If Dr. McCourt lives a long time, his son made a bad deal.

INSTALLMENT SALE

An installment sale is an alternative to the private annuity. Here you sell property to a family member (or outsider) for an installment note in which your family member agrees to pay principal and interest based on a fair market rate. Recognition of the gain can be in the year of sale or spread out over the term of the sale. The major differences between the installment sale and private annuity are as follows:

1. The installment note has a security interest.
2. Upon death, the remaining unpaid balance of the installment note (calculated on a present value basis) is an asset of the estate and subject to estate taxes.
3. The sale of stocks and bonds does not qualify for installment reporting. Hence, the installment sale is best used for the sale of real estate or tangible personal property.

An estate freeze is accomplished, similar to that of the private annuity, as postsale appreciation will benefit the new owner.

SELF-CANCELING INSTALLMENT NOTES

Self-canceling installment notes (SCINs) are a provision that may be added to the installment note specifying that no further payments will be made after your death. Inclusion of this provision requires an adjustment to the structure of the installment note, in the form of a higher annual payment. The benefit of the SCIN provision is that the value of the note is not included in the estate, which is the big negative of the installment note sale. However, the balance of the gain is reflected on the estate income tax return. This technique is aggressive and has only limited appeal.

GRANTOR-RETAINED TRUSTS

The primary motive for planning with grantor-retained trusts is to freeze the value of appreciating property without creating a gift. A variety of rules must be followed carefully, but with a properly drafted document it can be an excellent planning technique.

Often, the home is used in grantor-retained trust planning because it has likely increased in value and might be a significant portion of an estate. In a qualified personal residence trust (QPRT), an owner removes a home from an estate, passes it and its future appreciation to the children, and still lives there. The trust agreement is drafted and the house is deeded to the trust. At that point, a gift has been made to the children. This is a gift of a *future interest* and does not qualify for the $14,000 annual exclusion. In fact, the calculation of the amount of the gift is complicated because the owner retains the right to live in the home and the children will not receive full rights to the home until sometime in the future. In effect, the gifted value of the house is the remaining value after the grantor has used it for a period of years.

This is not to be confused with appraised value in the future. Several factors are used to determine the gifted value, including the following:

- The grantor's life expectancy as determined by the mortality tables
- The current interest rate environment as controlled by rates published by the IRS
- The number of years until the home is turned over to the children

This last factor is tricky. The grantor, wanting to live in the house for a long time, may pick 20 years. Unfortunately, if the grantor dies before the 20 years have elapsed, the house is brought back into the estate. This is not necessarily bad but it defeats the purpose of removing the house from the estate. A common choice of term is 10 years. If the grantor is 75 years old and has a home valued at $500,000, and the current interest rate is 6%, the remainder interest of the home is $130,500. Gift taxes will be paid on this amount, or the grantor can use the unified credit. In this case, the grantor has accomplished the following:

1. Your home is out of the estate, as long as the grantor lives 10 more years.
2. The future appreciation of the home is out of the estate.
3. The grantor may live in your house as long as he wishes.
4. The grantor has used a small part of the unified credit or paid a small gift tax.

There is a minor catch to the QPRT. At the end of the term, the children own the home and the grantor has to rent it back from them. However, this could be a useful way to help the children meet their financial needs.

Cost Basis

Under current law, when someone dies, the value of his or her property receives a stepped-up basis. That is, the new tax cost basis of all assets is equal to their date of death value.

Gift Tax

The exemption for gift taxes is at $5,340,000 for 2014; set to increase with inflation.

ETHICAL WILLS

An *ethical will is* a document designed to pass ethical values from one generation to the next (aka legacy or heritage will). It was first postulated in 1998 by Barry K. Baines, MD, in his *Ethical Will*

Resource Kit. He then founded the EthicalWill.com website, now known as Celebrations of Life. com. His hospice care experience provided the impetus for developing resources to help people write and preserve their legacy of values at any stage of life (personal communication).

ETHICAL WILLS FAQS

What form does an ethical will take?
Traditionally, it is a letter or collection of letters to one person or collective group. Audio, video, or multimedia versions are equally valuable.

Is an ethical will legally binding?
No. An ethical will is a personal message.

Who creates an ethical will?
Thoughtful, loving adults who wish to create an enduring message for their loved ones, born or unborn, and/or for their trustees or successors.

When should I create an ethical will?
Right now. Don't risk never getting it done. Get started with something short and think of it as a work in progress. Augment or change it as you and your audience age and change.

Source: Pinnacle Financial Advisors.

How long is an ethical will?
The average is two to 10 pages. Their brevity and thematic approach is an appealing alternative to a long, chronological autobiography. The idea is not to say everything, just a few very important things.

What should not go into an ethical will?
Negative, critical commentary. You will be remembered by your words.

Where should I keep my ethical will?
Make sure it can be easily found. Include it with your legal documents or indicate its location.

When should it be shared?
Sharing it during your lifetime can invite meaningful dialogue. You may prefer it be accessed only after your death. Either way, make sure it is dated and signed.

By 2005, Andrew Weil, MD, promoted ethic wills as a "gift of spiritual health" to leave family members. The goal is to link a person to both their family and cultural history, clarify ethical and spiritual values, and communicate a legacy to future generations.

Today, ethical wills are written by both men and women of every age, ethnicity, faith tradition, economic circumstance, and educational level. For FAs, an ethical will can open the door to start a bigger conversation about estate planning. Susan Turnbull, a principal with Personal Legacy Advisors in New Hampshire is the author of *The Wealth of Your Life: A Step By Step Guide for Creating Your Ethical Will*, a document that some financial advisors offer their clients as a template for creating them.

In recent years, the practice has been increasingly used by the general lay public and medical professionals. In fact, the American Bar Association (ABA) described it as an aid to estate planning in health care and hospice and as a spiritual healing tool.

DIGITAL ESTATE PLANNING

Did you know 25% of all life insurance policies go unclaimed and that 35% of living wills cannot be found when needed? A new Internet start-up company AfterSteps.com helps ensure you have completed and organized estate, financial, funeral, and legal planning documents with a step-by-step checklist to document wishes and ensure critical life decisions are made by you, not the government. And, they securely store important documents and information, and send alerts and reminders, when relevant legislation changes in your state, or if your documents are out-of-date. This helps ensure designated verifiers will receive complete end-of-life plans after death is confirmed.

WHEN TO REVIEW YOUR ESTATE PLAN

Your personal and financial life is constantly changing. Significant changes always necessitate the need to review your life. However, a few key events trigger the need to review your estate plan. If any of the events below have occurred since you reviewed your estate plan, see a competent advisor to help you achieve your goals.

1. Birth of a child or grandchild.
2. Death of a spouse, beneficiary, guardian, trustee, or personal representative.
3. Marriage of you or your children.
4. Divorce (review beneficiary designations and asset titling).
5. Move out of state. An estate is settled under the laws of the state in which the decedent resided. Certain provisions of a will that are valid in one state may not be in another.
6. Change in estate value. A large increase or decrease in the size of an estate may greatly affect some of the strategies that were implemented.
7. Changes in business. Starting, buying, or selling a medical practice or other business has an impact on your estate. The addition or death of a business owner will cause a review.
8. Tax law changes. EGTRRA has dramatically changed the way we plan for estate taxes. It is important to note that only planning for estate taxes has been effected. Estate planning involves much more than just the motivation to reduce or eliminate taxes. It is the assurance that your family is financially taken care of, that children have the opportunity to go to college, that your debts are paid, that charitable desires are achieved, provisions for a needy child, proper selection of a guardian, and the list goes on. Please do not use the new law as an excuse to not plan your estate.

OVERHEARD IN THE ADVISOR'S LOUNGE

From my perspective, estate planning is a team sport, and lawyers rely on financial advisers all the time to spot issues for clients. We do not share the opinion that non-lawyers are incapable of giving good advice.

J. Chris Miller, JD
Alpharetta, GA

ASSESSMENT

Estate planning is the process of anticipating and arranging for the disposal of an estate during your lifetime. It typically attempts to eliminate uncertainties over the administration of probate and maximize the value of an estate by reducing taxes and other expenses. Guardians are often designated for minor children and beneficiaries for incapacity. It overlaps to some degree with the retirement, asset protection, and insurance planning topics noted elsewhere in this textbook.

CONCLUSION

This chapter on estate planning addressed methods and strategies to reduce federal and state estate taxes. It may also help survivors clarify identity and focus life's purpose.

COLLABORATE

Discuss this chapter online with others at www.MedicalExecutivePost.com.

ACKNOWLEDGMENTS

To Hope Rachel Hetico, RN, MHA, CMP™ of iMBA Inc.; Eileen M. Sharkey, CFP® and Joel B. Javer, CLU, CFP® of Sharkey, Howes & Javer in Denver, Colorado; and J. Christopher Miller, JD, P.C., Alpharetta, Georgia.

FURTHER READING

Baines, BK: *Ethical Will Resource Kit*. Benedict Press, Charlotte, NC, 1998.
Baines, BK: *The Ethical Will Writing Guide Workbook*. Josaba Ltd, Burberry, Australia, 2001.
Christenson, P: A financial planner's guide to working with estate attorneys [a mutually beneficial relationship]. *Wealth Management*, March 17, 2014.
Clifford, D: *Estate Planning Basics*. Nolo Press, New York, 2013.
Clifford, D: *Plan Your Estate*. Nolo Press, New York, 2012.
Freed, R: *Your Legacy Matters*. Minerva Press, 2013. *Women's Lives, Women's Legacies: Passing Your Beliefs and Blessings to Future Generations*. Minerva Press, Minerva, Ohio, 2nd edition, 2012.
Friedman, SE and Alan, GW: *Reintroducing the Ethical Will: Expanding the Lawyer's Toolbox*. GP|Solo Law Trends & News, Washington, DC, 2(1), September 2005.
Howes, L, Sharkey, E and Javier, JB: Estate planning. In Marcinko, DE (editor). *Financial Planner's Library on CD-ROM*. Aspen Publishing, New York, 2003.
Jacobs, D: *Estate Planning Smarts*. DJ Working Unlimited Inc., New York, 2013.
Kador, J: The rep's guide to ethical wills. *Wealth Management*, page 58, March 2014.
Korn, DJ: Estate planning beyond the $10.68-M exclusion. *Financial Planning*, March 10, 2014.
Turnbull, S: *The Wealth of Your Life: A Step by Step Guide for Creating Your Ethical Will*. Benedict Press, Charlotte, NC, 2005.
Weil, A, MD: *Healthy Aging: A Lifelong Guide to Your Physical and Spiritual Well-Being*. Knopf, New York, 2005.
Welsh, A: Inheritance planning. *Financial Planning*. March 12, 2014.
Welsh, A: Estate planning: Don't miss digital assets. *Financial Planning*, March 26, 2014.

An intentionally defective grantor trust (IDGT) is an irrevocable trust for which one of the "grantor trust" provisions set forth in IRC Sections 671–679 is triggered. Transfers by the grantor to the IDGT will be complete for gift tax (and estate tax) purposes but incomplete for income tax purposes. Therefore, if the trust is drafted properly, the income and gains of the trust will be taxable to the grantor, but the assets transferred to the trust by the grantor will be excluded from the grantor's gross estate upon death. Further, the grantor's payment of income taxes attributable to the trust won't constitute a gift for federal gift tax purposes because the grantor is discharging personal legal obligations.

See IRC Section 734(b).
See IRC Section 1014.
United States v. Windsor, 570 U.S. ___, 133 S.Ct. 2675 (2013).
Rev. Rul. 2013-17, 2013-38 I.R.B. 201.

24 Selecting a Health Care Focused Financial Advisory Team

Providing Physician Centric—Not Advisor Centric—Holistic Financial Planning

David Edward Marcinko and Hope Rachel Hetico

CONTENTS

Most retail financial services products are designed to enhance the well-being of the Financial Advisor and/or vendor at the expense of clients.

The clients get only the leftovers.

Of course, no one tells them that secret.

They have to figure it out for themselves.

As the old line goes, "Where are the customers' boats?"

Rowland, M: Planning periscope [where advisors are the clients]
Financial Advisor Magazine, page 36, April 2014

Anyone following emerging healthcare trends and delivery models over the past few years has heard various permutations of the notion "team-based medical care," the "continuum of care," or "patient-centered care." All concerned hope that such high-performing holistic teams, with granular patient input, will improve health delivery and become essential to the advancement of coordinated, successful, and cost-effective healthcare and so too, the informed financial planning team process for physicians and medical professionals!

INTRODUCTION

Now, we introduce the related concept of team-based and client-centered financial planning advice for physicians and medical professionals. But the concept must be more than a tag line, marketing gimmick, or metaphor. And, there are several catches to this new team approach.

The first is doctor involvement to lead the team. Gone are the days of abrogating financial planning to some anointed "quarter-back," *uber-advisor* or planner coordinating inputs, team members, plans, advice, and financial products. Today, it is better to do-it-yourself (DIY) or pay the price, literally and figuratively. In other words, a philosophy of ME, Inc., not Financial Advisor, Inc.

The second is to ensure teams are, indeed, well educated and high-performing, using best practices, that demand the sort of whole-person and psychological attention discussed in the first chapter of this book and extending well beyond financial planning software for the general populace.

The third catch is full integration. In theory, everyone loves team-based medical care. But it is seldom used successfully and all must ensure the concept does not re-disintegrate into the disparate parts of traditional care, or the compartmentalized financial planning of the past. This is akin to the individual pieces of a scramble puzzle, which is never fully assembled, as a picture *in toto*. Complete—but not completed.

And, we must be absolutely sure of the team leader and of who is accountable—ME, Inc. or with a tour guide (FA *pro re nata*). Most importantly, who has responsibility with the needed authority. Team-based financial planning advice must not be a collective risk reduction mechanism for the involved consultants, as is often the case in medicine. And it must not be an invoice generating machine or revenue enhancing mechanism like some electronic medical records (EMRs). There must be fiduciary responsibility of all team members, collectively and individually, at all times.

Finally, the team must be more than an aspiration or theoretical model, it must be actual, executable, and real.

REAL NOTION OF TEAMS

In financial planning, there seems to be a fixation … that a team is a financial planner (certified, or not) and an attorney; nice, but not a couple (and not really a team in the true sense of group development as first proposed by Bruce Tuckman, in 1965).

In his model, Tuckman maintained that four phases are all necessary and inevitable in order for the team to grow, to face challenges, to tackle problems, to find solutions, to plan work, and to deliver results (*forming—storming—norming—performing*). Later, he added *adjourning* to successfully complete the task and break up the team. Timothy Biggs further added the *renorming* stage to reflect a period where the team reassembles, as needed. This puts the emphasis back on the ME, Inc. or physician team leader—as too many "diplomats" in a leadership role may prevent the team from reaching full potential. *Source*: http://infed.org/mobi/bruce-w-tuckman-forming-storming-norming-and-performing-in-groups/

This is why "team" must be more than a metaphor. It deserves more than lip service. Delivering client-centered, coordinated financial planning services and products demands true collaboration—a fully integrated team engaged in practices that involve each member at the top, highest, and best use of their licensure and education, optimizing their contributions and maximizing their impact on the well-being of the client.

In this context, board-Certified Medical Planners™ may play a lead role going forward, along with other like-minded and educated professionals. Unfortunately, the ranks of CMPs™, while growing, are still painfully small. But in addition to true expertise, they link physician–clients with appropriate providers and resources throughout the holistic professional life/practice planning continuum. They focus on the doctor–client's totality—emotional, financial, risk and business management, and psyche. They advocate for the doctor–client to connect him/her to the necessary resources, professional advisors, and consultants who need to have their voices heard. Such successful, high-functioning financial planning teams give each member a voice.

The medical professional must be an active participant, not a passive bystander. This is not the norm in financial planning today where doctors are urged to hire a team *quarterback*. But the NFL-QB is not a generalist at all; his arm is special and unlike all other teams players. He is unique, skilled, and exceptional. A franchise player!

Fortunately, past is not prologue in the era of transparency—tablet PCs, Skype®, and smart phones. To succeed in the hypercompetitive new era of health reform requires education, involvement, and active participation, in short, a new model of a physician-focused advisor. No longer is there a free lunch of passivity for medical professionals, either as doctors or advisory clients themselves. For financial planning in the new era of healthcare reform, successful doctors will assume the mantle of quarterback themselves.

ME, INC. OR GOING IT ALONE—BUT WITH A TEAM

The physician, nurse, or other medical professional should easily recognize that there are a vast array of opportunities, obstacles, and pitfalls when it comes to managing one's finances. Still, with some modicum of effort, the basic aspects of insurance, investments, taxes, accounting, portfolio management, retirement and estate planning, debt reduction, asset protection, and practice management can be largely self-taught. Yet, it is realized that nuances and subtleties can make a well-intentioned plan fall short. The devil truly is in the details. Moreover, none of these areas can be addressed in isolation; it is common for a solution in one area to cause a new set of problems in another.

Accordingly, most healthcare practitioners would be well served to hire (independent, hourly compensated, and *prn*) financial help. Unlike some medical problems, financial issues may not cause any "pain" or other obvious symptoms. Medical professionals tend to have far more complex financial situations than most lay people. Despite the complexities of the new world of health reform, far too many either do nothing or give up all control totally to an external *advisor*. This either/or mistake can be costly in many ways and should be avoided.

In reality, the medical professional needs a team composed of at least a financial analyst, lawyer, management consultant, risk manager (actuary, mathematician, or insurance counselor), and accountant at certain times in their career. At various points in time, each member of the team or significant others will properly assume a role of more or less importance, but the doctor must usually remain the "quarterback" or leader, in the absence of a truly informed other or Certified Medical Planner™.

This is necessary because only the doctor has the personal self-mandate with skin in the game to view the big picture. And, right or wrong, investments dominate the information available regarding personal finance and the attention of most physicians. One is much more likely to need or want to discuss the financial markets with their financial advisor than private letter rulings by the internal revenue service (IRS), or with their estate planning attorney, or tax accountant. While hiring for expertise is a good idea, there is a sinister way advisors goad doctors into using all their retail services, all of the time. That artifice is—the value of time.

Truely integrated physician-focused and financial planning is at its core a service business, not a product or sales endeavor. And, increasingly, money is more likely to be at the top of the list for providers as the healthcare environment is contracting. So, eschewing the quarterback model of advice and choosing to self-educate through this book and elsewhere may be one of the best efforts a smart physician can make.

RISKY WAYS TO SELECT ADVISORS

Financial advisors don't ascribe to the Hippocratic oath. People don't go to work on "Wall Street" for the same reasons other people become firemen and teachers. There are no essays where they attempt to come up with a new way to say, "I just want to help people."

FINANCIAL ADVISORS ARE NOT DOCTORS

Some financial advisors and insurance agents like to compare themselves to CPAs, attorneys, and physicians who spend years in training and pass difficult tests to get advanced degrees and certifications. We call these steps "barriers-to-entry." Most agents, financial product representatives, and advisors, if they took a test at all, take one that requires little training and even less experience. There are few barriers to entry (BTEs) in the financial services industry.

For example, most insurance agent licensing tests are 30 min in length. The Series #7 exam for stockbrokers is about 2 h, and the formerly vaunted CFP® test is only about 6 h. All are multiple-choice (guess) and computerized. An aptitude for psychometric savvy is often as important as real knowledge, and the most rigorous of these examinations can best be compared to a college freshman biology or chemistry test in difficulty. Most are the minimal threshold for entry.

Yet, financial product salesman, advisors, and stock brokers still use lines such as "You wouldn't let just anyone operate on you, would you?" or "I'm like your family physician for your finances. I might send you to a specialist for a few things, but I'm the one coordinating it all." These lines are designed to make us feel good about trusting them with our hard-earned dollars and, more importantly, to think of personal finance and investing as something that "only a professional can do." Unfortunately, believing those lines can cost you hundreds of thousands of dollars and years off retirement as "professional salesman" versus "amateur buyer" match units.

A more apt rejoinder, perhaps, would be something like this: "I don't need a professional to mow my lawn, why would I need one to manage my finances?" Just because there are people who would like you to overpay them to mow your lawn doesn't mean you must, or need, to hire one. It doesn't take much knowledge to run a lawnmower, set it to the right height, and make straight lines. Basic lawn care training, like the training of many financial advisors, lasts just a few minutes. And this seems to be the growing sentiment of an emerging subset of Internet-raised and astute new generation of enlightened physicians (http://whitecoatinvestor.com).

SO—WHAT DOES THE FINANCIAL SERVICES INDUSTRY THINK OF DOCTORS?

If you are still not sure what kind of relationship a typical financial "advisor" is seeking with you as a doctor, just consider what Dr. William Bernstein said in his classic work, *4 Pillars of Investing*:

- " ... Make no mistake about it, you are engaged in a brutal zero-sum contest with [the financial industry]—every penny of commissions, fees, [AUM percentages] and transactional costs it extracts is irretrievably lost to you ..."

- " ... Brokers do undergo rigorous training, sometimes lasting months in sales techniques. All brokerage houses spend an enormous amount of money on teaching their trainees and registered representatives what they need to know—how to approach clients, pitch ideas, and close sales. One journalist, after spending several days at the training facilities of Merrill Lynch, observed that most of the trainees had no financial background at all (Or, as one used car salesman/broker trainee put it, 'Investments were just another vehicle.') ...."
- " ... What do brokers think about almost every minute of the day? Sell, sell and selling! Because if they don't sell, they're on the next train home to Peoria. The focus on sales breeds a curious kind of ethical anesthesia. Like all human beings placed in morally dubious positions, brokers are capable of rationalizing the damage to their client's portfolios in a multitude of ways. They provide valuable advice and discipline. They are able to beat the market. They provide moral comfort and personal advice during difficult times in the market. Anything but face the awful truth: that their clients would be far better off without them. This is not to say that honest brokers that understand and manage the conflicts of interest inherent in the job do not exist. But in my experience, they are few and far between ...."
- " ... Stock Brokers will protest that in order to keep their clients for the long haul, they must do right by them. This is much less than half true. It's a sad fact that in one year a broker can make more money exploiting a client than in ten years of treating him honestly..."

Medical professionals still tend to have higher incomes and are an attractive target for most financial institutions and scam artists. We comprise 14% of the Tea Party's one-percenters ($307,000 earned income/year). Take caution when using the following as sources of advice.

Relying on Family and Friends

By far more people seek financial advice from trusted family members and friends than any other source. This is only natural. But beware of affinity scams that target a niche segment like high-earning physicians, dentists, certified registered nurse anesthetists (CRNAs), and so on.

Media

A few years ago the dominant media force in consumer-oriented financial matters was print, radio, and TV. But a recent iMBA Inc. study estimated that 80% of what the average physician knows about financial events comes from the Internet, PCs, tablets, and smart phones. There is nothing wrong with watching shows that cover the markets or subscribing to a consumer finance magazine. It is certainly a good idea to be informed. However, be wary of the quality and applicability of information put out by any media channel.

Internet

It is easy to run across an ad for prescriptions drugs on the Internet, about erectile dysfunction, low T-levels, and alopecia. Images prance across the screen followed by a litany of potential side effects and the obligatory "Ask your doctor about," With the expansion of the information superhighway, more and more companies are going direct to the consumer in some manner or another.

Financially speaking, this information can be of great benefit but should also generate more concern. It is very easy to project a particular image via the web. The webmaster controls the interaction from what you see to what you hear. One of the results of this is that the Internet has already garnered a reputation as a breeding ground for new scams. More prevalent, however, is the presentation of information meant to be useful that is simply wrong, misinterpreted, or misapplied.

The most terrifying source of misinformation on the net is blogs, video blogs, and chat rooms. Here, the entire interaction is clouded by anonymity, often disguised as amateurs but really scam artists. Some people enter chat rooms because there is a comfort in anonymity when asking a question. So, it is also essential that one understands the level of accountability a source may have.

Discount and Online Brokerages

- *True or false?* The key to investment success is to pay as little for a trade as possible.
- *True or false?* The higher the number of trades in an investment account, the better the investment results.
- *True or false?* The majority of revenue of a discount or online brokerage comes from trades.

The answers should be crystal clear. False, False, and True! It is almost entirely that simple.

Obviously, keeping costs down is an important objective of personal finance, but it is certainly not the key to success. There are many studies that show that active trading garners inferior results to a longer-term buy-and-hold type of strategy. One of the most publicized was conducted years ago by a UC-Davis team led by Dr. Terrance Odean. The study examined the actual tracing activity of thousands of self-directed accounts at a major discount brokerage over a 6-year period. The results were clear. Regardless of trading level, most of the accounts underperformed the market and showed that the higher the number of trades, the worse the result. Moreover, the U.S. stock market has again been on a tear since the incident of the 2011 crash and with continuing Federal Reserve expansionary policy. So, one would be wise to remember an old Wall Street saying—"Don't confuse brains with a bull market."

One cannot conclude that everyone is acting as his or her own investment advisor or financial planner. The advice business continues to thrive. Sales of load mutual funds, insurance, and financial products continue to grow, as has commission revenue at full-service firms. No-load funds have continued to grow as well and gain market share from the load funds. However, it would be inaccurate to tie all that growth to do-it-yourselfers. Much of the growth of no-load funds can be attributed to the advice of various types of advisors who are recommending the funds. They still get paid. In addition, several traditionally no-load fund families have begun to offer funds through brokers for a load, or revenue sharing relationship.

For clients, the primary attraction to a discounter is cost. Everyone loves a bargain. Once it is determined that it is a good idea to buy say 100 shares of IBM, the trade needs to get executed. When the trade settles, one owns 100 shares of IBM, regardless of what was paid for the trade. There is no harm in saving a few bucks. However, the decision to buy the IBM shares and when to sell those shares will have a far greater impact on the investment results than the cost of the trade as long as the level of trading is kept at a prudent level. The fact is that most good advisors use discount firms for custodial and transaction services. Some leading trading platforms to advisors are Schwab, Vanguard, DFA, and Fidelity, among others.

In addition to cost savings, discounters appeal to one's ego for business. Everyone wants to feel like a smart investor. Often, marketing materials will cite the IBM example and portray the cost difference as an example of how the investor is either stupid or being ripped off. There is also a strong appeal to one's sense of control. An investor is made to feel like they are the masters of their own destiny. All of this is a worthy goal. One should feel confident, in control, and smart about financial issues. Sporadically hiring a professional for a check-up should not result in losing any of these feelings, but rather, solidify them. Getting one's affairs in order is smart. The advisor works for the doctor–client, so a client should maintain control by only delegating tasks to the extent one is comfortable. Knowing that the particular circumstances are being addressed effectively should yield enhanced confidence.

The final reason people turn to discount and online brokerages is to avoid sales pressure. Unlike the stereotypical financial advisor, no one calls to push a particular stock. Instead, sales pressure is created within the mind of the investor. By maintaining a steady flow of information about stocks and the markets to the account holders, brokerages keep these issues in the forefront of the investor's minds. This increases the probability that the investor will act on the information and execute a trade. Add some impressive graphics and interfaces and the brokerage can keep an investor glued to the screen. The Internet has made this flow easier and cheaper for the brokerages to lower costs and increase the focus on trade volume to achieve profitability. This information flow, however, did little to protect investors during past bear markets. Moreover, it did not protect the professionals either.

Ironically, win or lose, this focus on trading is one of the very conflicts physician investors are trying to avoid by fleeing a traditional full-service broker.

Traditional Full-Service Brokers

It used to be that the only way to get investments and investment information was through paying commissions to a traditional broker. Then, on May-Day 1975, the brokerage industry went through significant deregulation, allowing for the discounting of commissions. Charles Schwab and Company, among others, was able to eliminate the advice component and offer trades at dramatically reduced rates. The full-service brokerage business responded by emphasizing the scope of their services, namely, research and advice in order to compete. The demand for both has continued to grow, even though research information is now readily available through many sources. These brokerage firms continue to thrive despite their poor performance in analyzing tech stocks, exemplified by the Enron and Global Grossing debacles, and crashes of 2007–2008 and 2011.

The fundamental flaw is the array of conflicts of interest between the firm and its customers. While the incentive to trade has been well chronicled as a conflict, these firms have not let consumer's demand for a better-aligned compensation arrangement go unnoticed. Fee-based versus fee-only account relationships have proliferated accordingly. In theory, this type of arrangement, usually a percentage of assets (1–2%), gives an incentive for performance, retention and service rather than trade activity. This certainly has merit. However, conflicts remain that should be considered.

The practice of paying brokers higher levels of compensation for in-house products was commonplace. Today, explicitly higher payouts still exist but are less common. Instead, firms may use the sale of proprietary mutual and index funds and other products as part of management's compensation. Other forms of nonmonetary compensation such as a better office, vacation trips, million-dollar (sales) roundtable dinners, and accolades can be used as incentive for the brokers. The greater profitability of these in-house offerings will keep this conflict around for some time.

Less obvious is the conflict between the investment banking arm, the research department, and the retail brokerage operations of a firm. Even firms with no proprietary funds to sell may grapple with this issue. Here, research is pressured to say favorable things about a particular company's stock by the investment bankers in hopes of obtaining more of that company's business. When a firm brings a company public, odds are great that a "strong buy" rating will come with the IPO. Of course, the lesson remains—consider the source.

Traditional stock brokers have a somewhat higher standard of accountability than the online firms as to their accountability. If you buy the stock of a company that goes bankrupt through an online broker, you have little recourse. After all, that was your choice. If a full-service broker recommended the stock to you, that broker will have to defend the recommendation. In turn, you may have signed an arbitration agreement in your contract that precludes litigation (gotcha)!

RIGHT ADVISORS

Hiring the "right" financial advisor when needed may put the medical professional in the position of being able to keep more of what you make and make more with what you keep. Further, it plugs up any gaps you may have overlooked. Often, there are risks to a person's financial security that you may not even know exists. A good advisor keeps clients from experiencing these nasty surprises.

The task of finding the right advisor is no different than the financial planning process itself. First, the characteristics desired must be identified. Second, information must be gathered about prospective advisors and analyzed in light of what is wanted. Then a selection of an advisor must be made and the results monitored relative to the original goals. There are lots of little things that make for a good working relationship with professionals in any field. They all seem to fall into three main categories: competence, ethics, and rapport. When all three are present, the relationship seems to work. Remove any of these and there may be a problem. With enough effort, a financial advisor with an adequate degree of all three can be found.

COMPETENCE

A hallmark of competence is experience. As with any endeavor, the more situations that are dealt with, the better the results with future work. At a minimum, 5–10 years of relevant advising experience should be required: absolutely no rookies. Financial planners come from all walks of life. Most have come into the business only after a bull market, and fade away with the next bear market. Corporate downsizing, the development of personal finance studies at major universities, online educational websites (Kahn Academy is nonprofit), and the general interest increase during bull market have drawn lots of people to the industry, to assist consumers, doctors, and DIYs, as well.

Most of these folks can make the case that their backgrounds make them a good choice. To a degree, they are correct. The laid-off engineer is probably blessed with good analytic skills and is used to following a proscribed disciplined process. A former teacher may have wonderful communication skills allowing for the translation of complex concepts into simple useable form. The CPA may be highly skilled with navigating the tax code.

However, the engineer may also be unable to carry on a conversation, getting so bogged down in analyzing things that he may fail to adequately manage and market his business. If he shuts down, the long-term relationship that was sought is gone. The teacher on the other hand may lack the necessary analytic and economic skills. Teachers also tend to make relatively modest salaries. Accordingly, it may take some time before an ex-teacher can get comfortable with the issues that face a higher-income client or the completely different tax structure that faces many medical professionals.

The CPA may initially know next to nothing about investments and financial planning, but be the chosen partner to run the newly formed planning and/or investment operations at the CPA firm. CPA firms are getting squeezed on the low end by H&R Block and computer software services and on the high end by the multinational consulting firms. As a result, the American Institute of Certified Public Accountants (AICPA) is pushing member firms to expand their sources of revenues and has declared financial planning as one of five core services CPA firms could provide. Many states have gone as far as allowing CPAs to collect commissions. To be sure, some CPAs make fine financial planners. For search purposes, however, a 20-year CPA that has been doing financial planning for a short time is potentially just as inadequate as anyone else with minimal experience. So, the search simply needs to go beyond that recommendation.

It is common for prospective clients to ask advisors to talk to current clients. Doing so has some value when assessing rapport and quality of service but only minimal value when assessing competence. No one has better knowledge of the quality of the relationship than does a client. Of course, it is unlikely that an advisor will put you in touch with anyone who is less than thrilled. Just as likely is that the advisor may decline to give you any names due to confidentiality issues and a respect for the clients' privacy; it doesn't hurt to ask, but do not expect much from this line of inquiry.

The persons most qualified to evaluate an advisor competence are other advisors. Once a few advisor names have been accumulated, these advisors should be asked whom they would recommend from outside of their own firm. Hopefully, some of the same names will come up.

There are several organizations that one can contact to assemble additional names and gather information regarding candidate's abilities. Some are merely membership organizations, others grant professional designations, and other credentials, and still others do both. The result is a ridiculous array of alphabet soup. Naturally, some credentials are good, while some, or even most, aren't.

The following is a brief list of the most significant:

- *CFP Board of Standards.* This is the intellectual property regulatory body that owns and licenses the Certified Financial Planner (CFP®) designation mark. Licensing is a strictly voluntary activity. Licensed CFPs® can perform no functions that a non-CFP® licensed advisor can perform (www.CFP-Board.org).

- *FPA—Financial Planning Association.* This group, officially formed on January 1, 2000, is the result of the merger between the Institute of Certified Financial Planners (ICFP) and the International Association of Financial Planning (IAFP.) This created a central organization for the financial planning profession (www.fpanet.org).

- *SFSP—Society of Financial Service Professionals.* This is the new name for what was the American Society for Chartered Life Underwriters® designation in the insurance community. But insurance agents work for the company, on commission, and not for you. Accordingly, its membership is dominated by insurance agents and is tied to The American College in Bryn Mawr, Pennsylvania, that grants the designation, and many others. Holding a designation is not a requirement for membership (610) 526–2500 (www.financialpro.org).

- *IMCA—The Investment Management Consultants Association.* Members must pass the Certified Investment Management Analyst (CIMA) course (800) 599–9462 (www.imca.org).

- *AICPA—American Institute of Certified Public Accountants.* The primary membership organization for CPA's (212) 596–6200 (www.aicpa.org).

- *NAPFA—National Association of Personal Financial Advisors.* A membership organization composed entirely of fee-only financial advisors (888) 333–6659 (www.napfa.org). Yet, Mark F. Spangler, former chairman (1996–1998), was convicted in 2013 of defrauding clients in Seattle, out of nearly $50 million. Spangler, who also managed assets for a number of wealthy Microsoft employees in the 1990s, was widely known in the RIA business.

CREDENTIALS

Among these organizations, one will find advisors with many different kinds of designations. A discussion of the merits of the most common credentials will follow their definitions.

- *CFP—Certified Financial Planner®.* To become licensed to use the marks in the past, one needed to complete an accredited educational course, subscribe to a code of ethics, show 3 years of full-time experience in addition to an undergraduate degree, and pass a comprehensive 2-day, 10-h examination. But recently, the CFP® Board announced that the exam would be reduced 40%, from 285 exam questions down to only 170, while the duration of the exam itself was reduced to a 6-h single-day exam. While the CFP® Board maintained the difficulty of the exam was not increased or decreased, many FAs wonder if the goal wasn't to at least create the perception that it will be easier and therefore more appealing, which in turn raised the question—did the CFP® Board lower the standards of the CFP® exam and try to make it easier to grow the ranks of CFP® certificants and garner recurring licensure fees? Maintaining the license requires adherence to the Code of Ethics and Practice Standards and fulfillment of the continuing education requirements. The continuing education requirement includes an ethics course once every 2 years. But the association was rocked by real or perceived unrest recently as the very definition of core terms such as fiduciary and stewardship responsibility, fee-based compensation, commission-only reimbursement definitions, kickbacks, and related CEU course and ethical improprieties have been alleged and challenged. The designation was created in 1974, and mark holders were not required to possess even a college degree until about 2008 (a HS diploma or GED was generally accepted).

- *CFA®—Chartered Financial Analyst®.* Currently, to become licensed to use the marks, one must sequentially pass three 6-h exams, show at least 3 years of full-time experience, and agree to adhere to a professional code of conduct. The CFA® designation has historically been considered a highly specialized program focused on the principles of investment management and financial analysis. However, in recent years, an increased number of CFAs have begun serving high net-worth individuals.

- *CLU—Chartered Life Underwriter.* This life insurance agent credential is conferred by the American College.
- *CPA/PFS—Personal Financial Specialist.* This designation can only be obtained by CPAs that are members of the AICPA. AICPA members must have at least 250 h of experience per year for 3 years preceding PFS application and pass a comprehensive examination. The examination requirement is waived for CPAs holding the CFP® marks.
- *MBA—Master of Business Administration.* An academic degree that may or may not have any bearing on one's ability to render sound personal financial advice. Typically, the MBA with a subspecialty in economics, finance, securities analysis, insurance, math, or accounting would add considerable value to the financial planning experience, especially if coupled with another degree or designation. A concentration in art history would not. Certainly, the MBA with a specific medical practice management background, perhaps as a former physician, or in conjunction with financial subdisciplines, or an MHA (Master in Healthcare Administration), would be very helpful in managing or consulting for the busy medical group. Similarly, the MSFS (Master of Science in Financial Services) is an academic degree that integrates the financial planning disciplines.
- *RIA—Registered Investment Advisor.* This is not a designation but a registration with either a state securities office or the Securities and Exchange Commission. Obtaining such requires the filing of a form called an ADV and the submission of a modest fee. There are no experience requirements or exams. On a side note, it is common for persons in the financial planning world to refer to the moniker RIA. However, it is actually illegal for an advisor to use the letters RIA on letterhead, business cards, and the like. The regulators believe that doing so gives the consumer the impression that it is some sort of designation and therefore an indication of competence—it is not.
- *Fee-Only.* This is an increasingly difficult term to describe as a method of compensation, not capability. It is supposed to be used to describe a service, an advisor, and/or a firm. Here, no portion of the compensation is derived based upon the purchase or sale of a financial product either directly or indirectly. Essentially, no commissions are received. In order to establish a fee-only practice, one need only register as an investment advisor as described above. Accordingly, fee-only has no relevance to the competence of the advisor in question whatsoever.

In the healthcare field, there are a variety of licenses and credentials that a consumer may encounter. From physicians, podiatrists, dentists, and nurse practitioners, each of these professional has varying degrees of competence, though ostensibly they all have met some minimal level of competence. Over the years, most patients have come to understand somewhat what is going on. Despite the years of evolution and the notoriously grueling road to becoming a doctor, there are still bad ones practicing medicine. It is not necessarily easy for the average patient to determine such with advanced education and training, fellowship and high state bars, for domestic medicine. The financial planning business (profession?) however is still in its infancy and akin to the wild west!

In the financial planning world, there is no magic license that shows the world that a particular advisor is a good one. Beyond those already mentioned, there is a plethora of designations that are narrow in scope, irrelevant to most family's needs, or thin on quality content. However, by compiling enough information, one can get an adequate handle on an advisor competence.

Too Many (Certifications) to Count Syndrome

In medicine, the abbreviation TMTC is well known. Sometimes, this term may be better applicable to the plethora of "credentials" and "certifications" in the financial services industry. A brief description for some of these so-called financial designations (not degrees) follows:

AAMS—Accredited Asset Management Specialist
AEP—Accredited Estate Planner
AFC—Accredited Financial Counselor
AIF—Accredited Investment Fiduciary
AIFA—Accredited Investment Fiduciary Auditor
APP—Asset Protection Planner
BCA—Board Certified in Annuities
BCAA—Board Certified in Asset Allocation
BCE—Board Certified in Estate Planning
BCM—Board Certified in Mutual Funds
BCS—Board Certified in Securities
C3DWP—3-Dimensional Wealth Practitioners
CAA—Certified Annuity Advisor
CAC—Certified Annuity Consultant
CAIA—Chartered Alternative Investment Analyst
CAM—Chartered Asset Manager
CAS—Chartered Annuity Specialist
CCPS—Certified College Planning Specialist
CDFA—Certified Divorce Financial Analyst
CEA—Certified Estate Advisor
CEBS—Certified Employee Benefit Specialist
CEP—Certified Estate Planner
CEPP—Chartered Estate Planning Practitioner
CFA—Chartered Financial Analyst
CFE—Certified Financial Educator
CFG—Certified Financial Gerontologist
CFP—Certified Financial Planner®
CFPN—Christian Financial Professionals Network
CFS—Certified Fund Specialist
CIC—Chartered Investment Counselor
CIMA—Certified Investment Analyst
CIMC—Certified Investment Management Consultant
CLTC—Certified in Long Term Care
CMFC—Chartered Mutual Fund Counselor
CMP—Certified Medical Planner
CPC—Certified Pension Consultant
CPHQ—Certified Professional in Healthcare Quality
CPHQ—Certified Physician in Healthcare Quality
CPM—Chartered Portfolio Manager
CRA—Certified Retirement Administrator
CRC—Certified Retirement Counselor
CRFA—Certified Retirement Financial Advisor
CRP—Certified Risk Professional
CRPC—Chartered Retirement Planning Counselor
CRPS—Chartered Retirement Plan Specialist
CSA—Certified Senior Advisor
CSC—Certified Senior Consultant
CSFP—Certified Senior Financial Planner
CSS—Certified Senior Specialist
CTEP—Chartered Trust and Estate Planner

CTFA—Certified Trust and Financial Advisor
CWC—Certified Wealth Counselor
CWM/S—Chartered Wealth Manager/Strategist
CWPP—Certified Wealth Preservation Planner
ECS—Elder Care Specialist
FAD—Financial Analyst Designate
FIC—Fraternal Insurance Counselor
FLMI—Fellow Life Management Institute
FRM—Financial Risk Manager
FSS—Financial Services Specialist
LIFA—Licensed Insurance Financial Analyst
MFP—Master Financial Professional
MSFS—Master of Science Financial Service Degree
PFS—Personal Financial Specialist
PPC—Professional Plan Consultant
QFP—Qualified Financial Planner
REBC—Registered Employee Benefits Consultant
RFA—Registered Financial Associate
RFC—Registered Financial Consultant
RFG—Registered Financial Gerontologist
RFP—Registered Financial Planner
RFS—Registered Financial Specialist
RHU—Registered Health Underwriter
RPA—Registered Plans Associate
WMS—Wealth Management Specialist

And there are more, current and emerging. Most only serve to confuse and obfuscate. This "professional" designation list is by no means inclusive of all financial professional designations. And, according to Bruce Spates, director FINRA Investor Education, representatives of organizations issuing professional designations may submit their securities or investment professional designation for possible inclusion in Financial Industry Regulatory Authority (FINRA)'s list of designations by completing their Professional Designation Form (personal communication).

Designation Fatigue

Another way to view the certification conundrum through this plethora of marks is to realize that according to Diana Britton of WealthManagement.com's 2013 survey *Advisor Benchmarking RIA Trend Report*, there was a percentage decline in all SEC Series licensers, except the #6, with the #65 getting attention from half of those surveyed. The survey of 381 RIAs also found that the number of those pursuing the CFP® marks was down to 36% in 2013, compared to 43% in 2011. Those seeking the CFA® charter were also down to 11%, from 16% in 2011. So, why the designation fatigue? It may be related to personal versus corporate goodwill. Or, the credibility of the advisor versus his/her sponsoring firm.

IOW: Are you just any Dr. Smith; or *the* Dr. Smith from Harvard University? This is the affiliation difference between hospital business goodwill that never dies, versus personal good will that dies with the doctor. Ditto for financial advisors.

Nevertheless, a list of members of an organization in your area can be obtained from the respective organizations. A good advisor will at the very least be a member of one of these groups, or have a designation or two or relevant focus. A bonus would be solid service to these organizations as a leader at a high level locally or nationally.

INVESTMENT POLICY STATEMENTS

As we have seen, if investing advice is one of the primary services desired by a medical professional, there is a shortcut question that should be asked of a financial advisor: "May I see an Investment Policy Statement?" If the advisor's answer is "What is that?" move on!

ETHICAL RESPONSIBILITIES

It does no good to hire a competent advisor if that advisor is not going to put their expertise toward the interests of a client. No one is going to tell a prospective client they are unethical. Everyone will say in some manner "Trust me." True trust is earned and the best way to earn trust is to be trustworthy. It may be impossible to determine if someone is going to do something wrong, but it is a simple minimum to perform a basic background check on a would-be advisor that would show any past indiscretions. Some of these require little more than a clean record and a "pulse."

Most financial advisors were regulated by the NASD, the National Association of Securities Dealers. Now, it is known as the FINRA. FINRA purports to be dedicated to investor protection and market integrity through effective and efficient regulation of the securities industry. FINRA is not part of the government. It is an independent, not-for-profit organization authorized by Congress to protect America's investors by making sure the securities industry operates fairly and honestly. They attempt to do this by

- Writing and enforcing rules governing the activities of more than 4190 securities firms with approximately 634,950 brokers
- Examining firms for compliance with those rules
- Fostering market transparency and educating investors

Moreover, FINRA says it works to ensure that

- Every investor receives the basic protections they deserve
- Anyone who sells a securities product has been tested, qualified, and licensed
- Every securities product advertisement used is merely "not untrue" and not misleading
- Any securities product sold is suitable for that investor's needs
- Investors receive complete written disclosure about the investment before purchase

In 2012, through aggressive vigilance, FINRA brought 1541 disciplinary actions against registered brokers and firms. They levied more than $68 million in fines and ordered $34 million in restitution to harmed investors. They also referred 692 fraud and insider trading cases to the SEC and other agencies for litigation and/or prosecution.

SALES LICENSE REVIEW

The NASD/FINRA self-regulatory organization (SRO) agency is composed of the nation's brokerage firms, despite the fact that SRO is often considered an oxymoron. Upon completion of a required exam, the FINRA will issue a variety of licenses. The most common are the Series 6, 7, and 24.

The Series 6 is essentially a license to sell packaged products, namely, mutual funds and variable annuities. It is most commonly held by insurance agents and bank representatives. Holding such a license allows the holder to collect commission income through its member firm.

The Series 7 exam includes issues relating to individual securities such as stocks, bonds, and limited partnership interests. This licensed stock broker is also known as a registered representative

(RR). But brokers no longer call themselves thusly, as the term has acquired a nefarious reputation over the years. Now, they are usually self-named as financial advisors (FAs), wealth managers, financial planners, financial translators, or similar.

The Series 24 covers issues of compliance and supervision and is required of branch managers of brokerage firms. All RRs (the proper name for a broker) must be supervised by someone with a Series 24, also known as a principal license.

Checking the background of an RR, a branch manager, or a member firm is easily done through FINRA/NASD Regulation Inc. (NASDR/FINRAR). NASD/FINRA maintains the Central Registration Depository (CRD). The CRD can be checked for a description of disclosable events by phone or by Internet. One should request information on an advisor's firm as well as the individual. A reputable advisor at a disreputable firm has its own set of potentially dangerous implications.

Many advisors are also registered as investment advisors or are solely registered either with their state or with the Securities and Exchange Commission. The appropriate body will have information as to whether there have been complaints or problems with an advisor or his firm. Advisors with less than $100 million in assets under management register at the state level; others with the SEC.

If the advisor in question is a CFP® licensee, the CFP Board of Standards will have information on any disciplines with regard to the Board's Code of Ethics or Practice Standards. However, this can be an infraction like the "improper" intellectual property use of their registered trademark or registration mark. And there is an emerging disgruntled cohort of CFP® mark holders who are leaving the designation as flaws are exposed in the entire licensing and intellectual property regulatory system.

Advisors who hold the CPA/PFS can be checked out with the AICPA with additional information obtained from the respective state's CPA licensing body. If an advisor is licensed to sell insurance products, information about regulatory infractions is to be obtained from the respective state insurance commissioner's office.

Beyond the records, there are other recognizable clues as to an advisor's ethics. First and foremost is the advisor's commitment to written disclosure. An advisor who hesitates to put the terms of one's engagement into writing is an advisor to be avoided. In practice, the best advisors go beyond the legal requirements for disclosure and provide information about such matters as compensation methods and potential conflicts of interest in an understandable form.

Advisors should disclose their educational and professional backgrounds readily. Ask for a CV or professional resume with schools, colleges, and university listings. Do not accept a marketing piece or sales accolade. It is important to ask the advisor directly about these matters in the interview process; however, written disclosures of such should be obtained and compared to the oral answers. Get suitability, fiduciary, and/or stewardship status in writing.

SUITABILITY RULE

A NASD/FINRA guideline that requires stock brokers, financial product salesmen, and brokerages to have reasonable grounds for believing a recommendation fits the investment needs of a client. This is a low standard of care for commissioned transactions without relationships, and for those "financial advisors" not interested in engaging clients with advice on a continuous and ongoing basis. It is governed by rules in as much as a Series 7 licensee is an RR of a broker-dealer. S/he represents the best interests of the firm, not the client.

And, last year, there were two pieces of legislation for independent broker-dealers—Rule 2111 on suitability guidelines and Rule 408(b)2 on ERISA. These required a change in processes and procedures, as well as mindset change.

Note: The Employee Retirement Income Security Act of 1974 (ERISA) codified in part a federal law that established minimum standards for pension plans in private industry and provides for extensive rules on the federal income tax effects of transactions associated with employee benefit plans. ERISA was enacted to protect the interests of employee benefit plan participants and their beneficiaries by

- Requiring the disclosure of financial and other information concerning the plan to beneficiaries
- Establishing standards of conduct for plan fiduciaries
- Providing for appropriate remedies and access to the federal courts

ERISA is sometimes used to refer to the full body of laws regulating employee benefit plans, which are found mainly in the Internal Revenue Code and ERISA itself. The responsibility for the interpretation and enforcement of ERISA is divided among the Department of Labor, Treasury, IRS, and the Pension Benefit Guarantee Corporation.

Yet, there is still room for commission-based FAs. For example, some smaller physician-clients might have limited funds (say under $100,000–$250,000), but still need some counsel, insight, or advice. Or, they may need some investing start-up service from time to time, rather than ongoing advice on an annual basis. Thus, for new doctors a commission-based financial advisor may make some sense.

PRUDENT MAN RULE

This is a federal and state regulation requiring trustees, financial advisors, and portfolio managers to make decisions in the manner of a prudent man, that is, with intelligence and discretion. The prudent man rule requires care in the selection of investments, but does not limit investment alternatives. This standard of care is a bit higher than mere suitability for one who wants to broaden and deepen client relationships.

PRUDENT INVESTOR RULE

The Uniform Prudent Investor Act (UPIA), adopted in 1992, by the American Law Institute's Third Restatement of the Law of Trusts, reflects a modern portfolio theory (MPT) and total investment return approach to the exercise of fiduciary investment discretion. This approach allows fiduciary advisors to utilize MPT to guide investment decisions and requires risk versus return analysis. Therefore, a fiduciary's performance is measured on the performance of the entire portfolio, rather than individual investments.

FIDUCIARY RULE

The legal duty of a fiduciary is to act in the best interests of the client or beneficiary. A fiduciary is governed by regulations and is expected to judge wisely and objectively. This is true for Investment Advisors (IAs) and RIAs, but not necessarily stock brokers, commission salesmen, agents, or even most financial advisors. Doctors, lawyers, CPAs, and the clergy are prototypical fiduciaries.

More formally, a financial advisor who is a fiduciary is legally bound and authorized to put the client's interests above his or her own at all times. The Investment Advisors Act of 1940 and the laws of most states contain antifraud provisions that require financial advisors to act as fiduciaries in working with their clients. However, following the 2008 financial crisis, there has been substantial debate regarding the fiduciary standard and to which advisors it should apply. In July 2010, The Dodd–Frank Wall Street Reform and Consumer Protection Act mandated increased consumer protection measures (including enhanced disclosures) and authorized the SEC to extend the fiduciary duty to include brokers rather than only advisors, as prescribed in the 1940 Act. However, as of 2014, the SEC has yet to extend a meaningful fiduciary duty to all brokers and advisors, regardless of their designation.

OVERHEARD IN THE ADVISOR'S LOUNGE: FIDUCIARY PLEDGE*

I, the undersigned, _____ ("financial advisor"), pledge to always put the best interests of _____ ("client") first, no matter what.

As such, I will disclose in writing the following material facts and any conflicts of interest (actual and/or perceived) that may arise in our business relationship:

- All commission, fees, loads, and expenses, in advance, client will pay as a result of my advice and recommendations;
- All commission and commissions I receive as a result of my advice and recommendations;
- The maximum fee discount allowed by my firm and the largest fee discount I give to other customers;
- The fee discount client is receiving;
- Any recruitment bonuses and other recruitment compensation I have or will receive from my firm;
- Fees I paid to others for the referral of client to me;
- Fees I have or will receive for referring client to any third-parties; and
- Any other financial conflicts of interest that could reasonably compromise the impartiality of my advice and recommendations.

Jeff Kuest, MBA, CFA, CFP®
(CounterPoint Capital Advisors)
Lake Oswego, Oregon

* © 2011–2015. All rights reserved. www.FiduciaryPledge.com Courtesy permission with personal communication from Jeff Kuest, MBA, CFA, CFP®

FIDUCIARY VERSUS NONFIDUCIARY

To understand the difference between fiduciaries and nonfiduciaries, examine the SEC conduct rules. Stock brokers (nonfiduciaries) are subject to FINRA Conduct Rule 2310(a), which reads:

> In recommending to a customer the purchase, sale or exchange of any security, a member shall have reasonable grounds for believing that the recommendation is suitable for such customer upon the basis of the facts, if any, disclosed by such customer as to his security holdings and as to his financial situation and needs.

A fiduciary follows a higher standard of conduct:

> A fiduciary duty is an obligation to act in the best interest of another party. A fiduciary obligation exists whenever the relationship with the client involves a special trust, confidence and reliance on the fiduciary to exercise his discretion or expertise in acting for a client. A person acting in a fiduciary capacity is held to a high standard of honesty and full disclosure in regard to the client and must not obtain a personal benefit at the expense of the client.

The five primary responsibilities as a fiduciary to clients are

- To always put clients' interest first
- To act with utmost good faith
- To provide full and fair disclosure of all material facts
- Not to mislead clients
- To expose all conflicts of interest and all compensation to clients

AIF® Designation

Investment fiduciaries and professionals are constantly exposed to legal and practical scrutiny—it comes from multiple directions and for various reasons. It is likely that complaints and/or lawsuits alleging investment mismanagement will continue to increase. Although some of these allegations may be justified, many can be avoided by having a clear knowledge of who constitutes a fiduciary and what is required of one.

The AIF Designation Training help mitigate this liability by instructing in practices that cover pertinent legislation and best practices. The AIF® designation represents a thorough knowledge of and ability to apply the fiduciary practices (www. fi360.com).

Stewardship

According to Donald Trone, of *LeaderMetrics*, there is an emerging body of thought and research aimed at getting an even better understanding of how a fiduciary standard is linked and impacted by leadership and stewardship. It is for decision-makers serving in critical leadership roles and governed principles (personal communication).

Three-Tiered Advisory Structure		
Title	**Standard**	**Governance**
1. Broker	Suitability	Rules
2. Advisor	Fiduciary	Regulations
3. Steward	Stewardship	Principles

In other words, the physician needs to know when to expect a recommended suitable brokerage transaction and when to expect a uniform fiduciary standard. Almost certainly, a uniform fiduciary standard will be preferred and is a daunting standard of care for RR and stock broker novices, while investment advisors, RIAs, CMP™, and fiduciary-focused financial advisors will master and embrace it for the good of the client.

UNIFORM PRUDENT INVESTOR ACT VERSUS FIDUCIARY ACCOUNTABILITY

More than a decade ago, Charles L. Stanley, CFP® gave an overview of the legislation and highlights areas of change for financial advisors and planners and to the financial services industry. To date, the UPIA has been enacted in most states. Essentially, the act changed the legal criteria for "prudent investing" for trusts. All assets owned by a trust are considered "investments" for purposes of the UPIA. Consequently, if a trust owns a life insurance policy or an annuity, it is considered an "investment" for purposes of the UPIA. Trustees and their advisors are subject to the act.

BACKGROUND REVIEW

The UPIA (California Probate Code Article 2.5) was adopted by the Uniform Conference of Commissioners on Uniform State Laws in 1994. When determining whether or not certain investing is "prudent," the standard is applied to the whole portfolio rather than to individual investments.

The UPIA radically changes the analysis of risk. The UPIA considers that risk is unavoidable. For example, fixed-income instruments carry the risk of loss of purchasing power, even though the principal may not be reduced in terms of real numbers. Risk is often desirable so long as it is sufficiently compensated. The UPIA seeks to compel the trustees to analyze the trade-offs between risks and returns, taking into consideration the needs and objectives of the trust, or client.

RESTRICTIONS REDUCED

The restrictions on what type of investments can be held in trust have been eliminated. The trustee can invest in anything that plays an appropriate role in achieving the risk/return objectives of the trust and that meets the other requirements of prudent investment. The trustee's duty to diversify trust assets is codified in the UPIA. It is now recognized that proper effective diversification may enhance returns and/or reduce risk at the same time.

The UPIA rejected the traditional trust rule that generally prohibited "delegation of duty" by trustees, especially the duty of investment for trust assets. Delegation is now permitted, subject to safeguards. Agents are now made liable if they do not follow the new law.

WHAT MUST A TRUSTEE DO TO COMPLY WITH THE ACT?

According to Stanley, to comply with the UPIA, trustees must review trust assets and make and implement decisions to either keep or discard assets in order to bring the trust portfolio into compliance with the purposes, terms, distribution requirements, and other circumstances of the trust:

- The trustee must diversify the assets of the trust unless it is prudent not to do so. For example, it would not be acceptable for the trust to hold all municipal bonds.
- The trustee must either comply with the Act in full or have the trust amended to restrict the requirements to diversify trust assets.
- The trustee must delegate if s/he believes that s/he doesn't have the expertise to perform certain functions; this is particularly anticipated in the area of investment management. The trustee is expected to document all of the above to be available for review by beneficiaries and/or courts should they become involved. This includes a written Investment Policy Statement. The act doesn't specifically require this, but how would one prove they had been acting as a prudent trustee without documentation?
- The trustee must periodically review the circumstances, assets and any professional delegates whom s/he has retained to assist him or her. The portfolio must be periodically rebalanced to maintain the established risk/reward characteristics identified in the Investment Policy Statement. This is not specifically stated, but is implied in 16047(b) and is a part of proper portfolio management under MPT. The act requires the costs of management to be "reasonable."
- The trustee must deal impartially with beneficiaries when there are two or more beneficiaries and must invest impartially, taking into account the differing interests of the beneficiaries, and the remainderman.

This essay is not a "final answer" in regard to compliance with the UPIA. Doctors and their financial advisors should consult with a competent attorney if questions remain.

VITAL QUESTIONS TO ASK A POTENTIAL FINANCIAL ADVISOR

Here are some important questions to ask at least three advisors that hold themselves out to be physician-focused financial planners. Then select the most suitable, based on your responses and gut feelings.

How Do You Get Paid?

All compensation methods are flawed in some manner. However, the advisor of choice will work using the desired method and will readily disclose compensation details. Vague is bad. It should be noted if disclosure has been lacking with previous dealings with brokers; for instance, one could take the information regarding compensation as evidence of gouging the consumer. Specifically, there have been many cases where two advisors are compared. One properly discloses costs and the other does not. To the unaware, the disclosing advisor may seem egregiously expensive. The advisor who failed to disclose may even encourage that line of thinking. In reality, the "more expensive" advisor is usually a better choice and the advisor who failed to disclose should be avoided.

Do You Receive Compensation for Referring Me to Others?

No is the desired answer. A good advisor might recommend a member best suited to serve the client when asked. There is no reason to cloud the picture with referral fees. A higher degree of confidence exists where no such payments are present. Of course, as a self-team leader this is nonproblematic. And, fee-only is supposed to be a fee-for-service model.

Can I Get Client and Professional References?

Confidentiality may yield a "No" to this question. Some advisors have lined up a few clients and allied professionals that have agreed to be used as a reference. Expect those to rave about the advisor. The more useful information gleaned from this question is how the advisor answers the question.

What Is Your Professional and Educational Background?

The answer provides some insight as to how the advisor got into the advising business and where the advisor is "coming from." No particular background is in-and-of-itself the best. A college education would at least indicate the ability to question conventional wisdom and think critically, rather than act as a trained spokesperson with stale ideas and no idea of the current healthcare ecosystem.

What Are Your Credentials?

No single credential will be the deciding factor as the doctor is best placed as the lead (ME, Inc.). Focused credentials for check-ups, however, are vital (CPA, JD, PhD, MBA, CFA®, etc.) And only the Certified Medical Planner™ has the professional mandate and education to integrate personal physician-focused financial planning with modern medical and business practice management principles within the context of fiduciary accountability at all times.

How Long Have You Been Rendering Personal Financial Advice to Medical Professionals?

Minimum 5–10 years (through bull and bears markets).

Do You Have Any Teaching or Writing Experience?

Ideally, they will have taught some and authored some peer-reviewed articles published in legitimate media, not trade magazine, ads, infomercials, ghost writers, or pay-for-play marketing campaigns.

Do You Have an Area of Specialization?

Obviously, the area of physician-focused, or health organization specialization is highly relevant.

What Services Do You Provide?

Some financial advisors do comprehensive financial planning; others only focus on investment management, insurance, estate or retirement planning, and so on. Others truly specialize in working with medical professionals and have made a commitment to them, such as Certified Medical Planners™. This is done by delivering financial planning advice alongside the investment management and other services for doctors, nurses, and so on. To a degree this makes sense. A great plan poorly executed with a faulty portfolio will likely fail. Likewise, a well-managed portfolio will not get one far if other areas of the financial picture are flawed. But the quantity of client–doctors in a practice does not always equate to quality advice.

Who Do I Send Money to and How Will I Keep Track of My Investments?

One can send a check or stock certificate to an advisor's office, but never ever make a check payable or sign over a certificate to the advisor for anything other than fees. Checks for investments and certificates (print and electronic) should be made out directly to the custodian, usually a brokerage firm. You should receive confirmations and statements directly from the custodian. Many advisors produce their own statements periodically. This can be a valuable service, but it should not replace confirmations and statements directly from the custodial firm. An advisor should never take possession of client funds.

When Do You Buy and When Do You Sell Investments?

This investment question needs to be answered decisively and clearly. Initially, the answer may be vague, but after some pressing the advisor should be able to outline a clear investment approach, though in general terms.

Do You Personally Research the Products You Recommend?

Yes was the correct answer to start with in the past, but a better response is that the advisor uses several sources of research to complement their own efforts. Be aware that many use Turn-Key Asset Management Programs (TAMPs) to charge a retail fee for a mass-customized, outsourced, and wholesale product. This is also a risk-reduction mechanism since an increasing number of FAs participate in these programs.

Can I See a Sample Comprehensive and Integrated Financial Plan for a Physician or Medical Professional?

This should be provided with no reference to the real client. Lack of such confidentiality is a deal killer. The work sample should give clues as to whether the advisor can communicate clearly in the written form. It might be for a new practitioner to review contemporaneous issues, as well as a mature physician, constructed a decade or more ago, to review past results.

Note: Three comprehensive life cycle physician-focused financial plan examples (.pdf format) are available from iMBA Inc., for only $99, by email delivery with *PayPal* invoice.

Request: AdviceForDoctors@OutLook.com or MarcinkoAdvisors@msn.com

Have You Ever Had Complaints Filed against You?

No is best, but a yes might be acceptable. Sometimes things simply do not work the way they were designed. You want the advisor's side of the story. Just because a client complained does not mean there really was a problem. Medical professionals frequently run across patients that do not necessarily repeat another medical professional's advice in a completely accurate manner. A bad medical outcome can result in a suit about whether the doctor acted improperly or not. Financial advisor clients sometimes do similar things. Obviously, if the advisor says there have been no complaints and the state securities office or CRD says something else, there will be no relationship.

Have You Appropriately Completed a U-4 Application?

The Form U-4 Application is a document financial advisors must complete to become registered in the appropriate jurisdictions. Upon completion of the registration process, advisors are assigned a CRD number from which they can be easily identified. Some certification-issuing organizations explicitly require that applicants answer "no" to all disclosure questions on the U-4 that discuss criminal and regulatory violations, civil judicial actions, and customer complaints, or else satisfactorily justify a "yes" answer. However, those that do not require it simply operate in such a way that applicants with inappropriate responses are not to be considered.

How Have These Complaints Been Resolved and What Has Been Done to Prevent Such Problems in the Future?

Even the best advisors can have a promising relationship go sour. Some clients say all the right things, but internally believe they are entitled to investments that only go up. Find out what lessons the advisor learned from the experience.

How Do I Complain or Seek Restitution?

The answer depends on the nature of the complaint. Make the advisor walk you through the process for a simple issue and for a more serious matter. If a check did not get deposited in a timely manner, the advisor should take responsibility for assuring that the office procedures are more efficient. A serious dispute is typically sent to arbitration or mediation instead of the courts. This is outlined in a contract with the advisor; negotiate it.

How Can I Terminate Our Relationship and What Costs Are Involved?

Ideally, one should be able to discontinue the relationship whenever deemed necessary without incurring more than nominal costs associated with transferring accounts to a new advisor. As competitive as this world has become, there is no benefit in being dramatically tied down to one provider either of advice or of product. A truly excellent advisor is willing to be held accountable and earn his fees each year, year after year. The advisor should assume the risks of a bad relationship. If one is asked to agree to significant exit fees, the risk rests with the client. This is not contrary to the long-term commitment required for successful investing. One should be able to maintain a long-term investment portfolio yet retain the ability to change advisors. If a change of advisors is desired, one will want to make sure that each and every security or other product is easily transferable in-kind to another institution. Most proprietary products will not transfer and must be liquidated. The client would be responsible for any resulting tax liability and liquidation fees. This lack of transferability is another negative involved with proprietary products. The brokerage firm, naturally, plans such as a client retention tool and thus a good thing.

Are You Subject to Noncompete Restrictions in Your Contract with Your Firm?

Most major full-service brokerage firms require a no-compete clause. By contract, the firm takes the position that they "own" the client. The broker is after all an RR. If an advisor has to deal with such, he will probably be barred from contacting clients if he goes to another firm. Clearly, this interferes with the advisor/client relationship. It is a good idea that if an advisor does change firms, one does not merely give him a free pass. He should be able to communicate how it will be of benefit to his clients.

There is a similar emerging problem in healthcare today when the patient asks a team: *Who is my doctor?* Or *to whom is the hospitalist or physician-owned hospital-based practitioner responsible?*

Who Is Your E&O Carrier and How Much Coverage Do You Carry?

E&O stands for errors and omissions and is an advisor's version of malpractice insurance. A smart independent advisor carries this coverage not only for protection but to level the playing field with the traditional brokerage firms somewhat. One of the drawing cards of the mega firms is the perception of the availability of deep pockets should a problem arise. Adequate E&O protects all parties by assuring that a mistake won't ruin the advisor or the client.

What Types of Technology Do You Use?

Many FAs are still very much in the paper-based manual world, mailing out monthly and/or quarterly reports that could be placed on a secure client portal of a website reports. Perhaps this is to justify asset management fee in some cases. So, ask about things like social media (personal preference). Does the FA advertise, and where? How credible are the marketing programs: hype, or PR? Remember, MDs and FAs may pay for marketing and advertising hype, but pray for good public and professional relations (PR). Ask about Skype, video chats, or webinars. Passwords and security questions are good, but biometric identification is even better. Or ask if they use a CRM (Client Retention and Management) system. This is akin to an eHR with e-forms filling and document imaging management and online signature processing capabilities to reduce the time to open, monitor, and end-out account information.

Rest assured, the next wave of technology and online advice platforms will be smarter and faster than what's come before. It won't put FAs out of business, but it will squeeze fees and give doctors and clients the tools to hold advisors more accountable. So, always consider what type of advice is given, and if their technology matches your thoughts on it.

What Happens When You Retire or If You Die or Become Disabled and Will Anyone Else Be Working with Me?

There should be a succession plan in place for each of these occurrences. It is fine, even desired, that the advisor be more than a one-person operation. At the very least, there should be some staff, with a sliding-scale fee structure. What is important here is that one understands who will be responsible for what and that an understudy is not the prime source of advice, and how each is charged. Better yet, assemble your own hand-picked integrated team.

Compensation Issues

The focal point of most disclosure is real or potential conflicts of interest, primarily compensation. There has been a torrential debate within the planning industry recently regarding which type of compensation is best. At times, the debate has gotten ugly within the industry. Definitions are blurred, fluid, and ill-defined, perhaps intentionally so. Those who receive some level of commission income have taken offense at the assertion made by some that they are somehow less ethical than fee-only advisors. The fee-only crowd has been accused of being holier-than-thou zealots. All the while, both sides of the debate seem to ignore the fact that how an advisor gets paid is completely irrelevant as to whether good advice is being rendered. It makes no more sense to pay a fee for bad advice than to pay a commission for bad advice. So how do financial planners get paid? Commissions, fees, or both.

Commissions

Commission income has been a cornerstone of the insurance industry financial advice business for decades. The primary advantage of paying on a commission basis is that one is paying on an as-needed basis. For instance, when a trade is executed, the commission is charged to facilitate the order. The rate paid will be higher than that charged strictly for execution and a portion of that additional charge goes to the advisor for helping decide whether to execute that trade. A commission is also usually higher for a financial product deemed less viable: think variable annuities, reverse mortgages, or whole life insurance; or, in healthcare, think subsidies (commissions) for the purchase of EMRs or meaningful use (MU) requirements. If a large subsidy or aggressive salesman is needed, the product itself may be suspect.

One of the significant disadvantages of this approach is the focus on transactions. The advisor, working in this capacity as a commissioned stock broker, has the financial incentive to either encourage a client to trade or spend his time with a client that will. It is not uncommon for the best course of action to be no action. This compensation arrangement does not give the advisor the financial incentive to render that advice.

In addition to the transactional bias, a common issue that arises is the use of incentive commissions to generate sales of particular products. The traditional place for this occurrence is with the development of in-house or proprietary products. Most major brokerage firms develop their own mutual funds, or variable annuity products, for instance. As mentioned previously, most major firms are no longer directly compensating brokers for such sales, but many continue to use the percentage of proprietary product in calculating bonuses. Further, much of the brokerage firm's management compensation in the United States is directly linked to proprietary product. Rather than pressuring the broker directly through their paychecks, the management team is given the incentive to push in-house products.

The discount brokerage firms are not immune to the proprietary product push. Instead of pro-actively pushing their products, they will put competing products at a disadvantage within their system. For instance, some online brokerages have their own version of an S&P Index fund. The in-house variety can be purchased without a transaction fee, whereas a competitor's version requires a purchase fee. Despite admonitions to review the prospectus before investing, the online firm is betting that the investor will elect the proprietary fund to save the transaction fee even though it typically carries a higher management fee.

Incentive compensation is not the sole domain of proprietary products by any stretch. Most mutual fund companies pay roughly the same level of commission to brokerage funds, but many will from time to time offer extra compensation to drive sales. This is common with funds that do not seem to attract much attention (and new investor money) usually due to poor performance.

Fees

The response to these conflicts has been the rapid growth of fees as the compensation method of choice. The three most common forms of fees are hourly, flat rate, and an annual percentage of assets or net worth. All eliminate the aforementioned problems but create their own potential conflicts of interest, though the conflicts inherent in a commissioned approach do not arise in a fee-only model. The four most common forms of fees are the following.

Hourly Rate

The hourly rate method ($100–250/h) has a similar advantage to a commissioned approach, namely, you only pay when you want to. This is an appropriate way to address a project need or to get a second opinion or spot check of a particular situation. It does not seem to foster good long-term relationships and few planners work exclusively on this basis. The obvious conflict arises from the incentive to take as much time as possible to do the work requested or to create work and the result-ing billable hours. A more subtle issue is that this method of compensation may not promote good communications between planner and client. At times, a client may be hesitant to call with questions or requests for fear of a bill. Conversely, the advisor may be hesitant to bill for time spent for fear of aggravating a client.

More problematic is the reliance on the doctor–client to determine when work is needed. Here, the client engages the advisor when the client perceives the need. The client may not be the best person to determine a need exists. Typically, the client will feel compelled to hire an advisor when there is a problem. This diminishes a significant benefit to hiring help—preventing problems from occurring in the first place.

Often, a well-designed financial plan is ineffective due to poor execution or the outright failure to implement. Without an ongoing compensation arrangement, there is not necessarily an incentive to assure proper implementation of the advice rendered. In a way, this is akin to the criticism of the commissioned approach. The advisor only has a financial incentive to spend his time on those that are ready to pay.

Flat Rate

The flat fee approach has many of the same advantages of the hourly method when applied to a project or second opinion situation. Again, however, ongoing attention is not in the cards. Annual retainers can address this flaw to a degree and ongoing service can be obtained.

There are two important downsides to this approach. First, is the opposite problem from that of hourly rates. With a flat fee, the incentive is to complete the work as quickly as possible and cut corners. The second downside comes into play with the delivery of investment management services. Here, performance has no bearing on the rewards to the advisor. It is this fact that has led to a percentage of assets as the most prevalent form of compensation in the planning community.

Annual Percentage of Assets

In theory, the percentage of assets method is the fairest when providing investment management services. Under this method, the advisor retains a percentage of the assets managed. With all of the fee approaches, it makes no difference which particular securities are selected, the compensation to the advisor is the same. The percentage method, however, changes this slightly in that the result of the selection does impact compensation. If the investments appreciate, the advisor gets a raise; if the values decline, the advisor gets a pay cut. Still h/she gets a percent on the original corpus for which s/he had no input. This is not really; share the gain, share the pain, as postulated. So, while many believe this is a better alignment of advisor and client interests, others do not and consider it ridiculously expensive. Financial advisors do love this model however, because it is like an annuity; cash keeps coming into the firm monthly which is good for cash flow, especially when provided by a TAMP. Moreover, the fees are automatically deducted from the client's account, often in a less than fully transparent fashion. This business model is also valued more than the traditional commission model, which must earn the fee on each and every transaction.

The most significant conflict arises from what to do with a particular sum of money. An advisor has an incentive to recommend that an inheritance be invested rather than applied to outstanding debts, pay off a home mortgage, or to start a business, for instance. Only if the advisor manages the money does s/he get paid.

EXAMPLE 24.1

A medical professional considering the DIY (ME, Inc.) approach (along with a proper education to do so with focused expert advice, *prn*) *versus* hiring an asset manager at the going rate (let's say 1% a year) ought to think of the long-term cost of this decision. A 7% return due to paying the adviser 1% a year versus 8% return makes a huge difference over an investing career.

For a doctor investing $100 K a year for 30 years, the difference is $1.9M ($11.3M vs. $9.4M). Some may suggest that this $1.9 million difference is awfully expensive handholding, even with quarterly meetings.

EXAMPLE 24.2

Here is how a TAMP might work:
One million dollars of investable assets managed for 1%/year = $10,000

- TAMP charges the FA 0.5% = $5000
- The FA receives $5000

The FA meets with the client quarterly, for a 1-h meeting, to discuss the same. The client is told to "stay the course" in bull or bear markets (good but expensive advice?). The FA earns the equivalent of $1250.00/h.

Percentage of Net Worth

Basing the fee on net worth instead of assets managed—the retirement of debt—for instance does not alter the fee as much because the effect on net worth is substantially equal to putting the funds in an investment account. This method is not free of conflict and shares two issues with the percentage of assets.

Both methods work against the use of funds on a current basis. The more a household spends or gives to family or charity, the less there is to manage and the lower the net worth.

To a degree, there is an incentive to be more aggressive in order to increase the value of an investment account or a household net worth. By being bold, a good result can increase the assets managed and the resulting fee income to the advisor. This potential problem is mitigated to a point by the fact that being bold in the investment world does not always pay off. Stocks in particular do go down substantially from time to time. Such an event translates to a pay cut.

Fees and Commissions (Fee-Based)

Finally, there is a large percentage of practitioners that use a combination of fees and commissions. Often, the term fee-based is used. The varieties of fee-based arrangements are vast. Investment accounts may be managed on a fee-only basis, yet the planner may receive a commission for placing an insurance policy. Here, we have a fee-only service (investment) but a fee-based planner. Confusing? It can be, but a good advisor will make clear disclosures to reduce confusion. Another common version is to charge a fee for the preparation of a financial plan with the implementation of the plan resulting in commissions. Also, some states allow a fee-offset where a fee is determined and any implementation commissions are rebated to the client up to the fee. Excess commissions are retained by the advisor.

The most common ethical abuse of the term fee-only, however, manifests itself in the arena of investment management. A client pays an annual fee but is not made aware that some investments that may be purchased, usually mutual funds, will also pay 12b-1 fees (trail commissions) to the brokerage firm. Despite the commission, the arrangement is presented as fee-only. Anytime the advisor has an FINRA/NASD license, one should ask and be told what role 12b-1s or revenue sharing arrangements will play in the relationship.

The ethical issue is not whether there are real or potential conflicts—there are. These conflicts can arise all by themselves. The ethical consideration is whether and how these issues are disclosed by the advisor and dealt with by both the client and the advisor. Ultimately, it is the client's responsibility to determine whether a conflict is clouding the advisor's recommendations.

Remember fee-based is not the same as fee-only.

Posting Website Fees

Many financial planning websites mention fees, as required, but still remain opaque to potential clients because the advisor wishes to control the discussion and understandably wishes to avoid the *website shopper* phenomenon. But s/he can still control the discussion, and still provide transparency, because posting up-front pricing information doesn't mean presenting information in a vacuum.

For example, a 1%/year fee doesn't have to just be 1%; it can be 1%, compared to an industry average cost of X%, where the average cost of an actively managed mutual fund is Y%. Similarly, it doesn't have to be a retainer fee of $1000/year; it can be a retainer fee for less than the cost of a monthly cable bill. And, a financial plan doesn't cost $2500; it costs 15 h of staff time to craft extensive, customized solutions, but saves the doctor so much more. And if services have a range of potential prices, they might be provided with some insight into the factors that impact the price/cost. Modern young and Internet-savvy doctors expect this sort of information.

For Whom Does an Advisor Work?

All advisors will claim to work for the client's benefit; not totally true. This is very different from actually working for the client. Most financial services marketing is focused on how a firm will help clients achieve goals. When one hires an advisor, in actuality, from a regulatory standpoint, most of the time the firm is being engaged but not the advisor directly.

According to securities regulations, an RR stock broker owes his allegiance to his firm. This is true regardless of whether the broker is an employee or an independent contractor. This is also true of insurance agents. And, as previously mentioned, more and more hospital-based physicians are beholden to their administrative masters, despite corporate practice of medicine legal prohibitions.

A registered investment advisor, on the other hand, has a fiduciary responsibility to his clients. This is a high standard under the law, despite the fact that there is no universal definition of the term. It is the same standard applied to trustees. A fee-only financial planner would be regulated as a registered investment advisor by his state or the SEC depending on the amount of assets managed, would be acting in a fiduciary capacity, and would not fall under the auspices of the FINRA/

NASD. That sounds fairly simple and explains to a degree the growth of the fee-only approach. The problem, of course, is that for all the benefits of the fee-only approach both to the client and to the planner, fee-only still has no bearing on the quality of advice.

In practice, most advisors are not fee-only. There has been some name calling within the advisory business because some in the fee-only camp have declared that they are more ethical. Many advisors who maintain FINRA/NASD licenses and receive some level of commission income take offense to this assertion! They contend that full and fair disclosure as well as the delivery of competent advice is the hallmark of ethical behavior.

To complicate matters for the consumer, a great number of advisors are dually registered as investment advisors and as representatives of an FINRA/NASD member firm and fall under both regulatory structures. So, it is possible for an advisor to deal with several regulatory bodies during the course of the day. Here's an example using three different client meetings:

- *Meeting one* is with a new male MD-client for whom the advisor has prepared a financial plan for a fixed fee. The advisor is likely to be working under the regulations applicable to investment advisors.
- *Meeting two* is with a female DDS who needs to buy some term life insurance. The advisor may have researched many companies and policies and recommended this policy to his client. In order to receive the applicable commission, the advisor must become appointed by the insurance company. The advisor is now an agent of the insurance company.
- *Meeting three* is a review for a long-time RN-client who purchased an array of mutual funds a few years ago. Here, if the advisor is collecting trail commissions from what are known as 12b-1 fees, s/he will be acting under the supervision of the FINRA/NASD.

If this advisor is a CFP® licensee, he would need to adhere to the CFP-Board of Directors Code of Ethics and Practice Standards in all three situations. CFP® licensees must act properly with every client, regardless of what other regulatory bodies may be involved. But what is "properly?"

Clearly, there is ample opportunity for confusion in regulating based on function; hence, the need for disclosure. It is important to understand what "hat" an advisor is wearing. Despite the complexities of the system in its current form, a client may seek restitution when a problem exists. Yet, practically this is very difficult. If an ME, Inc. client makes a mistake on their own, whether it was a bad investment through a discount brokerage or some noninvestment aspect of their financial lives, there is no recourse. So, take care.

This regulatory mess also gives some insight into why fee-only has become so popular. It is simpler for clients to understand and easier for advisors to deal with as well. However, it could be a mistake to focus a search solely within the fee-only community. There are thousands of truly outstanding advisors that maintain FINRA/NASD and/or insurance licenses. They do so for a myriad of reasons that have nothing to do with their ethics. The general rule should be to consider only competent advisors who practice full and fair written disclosure and will work on a fee basis. One should avoid any advisor whose only or primary claim to fame is that they are fee-only.

TEAM MEMBERS

Medical professionals frequently refer patients to specialists. No doctor can do it all and none should. In many ways, the medically focused financial planning world is similar. No advisor—not even a Certified Medical Planner™ charter holder—can or should try to be all things to all healthcare providers. Thus, at some point, a referral is in order.

As ME, Inc. team leader, your most common referrals will likely be to lawyers (estate planning and asset protection); CFAs®, securities analysts, and portfolio managers (investing, portfolio, retirement, and wealth management); actuaries, mathematicians, and insurance counselors (not necessarily insurance agents) for risk management needs; accountants (personal income tax planning and practice tax management endeavors and filings); qualified and nonqualified retirement plan experts for the same; corporate contract benefits experts for employed medical professionals; and MBA/PhD practice management consultants for the office.

FORM ADV: THE ESSENTIAL DOCUMENT

By law, financial planners and RIAs must provide you with a form ADV Part II or a brochure that covers the same information. Even if a brochure is provided, ask for the ADV. While it is acceptable, even desirable, for the brochure to be easier to read than the ADV, the ADV is what is filed with the appropriate state or SEC. If the brochure reads more like a slick sales brochure or the information in the brochure glosses over the items on the ADV to a high degree, one should consider eliminating the advisor from consideration.

Registering with a state or SEC gives an advisor a fiduciary duty to the client. This is a high standard under the law. There are several types of advisors who are exempt from registering and filing an ADV. First, there are RRs (brokers). Brokers have a fiduciary responsibility to their firms regardless of whether they are statutory employees or independent contractors. Second are attorneys and accountants whose advice is "incidental" to their legal or accounting practices. But why would one hire someone whose advice is "incidental" to his primary profession? A top-notch advisor is a full-time professional and should be registered. One should insist that their advisor be registered.

The ADV will describe the advisor's background and employment history, including any prior disciplinary issues. It will describe the ownership of the firm and outline how the firm and advisor are compensated. Any referral arrangements will be described. If an advisor has an interest in any of the investments to be recommended, it must be listed as well as the fee schedule. There is also a description of the types of investments recommended and the types of research information that is used.

A review of the ADV should result in an alignment of what the advisor said during the interview and what is filed with the regulators. If there is a clear discrepancy, choose another advisor. If it is unclear, discuss the issue with the advisor. (*Source:* SEC Headquarters, 100 F Street, NE, Washington, DC 20549, (202) 942-8088.)

ROLE OF TEAMWORK

The major players have been assembled. Will the team function together well enough to win the game? Getting all of the players on your advisory team to function well together may seem like a daunting task. In reality, it should be the easiest part of the process.

After taking the time to select the advisors, one should have a team composed of competent ethical professionals who have shown they communicate effectively. It is likely that, if these people are as good as they seem, they may already know each other and may have worked with each other. Moreover, good advisors want to learn more. They feed off good interaction with other advisors because it makes them better able to identify and address issues with their clients. This is not to say that merely hiring people adept in their particular field is all that is necessary for the development of good teamwork. The sports world is full of teams with loads of individual talent but no championship rings. There are steps that can be taken to help foster an appropriate level of teamwork.

1. Designate the quarterback-leader and preferably, *be* the *quarterback-leader*. In a world of ME, Inc., no one cares about your financial well-being more than you, nor should they. Only you have the personal mandate to coordinate your financial affairs from the big picture perspective.
2. Make sure the team knows each other. A collection of folks is not a team.

3. Define everyone's role and communicate your wishes to all the advisors.
4. Meet as a group on occasion.
5. Tolerate no arguments. The advisors should not debate the issues at hand in your presence in a manner that is of a personal nature. Such behavior should force reconsideration of the advisor(s) in question.
6. Make the advisors clarify confusing issues. Sometimes, a client, in a way that is not entirely accurate, may tell team member A what another team member B said regarding an issue. The inaccuracy might confuse A, who is now getting the information from the client. This happens frequently because the client is not an expert. A should call B directly to clarify. If instead A bad mouths B, there may be a problem with team chemistry. Call team member C for an opinion. If a change is desired, elicit the help of the remaining team members to find a replacement, perhaps your second choice originally. Maintain transparency.
7. Always remember, and remind if necessary, you, doctor client, are the boss.

The core members of the team preferably are the Certified Medical Planner™ (if available), lawyer, securities analysis and risk manager, and/or CPA. From time to time, however, other people will be needed. Bankers, real estate agents, and insurance agents or counselors are the most common. To assemble these other players, one should get feedback from the core advisors. All other things being equal an independent provider is usually better, the exception being the banker.

BANKER

As we have seen, doctors carry notoriously heavy debt loads. Beyond the costs of a medical education are substantial costs for equipping and staffing a practice. Technology changes fast these days and capital is required frequently.

Unfortunately, bankers are very conservative by nature. It may be increasingly difficult to borrow money, especially since modern bankers know that a medical degree is no longer the guarantee of a steady and high income that it once was in the past. As more than one banker has often opined, "We don't usually loan money to doctors who really need it." They may also not have a clue about what the practitioner can do to better compete in the managed care arena. Bankers do have a good concept of local community politics however, for those not familiar with a practice venue. They can frequently provide references to advisors (their internal profit generators). Bankers generally do not charge a fee for their "bank advice," but they do for products. The more business one does with a bank, the better the terms that can be obtained. But bankers are not fiduciaries.

REAL ESTATE AGENT

Real estate agents come in all sorts of forms. A good one shortens the sales cycle immensely. The choice of agent should consider both the size of the real estate agency and the experience of the agent. The agent desired is not a part-timer, nor someone with only a couple of year's experience. Further, the agent should be focused on the price range and type of property in question. A good agent asks lots of questions in order to try to keep buyers from looking at properties that do not match what is wanted, but like bankers, real estate agents are not fiduciaries.

When choosing *a listing agent,* the size and number of listings an agency maintains is an important consideration: the more the better. When interviewing an agent to sell a piece of property, ask about how they get and handle potential buyers. The essential question is, "Would someone buy from this person?"

PROPERTY AND CASUALTY AGENT

A good property and casualty (P&C) agent is needed to protect your home and business. The P&C agent should have an array of carriers with which the business can be placed. One should not hesitate to place different types of coverage with different insurers. Most insurance companies will offer a discount if you place multiple coverages with them. However, this may not be as beneficial as insuring each need with a specialist. Again, the P&C agent is not a fiduciary.

LIFE INSURANCE AGENT

Nobody likes to pay life and disability insurance premiums. Inadequate coverage, however, can completely devastate a family by quickly wiping out a lifetime of asset accumulation. Buying and maintaining the right amount and type of coverage from solid insurance companies at a reasonable price eliminates these risks in a very efficient manner. Unfortunately, an essential and relatively simple concept like this risk transfer has evolved into an area that makes many people downright queasy. The saying goes "insurance is sold; not bought."

The easiest way to handle this issue is to get consensus agreement from the core team members as to the amount and types of coverage. Once that is accomplished, appropriate agents can be contacted. The agents could be captive agents with insurance companies with policies known to be good for the coverage in question. Otherwise, independent agents with access to a large number of companies and products can be contacted. Regardless, in addition to the usual questioning regarding competence and a background check, the agent should be made aware that the core team will be reviewing all proposals. Proposals should include what is known as a ledger statement. Life insurance agents are not fiduciaries.

OVERHEARD IN THE ADVISOR'S LOUNGE: ON THE CERTIFIED FINANCIAL PLANNER BOARD-OF-STANDARDS ETHICS CONUNDRUM

When I became a CFP® in 1983, I decided to remove any potential conflict of interest and only accept fees for my financial planning services. Accordingly, I hold myself out as a "fee-only" planner. Over the years, "fee-only" has become the easiest way to be reasonably assured the financial planner is a true fiduciary.

However, a number of CFP®s have found a way to misuse this term, rearranging their compensation so they can brand themselves as "fee-only" without giving up lucrative commissions. Usually, they do this by owning two firms. One is a "fee-only" firm that charges consumers fees for planning advice. The other is a financial services company that earns commissions by selling the client financial products. The CFP® can take a salary or receive dividends from the financial services firm and thereby contend that he or she does not receive commissions. Slick…Too slick!

To stop this abuse, the CFP® Board recently passed a new requirement. It specifies that if CFP®s, or any party related to them, own any interest in a financial services company, they cannot call themselves fee-only. On the surface, this would appear to solve the problem and make it easier for potential clients to find planners who are true fiduciaries. The problem is, like all regulations, there are unintended consequences.

Those consequences have snared me, along with other fee-only planners who are careful to carry out their fiduciary duty to clients. In order to maintain my professional integrity, I'm even considering giving up the CFP® designation I have maintained with pride for 30 years.

Rick Kahler, MS, CFP®
(Kahler Financial Group)
Rapid City, South Dakota

COST OF HIRING AN ADVISOR

Hourly rates vary widely. In less affluent areas of the country, rates will start at about $100–250/h. In other circumstances, or for the complicated situations of some medical professionals, rates can go as high as several more hundred dollars per hour. Flat rates for producing a plan for a family with relatively simple needs should be a few hundred dollars. Households with estates in excess of $2 million should expect to pay about $1500–$2500 at a minimum.

For investment management services provided on a percentage of assets basis, the fee structures also vary widely. To gain a perspective on these costs, the average annual expenses of a mutual fund in the United States is around 1% but trending lower. As an average, there are many alternatives that cost more and many that cost less. High-quality advice and service should cost more than average. High-quality advice also dictates that the focus be on the complete picture including costs. A good advisor will opt for a low-cost alternative, all other things being equal.

It is true that it does not necessarily take as much effort to manage $5,000,000 as it does $500,000—just add another zero to each transaction. Accordingly, the fee should not be 10 times as great. It is also true that the tax consequences and the planner's liability exposure can be significantly greater with a larger portfolio, thus warranting a higher fee in terms of the actual dollars. As a result, one should expect that the percentage charged should decline as the amount of assets increases. For instance, one-half percent of $5,000,000 results in a $25,000 fee, whereas 1% of $500,000 yields a $5000 fee. The $5 million portfolio is 10 times as large, but results in a fee only five times as large as the half-million dollar portfolio.

Generally, try to limit the sum of the planner's fees and the underlying expenses of any mutual funds used to less than 1% per year. Assets in excess of $500,000 should be managed for a smaller percentage. Frequently, the fees on large accounts can be negotiated to a degree. Total expenses (advisor fee plus fund expenses) on portfolios of $2,000,000 or more should be less than 1%. For a TAMP, this is still considered very expensive automation, by informed physician investors and ME Inc. types.

If individual securities are used, there will be no fund expenses. However, it takes a higher level of research and attention to effectively manage a portfolio of individual securities. Therefore, add one-quarter percent to the maximums listed above. But most financial advisors do not do this anymore.

Following these guidelines in conjunction with other criteria for selecting an advisor will result in a total cost that is no more than slightly above "average" for smaller investment portfolios, yet yield the ongoing receipt of high-quality advice and service. For larger portfolios, the value only gets better, but still is retail expensive compared to ME Inc.

Some Stupid Things Financial Advisors Say to Clients

According to Lon Jefferies, MBA, CFP® of www.NetWorthAdvice.com, here are a few stupid things said by FAs to their doctor and other clients, along with some recommended *under-breath* rejoinders:

- *"They don't have any debt except for a mortgage and student loans."* OK. And I'm vegan except for bacon-wrapped steak.
- *"Earnings were positive before one-time charges."* This is Wall Street's equivalent of "Other than that Mrs. Lincoln; how was the play?"
- *"Earnings missed estimates."* No. Earnings don't miss estimates, estimates miss earnings. No one ever says "the weather missed estimates." They blame the weatherman for getting it wrong. Finance is the only industry where people blame their poor forecasting skills on reality.
- *"Earnings met expectations, but analysts were looking for a beat."* If you're expecting earnings to beat expectations, you don't know what the word "expectations" means.
- *"It's a Ponzi scheme."* The number of things called Ponzi schemes that are actually Ponzi schemes rounds to zero. It's become a synonym for "thing I disagree with."

- *"The (thing not going perfectly) crisis."* Boy who cried wolf, meet analyst who called crisis.
- *"He predicted the market crash in 2008."* He also predicted a crash in 2006, 2004, 2003, 2001, 1998, 1997, 1995, 1992, 1989, 1984, 1971…
- *"More buyers than sellers."* This is the equivalent of saying someone has more mothers than fathers. There's one buyer and one seller for every trade. Every single one.
- *"Stocks suffer their biggest drop since September."* You know September was only 6 weeks ago, right?
- *"We're cautiously optimistic."* You're also an oxymoron.
- *[Guy on TV]: "It's time to (buy/sell) stocks."* Who is this advice for? A 20-year-old with 60 years of investing in front of him, or an 82-year-old widow who needs money for a nursing home? Doesn't that make a difference?
- *"We're neutral on this stock."* Stop it. You don't deserve a paycheck for that.
- *"There's minimal downside on this stock."* Some lessons have to be learned the hard way.
- *"We're trying to maximize returns and minimize risks."* Unlike everyone else, who are just dying to set their money ablaze!
- *"Shares fell after the company lowered guidance."* Guys, they just proved their guidance can be wrong. Why are you taking this new one seriously?
- *"Our bullish case is conservative."* Then it's not a bullish case. It's a conservative case. Those words mean opposite things.
- *"We look where others don't."* This is said by so many investors that it has to be untrue most of the time.
- *"Is [X] the next black swan?"* Nassim Taleb's blood pressure rises every time someone says this. You can't predict black swans. That's what makes them dangerous.
- *"We're waiting for more certainty."* Good call. Like in 1929, 1999, and 2007, when everyone knew exactly what the future looked like. Can't wait!
- *"The Dow is down 50 points as investors react to news of [X]."* Stop it—you're just making stuff up. "Stocks are down and no one knows why" is the only honest headline in this category.
- *"Investment guru [insert name] says stocks are [insert forecast]."* Go to Morningstar.com. Look up that guru's track record against their benchmark. More often than not, their career performance lags an index fund. Stop calling them gurus.
- *"We're constructive on the market."* I have no idea what that means. I don't think you do, either.
- *"[Noun] [verb] bubble."* (That's a sarcastic observation from investor Eddy Elfenbein.)
- *"Investors are fleeing the market."* Every stock is owned by someone all the time.
- *"We expect more volatility."* There has never been a time when this was not the case. Let me guess, you also expect more winters?
- *"This is a strong buy."* What do I do with this? Click the mouse harder when placing the order in my brokerage account?
- *"He was tired of throwing his money away renting, so he bought a house."* He knows a mortgage is renting money from a bank, right?
- *"This is a cyclical bull market in a secular bear."* Vapid nonsense.
- *"Will Obamacare ruin the economy?"* No. And get a grip.

So, don't let these aphorisms blind you to the critical thinking skills you learned in college, honed in medical school, and apply every day in life (personal communication).

Direct to Investor Online Advisory Platforms ("Robo-Advisors")

Since the financial crisis in 2008, several start-up companies from Silicon Valley and Boston (Learn Vest, Betterment, Financial Guard, Quovo, WealthFront, Nest Egg Wealth, Wealth-Front, and

Personal Capital) have emerged with the mantra that individual investors, younger, and informed clients will receive portfolio strategies, financial advice, and performance metrics directly from various Internet and online advisory platforms. Termed robo-advisors by some, their existence heralds the doom of financial advisors, or at least drives down the value of FA guidance, reduces fees, and holds them more accountable to clients.

On the other hand, detractors say the financial advice may not be as good because the personalization will not be there, but pricing fees will be more competitive, at least initially. Going forward, price will get even lower and the service better. And ultimately, as consumers get more information online, product and service will improve and be delivered to them faster than through traditional human channels of distribution. The era of quarterly client meetings with TAMPs is fading. Clients will have access to their portfolios, in real time, all the time.

The growth of more traditional direct to investment platforms, such as E-Trade and Schwab, has outpaced FAs recently and human advisors must have the technology and niche space specificity to survive in the future. Realistically, *robo-advisors* and traditional flesh-and-blood FAs will seamlessly merge into a hybrid platform indistinguishable to almost everyone.

So, How Much Is a "Financial Advisor" Really Worth?

This chapter commenced with a rather uncomplimentary opinion of financial advisors, and the financial services and brokerage industry as a whole; deserved or not? The entire text hints at this attitude as well, in favor of going it alone or ME, Inc. investing when possible. Nevertheless, it is reasonable to wonder how much boost in net returns might an educated and informed, fee-transparent and honest, fiduciary-focused "financial advisor" add to a client's investment portfolio, all things being equal (*ceteris paribus*). And, can it be quantified?

Well, according to Vanguard Brokerage Services®, perhaps as much as 3%. In a recent paper from the Valley Forge, Pennsylvania-based mutual fund and ETF giant Vanguard said *financial advisors* can generate returns through a framework focused on five wealth management principles:

- *Being an effective behavioral coach:* Helping clients maintain a long-term perspective and a disciplined approach is arguably one of the most important elements of financial advice (potential value added: up to 1.50%).
- *Applying an asset location strategy:* The allocation of assets between taxable and tax-advantaged accounts is one tool an advisor can employ that can add value each year. (potential value added: from 0% to 0.75%).
- *Employing cost-effective investments:* This component of every advisor's tool kit is based on simple math: gross return less costs equals net return (potential value added: up to 0.45%).
- *Maintaining the proper allocation through rebalancing:* Over time, as investments produce various returns, a portfolio will likely drift from its target allocation. An advisor can add value by ensuring the portfolio's risk/return characteristics stay consistent with a client's preferences (potential value added: up to 0.35%).
- *Implementing a spending strategy:* As the retiree population grows, an advisor can help clients make important decisions about how to spend from their portfolios (potential value added: up to 0.70%).

But Vanguard notes that while it's possible all of these principles could add up to 3% in net returns for clients, it's more likely to be an intermittent number than an annual one because some of the best opportunities to add value happen during extreme market lows and highs when angst or giddiness (fear and greed) can cause investors to bail on their well-thought-out investment plans. And is the study applicable to doctors and allied healthcare providers? Also, recognize that the plethora of other *financial planning life cycle* topics addressed in this textbook were not included in the Vanguard investment portfolio-only study. *Source*: *Financial Advisor Magazine*, page 20, April 2014.

ASSESSMENT

Ultimately, physician-focused and holistic "financial lifestyle planning" is about helping some very smart people change their behavior for the better. But one can't help doctors choose which opportunities to take advantage of along the way unless there is a sound base of technical knowledge to apply the best skills, tools, and techniques to achieve their goals in the first place.

Most of the harms inflicted on consumers by "financial advisors" or "financial planners" occur not due to malice or greed but ignorance; as a result, better consumer protections require not only a fiduciary standard for advice but a higher standard for competency. The CFP® practitioner fiduciary should be the minimum standard for financial planning for retail consumers, but there is room for post-CFP® studies, certifications, and designations, especially those that support real medical niches and deep healthcare specialization like the Certified Medical Planner™ course of study (Michael E. Kitces, MSFS, MTax, CLU, CFP®, personal communication).

Being a financial planner entails life-long learning (LLL). One should not be allowed to hold themselves out as an advisor, consultant, or planner unless they are held to a fiduciary standard, period. Corollary—there's nothing wrong with a suitability standard, but those in sales should be required to hold themselves out as a salesperson, not an advisor.

The real distinction is between advisors and salespeople. Fiduciary standards can accommodate both fee and commission compensation mechanisms. However, there must be clear standards and a process to which advisors can be held accountable to affirm that a recommendation met the fiduciary obligation despite the compensation involved. Ultimately, being a fiduciary is about process, not compensation.

CONCLUSION

A medical practice, like a financial planning advisory firm, should be run as a business. Profit margins matter even when operating a patient-centric or client-centric business, as it represents better sustainability and is economically healthier for all parties.

In other words, you don't have to impoverish yourself as a doctor, or financial advisor, to have an effective business model. Thus, we share the philosophy that the fiduciary standard and personal financial success are not mutually exclusive. The information in this chapter will assist in the pursuit of this noble endeavor.

COLLABORATE

Discuss this chapter online with others at www.MedicalExecutivePost.com.

ACKNOWLEDGMENTS

To Daniel B. Moisand, CFP®, principal for Moisand Fitzgerald Tamayo, in Melbourne, Florida; Jeff Kuest, CFA, CFP®, founder and managing principal of Counterpoint Capital Advisers, Lake Oswego, Oregon and Thomas A. Muldowney MSFS, CFP®, CLU, AIF, CMP™ of Savant capital management, Rockford, Illinois.

FURTHER READING

Armstrong, D: Who oversees the overseers? *Wealth Management*, page 10, April 2014.
Barack, L: *Social Selling [Do's and Don'ts]*. *Wealth Management*, March 13, 2014.

Bernstein, W: *Deep Risk: How History Informs Portfolio Design (Investing For Adults) (Volume 3)*. Efficient Frontier Publications, McGraw-Hill, New York, 2013.

Bernstein, W: *The Investor's Manifesto: Preparing for Prosperity, Armageddon, and Everything in Between.* Wiley, New York, 2012.

Britton, D: Is the CFP board losing credibility in the eyes of advisors? *Wealth Management*, April 11, 2014.

Cimasi, RJ: The role of the Healthcare Consultant. In *ACOs [Value Metrics and Capital Formation]*. CRC [Productivity] Press, New York, 2014.

Coen, A: How to manage concierge services for HNW clients. *Financial Planning*, March 12, 2014.

Corbin, K: SEC to scrutinize advisor self-dealing. *Financial Planning*, March 7, 2014.

Egolf, D: *Forming Storming Norming Performing: Successful Communication in Groups and Teams (Third Edition)*. iUniverse Publishing, New York, 2013.

Front Line: Quantifying the high value of advisor advice. *Financial LAdvisors Magazine*, page 20, April 2014.

Jensen, MJ and Nir, M: *Six Secrets of Powerful Teams: A Practical Guide to the Magic of Motivating and Influencing Teams (The Leadership Series)*. CreateSpace Independent Publishing Platform from Amazon, New York, 2013.

Kitces, M: What Comes after CFP Certification? Finding Your Niche or Specialization with Post-CFP Designations. Kitces.com, March 24, 2014.

Marcinko, DE: *Financial Planner's Library on CD-ROM*. Aspen Publishing, New York, 2001, 2002, and 2003.

Marcinko, DE and Hetico, HR: *Business of Medical Practice [Transformation Health 2.0 Skills for Doctors]*. Springer Publishing Company, New York, 2010.

Moisand, D: Selecting Financial Advisors. *Financial Planning for Physicians and Healthcare Professionals.* Aspen Publishing, New York, 2003.

Odean, A and Shefrin, H: *Beyond Greed and Fear: Understanding Behavioral Finance and the Psychology of Investing (Financial Management Association Survey and Synthesis)*. Oxford University Press, USA, 2007.

Rasmussen, E: The rise of the robo-advisors. *Financial Advisors Magazine*, page 98, April 2014.

Roose, K: *Young Money: Inside the Hidden World of Wall Street's Post-Crash Recruits.* Grand Central Publishing, New York, 2014.

Trone, D: What sets them apart [fiduciary view point]. *Financial Advisor*, page 44, March 03, 2014.

Epilogue

In his dictionary, Webster defines the word *visionary* as "one who is able to see into the future." Unlike some pundits, prescience is not a quality we claim to possess. To the purveyors of economic gloom and doom, however, the financial future for physicians is a bleak *fait accompli*. If you were of this same philosophical ilk prior to reading this book, we hope that you now realize the bulk of financial planning and advisory activity may take place at the physician-executive level, as doctors take back their rightful place as maestro of their own ME Inc., symphony.

For this self-advisory migration to occur, MDs and FAs will need to consider the examples of our contributing authors to re-engineer their personal financial situations and practices with the tools of the new millennium. Hopefully, *Comprehensive Financial Planning Strategies for Doctors and Advisors: Best Practices from Leading Consultants and Certified Medical Planners*™ will prove useful in this regard and serve as a valuable resource for all involved in this often chaotic ecosystem of provider and advisor.

Do not be complacent, for as onerous as it seems, we may not survive autonomously as a profession without utilizing this sort of information, because the bar to a new level of financial planning acumen has been raised. Although many will still need professional advice on an as-needed basis, some believe that astute physicians will look back on 2016 and recognize it as the turning point in the current financial planning imbroglio as the growing sea-change becomes transparent to all concerned.

Therefore, please realize that our contributing authors face the same financial planning issues as you. And although the multi-degreed experts of this book may have a particular expertise, all financial advisors should never lose sight of the fact that, *above all else*, advice should be delivered in an informed manner with client interest, rather than self-interest, as a guiding standard.

Omnia pro medicus-clientis ("all for the doctor-client").

Fraternally,

David Edward Marcinko
Hope Rachel Hetico
Mackenzie Hope Marcinko
Ann Marie Miller
Contributing Authors

Appendix 1: Certified Medical Planner™ Chartered Professional Designation and Certification Program Descriptor and Curriculum: *Enter the Informed Voice of a New Generation of Fiduciary Advisors for Health Care*

As the financial planning industry grows, and quality information is available on the Internet, medical professionals have more access to information than ever before. At the same time, the growing number of consulting generalists leads to a troubling counter trend—more financial advisors mean less differentiation to being a financial advisor. Perhaps this is the reason for the embarrassing number of specious financial industry certifications in existence today. Enter the Institute of Medical Business Advisors, Inc. and its lifelong learning Certified Medical Planner™ initiative (Figure A.1).

THE INSTITUTE OF MEDICAL BUSINESS ADVISORS, INC.: FOCUS ON LIFELONG LEARNERS

The INSTITUTE OF MEDICAL BUSINESS ADVISORS (iMBA) INC. provides a team of experienced, senior level educators and consultants, led by Chief Executive and Medical Officer—*Dr. David Edward Marcinko*, FACFAS, MBA, CMP™, and Chief Academic Officer and Dean—*Eugene Schmuckler*, PhD, MBA, MEd, CTS, to construct individually focused curricula for life-long learners (LLLs). This curriculum is used throughout all phases of Certified Medical Planner™ program matriculation. iMBA Inc. and its staff of teaching professionals have decades of experience and didactic repute, supported by an unsurpassed in-bound research library, to augment knowledge of the integrated healthcare and financial services environment. Thus, the iMBA Inc. team provides superior online education in an asynchronous, cost-effective manner, by focusing on academic solutions for the unique needs of each adult learner. This vast niche network of cognitive and human resources ensures that the Certified Medical Planner™ instructional team maintains the highest level of current and future competence regarding industry trends to serve as the foundation for each adult-learner e-engagement.

A CRISIS OF INDUSTRY DIFFERENTIATION IN THE FINANCIAL PLANNING AND SERVICES SECTOR

The outcome of this trend is pressure on advisors to focus and find a niche to establish true differentiation from the competition. Realistically like doctors, no one advisor can be the best at everything for everyone; but it is possible to be the best for a special group of clientele, with a genuinely

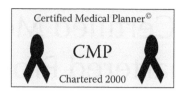

FIGURE A.1 Office of the Provost.

unique value proposition (UVP) not provided by other advisors. And, the efficacy of this approach increases as modern Internet search engines become better at helping to match people in need— with the providers who can offer them the best solutions.

By establishing a business focus, financial advisors create a scenario where the size of their targeted universe decreases, but the potential to capture the entire universe increases! This is marketing 101. Ultimately, the point is not to turn away prospective clients who don't fit the niche; it's to have a niche that's so well established that the only clients who contact the advisor are those who seek their advice. And so, there are so many clients seeking you; there isn't time to serve others, anyway!

Doctors, medical, and allied healthcare professionals are, for like-minded advisors, the perfect niche. *Why?* This space is full of educated and affluent, but often arrogant and challenging, participants who want and even desperately need informed- and physician-focused services. And, the space is in flux which is good for prospecting.

And consider this: medicine is made of specialists. The heart surgeon does not do brain surgery; the dermatologist does not deliver babies; and the podiatrist does not pull teeth. Moreover, the lowest paid physicians are generalists: family practice doctors, internists, gerontologists, pediatricians and general practitioners, and so forth. Medical niche super specialists earn the most money.

STIFFER COMPETITION FOR FINANCIAL PLANNERS

Unfortunately, most financial planners seem to still be operating under the old framework of faux differentiators like service-centricity, technology, and/or experience; rather than the real differentiator that comes from deep knowledge and specific wisdom. In marketing, this is known as the perceived *versus* real strategic competitive advantage dichotomy. *Want proof?* It is not unusual for the best/ busiest doctors to have a loathsome bed-side manner. Sad; but true! Any direction you look, quality

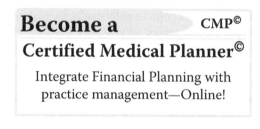

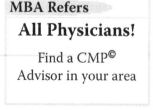
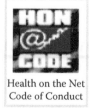

FIGURE A.2 The informed voice of a new generation of fiduciary advisors for healthcare. www.Certified MedicalPlanner.org

but generic financial advice is on the rise, and is quickly shifting from being a value-added differentiator to being the expected norm just to have a shot at attracting high value clients! (Figure A.2).

SPECIFIC INDUSTRY INSIDER KNOWLEDGE: THE NEW DIFFERENTIATOR

So what's the solution in a world where financial planners and their services are increasingly similar to each other (commoditized)? It's time for more advisors to establish a true Knowledge-Based Value Proposition (KBVP). Realize; retirement planning is not a niche.

Yes, the unique value proposition (UVP) marketing buzzword has been around for a long time, but few advisors seem to have truly internalized it. And, just being a financial advisor with sales "credentials" (Million Dollar Roundtable) and years of experience doesn't cut it anymore. Remember, clients appreciate two kinds of experience: good and bad. And, practice does not make perfect; only perfect practice makes perfect. So, experience is not an end point for differentiation anymore; now it's the minimum to get a foot in the door. Didn't 2000 smart but inexperienced Micro-Softies annihilate more than 400,000 experienced but traditional IBMers during the software operating systems (OS) wars three decades ago? *Masses of Asses* was the quip from Bill Gates. Instead, the key to differentiating is the education and knowledge you have, and the kind of clientele you work with. In other words, it's all about having a real niche; or a real KBVP; think UVP 2.0 for advisors serving, in our case, colleagues in the healthcare industrial complex.

In fact, in 2013, Cerulli Associates opined that financial advisors who keep a narrow niche focus are far better at convincing clients that they bring "incremental" or "quarterback value" to their relationships. "They have a deeper understanding of the client situation and pain points. Such a focus also helps them when competing against generalist advisors." *Source*: Megan Leonhardt—WealthManagement.com (November, 2013).

What's best in the new age is the increasing ability to build a narrow niche with a broad national clientele, relying on the power of both personal referrals and Internet search engines to help clients find YOU, the one best expert to help solve their problems!

UNDERSTANDING MARKET AND NICHE SIZE

Possessing KBPV and a clear niche market means, at least for that subset of clientele, you are the best advisor to offer a solution for their needs. In other words, the market itself might be smaller, but you can have the whole market because you're genuinely differentiated as the best provider of solutions for anyone tied to that market. This strategy can actually be far more successful than having a smaller slice of a larger market pie! *Why*? You can actually grow a smaller market niche faster and larger than a huge market. In any event, the bottom line is that as advice and credentials like the CFP® certification become increasingly main stream; the industry seems to be crossing a tipping point of no return. It is no longer a viable strategy to be a generalist for everyone and letting mere "experience" be your differentiator.

According to Michael E. Kitces, MSFS, MTAX, CFP®, CLU, ChFC, RHU, REBC, CASL, and many others, it is necessary for financial planners to have a niche to survive, flourish, and actually help clients more immensely than ever before (personal communication). A true win–win scenario!

INTRODUCTION

The elite CERTIFIED MEDICAL PLANNER™ charter designation program is a one year (four academic quarters), 500 h integrated, *live* and asynchronous, online course-of-study offered exclusively by the Institute of Medical Business Advisors, Inc. (iMBA). The program unites personal financial planning topics for healthcare professionals with modern medical practice management principles in the post managed care and PP-ACA era. It is an informed insider niche approach targeting advisors and consultants who wish to enter the ever-changing healthcare industrial complex ecosystem, which comprises almost 20% of domestic GDP. Adult learners spend 5–10 h per week reading, writing, and in instructor-led activities on both core topics and elective material.

CAREER LAUNCH FOR CERTIFIED MEDICAL PLANNERS™

As noted in a prior chapter, a 47-year-old doctor with $184,000 annual income needs about $5.5 million dollars for retirement at age 65. Although this average monetary corpus sounds daunting, it should serve as a wake-up call to all physicians to cut personal consumption, recognize liability risks, improve practice managerial efficiency, and save and invest more aggressively. And, to financial advisors and consultants, medical practice enhancement knowledge and health economics insight is now an integral part of the personal financial planning equation for all medical professionals. So, we believe the CERTIFIED MEDICAL PLANNER™ program stands alone.

> *CASE MODEL*: As a generic financial advisor, how would you answer this client prospect's inquiry?
> *QUESTION*: I'm a 47-year-old MD—Can you help me?
> *TRADITIONAL ANSWER*: I am a stock-broker (aka financial advisor) or insurance agent, and I sell financial products and insurance policies on a commission basis. *What do you want to buy?*
> *CURRENT ANSWER*: I am a financial planner, and I charge a percentage amount on the assets I "manage" for you. But, I have a minimum portfolio amount. *So how much money do you have to invest?*
> *NICHE ANSWER*: Yes! I am a fully CERTIFIED MEDICAL PLANNER™ practitioner. I understand holistic financial planning for medical professionals and current health industry tumult. And, as an informed fiduciary—with transparent fees—I can help with your medical practice, business, and/or personal financial planning matters. *When can we meet to discuss your needs?*

INDUSTRY HISTORY AND IDENTITY CRISIS

During the 1963–1972 time period, Nobel Laureate Kenneth J. Arrow, PhD, shocked academe by identifying health economics as a distinct field of study! Yet, the seemingly disparate insurance, asset allocation, econometric, statistics, portfolio management, taxation, and financial planning principles he studied have remained invisible and transparent to most participants. And so, an industry identity crisis was born that continues today. The generalist versus the niche health economics expert!

Nevertheless, to informed cognoscenti, this educational dichotomy served as predecessor to the modern healthcare advisory era. In 2004, Arrow was awarded the National Medal of Science for his innovative views, and is now considered the *father* of health economics.

Now, financial service professionals realize the obvious; that the healthcare industrial complex is quickly changing. This milieu has prompted physicians to frantically search for new ways to improve office revenues and grow personal assets. And, the current generation of Health 2.0 savvy young medical professionals is no longer content with traditional *Monte Carlo*, software driven, or de-rigueur financial planning advice for the masses! As medical providers, they seek information like themselves: for *the vital few—not the trivial many*. They want an educated, modern and accountable advisor, or Certified Medical Planner™ on their side; or many will—and should—go it alone (ME, Inc.). This very text is an attempt to show them the way; not sell them on the traditional FA model.

Moreover, the largest transfer of wealth in the U.S. history is taking place as mature doctors sell their practices or inherit parents' estates. Increasingly, the artificial boundary between traditional financial planning, modern health economics, and contemporaneous medical practice management is … *blurring*.

This disruption was noted by the Institute of Medical Business Advisors Inc. (iMBA, Inc.) a decade ago. A research and development program with corpus of work resulted in publications in the Library of Medicine, National Institute of Health, and the Library of Congress, along with related trade industry publications, a dozen textbooks, essays, magazine articles, and working white papers.

Note: The Vilfredo Pareto principle (also known as the 80–20 rule, the law of the vital few, or the *principle of sparsity*) states that for many events, roughly 80% of the effects come from 20% of the causes.

THE INSTITUTE OF MEDICAL BUSINESS ADVISORS, INC.

And so, from 2002 to 2007, the R&D efforts of a governing board of multi-degreed and designated physician–advisors–educators from iMBA Inc. identified the need for integrated personal financial planning and medical practice business management as an effective first step in the business survival and wealth building life cycle for healthcare providers. Now—more than ever—desperate doctors of all ages are turning to financial advisors and medical management consultants for help. Symbiotically, generalist advisors are finding the mutual need for extreme niche knowledge is obvious.

But, there was no established curriculum or educational program; no corpus of knowledge or codifying glossary; no terms-of-art; no academic accreditation, *gravitas* or fiduciary accountability; and certainly no identifying professional designation that demonstrates integrated subject matter expertise for the increasingly unique healthcare-focused financial advisory niche ... *Until Now*!

Identity Crisis Solved!

Enter a formalized online virtual curriculum and charter designation program that promotes and identifies educated advisors in one of the fastest-growing, lucrative, and challenging modern niche markets, today.

DISTINCTIVE FEATURES OF ONLINE EDUCATION

The Electronic Classroom

The intellectual model for iMBA's online CERTIFIED MEDICAL PLANNER™ program is the Electronic Classroom (EC). In the EC, a small group of 1–5 students interact personally with a living instructor. With this low student/faculty ratio, the environment is intimate, although virtual. Some students/faculty find that they are more comfortable communicating via their computers, tablets, or smart phones than others; but many who try online learning find that they are surprised by the genuinely personal level of communication. This is known as an *Electronic Discussion Activity* (EDA) and represents the core of any online asynchronous learning experience.

Asynchronous Education

The EC is conducted in an *asynchronous* mode, meaning that CERTIFIED MEDICAL PLANNER™ program participants can sign-on and access a class whenever it's most convenient to them. Three classes are typically available over the course of a week. This helps busy consultants, FAs, and working adult-learners avoid the time constraint problems they would face with a "real time" exchange.

Live Interactive Education

Electronic Classes can require intense interaction between *live* faculty members and adult learners, often more so than in many traditional on-ground courses; and most automated computer-based training (CBT) programs. Students are typically expected to log in and contribute three to five times each week. With this frequency of interaction, students and faculty all get to know one another, well. There are few opportunities for passivity. In fact, in the EC of the CERTIFIED MEDICAL PLANNER™ program, students tend to interact with instructors much more than in traditional settings; thus promoting future peer-based discussions and real-world applications. Moreover, in the electronic classroom, everyone must write; particularly for the R&D loaded CERTIFIED MEDICAL PLANNER™ program. All assignments are typed, creating a permanent record of each person's contribution. Faculty members find this promotes careful, reflective submissions from most students. Additionally, instructors can easily monitor student progress and communicate with those who need help, or who have trouble keeping up. This is usually done privately by e-mail, Skype®, or phone after certain online expectations have been clarified.

FLEXIBLE ANYTIME–ANYWHERE EDUCATION

Because of the extreme flexibility of the iMBA virtual classroom, punctuality is not a problem, and adult-learners don't lose valuable class time due to weather, traffic, or unforeseen scheduling conflicts; the bane of all working financial services professionals or medical management consultants. Also, students who travel can log in from anywhere and therefore will not fall behind in their CERTIFIED MEDICAL PLANNER™ class work. This is known as *anytime–anywhere* education. For these reasons and many others, online distance learning is quickly earning adherents among adult learners, faculty, and the profession both nationally and internationally. Some virtual students may find that they learn even more in this environment, augmenting state-of-the-art prestige of the CERTIFIED MEDICAL PLANNER™ program from iMBA, Inc.

EDUCATION MODEL NOT FOR EVERYONE

There are some important caveats to this almost idyllic picture of the online learning model.

First, students and instructors must be fully trained and supported in the use of computer technology. They must be exposed to examples of "good practice" and mentored by colleagues with extensive prior experience in the electronic teaching and learning classroom. Successful online teaching requires much more than simply placing one's lectures online; it mandates the careful rethinking of an entire course and the "way" of teaching.

Second, online learning requires much more than simply reading chapter material and answering a few questions. It mandates the careful thinking and the application of learned material to solve real-world problems, for future physician clients. All assignments and responses are reviewed and, if necessary, corrected and redesigned. For students; discipline, reading, and writing skills are prerequisites.

For example, like most iMBA faculty members, Dr. Paul Edelson, author of Complete Book of Distance *Learning Schools*, teaches courses online and has determined that for his classes to be successful, each element must be carefully spelled out in greater detail than in courses with conventional syllabi, where ambiguities can be "talked out" in class. He has also discovered that without the visual cues that are commonly taken for granted in the face-to-face classroom, he must pay greater attention to written comments and ask probing questions that require students to respond and follow-up in greater detail. In the end, he found the results of adult learning and teaching online may be comparable to what students experienced in the online classroom. We could not agree more.

Finally, the growth of online learning attests to its increasing acceptance by students, faculty, and the financial, educational, and healthcare industrial complex. All groups have discovered that the many positive features of the electronic classroom can outweigh the negative effects of not physically meeting in an on-ground class. Hence, the CERTIFIED MEDICAL PLANNER™ program strives to be a leader, not a follower, in contemporary education.

In academic summary, those comfortable with "fill-in-the-bubble-blank" written tests of the past; or the "rote-sales training" and "multiple guess" formats of automated CBT programs of the early pioneering years (without critical thinking ability); need not apply for CERTIFIED MEDICAL PLANNER™ matriculation. The revolutionary "live" program is nothing less than exceptional health industry education for professional financial advisors, and medical management consultants.

ENTER THE CERTIFIED MEDICAL PLANNER™ PROGRAM CURRICULUM

The CERTIFIED MEDICAL PLANNER™ charter designation program is a live instructor led and online asynchronous educational program. An intimate and personalized team approach is used to increase health industry management experience, business knowledge, and financial advisory affinity for physicians in an honest and ethical fashion. And, as these educated advisors climb their respective career hills, even the most demanding doctors seem attainable and in reach, as valued clients!

PROGRAM TOPICS AND SUBJECT AREAS

1. Financial Planning for Healthcare Professionals (3 months, 6 class modules)
2. Healthcare Administration and Medical Practice Management (6 months, 12 class modules)
3. Risk Management and Insurance Strategies for Healthcare Professionals (3 months, 6 class modules)

CMP™ Program Course Curriculum

The Certified Medical Planner™ curriculum follows these three textbooks and chapter contents, for each "chapter-class module" of study. Each chapter module involves two weeks of study with six live instructor led E-mail Discussion Activities (EDAs). The 48 weeks of study, with 24 topics in the curriculum, are subject to change without notice because of the ever-evolving healthcare industrial complex and diverse background of each adult learner.

1. Financial Planning for Healthcare Professionals
   - The Psychology of Money, Behavioral Economics, and Finance
   - Macro- and Micro-Economics of Healthcare Finance
   - Cash Flow Management and Financial Statement Analysis
   - Personal, Business, and Medical Practice Insurance Concepts
   - Medical Office and Personal Income Tax Principles and Reduction Strategies
   - Investing Principles, Vehicles, and Asset Allocation-Gen X and Y
   - Malpractice Insurance and Risk Management
   - The ACA and Health Reform
   - Modern Portfolio Theory, CAP-M, and APM Construction
   - Hedge Funds, M-N Funds, Crypto-Currency, and Alternative Investments (AIs)
   - Investment Policy Statement (IPS) Creation and Analysis
   - Retirement and Practice Succession Planning
   - Asset Protection and Trust Principles
   - Estate Planning, Wills, and Charitable Giving
   - Medical Practice Valuation
   - Fiduciary Responsibility
   - Types of Advisors and Consultants
2. Healthcare Administrate and Medical Practice Management
   - The Healthcare Industrial Complex
   - Emerging Healthcare Markets
   - Health Economics and Finance
   - Medical Practice Business Planning

- Office Launch and Development
- Staffing and Management Human Resources and Outsourcing
- Patient Resources Management
- Health Information Technology
- eMRs, eDRs, eHRs, PHRs, and MU
- Professional Medical Relations
- Practice Decision Management
- Medical Clinic Cash Flow Analysis
- Office Expense Costing and Modeling
- Accounting for Mixed Practice Costs
- Medical Activity-Based Costing
- CPT® and ICD9-10 Codes; Capitation Reimbursement Economics
- Health Law and Policy
- Negotiating Contract Cost Volume Profit Analysis
- Revenue Cycle Performance
- IBNRs Healthcare Claims
- Internal Controls and Fraud Prevention
- Physician Compensation and Salary
- Financial Accounting, Banking, and Practice Benchmarks
- Concierge Practice, Private Pay, and other Medical Business Models
- Appraisals and Business Valuations
- Medical Practice Sales and Contracts
- Patriot Act and SAR-BOX Act
- Physician Recruitment and Retention
- Medical Ethics, Munificence, and Sovereignty
- Career Development and Leadership
3. Risk Management and Insurance Strategies for Healthcare Professionals
   - Health, PP-ACA Risks, and Life Insurance for Medical Professionals
   - Property and Possession Insurance
   - Medical Practice Business Insurance
   - Noncompetition and Practice Agreements
   - Medical Employment Restrictive Covenants
   - Paper and Electronic Medical Records and Recording Risks
   - Medical Billing and Coding Issues
   - Sexual Harassment in Healthcare
   - Medical Workplace Violence
   - Medical Malpractice, Liability, and Tort Reform Risks
   - Capitation Liability Theory
   - Medical Malpractice Trial Risks
   - On Call and Expert Witness Risks
   - Social Media, Twitter, TM, and Futuristic Risk Management
   - Unrecognized New-Wave and Next-Gen Risk Management Issues
   - Financial and Operative Risks of Divorce and Special Situations
   - Types of Insurance Agents, Advisors, and Consultants

Note: The program may be *crashed* under special situations and/or delivered *on-ground*, in groups of motivated learners, upon request. The formal curriculum is outlined in course textbooks and may be modified based on prior applicant education and experience. Generally, course topic substitutions, rather than advanced credit, is given for other certification or degree holders. The body of knowledge is just too vast, and changing too omit. So, topics and requirements are subject to change without notice mirroring modernity.

A GROWING OEUVRE OF TEXT BOOKS AND INDUSTRY STATURE

iMBA Inc. recognized that some adult learners appreciate reading current medical business management theory, healthcare economics, technology or financial planning information privately, prior to matriculation. However, there is a virtual information overload out there, little of which addresses the pragmatic concerns of the modern medical provider or healthcare industry participant. Little imparts the wisdom to become a better financial advisor or medical management consultant. Most seems designed to sell and motivate the purchase of financial products.

Therefore, as part of the iMBA Research Library for the Certified Medical Planner® program, the following *in-house* produced books (and white-papers) are used. Readers may recognize some nationally known contributing authors and Certified Medical Planner™ charter holders.

REQUIRED FINANCIAL PLANNING TEXTBOOKS

- *Comprehensive Financial Planning Strategies for Doctors and Advisors: Best Practices from Leading Consultants and Certified Medical Planners™*
- *Risk Management, Security and Insurance 2.0 Strategies for Doctors and Advisors: Best Practices from Leading Consultants and Certified Medical Planners™*

REQUIRED PRACTICE MANAGEMENT TEXT BOOK

- *The Business of Medical Practice: Transformation Health 2.0 Skills for Doctors*; 3rd edition.

REQUIRED DICTIONARIES*

- Dictionary of Health Economics and Finance.
- Dictionary of Health Insurance and Managed Care.
- Dictionary of Health Information Technology and Security.

SUGGESTED HEALTH INSTITUTION TEXTBOOKS

- *Hospitals and Healthcare Organizations*: *Management Strategies, Operational Techniques, Tools, Templates, Checklists, and Case Studies.*
- *Financial Management Strategies for Hospitals and Healthcare Organizations: Tools, Techniques, Checklists, and Case Studies.*

PROGRAM OPERATIONS AND LOGISTICS

To maximize development opportunities with the latest technologies, CMP™ books, white-papers, and course content are built around three key principles:

1. *Interactivity*—Course content using books, real-world case studies, glossaries, online content, and web blogs to enhance the learner's role as an engaged participant.
2. *Flexibility*—Material offered in short e-learning chapter modules to support professional goals. The content is delivered in print, or electronically, to suit differing learning styles.
3. *Access*—A "live" instructor is available 24/7/365 to minimize time away from job responsibilities, family, or scheduling difficulties, with thrice/weekly virtual classrooms.

---

* *Note:* Designated Doody's Core Academic Title!

IDEAL CERTIFIED MEDICAL PLANNER™ CANDIDATES

Matriculation acceptance is selective and a BS/BA degree with background check and/or CRD/FINRA check is required. Typically accepted students include multiple derivations of the following medical degrees and financial industry certifications:

BS/BA
MSHA
CFP®
PhD
MBA/DBA
MS
CFA®
CPA/EA
JD/LLM
CLU/ChFC
MD/DO
RN/PA/NP
DDS/DMD
CMO/CIO
MPH/DPH
DPM
CIMA
CXOs, etc.

ACADEMIC LEVELS OF THE CERTIFIED MEDICAL PLANNER™ MARK

1. *Certified Medical Planner™ (Honorary):* Granted to the original Certified Medical Planner™ Board of Director (CMP-BOD) members due to their deep integrated and proven subject matter expertise, ethics, and national notoriety (*grandfathered designation;* without formal course work or testing). This level is no longer available.
2. *Certified Medical Planner™ (Candidate):* Granted to an adult-learner whose course of work is satisfactory and currently *in-progress.*
3. *Certified Medical Planner™ (Practitioner):* Granted to a charter-holder who has completed the full course of study (500 h) and is in current compliance with all continuing Maintenance of Certification (MOC) requirements!

HOW TO BECOME A CERTIFIED MEDICAL PLANNER™

A six step approach is used:

1. *Professional Experience*—A successful CMP™ candidate must have 5–10 years of financial advisory or management and consulting industry experience within the medical community. One physician or medical client letter of professional recommendation is required.
2. *Coursework*—A candidate must complete the entire online education program in 12 months. An estimated 5–10 h per week of study, for a total of 500 h/year, is expected. But, the program may be accelerated, or "crashed" to expedite graduation completion in some cases. Group discussions and Skype® teleconferences are also possible.
3. *Examination*—Admission and classes matriculation is provided on a rolling monthly basis in an asynchronous fashion; *via* secure PC, anytime or anywhere. No multiple-choice tests

or mega examinations are required for the thrice weekly class format; 2 week courses/12 courses per semester; four semesters per year; 48 week total program length. Instead of *fill-in-the-blank tests*, E-mail Discussion Activities (EDAs) are used with 250-word essay responses for deep subject matter understanding, not just lucky guesses. Class expectations, and real-world performance, is high. English language, typing, and writing proficiency are required.

4. *Signed Ethics Statement*—Each CMP™ candidate must sign a Standard Code of Ethics to verify an individual pledge to maintain a high standard of conduct, competence, knowledge, professionalism, integrity, objectivity, and fiduciary responsibility in the practice of his/her specialty.

5. *Maintenance of Certification (MOC)*—During each two-year cycle, a CMP™ designee must write an original peer-reviewed and accepted textbook chapter, published essay, white-paper or related treatise in Modern Language Association (MLA) or AMA (American Management Association) format that is approved by iMBA Press. Editorial assistance is available. No ghost-writing, vanity, self-publications, trade magazine articles, or purchased content are allowed. This innovative requirement allows the academic dean to continually create and update the iMBA library of textbooks, dictionaries, working white papers, handbooks, and so on. The iMBA Inc. targeted library stays current and grows in this manner. And, there is NO recurring CEU fee, or required annual dues; a very unique model in the industry. The program seeks insight and cognitive power, not practitioner lucre.

6. *Matriculation Application and One-Time Nonrefundable Due Diligence Fee*—Course acceptance is selective and not automatic and a telephone interview may be required. An undergraduate (bachelor) degree is required. An educational, criminal, and financial background check is performed. The program is focused, competitive, and selective.

ADULT LEARNER EXPERIENCES

The following opinions are from actual Certified Medical Planner™ *candidates*:

"I really like the supportive approach to learning. The limited number of Certified Medical Planner™ students each semester allows the staff to take an evident, genuine interest in the success of learners. I also agree with the program's premise that specialization is necessary for success as a financial advisor, and for providing the best advice to clients. I also appreciate that I had the opportunity to submit my first published work."

"The online Certified Medical Planner™ program has shined a harsh light on how much I still have to learn. I would like for part of the program to include suggestions for continued professional development and practice growth."

"I would incorporate some form of case study for each semester that examines some particular topic. I envision almost a quarterly thesis that would be based upon a prearranged list of topics.

For example, one thesis may involve the analysis of a set of medium sized practice financials and operating results. As an alternative, the program could incorporate a juried presentation designed to incorporate a wide spectrum of the knowledge gained during the program. Perhaps this presentation could begin late in the second quarter with subsidiary presentations designed to allow the faculty to gauge progress and suggest revisions. This would likely increase the rigor of the program and make it more difficult for some professionals to undertake it."

"You will be more able to talk-the-talk of physicians if you have completed the Certified Medical Planner™ program."

WHITHER THE CMP™ PROFESSIONAL DESIGNATION MARK

The Certified Medical Planner Board of Standards and iMBA Inc. owns the terms, copyright, and certification mark CMP™ CERTIFIED MEDICAL PLANNER™, CMP™ (with license plate design), which it awards to individuals who successfully complete the Board's initial course work and ongoing certification requirements. The copyright, and then trademark, has been confirmed by CACI International. A public company since 1962, CACI is a member of the Fortune 1000s Largest Companies and Russell 1000 index. The chairman and CEO of CACI Inc. is Dr. JP (Jack) London. All rights reserved. USA. A Federal Registered Mark® is pending.

How to Use the CMP™ Marks

When used, the CMP™ mark must be displayed under strict use and reproduction guidelines, or their value as trademarks could be lost.

- Use either lower case *or* capital letters, but be consistent.
- Never use periods.
- Always use the trade-mark (™) symbol.
- Always associate with the individual(s) certified by the CMP™ Board.
- If possible, use three components of the design (license plate, "CMP" and ™).
- Always reproduce the logo design from original artwork.
- Always associate with the individual(s) certified by the CMP Board.
- Never alter or modify the license plate design.

OVERHEARD IN THE ADVISOR'S LOUNGE: ON FINANCIAL CERTIFICATIONS AND DESIGNATIONS

I will rank the designations I have earned, or have made progress in earning:

1. CFA (really tough unless you work in securities valuation every day).
2. CPA (this was a very tough exam and required a lengthy process of learning. However, I think that much of the CPA exam was rote—without a full understanding of the content).
3. CFP® (this is a little more difficult than the CMP™ mainly because of the time constraints and structure of the exam). It is less difficult than the CPA because it incorporates some of the knowledge that CPAs typically already possess (prior to November 2014 Exam).
4. CMP™—Certified Medical Planner™ program 12-month course.
5. CLU (these exams were not very difficult but mainly required time and some limited reading).
6. Securities Licensure (Series #7).
7. Insurance Licensure.

Wayne Firebaugh, CPA, CLU, CFP®, CMP™
Private Practitioner-Registered Investment Advisor
[Roanoke, VA]

CERTIFIED MEDICAL PLANNER™ DESIGNATION VERIFICATION AND COMPLIANCE SERVICE

Sherry Cooper
National Compliance Services, Inc.

Verification Supervisor
561.330.7645 ext 208
561.330.7044 (fax)
scooper@ncsonline.com

Bruce Spates – Director, FINRA Investor Education
240-386-4962 office
240-386-4964 fax
http://www.finra.org

FINRA does NOT approve of the Certified Medical Planner™ designation nor does it endorse *any* professional designation, such as the more widely known CERTIFIED FINANCIAL PLANNER®. Inclusion/omission of the marks in their database imply that FINRA considers the designation to be acceptable for use by a registered representative (stock-broker). Furthermore, state securities regulators may prohibit or restrict the use of certain listed designations by registered persons and investment adviser representatives. *Why?*

Scenario: Bernie Madoff, a past vice chairman of FINRA wasn't merely a name associated with FINRA … in some sense Madoff was FINRA. Madoff joined FINRA (then NASD) in 1994 and was vice chairman while his Ponzi scheme was under way. Peter Madoff made it to that same office at one point. Mark Madoff was on the National Adjudicatory Council, another regulatory body that reviews disciplinary decisions made by FINRA. It was an appointed position courtesy of CEO Mary Schapiro, who as chairman of the SEC until December 14, 2012. Finally, Shana Madoff, a compliance officer until the firm's collapse, was a member of a compliance advisory committee of FINRA. *Source*: http://www.fpanet.org/journal/CurrentIssue/TableofContents/AskingtheWrongQuestionsofFINRA/

Note: iMBA Inc. and the CMP™ program are an educational and academic, not state or FINRA/SEC affiliate.

DISCIPLINARY PROCESS

If any medical professional client has a complaint against a *Certified Medical Planner*™ charter-holder, they may submit a complaint to initiate investigation the matter. All *Certified Medical Planner*™ designees should act in accordance with the *Code-of-Ethics*, along with applicable state and federal governing regulatory bodies. Investigation costs are incurred by the designee. Complaints are submitted in writing, and must include supporting documents, to this address:

The Institute of Medical Business Advisors, Inc.
Peachtree Planatation West—Office Park
Suite #5901 Wilbanks Drive
Norcross, GA 30092-1141
www.CertifiedMedicalPlanner.org

THE FUTURE

We imagine a customized network of learning centers electronically linked and globally functioning as academic centers-of-excellence and operating 24/7/365. For example, MOOC is a *massive open online course* aimed at large-scale interactive participation. In addition to traditional course materials, MOOCs provide interactive user forums that help build a community for doctors and nurses, students and adult-learners, professors, instructors, and online teaching assistants (TAs), and so forth.

Why? Medical, business and graduate schools, and allied healthcare educators, are *finally* beginning to identify students who are adept at learning online and reward the top achievers and professors. And, employers and recruiting firms are beginning to troll MOOCs seeking viable job candidates. In fact, when last checked, the nation's graduate students were enrolled in more than

118 online graduate level programs in business management, IT, and the health sciences. MOOCs offer greater access for a larger number of students, at significantly lower costs than on-site programs. And, the irony is that traditional healthcare management programs have only begun to consider these broader implications.

By the same token, technology such as Blackboard®, Cernage, eXplorance, Kalture, and related must be used to full potential. Smart phones, laptop, desk PCs and tablets, videos, interactive games, simulations and related apps with Skype-like virtual classrooms and cloud storage are obvious embellishments to our online Certified Medical Planner™ educational initiatives.

We look forward to this didactic journey of the future.

ACKNOWLEDGMENTS

To Mackenzie Hope Marcinko, Ann Marie Miller, RN, MHA, Professor Hope Rachel Hetico, RN, MHA, CHQ, CMP™, Rachel Pentin-Maki, RN, MHA, and Eugene Schmuckler, PhD, MBA, MEd, CTS Academic Dean, consulting psychologist, and senior psychometrist for the Institute of Medical Business Advisors Inc., and the Certified Medical Planner™ online professional designation and certification education program. To Dr. William P. Scherer, MS, chief technology officer, and Parin Kothari, MBA, chief marketing officer; and to the Princeton Review™ modified by iMBA Inc. and adapted from the Complete Book of Distance Learning Schools by Dr. Jerry Ice and Dr. Paul Edelson.

FURTHER READING

Bowen, WG: *Higher Education in the Digital Age*. Princeton University Press, New Jersey, 2013.

Cimase, RJ: *Accountable Care Organizations [Value Metrics and Capital Formation]*. Productivity Press, Boca Raton, FL, 2013.

Collins, A: *Rethinking Education in the Age of Technology: The Digital Revolution and Schooling in America (Technology, Education—Connections) [Technology, Education-Connections, the Tec Series]*. Teacher College Press, New York, 2011.

Cook, K: *Online Education 2.0: Evolving, Adapting, and Reinventing Online Technical Communication* [Paperback]. Baywood Publishing Company Inc., Amityville, NY, 2013.

Kitces, M: Are financial planners experiencing a crisis of differentiation? www.Kitces.com, August 5th, 2013.

Kitces, M: What Comes after CFP® Certification? Finding Your Niche Or Specialization With Post-CFP® Designations Kitces.com, March 27, 2014.

Marcinko, DE and Hetico, HR: *The Business of Medical Practice [Transformation Health 2.0 Skills for Doctors]*. Springer Publishing, New York, 2000, 2005 and 2010.

Marcinko, DE and Hetico, HR: *Dictionary of Health Economics and Finance*. Springer Publishing, New York, 2008.

Marcinko, DE and Hetico, HR: *Dictionary of Health Information Technology and Security*. Springer Publishing, New York, 2008.

Marcinko, DE and Hetico, HR: *Dictionary of Health Insurance and Managed Care*. Springer Publishing, New York, 2007.

Marcinko, DE and Hetico, HR: *Financial Management Strategies for Hospitals and Healthcare Organizations [Tools, Techniques, Checklists and Case Studies]*. Productivity Press, Boca Raton, FL, 2014.

Marcinko, DE and Hetico, HR: *Financial Planner's Library on CD-ROM*. Aspen Publishers, New York, 2001, 2002, and 2003.

Marcinko, DE and Hetico, HR: *Financial Planning for Physicians*. JB Publishers, Sudbury, MA, 2006.

Marcinko, DE and Hetico, HR: *Hospitals and Healthcare Organizations [Management Strategies, Operational Techniques. Tools, Templates, and Case Studies]*. Productivity Press, Boca Raton, FL, 2013.

Marcinko, DE and Hetico, HR: *Insurance and Risk Management Strategies for Physicians and Advisors*. JB Publishing, Sudbury, MA, 2008.

Moore, M: *Distance Education: Cengage Learning*. New York, 2011.

Shattuck, K: *Assuring Quality in Online Education: Practices and Processes at the Teaching, Resource, and Program Levels (Online Learning and Distance Education)*. Stylus Publishing, Sterling, VA, 2014.

Vai, M: *Essentials of Online Course Design: A Standards-Based Guide (Essentials of Online Learning)*. Routledge Press, New York, 2011.

Appendix 2: Sample Transformational Physician Financial Life Style Plans: *Did They Stand the Test of Time Since Creation in 2000?—You Decide*

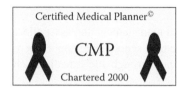

We are often asked by physicians and colleagues: medical, nursing, and graduate students; and/or prospective clients or their financial advisors (FAs), to see an actual "comprehensive" financial plan. This is a reasonable request. And, although most doctors and healthcare professionals have a general idea of what's included, many have never seen a professionally crafted and well-integrated financial plan. This not only includes the outcomes, but the actual input data and economic assumptions, as well.

And so, we thought it novel to present such a treatise for hindsight review by using a real life but traditional plan constructed more than 15 years ago (circa: FY 2000) and letting reader's review, evaluate, and critique the same. Certified Medical Planner™ input was then made more than a decade later.

- Part I is for a married drug-rep, then medical school student (about 51 pages) with no children.
- Part II is for the same mid-career practicing physician (about 28 pages) with 2 children.
- Part III is for the same experienced practitioner at his professional zenith (about 56 pages).

And, we challenge all financial advisors to do the same and compare their results with us.

SAMPLE PHYSICIAN FINANCIAL LIFE STYLE PLANS

DID THEY STAND THE TEST OF TIME SINCE CREATION IN 2000?—YOU DECIDE

- Comprehensive Financial Mega Plan Example—Physician Age 30
- Comprehensive Financial Mega Plan Example—Physician Age 40
- Comprehensive Financial Mega Plan Example—Physician Age 55

Note: All three financial plan examples [.pdf format] are available from iMBA Inc., for only $99, by email delivery with secure *PayPal* invoice. Suggested revisions and updates by a Certified Medical Planner™ for 2015 are included.

Request: AdviceForDoctors@OutLook.com OR MarcinkoAdvisors@msn.com

KEY INPUTS AND ASSUMPTIONS

SAMPLE MEGA PLAN FOR A NEW PHYSICIAN

Joe Good, a 30-year-old pharmaceutical sales representative, and his pregnant wife Susie Good, a 30-year-old accountant, sought the services of a financial advisor (FA) because of a $150,000 inheritance from Joe's grandfather. The insecurity about what to do with the funds was complicated by their insecurity over future employment prospects, along with Joe's frustrated boyhood dream of becoming a physician, along with only a fuzzy concept of their financial future. After several information-gathering meetings with the FA concrete goals and objectives were clarified, and a plan was instituted that would assist in financing Joe's medical education without sacrificing his entire inheritance and current lifestyle. They desired at least one more child, so insurance and other supportive needs would increase and were considered, as well. Their prioritized concerns included the following:

1. What is the proper investment management and asset allocation of the $150,000?
2. Is there enough to pay for medical school and support their lifestyle?
3. Can Susie be the bread winner through Joe's medical school, internship, and residency years?
4. Can they afford another child?
5. Can they indemnify insurance through this transitional phase of life, including survivorship concerns of premature death or disability?

Current income was not high, and current assets were below the unified estate tax credit. Therefore, income and estate-planning concerns were not significant at that time.

After thoroughly discussing the gathered financial data, and determining their risk profile several years later, a Certified Medical Planner™ professional made the following suggestions to the original FA's plan:

1. Reallocate the inheritance based on risk tolerance, from conservative to long-term growth.
2. Maximize group health, life, and disability insurance benefits.
3. Supplement small quantities of whole life insurance with larger amounts of term insurance.
4. Create simple wills, for now.

SAMPLE MEGA PLAN FOR A MID-LIFE PHYSICIAN

A second plan was drawn up 10 years later, when Joe Good was 40 years old and a practicing internist. Susan, age 40, had been working as a consultant for the same company for the past decade. She was allowed to telecommunicate between home and office. Daughter Cee is nine years old, and her brother Douglas is seven years old. The preceding suggestions had been implemented. The family maintained their modest lifestyle, and their investment portfolio grew to $392,220, despite the withdrawal of $10,000 per year for medical school tuition. The financial planning aspects of the family's life went unaddressed. Educational funding needs for Cee and Douglas prompted another frank dialogue, but with a new FA, as the original advisor had left the firm.

After thoroughly discussing the gathered financial data, and again determining their risk profile, a Certified Medical Planner™ professional made the following suggestions to the original plan:

1. Reallocation of the investment portfolio.
2. Educational funding for both children.
3. Tax reduction strategies.
4. Medical partnership buy-in concerns.

5. Maximization of their investment portfolio.
6. Review of risk management needs and long-term care insurance.
7. Retirement considerations.
8. Grow the $392,220 nest egg indefinitely.
9. Project future educational needs with current investment vehicles.
10. Maximize qualified retirement plans with tax-efficient investments.
11. Retain a professional medical practice valuation firm for the practice buy-in.
12. Update wills for bypass marital trust-testamentary planning; including guardians for the kids.

SAMPLE MEGA PLAN FOR A MATURE PHYSICIAN

At age 55, Dr. Joseph B. Good was a board-certified and practicing internist and partner of his group. Susan, age 55, was the office manager for Dr. Good's practice, allowing her to provide professional accounting services to her husband's office and thereby maximizing benefits to the couple from the practice. Daughter Cee was 24 years old, and her brother Douglas was 22 years old. The preceding suggestions had been implemented. They upgraded their home and modest lifestyle within the confines of their current earnings. They did not invade their grandfather's original inheritance, which grew to $1,834,045. Reallocation was needed. The other financial planning aspects of their lives had gone unaddressed. Retirement and estate planning issues prompted another revisit of their plan. Their prioritized concerns at this point were as follows:

1. Long-term care issues
2. Retirement implementation
3. Estate planning
4. Business continuity concerns

After thoroughly discussing the gathered financial data and determining their risk profile, the Certified Medical Planner™ professional made the following suggestions to the original plan:

1. Analyze the cost and benefits of long-term care insurance, funded with current income.
2. Reallocate portfolio assets and plan for estate tax with offspring and charitable considerations.
3. Retain a practice valuation firm for sale, with proceeds to maintain their lifestyle until age 70.

$99: ORDER TODAY: AdviceForDoctors@OutLook.com OR MarcinkoAdvisors@msn.com

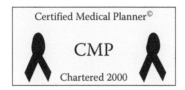

Certified Medical Planner©
CMP
Chartered 2000

(The informed voice of a new generation of fiduciary advisors for healthcare. www.Certified MedicalPlanner.org)

Appendix 3: Financial Investing and Economics Terminology: *Glossary of Important Definitions*

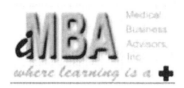

Much has been written and much has been opined on the topic of personal financial planning for physicians and healthcare providers in this textbook. But occasionally, we all still get lost in a wide array of acronyms, jargon, and terms that are constantly changing in this ecosystem. And so, this glossary serves as a ready reference for those who want to know about these definitions in a quick and ready manner.

accounting equation: assets equal liabilities plus owner's (stockholder's) equity.

accounts payable: the amount of money a healthcare organization is obligated to pay vendors. A liability backed by general reputation and credit of the debtor.

accounts receivable: the amount of money a healthcare organization is due from insured patients, payers, vendors, or other sources.

accretion: the difference between bond price at original discount purchase and current par value; asset increase through internal growth and expansion.

accrual basis of accounting: a method of accounting which attempts to match health entity revenues with expenses and claims by recognizing revenue when a service is rendered and expense when the liability is incurred irrespective of the receipt or disbursement of cash.

accrued interest: the interest earned, but not received, when a buyer purchases a hospital or other bond (debt) from a bondholder. The buyer owes the bondholder interest for the period of time the bondholder held the bond. Because interest is paid semi-annually, the period of time that has elapsed is the accrual period.

acid test ratio: a liquidity ratio that measures how much cash and marketable securities are available to pay all current liabilities of a healthcare business organization (i.e., cash and marketable securities/current liabilities).

additional paid-in capital: common stock plus donated capital or paid-in-capital excess of par value.

ADV: a two-part form filed by investment advisors who register with the Securities and Exchange Commission (SEC), as required under the Investment Advisers Act. ADV part ii information must be provided to potential investors and made available to current investors.

after market: a marketplace for a security either over-the-counter (OTC) or on an exchange after an initial public offering has been made.

alpha: the measure of the amount of a stock's expected return that is not related to the stock's sensitivity to market volatility. It measures the residual non-market influences that contribute to a securities risk unique to each security. Alpha uses beta as a measure of risk, a benchmark, and a risk-free rate of return (usually T-bills) to compare the actual performance with the expected performance. For example, a fund with a beta of .80 in a market that rises 10% is expected to rise 8%. If the risk-free return is 3%, the alpha would be—0.6%, calculated as follows:

$$(Fund\ return - Risk\text{-}free\ return) - (Beta \times Excess\ return) = Alpha$$

$$(8\% - 3\%) - [0.8 \times (10\% - 3\%)] = -.6\%$$

A positive alpha indicates out performance while a negative alpha means under performance.

American depository receipt (ADR): a receipt evidencing shares of a foreign corporation held on deposit or under the control of a U.S. banking institution; it is used to facilitate transactions and expedite transfer of beneficial ownership for a foreign security in the United States. Everything is done in dollars and the adr holder doesn't have voting rights; essentially, the same as an American depository share (ADS).

amortize: to pay-off or liquidate a debt on an installment basis.

angel: a wealthy private investor.

annuity: a series of equal periodic payments. An investment product in which an investor contributes money into a plan and then elects to receive pay-out in a fixed or variable amount, usually at retirement. Two important features of this product: (1) Tax deferred growth of earnings during the accumulation period. However, it is important to note that when you elect to receive payment you will be taxed at ordinary income rates on everything exceeding the cost basis. (2) The annuity will provide lifetime retirement income for the annuitant through the mortality guarantee.

arbitrage: the simultaneous purchase and sale of the same or equal securities, such as convertible securities, in such a way as to take advantage of price differences prevailing in separate markets. the risk is usually minimal and the profit correspondingly small.

arbitrage price theory (APT): a multivariable systematic risks method to estimate the cost of equity capital.

ask price: (1) the price at which a healthcare security, stocks, bonds, or mutual fund's shares can be purchased. The asking or offering price means the net asset value per share plus sales charge. (2) The offer side of a quote.

at-the-money: an option is at-the-money if the underlying security is selling for the same price as the exercise price of the option.

auction market: a market for securities, typically found on a national securities exchange, in which trading in a particular security is conducted at a specific location with all qualified persons at that post able to bid or offer securities against orders via outcry.

average annual total return: the average annual profit or loss realized at the end of a specified calendar period, assuming all dividends and capital gains, stated as the percentage gained or lost per dollar invested.

back-end load: a surrender charge deducted in some financial and insurance products. Most have a decreasing back-end load that generally disappears completely after a certain number of years.

balanced fund: investment companies that strive to minimize market risks while at the same time earning reasonable current income with varying percentages of bond, preferred, and common stocks.

balance sheet: one of four major financial statements for a healthcare organization. It presents a summary of assets, liabilities, and net assets for a specific date. A condensed statement showing the nature and amount of assets and liabilities, shown in dollar amounts what the company owns, what it owes, and the ownership interest (shareholders' equity).

balance sheet equation: Assets = Liabilities plus Stockholder's (owner's) Equity.

barbell portfolio: bond distribution where most maturity dates either fall at the short-term or long-term end of a given time period, with few intermediate maturity bonds.

basis: property basis is the original cost adjusted by charges (such as deductions for depreciation) or credits (such as capitalized expenditures for improvements); it sets the base for calculating depreciation and assists in establishing the gain or loss on sale of the property. An investor's basis establishes the gain or loss on sale of the investor's unit(s) and sets an upper limit on his ability to take any losses generated by a property.

basis point: one tenth, of 1% of yield. If a yield increases from 8.25% to 8.50%, the difference is referred to as a 25 basis point increase. The exchange rate where: one percentage point equals 100 basis points (bps).

bear market: a declining securities market in terms of prices.

beta: systemic risk measurement benchmark correlating with a change in a specific index. the measure of a stock's volatility relative to the market, where a beta lower than 1 means the stock is less sensitive than the market as a whole; higher than 1 indicates the stock is more volatile than the market. The healthcare industry is considered to be increasingly volatile and hence possess a higher beta.

bid price: the price at which a buyer is willing to buy an option or stock.

Black–Scholes model: a sophisticated options pricing method.

blue chip: the common stock of a large, well-known corporation with a relatively stable record of earnings and dividend payments over a period of many years.

book-value: cost of capital assets minus accumulated depreciation for health care, or other organization. The net asset value of a healthcare companies common stock. This is calculated by dividing the net tangible assets of the company (minus the par value of any preferred stock the company has) by the number of common shares outstanding.

bucket shop: illegal brokerage firm that is slow to execute client orders to augment profits.

bull market: a rising securities market in terms of price.

capital asset: all assets except property held for resale in the normal course of business (inventory), trade accounts and notes receivable, and depreciable property and real estate used in a trade, healthcare, or other business.

capital asset pricing model (CAPM): an economic model that uses beta and market return to help investors evaluate risk return trade-offs in investment decisions.

capital structure: the permanent and long-term financing structure of a healthcare or other organization including long-term debt, preferred stock, and net worth; but not including short-term debt or reserve accountants.

Chinese wall: artificial and imaginary separation between investments, research, and financial departments of a brokerage house.

churning: the practice of a provider seeing a patient more often than is medically necessary, primarily to increase revenue through an increased number of visits. A practice, in violation of SEC rules, where a salesperson affects a series of transactions in a customer's account which are excessive in size and/or frequency in relation to the size and investment objectives of the account. An insurance agent who is churning an account is normally seeking to maximize the income (in commissions, sales credits, or mark-ups) derived from the account.

circuit breakers: exchange methods to temporarily stop trading following pre-specified market drops.

clone fund: a mutual fund that mimics or attempts to match another, with reduced fees and expenses.

convertible preferred stock: preferred stock that can be exchanged for common stock.

correction: sharp reverse or downward movement in securities or commodities, prices, usually greater than 10%.

coupon: (1) a detachable part of a bond which evidences interest due. The coupon specifies the date, place, and dollar amount of interest payable, among other matters. Some older coupons may be redeemed semi-annually, by detaching them from bonds and presenting them to the paying agent or bank for collection. (2) The term is also used colloquially to refer to a security's interest rate.

covered call: an option strategy in which a call option is written against a long stock (stock held in a client's portfolio).

covered put: an option strategy in which a put option is written against a sufficient amount of cash (or T-bills) to pay for the stock purchase if the short position is assigned.

covered short: the purchase of commodities or securities to cover a short position.

cram down: slang term for the forced acceptance by stockholders of unfavorable terms in a corporate merger or acquisition.

current assets: assets used or consumed within 12 months. Cash plus any other assets that will be sold, converted into cash, or used during a hospital's "cash conversion cycle," or the cycle of cash to medical services, to third-party insurance payer, and back to cash, again. Most commonly included with cash are marketable securities, patient accounts receivable, and inventory.

current liabilities: as a rule, debts or obligations that must be met within a year. On a stock, the annual dividend divided by the current ask price; on a bond, the annual interest dividend by the current market value. "What you get, divided by what you pay."

current ratio: a liquidity measure to determine how easily current debt may be paid (current assets/current liabilities).

current yield: on a stock, the annual dividend divided by the current ask price; on a bond, the annual interest dividend by the current market value. "What you get, divided by what you pay."

debentures: a type of bond that is issued by hospital or other corporations. Debentures do not have a special lien on the corporation's property, but the bondholders do have first claim on all assets not already pledged. Next are subordinated debentures, which have a claim on assets after the more senior debt is satisfied.

deflation: a sustained period of falling interest rates, prices, and economics.

delta: relationship between the price of an option and its underlying futures contract or stock price.

derivative: derivatives are financial arrangements between two parties whose payments are derived from the performance of an agreed-upon benchmark. They can be issued based on currencies, commodities, government or corporate debt, home mortgages, stocks, interest rates, or any combination of the above. The primary purpose of derivatives is to hedge investment risk. In the case of debt securities, derivatives can swap floating interest-rate risk for a fixed interest rate. Because the possibility of a reduced interest rate is the most important risk to the investor's capital, coupled with changes in currency values, derivatives can be an important investment tool. Derivatives can be risky if they involve high leverage: both parties to the transaction are exposed to market moves with little capital changing hands. Remember, when the market moves are favorable, the leverage provides a high return compared with the relatively small amount of investment capital actually at risk. However, when market moves are unfavorable, the reverse is true: enormous losses may be incurred. International healthcare corporations are major investors in derivatives, because exports can suffer upon currency fluctuations or the corporations want to change a floating rate liability to a fixed-rate obligation. However, even though corporations were originally the main purchasers of derivatives (primarily because of the high minimum transaction size), the opportunity is now available for some individuals to take advantage of the benefits of derivatives. This is done primarily through private partnerships (not generally available to the public).

dilutive effect: the lowering of the book or market value of the shares of a company's stock as a result of more shares outstanding. A company's initial registration may include more shares than are initially issued when the company goes public for the first time. Later, an issue of more stock by a company (called a "primary offering," distinguished from the "initial public offering") dilutes the existing shares outstanding. Also, earnings-per-share calculations are said to be "fully diluted" when all common stock equivalents (convertible securities, rights, and warrants) are included. "Fully diluted" numbers are used in analysis when there is a likelihood of conversion or exercise of rights and warrants.

divided account (Western account): a method for determining liability stated in the agreement among underwriters in which each member of an underwriting syndicate is liable only for the amount of its participation in the issue, and not for any unsold portion of the participation amounts allocated to the other underwriters.

dividends: distributions to stockholders earned and declared by a corporate healthcare or hospital board of directors.

duration: the average time to collect a bond's principal and interest payment. A measure of volatility, expressed in years, taking into consideration all of the cash flows produced over the life of a bond. For example, if the duration of a bond is five years, then the price of the bond changes 5% for every 1% change in interest rates.

Dutch auction: auction market where price is reduced until sold (the U.S. T-bill system).

earnings per share (EPS): the amount of a company's profit available to each share of common stock. EPS = net income (after taxes and preferred dividends) divided by number of outstanding shares.

Eastern account: an undivided brokerage account.

economic profit: the difference between total healthcare revenue and the cost of all related inputs used by an entity over time; net present value (NPV).

efficient market hypothesis (theory): belief that all market prices and movements reflect all that can be known about an investment. If all the information available is already reflected in stock prices, research aimed at finding undervalued assets or special situations is useless.

either/or order: an order consisting of a limit and a stop for the same security at different prices. Execution of one order will cancel the other.

elastic demand: occurs when the price of elasticity of demand for healthcare goods, products, or services exceed one (1) unit.

equity risk premium: the risk-free rate-of-return, plus the rate-of-return to reflect the risk of the healthcare business entity over the risk-free-rate.

equivalent pretax yield on taxable bond (EPYTB): municipal bond yield/1−tax rate.

European option: an option that can be exercised only on the expiration date.

ex-dividend: occurs when dividends are declared by a company's board of directors, they are payable on a certain date ("payable date") to shareholders recorded on the company's books as of a stated earlier date ("record date"). Purchasers of the stock on or after the record date are not entitled to receive the recently declared dividend, so the ex-dividend date is the number of days it takes to settle a trade before the record date (currently one business days). A stock's price on its ex-dividend date appears in the newspaper with an x beside it.

factoring: the sale of medical accounts receivable at a discount.

fair market value (FMV): a legal term variously interpreted by the courts, but generally meaning the price at which a willing buyer will buy and a willing seller will sell an asset, in an open free market with full disclosure.

fill-or-kill (FOK) order: an order that requires immediate purchase or sale of a specified amount of stock. If the order cannot be filled immediately, it is automatically canceled (killed).

fixed budget: a financial plan in which specifically allocated amounts do not vary with level of activity or volume; static budget.

flip: the purchase of stock shares, especially in an IPO, and immediately selling them for profit.

float: time delay in the billing and collect cycle.

fourth market: direct institutional trading without the use of an intermediary or brokerage firm.

front-end load: funds paid at the outset of the direct participation program that does not contribute materially to the actual investment vehicle. Front-end load typically consists of distributions to general partners, organizational fees, or acquisition fees.

front-running: form of market manipulation where a broker/dealer delays processing of a large customer trade in an underlying security until the firm can execute an option's trade in that security in anticipation of the client's trade impacts on the underlying security.

fundamental analysis: this type of analysis uses a quantitative (using numbers) approach to market forecasting based on an analysis of corporate balance sheets and income statements. A corporation's strengths and weaknesses, as shown by arithmetic formulas and other measurements of economic and industry trends, are used to predict future price movements of its stocks and bonds.

futures contract: a contract calling for the delivery of a specific quantity of a physical good or a financial instrument (or the cash value) at some specific date in the future. There are exchange-traded futures contracts with standardized terms, and there are OTC futures contracts with negotiated terms.

geometric mean: the Nth root of the product of "n" numbers.

ghost: one who works with two or more market makers to manipulate stock prices; unethical behavior.

glamor stock: equities with wide public exposure, owned by institutions, and followed by many stock analysts with high growth rate potential.

GNP deflator: the ratio of real to nominal GNP as an index of average prices used to deflate GNP.

going long: purchasing and owning securities outright for potential profit.

going short: selling securities otherwise not owned.

good till canceled order: a limit securities order that remains valid indefinitely, until executed or canceled by the customer.

gross domestic product (GDP): the total current market value of all goods and services produced domestically during a given period; differs from the gross national product (GNP) by excluding net income that residents earn abroad.

growth fund: a mutual fund whose primary investment objective is long-term growth of capital. It invests principally in common stocks with growth potential.

growth income fund: a mutual fund whose aim is to provide for a degree of both income and long-term growth.

gunslinger: an aggressive portfolio manager prone to risk taking in order to achieve higher investment returns.

haircut: slang term for a very steep broker-commission.

hammering the market: an intense stock market sell-off period.

hostile takeover: corporate shareholder transfer (takeover) against the wishes of management and directors, and usually financed by debt, such as junk bonds (low investment grade debt), and as in a leveraged buy-out (LBO) situation.

hot issue: a security that is expected to trade in the aftermarket at a premium over the public offering price.

illiquid: a dearth of cash flow to meet current obligations and/or maturing debt.

imputed interest: rate or amount of interest considered to have been paid; although not actually paid.

income elasticty of demand: a patient-consumer purchase-sensitivity measurement compared to each 1% change in income.

income in-respect-of-a-decedent: amounts due and payable to a decedent at his or her death because of some right to income. [IRC §691(c)(2)]

income stock: stock purchased for its income and dividend producing ability rather than its growth potential.

indenture: a written agreement between the issuer and creditors by which the terms of a debt issue are set forth, such as rate of interest, means of payment, maturity date, terms of prior payment of principal, collateral, priorities of claims, trustee.

index: a stock market indicator, derived in the same way as an average, but from a broader sampling of securities.

inefficient markets: securities or commodities that do not reflect the risk–return relationship, allowing for profit or loss.

inelastic demand: occurs when the price elasticity of demand for healthcare services is equal to, or greater than zero but less than 1.

inelastic supply: occurs when the price elasticity of supply for healthcare services is equal to, or greater than zero but less than 1.

inflation factor: a premium loading to provide for future increases in medical costs and loss payments resulting from inflation. A loading to provide for future increases resulting from inflation in medical costs and loss payments.

insider: technically, an officer or director of a company or anyone owning 10% of a company's stock. the broader definition includes anyone with nonpublic information about a company.

insider trading: the act, in violation of sec rule 10b-5 and the insiders trading act of 1988, of purchasing or selling securities (or derivative instruments based on those securities) based on information known to the party purchasing or selling the securities in his capacity as an insider (i.e., as an employee of the issuer of the securities) or as a result of information illicitly provided to him by an insider. Extensive case law exists concerning the varieties of acts that may be considered to be insider trading or the circumstances in which a person may be considered to be an insider or to be trading illegally on the basis of inside information.

inverted yield curve: long-term interest rates that are lower than short-term rates; unusual graphical situation.

January effect: the historic tendency of smaller stocks to rise in early January each year.

Jesen index: performance measurement comparing absolute realized investment returns with risk-adjusted returns.

junk bond: a speculative security with a rating of BB or lower. Sometimes called a "High Yield" security.

kappa: volatility measurement and pricing model for financial derivatives.

kiting: to drive securities prices higher through financial market manipulations or to take advantage of check cashing float time; unethical.

Kondratief, Nikolai; wave: Russian economist who suggested that financial markets can be very long; up to 50 years in length.

ladder: a series of increasingly longer and revolving debt issues to accommodate interest rate risks and changes regardless of economic cycle.

Laffer, Arthur; curve: suggestion that domestic economic output grows with decreased marginal income tax rates.

lagging economic indicator: an economic benchmark such as the unemployment rate, which changes after the economy has started to follow a particular trend.

law of supply: principle suggesting that the higher the price of a healthcare good or service, the greater the quantity that sellers are willing and able to make over time.

leading economic indicator: an economic benchmark such as new housing starts, which changes before the economy has started to follow a particular trend.

levels: level of service for NASDAQ trading firms:

> Level 1—A single average price quote for those not trading OTC.
>
> Level 2—Level 1 plus trade reports, executions, negotiations, networks, clearing; and bid–ask price quotes for all firms and customers.
>
> Level 3—Levels 1 and 2, plus the ability to enter quotes, execute orders, and send information, for and by market makers.

LIBOR: London interbank offered rate is the rate international banks charge each other and varies throughout each business day reflecting global economic conditions. CX.

liquid asset: asset easily and quickly converted into cash without price loss.

liquidity ratios: relationships of short-term obligation payment abilities (i.e., quick ratio, current ratio, etc.).

load: the amount added to net premiums (risk factor minus interest factor) to cover the company's operating expenses and contingencies. The loading includes the cost of securing new business, collecting premiums, and general management expenses. Precisely, it is the excess of the gross health insurance premiums over net premiums.

long bond: government bonds with a maturity time frame greater than 10 years; usually 30-year U.S. treasuries, which suspended issuance in 2001, but was reinstituted on February 9, 2006.

long position: a term used to describe either an open position that is expected to benefit from a rise in the price of the underlying stock (such as long call, short put, or long stock) or an open position resulting from an opening purchase transaction such as long call, long put, or long stock; securities bought or owned outright.

maintenance call: sometimes called a "margin call"; a demand on a customer with a margin account to deposit cash or securities to cover account minimums required by regulatory agencies and the brokerage firm. Because these minimums are based on the current value of the securities in the account, maintenance calls can occur as a result of movements in the market price of securities.

margin: the amount of equity required in an account carried on credit, presently 50% of total cost for eligible stock under federal reserve regulations, OR, corporate revenues less expenses. An amount, usually a percentage, is added to an index to determine the interest rate for a variable loan at each adjustment period. For example, if the index is at 5.0, and the margin is 1.5, the interest rate is 6.5%.

mark-to-the market: as the market value of a margined security declines, the broker/dealer will demand more in cash to maintain the minimum requirement. The written notice for such demand is a mark to the market.

mark-up: the fee charged by a broker/dealer acting as a dealer when he buys a security from a market maker and sells it to his customer at a higher price. The markup is included in the sale price and is not itemized separately in the confirmation except on a simultaneous (risk less) transaction.

mezzanine level: the time period just prior to the initial public offering (IPO) of a healthcare organization or other company.

money market account: a checking account that earns interest generally comparable to money market funds, although the rates paid by any particular bank may be higher or lower.

money supply: the amount of money in circulation. The money supply measures currently (1985) used by the Federal Reserve System are

- M1 – Currency in circulation + demand deposit + other check-type deposits.
- M2–M1 + savings and small denomination time deposits + overnight repurchase agreements at commercial banks + overnight Eurodollars + money market mutual fund shares.
- M3–M2 + large-denomination time deposits (Jumbo CDs) + term repurchase agreements.
- M4–M3 + other liquid assets (such as term Eurodollars, bankers acceptances, commercial paper, Treasury securities, and the U.S. Savings Bonds).

multiplier effect: money supply expansion from Federal Reserve member banks that lend money enhancing their supply.

mutual company: a company that has no capital stock or stockholders. Rather, it is owned by its policy owners and managed by a board of directors chosen by the policy owners. Any earnings, in addition to those necessary for the operation of the company and contingency reserves, are returned to the policy owners in the form of policy dividends.

mutualization: the process of converting a stock insurance company into a mutual insurance company, accomplished by having the company buy in and retire its own shares.

naked option: an uncovered option position. When the writer (seller) of a call option owns the underlying stock (said to be "long" the stock), the option position is a "covered call." if the writer (seller) of a put option is short the stock, then the position is a "covered put." Writing a covered call is the most conservative options strategy, but writing a covered put is the most dangerous because there is no limit to how high the stock can go and thus to how great the loss can be on the short sale.

negative yield curve: graphical illustration where long-term interest rates are less than short-term interest rates.

negatively correlated: two financial securities that move in opposite directions.

net working capital: the difference between current asset and current liabilities for a health care or other entity.

net worth: the surpluses and capital of a healthcare entity; but may occasionally refer to the common shareholder's position, or assets minus liabilities plus stockholders equity.

no-load mutual fund: mutual funds offered directly to the public at net asset value with no sales charge.

nominal: expressed in current dollars or actual money amounts.

notes payable: a legal obligation to pay creditors or holders of a valid lien or claim.

notes receivable: a written promise for the future collection of cash.

off balance sheet financing: the acquisition of assets or services with debt that is not recorded on the balance sheet, but may appear as a small footnote.

open-end fund: a mutual fund formed to continuously issue and buy back shares to meet investor demand. The share price is determined by the market value of the securities held by the fund's portfolio, and it may be higher or lower than the original purchase price. Open-end funds can range from load to no-load.

orphan stock: stocks neglected by research analysts.

out-of-the-money: an option that has no intrinsic value. A call option is out-of-the-money when the exercise price is higher than the underlying security's price. A put is out-of-the-money when the exercise price is lower than the underlying security's price.

over-the-counter (OTC) market: a market for securities made up of securities broker/dealers who may or may not be members of securities exchanges. Over the counter is a market conducted anywhere other than on an exchange.

paid-in-capital: money received by a corporation from investors, for equity.

par value: for common stocks, the value on the books of the corporation. It has little to do with market value or even the original price of shares at first issuance. The difference between par and the price at first issuance is carried on the books of a corporation as "paid-in capital" or "capital surplus." Par value for preferred stocks is also liquidating value and the value on which dividends (expressed as a percentage) are paid, generally $100 per share.

payment-in-kind: securities that pay interest or dividend payment in additional securities of the same kind.

penny stocks: stocks selling for under $1; usually highly speculative.

Phantom stock plan: an arrangement under which an employee is allowed the benefits of owning employer securities even though shares are not actually issued to the employee.

Phillips curve: relationship between interest rates and unemployment levels.

pink sheets: daily publication of wholesale prices of OTC stocks that are generally too small to be listed in newspapers; historically named for the color of the paper used. A list issued by the National Quotation Bureau identifying market makers dealing in corporate equity securities in the OTC market.

plow back: reinvesting profits back into a business, rather than distributing it as dividends or profit to shareholders, investors, or capital suppliers.

plus tick: a transaction on a stock exchange at a price higher than the price of the last transaction.

prime rate: the cost of capital or interest rate a bank charges its most credit worthy customer or institutions.

put bonds: put bonds allow bondholders to give bonds (put) back to the issuer at par on specified dates prior to maturity. Put bonds have either a fixed or variable interest rate and may have single or multiple tender dates. They can also be either mandatory (in which case the investor has a specified period of time to keep the bonds at the new rate) or optional (in which case the investor has a specified time period to tender the bonds).

put option: an instrument that grants the holder the right to sell a stated number of shares (typically 100) of the underlying security within a stated period of time at the exercise price.

put writer: one who receives a financial premium and accepts for a time period, the obligation to buy an underlying security for a specific price at the put buyer's discretion.

qubes (QQQQ): NASD technology-laden tracking exchange-traded fund (ETF) index on the American Stock Exchange (AMEX).

quick asset ratio: the ratio of cash, accounts receivable, and marketable securities to current liabilities.

quick assets: cash or those assets that can quickly be converted into cash.

quick ratio: a measure of healthcare entity financial liquidity: (cash + marketable securities + ARs/current liabilities); acid test.

raider: one who buys controlling stock in a company and instills new senior management.

ratio analysis: a method of analyzing a healthcare or other entities' financial condition calculated from line items in the financial statements. There are four major categories: liquidity, profitability, capitalization, and activity.

real estate investment trust (REIT): a company that manages a portfolio of real estate holdings for capital appreciation, income, or both; type of mutual fund.

real GNP: gross national product calculated from a base, nominal or reference year.

rebalance: to sell or buy securities in a portfolio in order to return to prescribed set allocation or proportional constraints.

registered representative examination: the series seven (7) securities licensing examination for stock brokers [aka FAs].

Regulation D: the part of the Securities Act of 1933 that deals with private securities placements. The major provisions deal with accredited investors and both dollar limits (aggregation) and investor limits (integration). Under this regulation, private placements meeting the stipulations are exempt from registration with the sec.

Regulation T: Federal Reserve Bank (FRB) regulation that explains the conduct and operation of general and cash accounts within the offices of a securities broker/dealer firm, prescribing a code of conduct for the effective use and supervision of credit. According to Regulation T, one may borrow up to 50% of the purchase price of securities that can be purchased on margin. This is known as the initial margin. Also, it dictates that payment must be received no later than 1-business day after the trade and what happens if you do not pay on time.

re-hypothecation: stocker–broker–dealer pledge of securities in a margin account as collateral for a loan.

restricted security: a portfolio security not available to the public at large, which requires registration with the Securities and Exchange Commission before it may be sold publicly; a "private placement" frequently referred to as a "letter stock."

risk arbitrage: a purchase and/or short sale of the same or potentially equal securities at prices that do not immediately guarantee a profit. Alternatively it is to play one security against another to take advantage of a disparity in price. Usually used during corporate takeover attempts.

round lot: a unit of trading or a multiple thereof. On the New York Stock Exchange, stocks are traded in round lots of 100 shares for active stocks and 10 shares for inactive ones. Bonds are traded as percentages of $1000, with municipal bonds traded in minimum blocks of five bonds ($5000 worth).

rule of 72: 72 divided by interest rate equals the time period in years for a doubling of a principle sum.

Santa Claus rally: historic rise in stock market prices between New Year and Christmas Day.

Sarbanes–Oxley Act (SARBOX): 2002 Corporate Responsibility Act (CRA), covering financial, accounting, certification, and new protections governing securities fraud.

secondary market: (1) the aftermarket for securities; the resale of outstanding securities. (2) A public offering by selling stockholders. If listed on the NYSE, a member firm may be employed to facilitate such an offering in an OTC net transaction for a purchaser, with prior approval of the Exchange. Both member and nonmember broker/dealers can participate in this distribution.

secondary offering: a sale of a large block of securities already issued by a corporation and held by a third party. Because the block is so large, the sale is usually handled by "investment bankers" who may form a "syndicate" and peg the price of the shares close to current market value.

Securities Investor Protection Corporation (SIPC): a government-sponsored, private corporation that guarantees repayment of money and securities in customer accounts valued at up to $500,000 per separate customer ($100,000 cash), in the event of a broker/dealer bankruptcy.

securitization: the act of aggregating debt or companies in a risk pool, as with Physician Practice Management Corporations (PPMCS), and then floating new securities with reduced risk backed by the pool.

seller's market: situation when there is more demand for a healthcare good, product, or service, than available supply.

sell-stop order: a securities order that becomes a market order to sell if and when someone trades a round-lot at or below the stop price used to protect a long position.

series 3: sales license for commodities futures.

series 6: sales license for mutual funds and variable annuities.

series 7: sales license for all types of securities products, with the exception of commodities futures.

series 26: supervisory license for investment company and variable annuity products.

series 63: license to sell securities and render investment advice.

Sharpe, William; index: a risk-adjusted ratio measure of financial performance correlates the return-in-excess of the risk-free-rate of return, by a portfolio's standard deviation.

shelf registration: corporate ability to sell pre-SEC registered shares under favorable economic climates with a minimum of paperwork.

short: selling a security not owned.

short-against-the-box: a short sale made when the investor owns securities identical to those sold short. The purpose is to defer, for tax purposes, recognition of gain or loss with respect to the sale of securities "in the box."

short cover: long (owned) purchase of securities by a short seller investor to replace those borrowed short (un-owned) sale.

short sale: the sale of a security (i.e., stocks and bonds) before it has been acquired. An investor anticipates that the price of a stock will fall, so he sells securities borrowed from the brokerage firm. The securities must be delivered to the firm at a certain date (the "delivery date"), at which time the investor expects to be able to buy the shares at a lower price to "cover his position."

skimming: the practice in health programs paid on a prepayment or capitation basis, and in health insurance, of seeking to enroll only the healthiest people as a way of controlling program costs.

sleeper: security with little investor interest but with great potential.

small firm effect: the tendency of securities of smaller corporations to outperform larger ones.

spot price: the currency price of a commodity.

spread: (1) the difference in value between the bid and offering prices. (2) The difference between the public offering price and the amount received by the issuer.

spread (option): purchase and sale of option contracts of the same class with different expiration dates and/or strike prices.

stagflation: a time of inflation without GNP growth.

street name: the registration of securities in the name of a brokerage firm, rather than the buyer.

stochastic index: technical tool to determine a financial market's over-sold or over-bought condition; risk dampening method.

stock buyback: a corporation may repurchase shares outstanding on the open market and retire them as "treasury shares." this antidilutive action increases earnings per share, which consequently raises the price of the outstanding shares. Companies often announce a "share repurchase plan" when insiders feel the company is undervalued; the action strengthens the company and helps preclude a takeover.

stop-limit order: an order that becomes a limit order to sell when someone creates a round lot transaction at, or below, the stop price.

stopp-loss: insuring with a third party against a risk that an MCO cannot financially and totally manage. For example, a comprehensive prepaid health plan can self-insure hospitalization costs with one or more insurance carriers.

stop order: a sale or purchase in order to preserve gains or limit securities losses.

stop payment: a request to a bank not to honor or allow the payment of a check after it has been delivered but before it has been presented.

street: the slang term for Wall Street.

suicide pill: any anticorporate takeover strategy that puts itself (company) in jeopardy.

supply curve: illustration of how quantity supplied varies with the price of a healthcare good or service.

supply side economics: financial incentives used to influence the aggregate supply curve.

supply side shock: an abrupt change in aggregate supply.

support level: security price level bottom caused by investor demand.

SWAP: a sale of a security and the simultaneous purchase of another security, for purposes of enhancing the investor's holdings. The swap may be used to achieve desired tax results, to gain income or principal, or to alter various features of a bond portfolio, including call protection, diversification or consolidation, and marketability of holdings.

sweetner: any feature added in addition to-a-securities offering to make it more attractive to investors, for purchase.

synthetic position: a strategy involving two or more instruments that has the same risk/reward profile as a strategy involving only one instrument. The following list summarizes the six primary synthetic positions.

> **Synthetic long call**—A long stock position combined with a long put.
> **Synthetic long put**—A short stock position combined with a long call.
> **Synthetic long stock**—A long call position combined with a short put.
> **Synthetic short call**—A short stock position combined with a short put.
> **Synthetic short put**—A long stock position combined with a short call.
> **Synthetic short stock**—A short call position combined with a long put.

tactical asset allocation: active portfolio rebalancing based on relative market attractiveness.

takeover: usually a hostile change in the controlling interest of a corporation with a new management team; typically financed by debt, as in a leveraged buyout (LBO).

technical analysis: an approach to market theory stating that previous price movements, properly interpreted, can indicate future price patterns, too. A technical analyst watches the market, not the company, and is sometimes called a chartist, for obvious reasons.

Ted spread: commodity money price difference that occurs with interest rates between European denominated dollars (Euros) and the U.S. Treasury bills; slang for *Treasury over Euro Dollars.*

ten-bagger: an equity that grows in price by a factor of 10.

thin issue: a small number or volume of securities transactions.

third market: OTC transactions in listed stocks.

tick: a transaction (up or down) on the stock exchange.

ticker symbol: stock symbol used on the ticker tape, in newspapers, or electronically, and so on.

time value of money: money received in the present can earn money over a period of time (making the amount ultimately larger than if the same initial sum was received later). Therefore, both the amount of investment return and the length of time it takes to receive that return affect the rate of return (i.e., the value of the return).

tombstone ad: an ad announcing securities offering which merely gives the size of the offering, the name of the firm or underwriting group from which a prospectus is available, and a disclaimer that the ad is not an offer to sell nor a solicitation of an offer to buy.

ton: slang for $100 million dollars.

Treynor index: a risk-adjusted measure of financial performance that correlates the return-in-excess of the risk-free-rate of return, by a portfolio's systemic risk-of-the-market.

twisting: inducing the termination of a health or life insurance policy in order to purchase a new one, and/or the rapid turnover of securities to generate sales commissions for the agent or broker.

two-sided market: a market with firm bid and ask prices; often requiring a *specialist* to maintain a fair and orderly market.

uncovered option: a short securities option position that is not fully collateralized if notification of assignment should be received. A short call position is uncovered if the writer does not have a long stock position to deliver. A short put position is uncovered if the writer does not have the financial resources available in his or her account to buy the stock.

uncovered put writer: a put writer is uncovered (naked) when that writer does not hold a long put of the same securities class, with an equal or higher exercise price.

undivided account (Eastern account): a method for determining liability stated in a securities underwriting agreement in which each member of the underwriting syndicate is liable for any unsold portion of a securities issue according to each member's percentage participation in the syndicate.

value investing: a style of investing which searches for undervalued companies in hope of sharing in the future gains.

velocity of money: the rate at which the money supply is used to make transactions for final goods and services.

venture capital: private capital supplied for a risky start-up business; usually in return for an equity share of the corporation.

vulture fund: a fund of depressed or below market rate securities or other assets.

wallaper: worthless or near worthless securities.

warrants: certificates that allow the holder to buy a security at a set price, either within a certain time period or in perpetuity. Warrants are usually issued for common stock, at a higher price than current market price, in conjunction with bonds or preferred stock as an added inducement to buy. An inducement attached to new securities giving the purchaser a long-term (usually 5–10 years) privilege of subscribing to one or more shares of stock reserved for him by the corporation from its unmissed or treasure stock reserve.

wash sale: when an investor sells a security at a loss, he can use that realized loss to offset a realized gain in order to reduce his tax liability on that gain. If the seller reacquires that or a substantially identical security within a 30-day period prior to or after the sale, he will lose the tax benefit of that realized loss.

whisper numbers: unofficial projected corporate earning estimates by Wall Street analysts; Wall Street financial performance gossip.

white knight: friendly investor sought to save a company from a hostile takeover.

Wilshire index: an equity stock index composed as a surrogate for 5000 firms.

window dressing: portfolio manager year-end buying or selling for shareholder presentations.

wirehouse: a stock brokerage firm; usually retail or boutique and/or national or regional in nature.

wrap account: a discretionary brokerage securities account where all sales, administrative fees, and commissions are included in an annual percentage-based management fee (1–3%).

yellow sheets: pink-sheet "bid" and "ask" OTC price listings for a market maker in corporate bonds.

yield (rate of return): the dividends or interest paid by a company on its securities, expressed as percentage of the current price or of the price of original acquisition.

yield curve: curvilinear relationship between time to maturity, and yield, for a specific asset class. a graph that plots market yields on securities of equivalent quality but different maturities, at a given point in time. The vertical axis represents the yields, while the horizontal axis depicts time to maturity. The term structure of interest rates, as reflected by the yield curve, will vary according to market conditions, resulting in a variety of yield curve configurations:

> **Normal or positive yield curve**—Indicates that short-term securities have a lower interest rate than long-term securities.
>
> **Inverted or negative yield curve**—Reflects the situation of short-term rates exceeding long-term rates.
>
> **Flat yield curve**—Reflects the situation when short- and long-term rates are about the same.

yo-yo-stock: an equity whose price fluctuates in an often wild manner.

zero coupon bond: a bond that pays both principal and interest at maturity. These debt instruments pay interest only at maturity, as compared with semi-annual interest payments on treasuries. Zero coupon bonds generate no coupon payments whatsoever throughout the life of the security. They are sold at a discount to the face value of the bond, and as the maturity date moves closer, the price of the bond will move toward par. Therefore, the investment return comes entirely from the price increase between the time of purchase and the maturity date (or redemption date, if it is sold prior to maturity). The coupon income is not reinvested and thus the potential income derived from reinvestment is not considered in valuing the zero's investment performance. Zero coupon bonds can be applied in a variety of ways:

- STRIPS is an acronym for Separate Trading of Registered Interest and Principal Securities. STRIPS consists of either the interest or principal on the U.S. Treasury bonds. They are direct obligations of the U.S. government and are considered the safest and most liquid of all zero coupon bonds. They have maturities from 6 months to 30 years.
- CATS are an acronym for Certificates of Accrual on Treasury Securities. These are physical certificates representing cash flows of the U.S. Treasury bonds that are held in a separate trust. Because CATS represent cash flows of treasury bonds, they are considered to be backed by the government. They have maturities from 1 to 22 years.

zero-minus tick: a transaction on the Stock Exchange at a price equal to that of the preceding transaction but lower than the last different price.

zero-plus tick: a transaction on the Stock Exchange at a price equal to that of the preceding transaction but higher than the last different price.

zeta: a type of volatile derivative pricing model; vega, kappa, omega, or sigma.

zombies: insolvent or bankrupt companies that are still in operation (i.e., dot com zombies).

ACKNOWLEDGMENTS

To James Nash of the Investment Training Institute in Tucker, Georgia and Jeff Kuest, CFA, CFP®, founder and managing principal of Counterpoint Capital Advisers, Lake Oswego, Oregon.

FURTHER READING

Marcinko, DE and Hetico, HR: *The Business of Medical Practice*, 3rd edition. Springer Publishing, New York, 2010.

Marcinko, DE and Hetico, HR: *Dictionary of Health Economics and Finance*. Springer Publishing, New York, 2007.

Marcinko, DE and Hetico, HR: *Dictionary of Health Information Technology and Security*. Springer Publishing, New York, 2008.

Marcinko, DE and Hetico, HR: *Dictionary of Health Insurance and Managed Care*. Springer Publishing, New York, 2006.

Marcinko, DE and Hetico, HR: *Financial Management of Hospitals*. Productivity Press, Boca Raton, FL, 2014.

Marcinko, DE and Hetico, HR: *Hospitals and Healthcare Organizations*. Productivity Press, Boca Raton, FL, 2013.

Appendix 4: Sources of Medical Practice Management and Health Care Financial Planning and Consulting Information: *Granular Data with Deep Subject Matter Statistics Required*

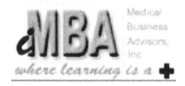

According to Robert James Cimasi, MHA, ASA, FRICS, MCBA, CVA, CM&AA, Certified Medical Planner™, the following are widely accepted sources for medical practice management and health economics and financial planning consulting information, data, and advice [personal communication Health Capital Consultants LLC, St. Louis, MO (www.HealthCapital.com)].

PART I: FINANCIAL AND HEALTH ECONOMICS BENCHMARKING

Financial benchmarking can assist healthcare managers and professional financial advisors (FAs) in understanding the operational and financial status of their organization or practice. The general process of financial benchmarking analysis may include three elements: (1) historical subject benchmarking; (2) benchmarking to industry norms; and (3) financial ratio analysis.

Historical subject benchmarking compares a healthcare organization's most recent performance with its reported performance in the past in order to: examine performance over time; identify changes in performance within the organization (e.g., extraordinary and nonrecurring events); and to predict future performance. As a form of internal benchmarking, historical subject benchmarking avoids issues such as differences in data collection and the use of measurement tools, and benchmarking metrics that often cause problems in comparing two different organizations. However, it is necessary to common size data in order to account for company differences over time that may skew results [1].

Benchmarking to industry norms, analogous to Fong and colleagues' concept of industry benchmarking, involves comparing internal company-specific data to survey data from other organizations within the same industry [2]. This method of benchmarking provides the basis for comparing the subject entity to similar entities, with the purpose of identifying its relative strengths, weaknesses, and related measures of risk.

The process of benchmarking against industry averages or norms will typically involve the following steps:

1. Identification and selection of appropriate surveys to use as a benchmark, that is, to compare with data from the organization of interest. This involves answering the question, "*In which survey would this organization most likely be included?*"
2. If appropriate, recategorization and adjustment of the organization's revenue and expense accounts to optimize data compatibility with the selected survey's structure and definitions (e.g., common sizing).
3. Calculation and articulation of observed differences of organization from the industry averages and norms, expressed either in terms of variance in ratio, dollar unit amounts, or percentages of variation.

Financial ratio analysis typically involves the calculation of ratios that are financial and operational measures representative of the financial status of an enterprise. These ratios are evaluated in terms of their relative comparison to generally established industry norms, which may be expressed as positive or negative trends for that industry sector. The ratios selected may function as several different measures of operating performance or financial condition of the subject entity.

Common types of financial indicators that are measured by ratio analysis include

1. *Liquidity. Liquidity ratios* measure the ability of an organization to meet cash obligations as they become due, that is, to support operational goals. Ratios above the industry mean generally indicate that the organization is in an advantageous position to better support immediate goals. The *current ratio*, which quantifies the relationship between assets and liabilities, is an indicator of an organization's ability to meet short-term obligations. Managers use this measure to determine how quickly assets are converted into cash.
2. *Activity. Activity ratios*, also called *efficiency ratios*, indicate how efficiently the organization utilizes its resources or assets, including cash, accounts receivable, salaries, inventory, property, plant, and equipment. Lower ratios may indicate an inefficient use of those assets.
3. *Leverage. Leverage ratios*, measured as the ratio of long-term debt to net fixed assets, are used to illustrate the proportion of funds, or capital, provided by shareholders (owners) and creditors to aid analysts in assessing the appropriateness of an organization's current level of debt. When this ratio falls equal to or below the industry norm, the organization is typically not considered to be at significant risk.
4. *Profitability.* Indicates the overall net effect of managerial efficiency of the enterprise. To determine the profitability of the enterprise for benchmarking purposes, the analyst should first review and make adjustments to the owner(s) compensation, if appropriate. Adjustments for the market value of the "*replacement cost*" of the professional services provided by the owner are particularly important in the valuation of professional medical practices for the purpose of arriving at an "*economic level*" of profit.

The selection of financial ratios for analysis and comparison to the organization's performance requires careful attention to the homogeneity of data. Benchmarking of intra-organizational data (i.e., internal benchmarking) typically proves to be less variable across several different measurement periods. However, the use of data from external facilities for comparison may introduce variation in measurement methodology and procedure. In the latter case, the use of a standard chart of accounts for the organization or recasting the organization's data to a standard format can effectively facilitate an appropriate comparison of the organization's operating performance and financial status data to survey results.

OPERATIONAL PERFORMANCE BENCHMARKING

Operational benchmarking is used to target noncentral work or business processes for improvement [3]. It is conceptually similar to both process and performance benchmarking, but is generally classified by the application of the results, as opposed to what is being compared [4]. Operational benchmarking studies tend to be smaller in scope than other types of benchmarking, but, like many other types of benchmarking, are limited by the degree to which the definitions and performance measures used by comparing entities differ [5]. Common sizing is a technique used to reduce the variations in measures caused by differences (e.g., definition issues) between the organizations or processes being compared [6].

Common sizing is a technique used to alter financial operating data prior to certain types of benchmarking analysis and may be useful for any type of benchmarking that requires the comparison of entities that differ on some level (e.g., scope of respective benchmarking measurements, definitions, business processes). This is done by expressing the data for differing entities in relative (i.e., comparable) terms [7].

For example, common sizing is often used to compare financial statements of the same company over different periods of time (e.g., historical subject benchmarking), or of several companies of differing sizes (e.g., benchmarking to industry norms). The latter type may be used for benchmarking an organization to another in its industry, to industry averages, or to the best performing agency in its industry [8]. Some examples of common size measures utilized in health care include

1. Percent of revenue or per unit produced, for example, relative value unit (RVU)
2. Per provider, for example, physician
3. Per capacity measurement, for example, per square foot
4. Other standard units of comparison

As with any data, differences in how data are collected, stored, and analyzed over time or between different organizations may complicate the use of it at a later time. Accordingly, appropriate adjustments must be made to account for such differences and provide an accurate and reliable dataset for benchmarking.

PART II: MEDICAL PRACTICE MANAGEMENT DATA SOURCES

AMERICAN MEDICAL ASSOCIATION SURVEYS

Physician Characteristics and Distribution in the United States

The AMA maintains a comprehensive database of information on physicians in the United States. The Physician Masterfile is updated annually through the Physicians' Professional Activities questionnaire and the validation efforts of AMA's Division of Survey and Data Resources. The publication "Physician Characteristics and Distribution in the US" is based on a variety of demographic information from this source. This database contains the largest sample of solo and small group practitioners.

PHYSICIAN SOCIOECONOMIC STATISTICS

This AMA survey publication is the result of the merger of two AMA annuals: *Socio-economic Characteristics of Medical Practice;* and *Physician Marketplace Statistics.* The merged survey is based on the AMA's annual core survey of the Socioeconomic Monitoring System. Random samples of physicians from the Physician Masterfile are given a questionnaire and interviewed by telephone concerning a wide range of economic and practice characteristics. The annual publication reports data on the following categories:

- Age profiles of physicians
- Weeks and hours of practice
- Utilization of physician services
- Fees for physician visits
- Professional expenses
- Physician compensation
- Distribution of revenue by payer
- Managed care contracts
- Other physician marketplace statistics

GROUP PRACTICE ASSOCIATIONS COMPENSATION AND PRODUCTION SURVEYS

MEDICAL GROUP COMPENSATION AND PRODUCTIVITY SURVEY (AMGA—AMERICAN MEDICAL GROUP ASSOCIATION)

AMGA, formerly the American Group Practice Association, has conducted compensation and production surveys for more than 20 years. These surveys are co-sponsored by McGladrey & Pullen who surveys almost 3000 group practices nationally. Compensation and production data are provided for medical specialties by size of group, geographic region, and whether the group is single or multispecialty.

PHYSICIAN COMPENSATION AND PRODUCTION SURVEY (MGMA—MEDICAL GROUP MANAGEMENT ASSOCIATION)

MGMA's membership compensation and production survey is one of the largest with approximately 2000 practice respondents. Data are provided on compensation and production for more than 100 specialties with detailed summaries on the 20 largest, including breakdowns for years in specialty, single, or multispecialty practice, geographic regions, and percent of at-risk managed care revenues. The survey data are also published on CD-ROM by John Wiley & Sons ValueSource®. Additional levels of detail available in this media provide enhanced benchmarking capabilities.

MEDICAL PRACTICE EXPENSE SURVEYS

1. *Cost Surveys (MGMA):* MGMA's Cost Survey is one of the best-known surveys of group practice income and expense data. It currently has over 2000 respondents. Data are provided for a detailed listing of expense categories and are also calculated as a percentage of revenue and per FTE (full-time equivalent) physician, FTE provider, patient, square foot, and RVU (relative value units). The survey provides information on multispecialty practices by performance ranking, geographic region, legal organization, size of practice, and percent of capitated revenue. Detailed income and expense data is provided for single specialty practices in 19 different specialties. John Wiley's ValueSource® division also publishes this survey on CD-ROM.
2. *Medical Group Financial Operations Surveys (AMGA):* This survey was created through a partnership between RSM McGladrey and AMGA. The financial operations survey provides critical benchmark data on support staff salaries and benefits, physician salaries, staffing profiles, and other key financial indicators. The information, including data as a percent of managed care revenues, per full-time physician, and per square foot, is subdivided by specialty mix, size of practice, and geographic region with detailed summaries of

single specialty practices in more than 30 specialties. These specialty summaries provide compensation and expense data per full-time physician and per square foot.

3. *National Association of Healthcare Consultants' Statistical Surveys (Medical and Dental Income and Expense Averages)*: Produced by the Practice Asset Management, LLC & SH Systems, Inc., this survey is developed through a joint service agreement between the Society of Medical Dental Management Consultants (SMD) and NAHC. It has been published annually for a number of years and includes detailed income and expense data from more than 2800 practices in 56 specialties. The data are divided into four geographic regions and by solo or group practice.

AMBULATORY SURGERY CENTER SURVEYS

AMBULATORY SURGERY CENTER PERFORMANCE SURVEY

These reports are based on the prior years' data published by MGMA. The American Association of Ambulatory Surgery Centers (AAASC) collaborates and provides support for each year. The report provides financial and operating data that is very similar to MGMA's medical group "Cost Survey." Data are presented in the following divisions: As a Percent of Total Medical Revenue; Per Square Foot; Per Case; Per Procedure; and Per Operating Room. Each of these data points is reported by a range of statistical measures of central tendency including: mean, median, upper quartile, lower quartile, 10th percentile, and 90th percentile. Data are further classified by size of ASC (by number of annual cases); by type of ownership; and, by selected specialties.

OUTPATIENT SURGERY CENTER MARKET REPORT

Since 1990, SMG Marketing Group, now owned by Verispan, has compiled and maintained a database of U.S., freestanding ASCs (not hospital-owned facilities). Until 2004 when the title changed, the survey was published as the "Report and Directory: Freestanding Outpatient Surgery Centers." This report contains a directory of facilities and chains with contact and ownership information as well as specialty and number of operating rooms. It is accompanied by a statistical report on the ASC industry, which includes data on demographics including utilization and patient volumes and also surgical specialty and procedure analysis; managed care and other contracting; and growth and revenue trends and projections for 2015 and beyond.

MANAGEMENT SERVICES ORGANIZATION SURVEYS

COST SURVEY FOR INTEGRATED DELIVERY SYSTEM PRACTICES

This survey began as A National Initiative: The Survey of Hospital-Sponsored Management Services Organizations conducted and published by the consulting firm Medimetrix in 1997. MGMA then took over and the survey was expanded to include data on integrated delivery system practices, as well as MSOs. The report was renamed again, as the Cost Survey for Integrated Delivery System Practices. Today, the first part of the report provides financial and operating data on medical practices similar to MGMA's medical group "Cost Survey." The second part is devoted to MSOs with similar types of financial and operating data (not their member practices). In both sections, data are presented in the following divisions: Per FTE Physician; As a Percent of Total Medical Revenue; Per Square Foot; Per Total RVU; Per Work RVU; and Per Patient. Each of these data points is reported by a range of statistical measures of central tendency including: mean, median, upper quartile, lower quartile, 10th percentile, and 90th percentile.

MANAGED CARE DIGEST SERIES® [WWW.MANAGEDCAREDIGEST.COM]

The Sanofi-Aventis Managed Care Digest Series® is part of a continuing commitment to provide medical professional with the latest, most essential information on the evolution of health care. The Series, available freely online or in print, provides key benchmarking data that can help assess value, control costs, and develop business strategies for

- Hospitals
- Nursing homes
- Healthcare agencies
- Integrated health systems
- HMOs/PPO and MCOs, etc.
- Medicare, Medicaid, and medical groups

The Series acknowledges Verispan LLC, Yardley, PA as the research and reporting source for data based on information gathered by mail, email, and telephone surveys effective each quarter. It was commissioned, sponsored, and underwritten in an arm's length fashion, developed and produced by Forte Information Resources, LLC, Denver, Colorado, by Richard Frye; PhD (personal communication).

THE SHERLOCK COMPANY WWW.SHERLOCKCO.COM

The Sherlock Company assists healthcare organizations and health plans, their business partners and their investors in the treasury, strategic, and control functions of finance. The company provides benchmarking data and analysis for the management of administrative health functions. It performs valuation and due diligence for business combinations and other capital transactions and offers financial research publications concerning managed care. The company also provides informed solutions for health plan finance. Products include the Sherlock Expense Evaluation Report, Pulse, Health Plan Navigator and Corporate Finance Services. Since its founding in 1987, by Douglas B. Sherlock, CFA, MBA, the Sherlock Company is known for its impartiality and technical competence in service to its clients (personal communication).

SUMMARY

Whether the PP-ACA and other current or proposed healthcare reform efforts continue to gain momentum or deteriorate going forward, the demand for a uniform standard for benchmarking physicians, and healthcare enterprises that includes quality, performance, productivity, utilization, and compensation measures seems to be increasing. Benchmarking will be used progressively more by medical providers and healthcare organizations in order to facilitate reductions in healthcare expenditures while simultaneously improving products, service quality, and personal resources and financial stability.

From a medical management perspective, the use of benchmarking as a performance indicator will become increasingly important in health care as quality assurance and effectiveness research becomes more pronounced through pay-for-performance (P4P) initiatives and increasingly stringent fraud and abuse laws.

From a financial planning standpoint, as managerial consulting firms, FAs and the IRS initiate cost, managerial and financial accounting audits, valuations and reviews, physicians, and other practitioners through benchmarking data will become progressively more important; especially for personal planning endeavors and nonprofit healthcare organization wishing to maximize revenues and/or retain their tax exempt status [9].

Additionally, if healthcare spending continues to rise, patients and regulators will increasingly view medical providers with scrutiny, further emphasizing the importance of standardizing comparative measures to benchmark utility and productivity of all healthcare provider enterprises; and to prepare innovative, comprehensive, integrated and highly specific financial plans for modernity.

ACKNOWLEDGMENTS

To Todd A. Zigrang, MBA/MHA, ASA, FACHE and Anne P. Sharamitaro, Esq., executive vice president and general counsel at Health Capital Consultants (HCC), LLC, St. Louis, Missouri (www.HealthCapital.com).

REFERENCES

1. "Common Size Financial Statements," by NetMBA.com, 2007, http://www.netmba.com/finance/statements/common-size/ (Accessed 8/13/2009), p. 3.
2. See "Benchmarking: A general reading for management practitioners," by Sik Wah Fong, Eddie W.L. Cheng, and Danny C.K. Ho, *Management Decision*, 36(6), 1998, 410.
3. "A perspective on benchmarking," Gregory H. Watson in conversation with the Editor, *Benchmarking for Quality Management & Technology*, 1(1), 1994, 6.
4. "A perspective on benchmarking," Gregory H. Watson in conversation with the Editor, *Benchmarking for Quality Management & Technology*, 1(1), 1994, 6.
5. "A perspective on benchmarking," Gregory H. Watson in conversation with the Editor, *Benchmarking for Quality Management & Technology*, 1(1), 1994, 6.
6. "*Principles of Financial & Managerial Accounting,*" Carl S. Warren, Philip E. Fess, 3rd edition, South-Western Publishing Co., Cincinnati, Ohio, 1992, p. 1169.
7. "*Principles of Financial & Managerial Accounting,*" Carl S. Warren, Philip E. Fess, 3rd edition, South-Western Publishing Co., Cincinnati, Ohio, 1992, p. 1169.
8. "*Principles of Financial & Managerial Accounting,*" Carl S. Warren, Philip E. Fess, 3rd edition, South-Western Publishing Co., Cincinnati, Ohio, 1992, p. 1169.
9. "Enforcement efforts take aim at executive compensation of tax-exempt health care entities," by Candace L. Quinn and Jeffrey D. Mamorsky, 18 Health Law Reporter 1640, Dec. 17, 2009; "An Introduction to I.R.C. 4958 (Intermediate Sanctions)," by Lawrence M. Brauer, Toussaint T. Tyson, Leonard J. Henzke, and Debra J. Kawecki, Internal Revenue Service, 2002 EO CPE Text, http://apps.irs.gov/pub/irs-tege/eotopich02.pdf (Accessed 12/28/09), p. 275–276.

FURTHER READING

Cimasi, RJ, Alexander, T and Zigrang, TA: Update on research and financial benchmarking in the healthcare industry. In: Marcinko, DE and Hetico, HR [Editors]: *Financial Management Strategies for Hospitals and Healthcare Organizations [Tools, Techniques, Checklists and Case Studies]*. Productivity Press, Boca Raton, FL, 2014.

Firebaugh, JW and Marcinko, DE: Hospital endowment fund management. In: Marcinko, DE [Editor]: *Healthcare Organizations [Financial Management Strategies]*. Productivity Press, Boca Raton, FL, 2013.

Marcinko, DE and Hetico, HR: *Dictionary of Health Economics and Finance*. Springer Publishing, New York, 2007.

Marcinko, DE and Hetico, HR: *Selecting Practice Management Consultants Wisely*. Springer Publishing, New York, 2010.

Index

A